BIOPSY INTERPRETATION SERIES

BIOPSY INTERPRETATION OF THE LUNG

Third Edition

BIOPSY INTERPRETATION SERIES

BIOPSY INTERPRETATION OF THE LUNG

Third Edition

David Ilan Suster, MD
Associate Professor
Director of Surgical Pathology
Department of Pathology, Immunology and Laboratory Medicine
Rutgers University, New Jersey Medical School
Newark, New Jersey

Saul Suster, MD
Professor and Chair Emeritus
Department of Pathology and Laboratory Medicine
Medical College of Wisconsin
Milwaukee, Wisconsin

Wolters Kluwer

Philadelphia • Baltimore • New York • London
Buenos Aires • Hong Kong • Sydney • Tokyo

Acquisitions Editor: Nicole Dernoski
Development Editor: Ariel S. Winter
Editorial Coordinator: Sunmerrilika Baskar
Marketing Manager: Kirsten Watrud
Production Project Manager: Matthew West
Design Coordinator: Steve Druding
Manufacturing Coordinator: Lisa Bowling
Prepress Vendor: Straive

Third edition

9 8 7 6 5 4 3 2 1

Printer in Mexico

Cataloging-in-Publication Data available on request from the Publisher

ISBN: 978-1-9752-4067-7

---

shop.lww.com

QUADM0925

DEDICATION

To my family for their endless support on this journey.

D.I.S.

To my wife, Jenny, and to our children, David and Dana.

S.S.

PREFACE

The topic of the interpretation of lung biopsies has continued to acquire increased significance as diagnosis of disease progressively relies on minimally invasive techniques that cause the least harm to patients. With the increase in the use of limited lung biopsies for the diagnosis of lung disease, pathologists have been called to "do more with less" and provide the answers needed by the clinicians to spare the patients a major procedure. We have been enormously gratified by the enthusiastic reception by our readers of the second edition of this book and have been called to work on this third edition due to the many advances in the understanding of lung disease accrued over the past few years. This new edition has been expanded to include several new advances, in particular regarding our understanding of the genetic events underlying lung diseases, and the role of emerging new markers and molecular abnormalities for the diagnosis of such conditions. Additional color illustrations have been added to the text to expand on the various aspects of some of the described conditions, and the references have been updated with the newest information currently available. Changes in terminology, updated diagnostic criteria, and molecular advances for the various entities have also been incorporated into this new edition. Although the text incorporates the current terminology and criteria espoused by the World Health Organization for the diagnosis of neoplastic diseases of the lung, we have also presented our approach and understanding on many of these processes where appropriate based on our personal experience. We are grateful to all the colleagues who have contributed with their interesting consultation cases to the material in this volume and to our residents and students who challenge us every day with questions that test the limit of our understanding. We hope you will find this new edition to be helpful in guiding you to the correct interpretation of lung biopsies and a valuable adjunct to your diagnostic armamentarium.

David Ilan Suster, MD
Saul Suster, MD

CONTRIBUTOR

Michael E. Kallen
Associate Professor
Department of Pathology
University of Maryland School of Medicine
Baltimore, Maryland
Chapter 10. Lung Transplant Pathology
Chapter 11. Lymphoid Lesions of the Lung

CONTENTS

1

METHODS FOR OBTAINING LUNG BIOPSIES

Lung biopsies represent an important and often definitive method for establishing a diagnosis in patients afflicted with pulmonary disorders. Various methods are currently routinely employed for the evaluation of lung tissue: endoscopic biopsies, transthoracic (percutaneous) core needle biopsies, cryobiopsies, robotic-assisted thoracoscopic surgery (RATS), and video-assisted thoracoscopic surgery (VATS) lung biopsy. The older method of open lung biopsy via thoracotomy was associated with significant morbidity and has been largely abandoned in favor of VATS or other newer techniques. Techniques based on the cytologic examinations of specimens obtained through fine needle aspiration (FNA) or bronchial brushings and washings also play a role in the evaluation of patients with lung disorders but will not be a subject of discussion in this book. The selection of the biopsy method employed will be dictated by the clinical circumstances and the level of experience and skill of the thoracic surgeon, pneumonologist, or interventional radiologist. Obviously, the diagnostic yield for a focalized endobronchial lesion will be much higher on endobronchial biopsy than for a diffuse or peripheral lung process. However, lung diseases with predominant peribronchial distribution such as sarcoidosis are amenable to diagnosis on transbronchial biopsy. Conditions in which diagnostic features depend on demonstration of temporal heterogeneity and variations in the histopathologic features from site to site, such as idiopathic interstitial pneumonias, will require a VATS approach and will yield only extremely limited results on endoscopic biopsies. Correlation of the clinical information and radiographic findings is indispensable for a correct interpretation. It is important that the pathologist be provided with a full clinical history, results of imaging studies, and other clinical test results, as well as a provisional or suspected differential diagnosis by the surgeon or clinician at the time the biopsy specimen is submitted.

BRONCHIAL ENDOSCOPIC BIOPSY

Endoscopic bronchial or transbronchial biopsy constitutes a technique whereby biopsy material is generally obtained through a flexible tube that is inserted into the airways (fiberoptic bronchoscopy). It is the most commonly used invasive technique currently available for obtaining lung tissue biopsies. Although rigid bronchoscopes were used for obtaining biopsy material as far back as the 1940s,[1,2] it was not until the development of fiberoptic technology that this technique truly came of age. The first flexible fiberoptic bronchoscope was developed and introduced into clinical practice by Ikeda[3] in 1970. Since then, further refinements and additional experience with this instrument have firmly established this modality as a highly valuable technique for obtaining lung tissue biopsies for diagnosis. The development of videobronchoscopy has further refined our capabilities for diagnosis and currently permits capturing digital images using an embedded camera that transmits them to a digital monitor. The latter technique provides the advantage of capturing images and storing them in various formats for teaching and research in addition to procuring the biopsy samples.

Rigid bronchoscopy is more limited in terms of the depth of airways examination and is usually used for evaluation of proximal lesions in the upper airways and for the extraction of foreign bodies or the management of hemoptysis. It is limited by the inability to properly visualize terminal bronchi and the need for general anesthesia.

Bronchoscopy is generally carried out with light sedation and topical anesthesia in an outpatient setting. The bronchoscope can be introduced by either a transnasal or transoral approach. The field of vision is usually 80°, with the angle of deflection usually 160° to 180°. The scope is equipped with a light source, camera, suction and irrigation ports, and biopsy tools. The size and width of the instrument will depend on the number of fiberoptic bundles; the larger the number of fiberoptic bundles, the greater the light transmitted by the scope. Most scopes have the ability to permit examination of segmental and subsegmental bronchi up to sixth-order bronchi.[4] Diagnostic yield can be enhanced in certain settings when the results of bronchial biopsy are combined with the findings of bronchial washings, brushings, and alveolar lavage.[5,6]

There are very few contraindications for fiberoptic bronchoscopy. They mostly involve coagulopathy, recent myocardial ischemia, or high-risk patients with increased intracranial pressure. The main risk of bronchoscopy is compromising the patient's airway, particularly in cases of tracheal stenosis or tumor. Rare complications include bradycardia, hypotension, syncope, and arrhythmias. Morbidity in most large studies has varied from 0.05% to 1%, and mortality is around 0.01%.[7] The biopsy samples can be either endobronchial, comprising only the superficial mucosal surface (Figs. 1.1 and 1.2; eFig. 1.1), or transbronchial for deeper lesions within the parenchyma of the lung or lesions lying beneath the bronchial surface (Fig. 1.3). Biopsy of the bronchial mucosa is accomplished using a cupped forceps that is introduced through the flexible shaft of the bronchoscope. This allows visualization of the mucosa, lamina propria, muscle layer, and peribronchial lymphovascular network. The transbronchial technique uses a different kind of forceps that is generally advanced into a distal airway

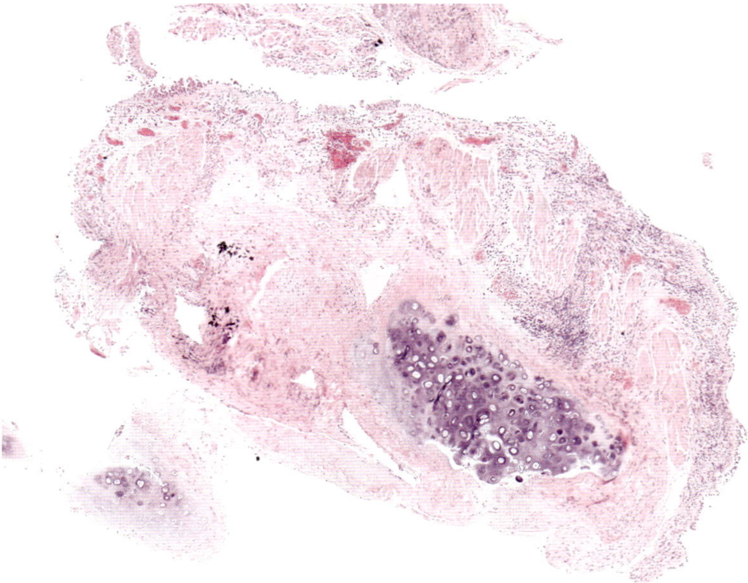

FIGURE 1.1 **Endobronchial biopsy showing normal bronchial mucosa.** Notice surface mucosa overlying hyaline bronchial cartilage and smooth muscle in the lamina propria.

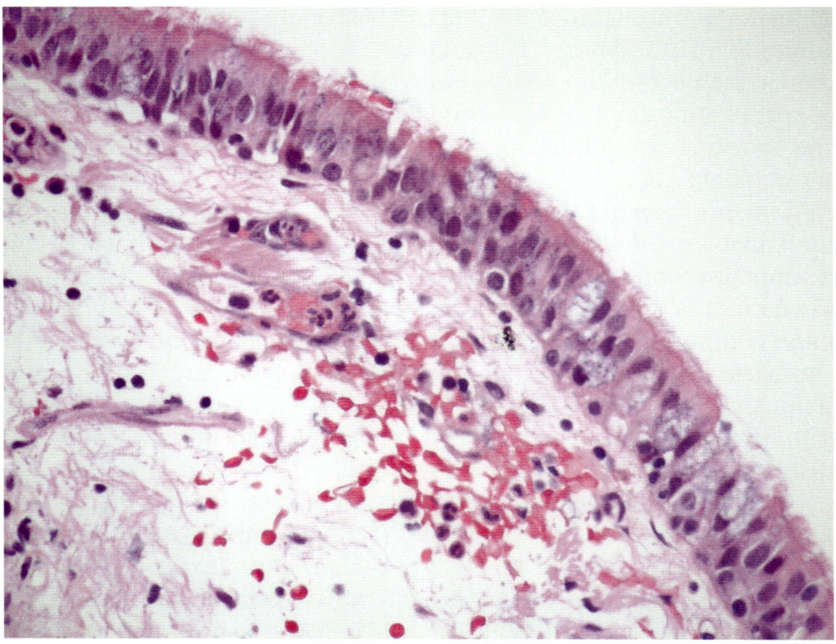

FIGURE 1.2 **Higher magnification of endobronchial biopsy showing normal columnar-ciliated surface epithelium.**

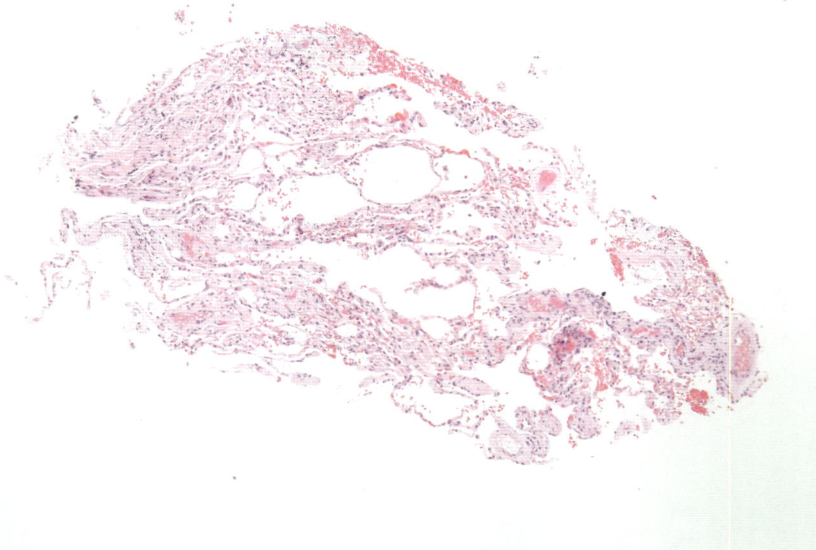

FIGURE 1.3 **Transbronchial biopsy showing normal lung parenchyma with preserved alveolar spaces.** Notice the dilated capillaries within the interstitium in the alveolar walls.

and forces the bronchiolar wall and peribronchial lung parenchyma into the mouth of the device. The material sampled usually comprises lung parenchyma beyond the cartilaginous plate and includes alveolar spaces.

Although bronchial biopsies can be highly effective for the diagnosis of certain lung conditions, they may have serious limitations in many instances (Table 1.1).

The most useful role for bronchial biopsies is in the diagnosis of lung tumors involving the bronchial tree. Tumors most commonly accessible to the bronchoscope in the major airways include bronchogenic squamous cell carcinoma, small cell carcinoma, low-grade neuroendocrine carcinoma ("carcinoid" tumor), and certain salivary gland–type tumors such as mucoepidermoid carcinoma and adenoid cystic carcinoma (Fig. 1.4). Adenocarcinomas, particularly those in peripheral locations or not involving the bronchial tree, may not be easily detected by endobronchial or transbronchial biopsies.

Bronchoscopy has become increasingly used for the diagnosis and staging of lung cancer in recent years.[8] Endoscopic evaluation of early-stage squamous cell carcinoma can provide a basis for the determination of therapeutic strategies depending on the gross configuration of the tumor (ie, polypoid, diffuse).[9] Ultrasound-guided transbronchial endoscopic biopsies have also increased the yield of positive diagnosis for solitary pulmonary nodules less than 3 cm in diameter that cannot be normally

TABLE 1.1 Limitations and Indications of Bronchial Endoscopic Biopsies

High Diagnostic Yield	Moderate Diagnostic Yield	Poor Diagnostic Yield
Squamous cell carcinoma	Alveolar hemorrhagic syndromes	Adenocarcinoma
Carcinoid tumor	Capillaritis	Metastatic tumors
Small cell carcinoma	Collagen vascular diseases	Sarcomas
Mucoepidermoid carcinoma	Alveolar proteinosis	Other unusual tumors
Adenoid cystic carcinoma	Lymphangioleiomyomatosis	Interstitial lung diseases
Opportunistic infections	Sarcoidosis	Acute pneumonias
Lung transplant patients	Lymphoproliferative disorders	Granulomatosis with polyangiitis

visualized under conventional fluoroscopy.[10] Diagnosis of endobronchial metastases can also be successfully accomplished in many instances by bronchoscopic biopsy techniques.[11] Clinical correlation and a thorough patient history, however, are required in most instances to distinguish these tumors from primary cancers.

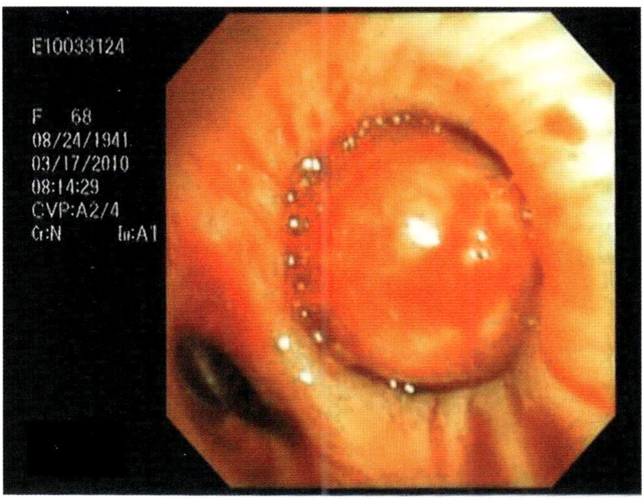

FIGURE 1.4 Bronchoscopic examination reveals a polypoid, intraluminal endobronchial mass with smooth contours occluding the lumen corresponding to a bronchial "carcinoid" tumor (low-grade neuroendocrine carcinoma). (Courtesy of Dr. George Haasler, M.D., Thoracic Surgery, Medical College of Wisconsin.)

Another indication for endoscopic biopsy is for the diagnosis of opportunistic infections, including fungal infections (such as *pneumocystis jirovecii*) and viral infections (such as cytomegalovirus). The diagnostic yield for opportunistic infections in AIDS patients can be as high as 90% when cytologic and biopsy methods are combined.[12,13] Bronchial biopsy is also very useful for the evaluation of lung transplant patients, particularly in the diagnosis of acute allograft rejection.

Conditions in which transbronchial lung biopsies may yield diagnostic information in certain circumstances include diffuse alveolar hemorrhage with necrotizing capillaritis in patients with granulomatosis with polyangiitis and other antineutrophil cytoplasmic antibody–related conditions. Bronchial biopsy may also yield diagnostic tissue in cases of pulmonary alveolar proteinosis or lymphangioleiomyomatosis, particularly when there is extensive disease. The same applies to cases of sarcoidosis in which transbronchial biopsy may yield well-formed epithelioid granulomas, although the latter remains strictly a diagnosis of exclusion and requires clinical correlation. Diagnostic information can also be obtained from limited bronchial biopsy material containing dense lymphoid infiltrates, particularly when utilizing modern molecular techniques for the study of clonal gene rearrangements, specific translocations, and detection of light chain restriction using paraffin-embedded tissue biopsies with polymerase chain reaction (PCR), fluorescence in situ hybridization (FISH), next-generation sequencing (NGS), or other techniques.

Conventional transbronchial biopsies may be of very limited or no value in the evaluation of various lung conditions, including peripheral tumors that are not accessible via conventional fiberoptic bronchoscope, metastatic tumors that do not involve the major airways, and sarcomas and other rare tumors in which a limited sample may not supply the necessary information for a definitive diagnosis. In acute pneumonias, the findings will be so nonspecific that anything beyond a generic diagnosis of diffuse alveolar damage may not be possible. The size and number of tissue fragments obtained for evaluation may also influence the diagnostic yield of the procedure; the smaller the size of the biopsy and the fewer the tissue samples obtained, the lower the yield (Fig. 1.5).[14,15]

Some of the aforementioned sampling-related issues may be ameliorated by the use of newer technologies. For example, newer techniques such as electromagnetic-guided bronchoscopy allow for minimally invasive sampling of peripheral lung lesions though this comes at the cost of pneumothorax rates ranging from 4% to 62% (averaging 20%).[16-18]

One of the least practical uses of endoscopic lung biopsies is for the evaluation of interstitial lung disease.[19] Criteria for the diagnosis of these conditions are currently based on the examination of surgical lung biopsies.[20] Because the diagnosis of interstitial lung disease is heavily dependent on the temporal and spatial relationship of the changes requiring comparison from various areas of the lung (often from separate lobes), results obtained from transbronchial biopsies will be of extremely limited value for the diagnosis

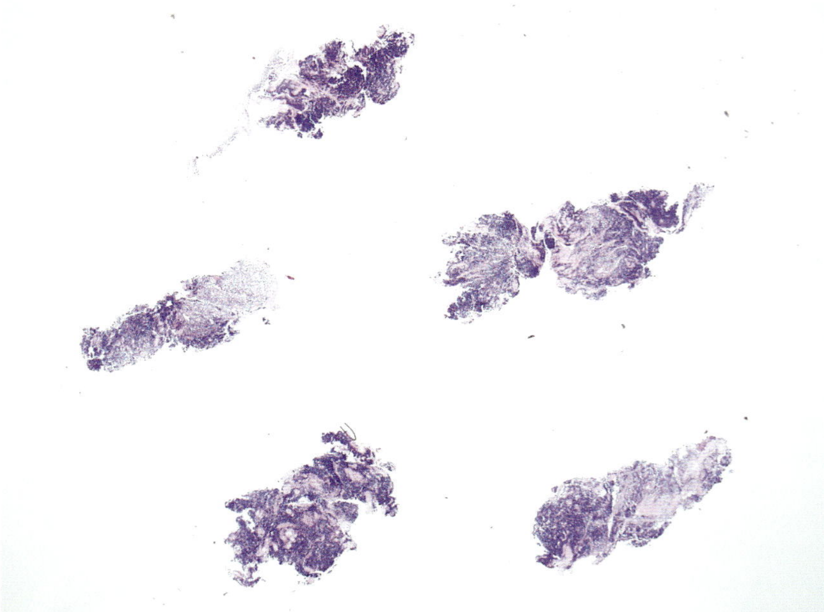

FIGURE 1.5 **Appropriate tissue sampling on transbronchial lung biopsy.** Notice in this sample there are multiple small tissue fragments. This dramatically improves the chances for a definitive diagnosis as compared to a biopsy with a single small fragment.

of usual interstitial pneumonia, desquamative interstitial pneumonia, respiratory bronchiolitis–associated interstitial lung disease, nonspecific interstitial pneumonia, hypersensitivity pneumonitis, autoimmune disease, and others. Attempting to establish a definitive diagnosis of a specific interstitial lung disease on a transbronchial biopsy may often be misleading and nearly impossible in most cases. The bulk of the literature has demonstrated that the diagnostic yield and accuracy of endoscopic bronchial biopsy for the diagnosis of diffuse interstitial lung disease is much less than that of other techniques such as open biopsy, RATS, and VATS.[21,22] Assisted thoracoscopic procedures have become increasingly favored over open lung biopsy for the diagnosis of interstitial lung disorders owing to the decreased morbidity and hospital stay associated with the former.[23-25]

Use of transbronchial biopsy in patients with interstitial lung disease to rule out certain conditions that present with a similar clinical and radiographic picture, such as sarcoidosis and lymphangitis carcinomatosa, may be justified and indicated in selected instances. The appropriate approach by the endoscopist who submits a biopsy in such instances would be to provide the pathologist with a pertinent clinical history, provide information regarding the existence of interstitial lung infiltrates in the requisition form, state the differential diagnosis, and request that alternative conditions such as sarcoidosis, lymphangitis carcinomatosa, or others be ruled out.

Endoscopic biopsy procedures of the bronchial tree are often complicated by artifacts and nonspecific changes that can obscure the underlying process and create pitfalls for diagnosis. These include tissue compression with crushing artifact or collapse of the lung parenchyma and bleeding. Compression of lung parenchyma may superficially simulate interstitial fibrosis on scanning magnification owing to the apposition of alveolar walls against one another. Closer examination will demonstrate that the alveolar septa are of normal thickness and that only their close proximity creates an illusion of fibrosis (Fig. 1.6). Tangential sectioning of medium and large caliber vessel walls may also contribute to the impression of interstitial fibrosis in endoscopic biopsies. Crushing of lymphocytes may create a picture suggestive of small cell bronchogenic carcinoma (Fig. 1.7; eFig. 1.2); use of immunostains may be warranted under such circumstances to identify CD45-positive cells versus keratin-positive cells in these areas (Fig. 1.8). Bleeding is a common complication of the biopsy procedure and may be confused for pathologic hemorrhage. In most instances of pathologic pulmonary bleeding, however, the lung parenchyma will also contain fibrin and hemosiderin-laden macrophages (Fig. 1.9; eFig. 1.3).

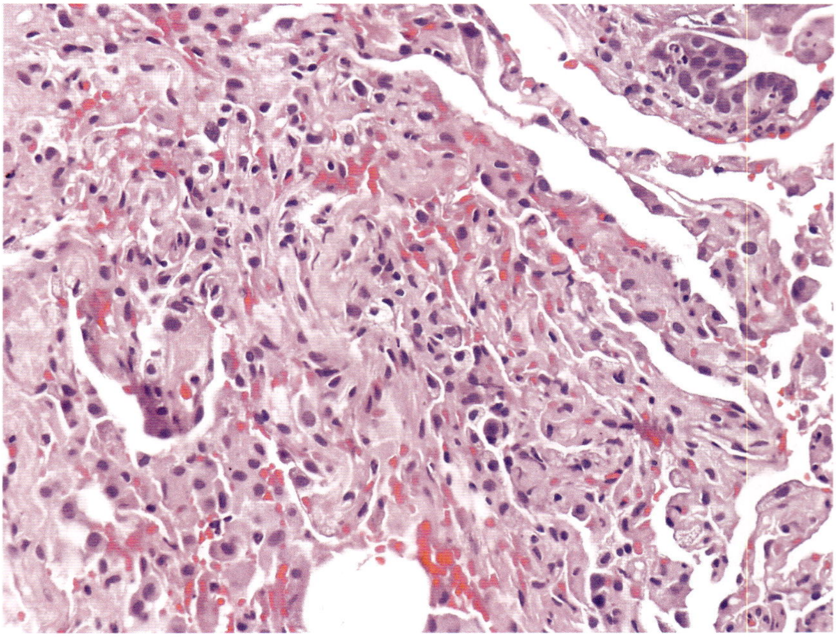

FIGURE 1.6 Collapse of alveolar walls with close apposition of alveolar septa may give an initial impression of interstitial fibrosis; closer examination shows that alveolar septa are of normal thickness.

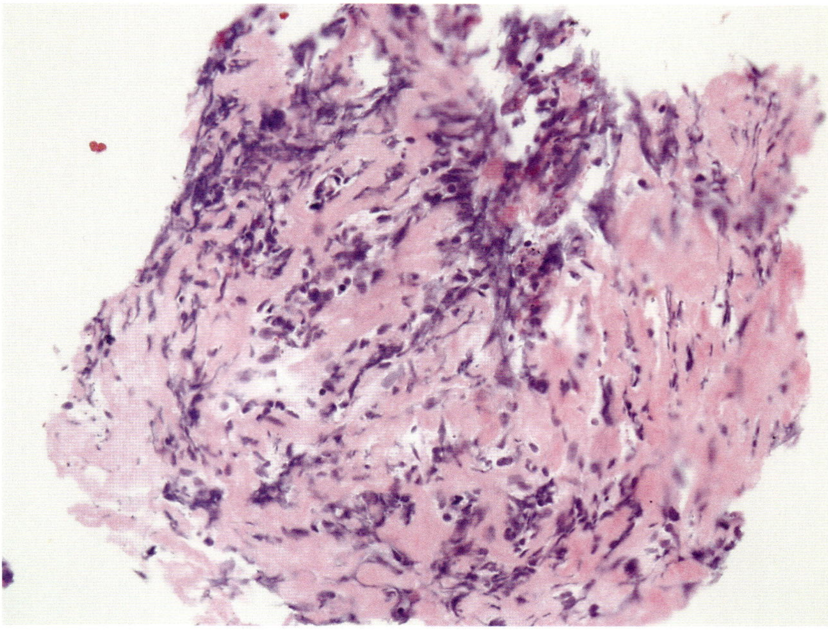

FIGURE 1.7 **Transbronchial biopsy with extensive crushing of lymphocytes may suggest the possibility of small cell carcinoma.**

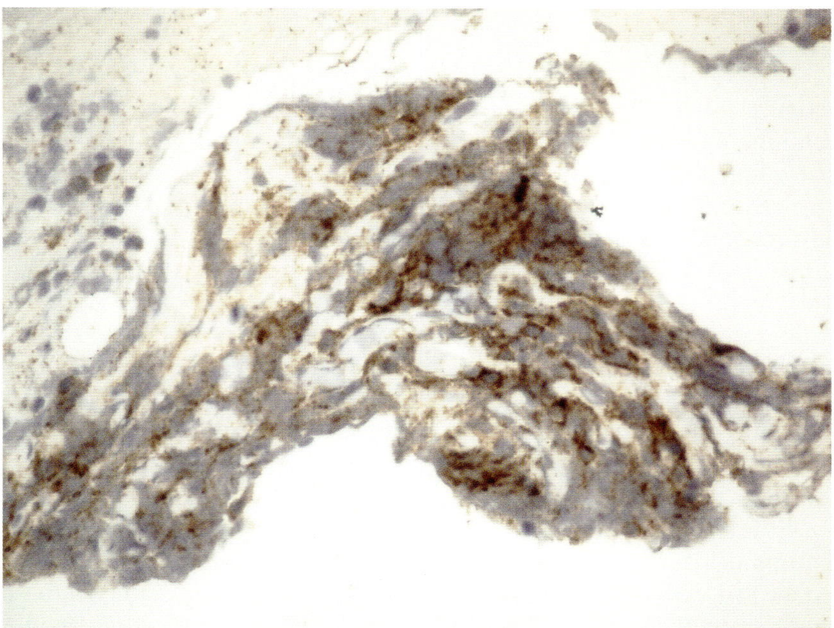

FIGURE 1.8 **Immunohistochemical stain for CD45 (leukocyte common antigen) shows a positive reaction, indicating that the crushed cells correspond to lymphoid cells.** A keratin stain was negative.

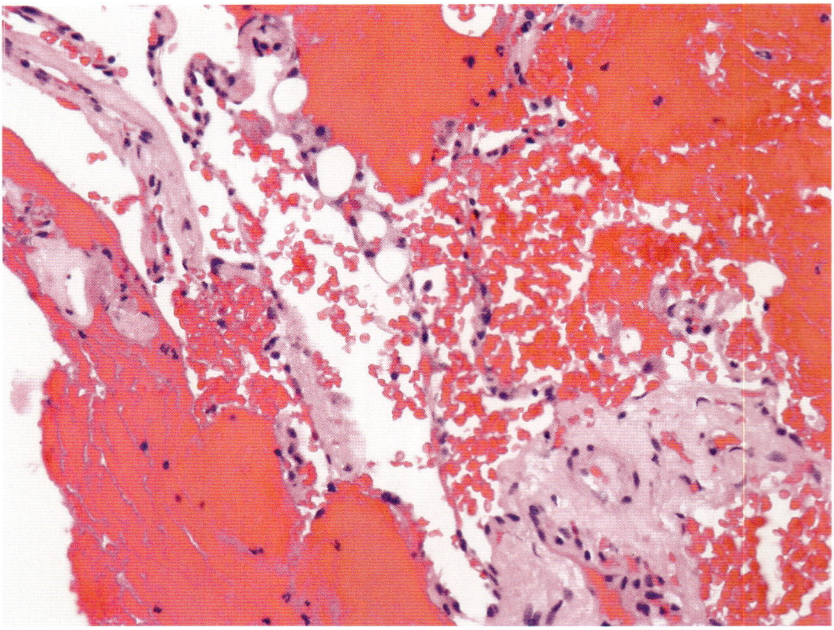

FIGURE 1.9 **Bleeding caused by the biopsy procedure in transbronchial lung biopsy.** Notice the absence of hemosiderin-laden macrophages and fibrin; this should not be confused for actual pathologic bleeding caused by bleeding disorders.

CRYOBIOPSY

Cryobiopsy was first used in thoracic diseases in 1978 and was used for debulking larger tumors.[26] In the last decade and a half, the technique was reintroduced as an additional method of procuring lung tissue including improved performance for diffuse parenchymal (interstitial) lung diseases. The procedure is based upon the Joule-Thomson effect that describes the change in temperature that accompanies the expansion of a gas. During cryobiopsy, the sharp temperature drop around the tip of the probe leads to adherence of surrounding moist lung tissue to the probe itself which is then retracted with the biopsy material. The diameter of the cryoprobe and the freezing time are the two key determinants of the size of the biopsy specimens obtained.[27] The two primary complications of this technique are bleeding and pneumothorax, though other rare complications have been reported.[28-31]

Studies have identified that cryobiopsy is able to procure larger amounts of tissue, often with less artifact (particularly less crush artifact) compared to forceps biopsy. In one study, the mean specimen area procured using the cryoprobe was 15.11 mm^2, while the mean specimen area obtained using forceps was 5.82 mm^2 (Figs. 1.10 and 1.11).[32] This technique has demonstrated promise including increased diagnostic yields and increased diagnostic accuracy both for tumors and for diffuse parenchymal

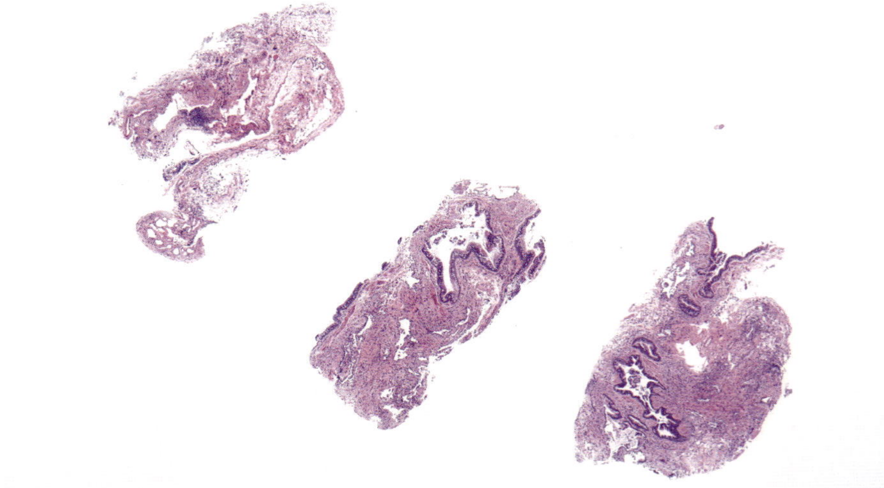

FIGURE 1.10 **Example of tissue acquired by cryobiopsy.** There are multiple relatively large fragments of peribronchial and alveolated lung tissue present with minimal artifact. This particular biopsy was taken for the evaluation of fibrosing lung disease and demonstrates areas of the lung parenchyma involved by fibrosis.

diseases and has been incorporated into several guidelines.[33-37] In addition to serving as a viable alternative for the management of patients with lung tumors or interstitial lung disease, cryobiopsy has been demonstrated to be effective in the management and evaluation of lung transplant patients (Figs. 1.12-1.14).[38-41] The lack of significant crush artifact on cryobiopsies

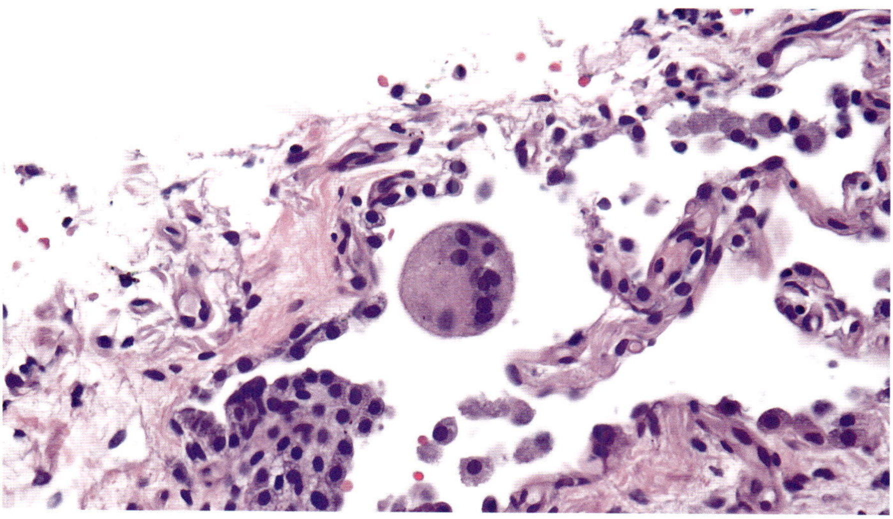

FIGURE 1.11 **Higher-power magnification from a cryobiopsy shows extremely clean histology with good nuclear detail and no evidence of crush artifact.**

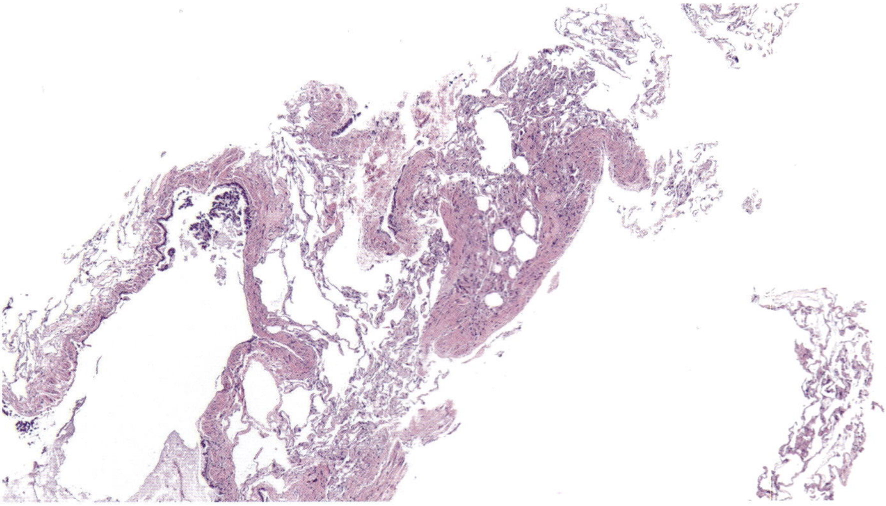

FIGURE 1.12 **Low-power magnification of a cryobiopsy taken from a lung transplant recipient.** The image shows a nice area of evaluable lung parenchyma on the biopsy with good histology.

is also of particular benefit in the evaluation of lymphoid lesions or neuroendocrine lesions of the lung that have a tendency to easily crush and become distorted (Figs. 1.15 and 1.16).

Cryobiopsy is a welcome advance in bronchoscopic technology; however, it has not yet become the de facto method for lung biopsies. The procedure

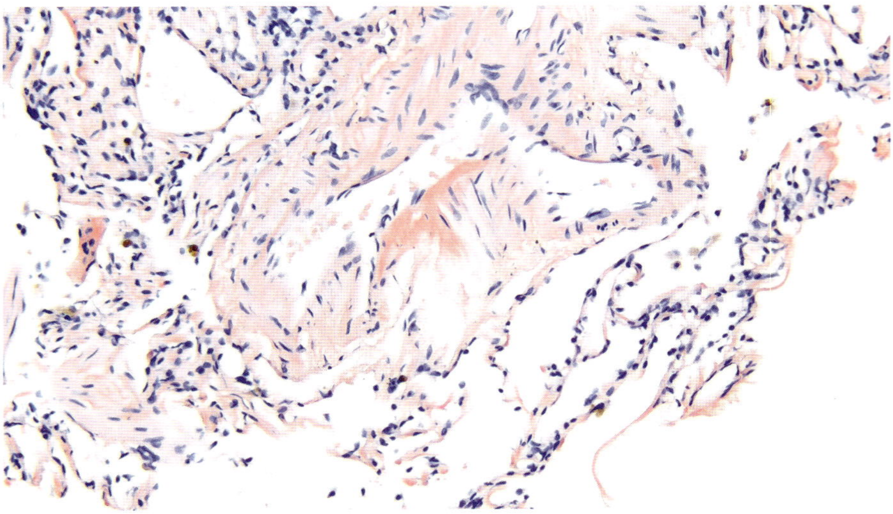

FIGURE 1.13 **Congo red special stain in the same case identified focal areas of amyloid deposition seen as a slight orangeophilic blush on the sidewall of a blood vessel.**

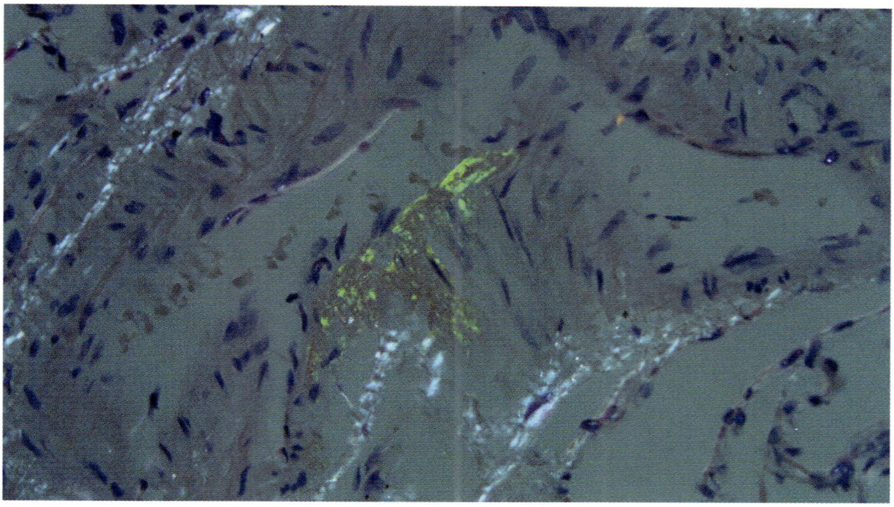

FIGURE 1.14 **Polarized light examination of the same area demonstrates the classic apple-green birefringence of amyloid.** This finding was extremely focal and may not have necessarily been sampled or been evaluable with traditional forceps biopsy.

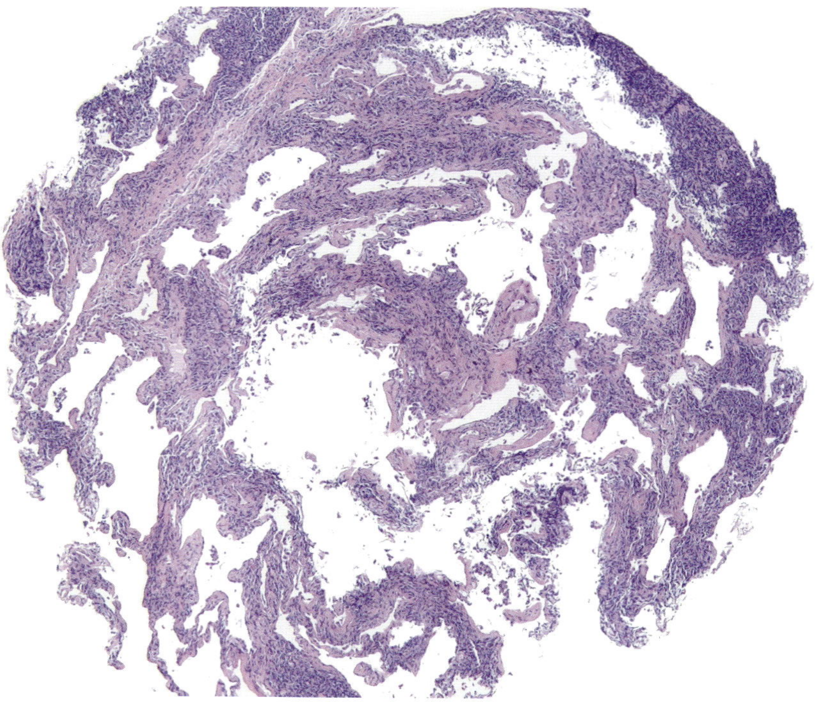

FIGURE 1.15 **Cryobiopsy performed in a patient with diffuse lymphoid infiltrates.** The fragment of sampled lung parenchyma is ample and demonstrates a diffusely infiltrative lymphoid cell population with minimal crush artifact.

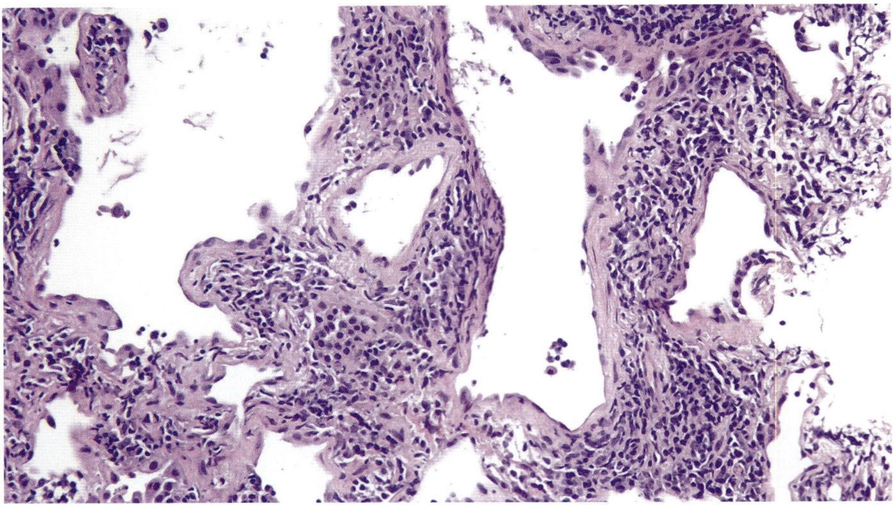

FIGURE 1.16 **Higher-power magnification of the lesion demonstrates sheets of lymphocytes and plasma cells expanding the alveolar septal walls and was highly suggestive of a diagnosis of diffuse lymphoid hyperplasia.** Note that the histology is relatively well preserved with minimal crush artifact allowing for easier interpretation.

is heavily dependent on operator experience and technical skill. It also in most cases requires intubation and sedation and thus can be a more complicated procedure to schedule and set up compared to some types of conventional bronchoscopy that can be performed under conscious sedation. In addition, the technology and methodology has not been completely standardized across all centers with variation in the types of cryoprobes used, number of biopsies taken, and clinical scenarios in which it is used.[40]

TRANSTHORACIC PERCUTANEOUS CORE NEEDLE BIOPSY

Transthoracic percutaneous biopsies under computerized tomography (CT) guidance or using ultrasound techniques have been employed during the past three decades with great success for the evaluation of pulmonary pathology. The technique is typically employed in the radiology department because it requires advanced radiologic equipment and expertise. This approach is particularly well suited to the evaluation of peripheral lung lesions, in particular pleural-based tumors.[42] Ultrasound-guided percutaneous biopsies offer the advantage of real-time visualization of the path of the needle, thus allowing a more rapid examination than that possible under CT guidance.[43] Advances in CT technology, however, now also allow real-time visualization of the procedure using continuous CT fluoroscopy.[44] A survey of transthoracic needle biopsies of lung masses disclosed that approximately 70% of participating medical centers in the United States and Canada performed the procedure under CT guidance,

8% under fluoroscopy, and 22% used a combination of CT and fluoroscopy. FNA was the procedure of choice in 73% of centers, whereas 14% preferred core biopsies, and 13% employed a combination of both techniques.[45] Core biopsies have had wider acceptance in the United Kingdom than in the United States, where more than 30% of centers utilize it as their sole technique.[46] The combined use of FNA and core biopsy, however, appears to yield the best results.[47,48] There may be specific indications, advantages, and disadvantages to both techniques. The role of FNA in the evaluation of pulmonary processes is beyond the scope of this book and will not be dealt with here. The reader is referred to the various specialized texts addressing this issue in the literature.

The main indications for transthoracic core needle biopsy are listed in Table 1.2. These include evaluation of a patient with a new or enlarging solitary pulmonary nodule, especially in peripheral locations; a patient with a hilar mass in whom bronchoscopy was negative; for the staging of patients with intrathoracic malignancy; in patients with consolidation of lung parenchyma in whom an infectious organism has not been isolated; and in patients with pleural thickening suspicious for malignancy (Fig. 1.17; eFig. 1.4). Although there are no absolute contraindications to transthoracic needle biopsy, a few relative contraindications do exist, including patients with bleeding diathesis, on mechanical ventilation, with moderate or severe obstructive lung disease, pulmonary hypertension, or patients with a history of contralateral pneumonectomy. Some studies have also suggested that there is a possible association between percutaneous needle biopsy and risk of pleural recurrence among patients with

TABLE 1.2 Indications for Percutaneous Core Biopsy

Indications
Patient with a peripheral pulmonary nodule
Patient with a hilar mass with negative bronchoscopy
Staging of intrathoracic malignancies
Patient with suspected lung infection in whom other techniques failed to identify the organism
Patient with pleural thickening suspicious for malignancy
Relative Contraindications
Bleeding disorders
Obstructive lung disease/mechanical ventilation
Pulmonary hypertension
Patients on mechanical ventilation
Patients with subpleural bulla, vascular lesions, or possible echinococcal cyst

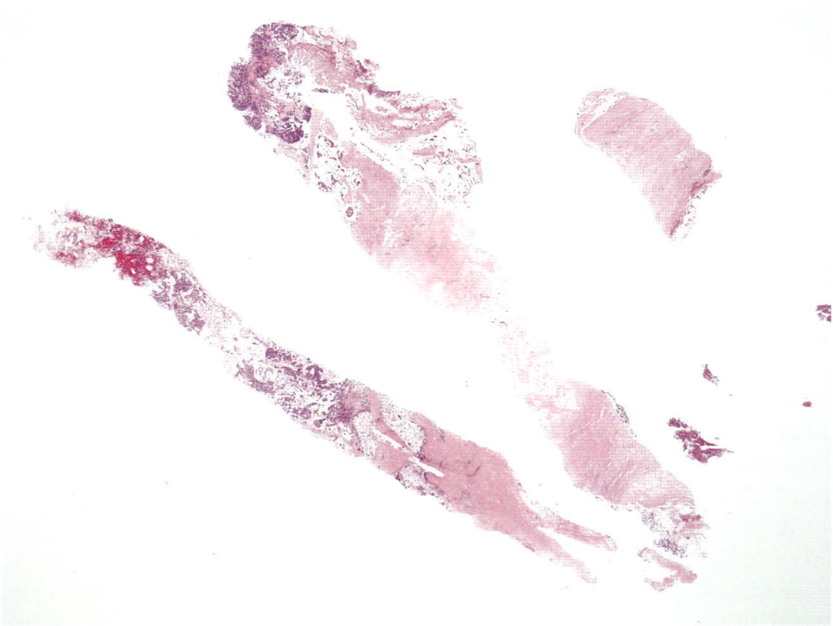

FIGURE 1.17 **Percutaneous needle core biopsy of peripheral lung nodule demonstrating tumor identifiable as an adenocarcinoma.**

low-stage, subpleural, lung cancers.[49,50] Also, patients with a history of or clinical circumstances suspicious for subpleural bulla, vascular lesions, or echinococcal cyst should be approached with great caution to avoid unnecessary complications. All patients undergoing transthoracic core biopsy should have a blood coagulation profile prior to the procedure, including platelet count and prothrombin time. Patients with central lesions in whom intravenous contrast is required for CT-guided biopsy should have renal function tests done prior to the procedure.

Percutaneous core biopsy is performed under local anesthesia and involves the introduction of a large-bore cutting needle through the pleura into the chest cavity. Obviously, the patients need to have the ability to cooperate with the procedure; patients who cannot maintain a prone or decubitus position, who cannot hold their breath, or who cannot lie still are poor candidates for this procedure. The main complication is the development of pneumothorax, the majority of which can usually be detected immediately following the procedure. The second most common complication is hemorrhage, with or without hemoptysis. Hemorrhage from transthoracic biopsies, however, is usually self-limited. In addition, there is a small chance of pleural-based hematoma development.[51] Widely used guidelines for percutaneous core biopsy have been developed.[52] The majority of published studies demonstrate that the technique is safe with a low incidence of complications, morbidity, and mortality. Trucut (14G) and Surecut (15G or 16G, modified Menghini) needles are the types most commonly used.[53,54]

The use of large-bore cutting needles has been found to be superior to FNA sampling in terms of providing more specific diagnoses, particularly for the characterization of neoplastic processes.[53] FNA, although yielding a high rate of positive diagnosis of malignancy, has been found to have a limited capability for accurately identifying the cell type in up to one-third of cases, thus limiting management options for the treatment of the tumors.[55] Moreover, diagnosis of benign lesions is made more difficult on FNA material than with core biopsies.[53,56] CT-guided core needle biopsy has also been found to be associated with a higher diagnostic accuracy for the evaluation of pneumonia and its mimics than FNA.[57] In a study from the United Kingdom,[58] significantly more core biopsies than fine needle aspirates were diagnostic (93% vs 78%; $P < .005$). No differences were found in the frequency of complications between the two groups.

VIDEO-ASSISTED THORACOSCOPIC SURGERY LUNG BIOPSY

VATS offers the opportunity for obtaining multiple, relatively large tissue samples from lesions of the lung using a minimally invasive approach that involves the use of small incisions without spreading the ribs. This approach reduces the morbidity and mortality and allows a quicker return to normal activities with minimal hospitalization. The technique involves the use of trochars and a thoracoscope that is usually inserted through a 2-cm incision in about the sixth or seventh intercostal space along the midclavicular line. Two additional 2-cm incisions are made in about the fifth intercostal space, one anteriorly and the other posteriorly, creating a triangular configuration that facilitates access to various parts of the chest. VATS is generally performed under general anesthesia, although relatively limited procedures such as pleural biopsies can also be performed under local anesthesia. The procedure is accomplished by ventilating the opposite lung through a double-lumen endotracheal tube and allowing the affected lung to collapse. Following insertion of the thoracoscope, the lung collapses and quickly separates from the chest wall, allowing clear visualization of all the major structures in the chest cavity.

A large number of thoracic operations can now be performed with VATS, including wedge resection and lobectomy. Lung biopsy is the most common procedure performed by VATS (eFig. 1.5).[59] The morbidity and mortality are very low, and patients are usually discharged on the first or second postoperative day. The procedure can even be performed on an outpatient basis.

VATS is particularly well suited to the evaluation of diffuse interstitial lung disease. The technique allows for generous sampling of multiple sites without the need for an open thoracotomy incision and permits adequate evaluation of lung tissues (Fig. 1.18). VATS has been shown to be as effective as open lung biopsy for the diagnosis of interstitial lung

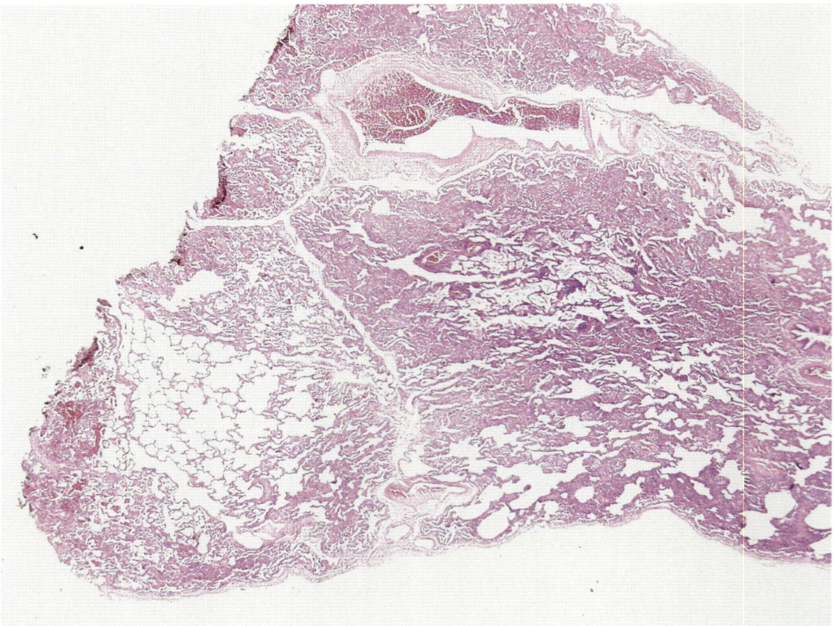

FIGURE 1.18 **Video-assisted thoracoscopic surgery biopsy for evaluation of interstitial lung disease.** Notice wedge-shaped contour of the biopsy with the apex opposite to the pleural surface.

disease, resulting in shorter hospital stays and fewer complications.[60] The procedure is considered safe in most patients; however, one study found a 4.4% mortality rate (3 of 68 patients) in a retrospective analysis of patients undergoing VATS biopsy for interstitial lung disease.[61]

VATS is also useful for the evaluation of peripheral lung lesions, in particular, indeterminate solitary pulmonary nodules.[62,63] This technique is particularly valuable for those cases in which endoscopic biopsy or core needle biopsy yields equivocal results. It has been shown that as many as 29% of patients whose condition was not diagnosed as malignant on transthoracic needle biopsy are ultimately found to have carcinoma.[64] VATS is not suitable for centrally located lesions because they generally cannot be reached by a thoracoscopic approach. Also, new lesions larger than 3 cm in greatest diameter are more likely to be malignant and may require thoracotomy.

The only absolute contraindication to VATS lung biopsy is a patient's inability to tolerate a general anesthetic with single-lung ventilation. This situation, however, is extremely unusual, except among mechanically ventilated patients with severe respiratory failure. VATS is also not feasible in patients who have previously undergone a pneumonectomy and thus do not have an opposite lung to ventilate. Prior thoracotomy with the development of adhesions can also make VATS difficult; however, in most instances, the adhesions can be lysed under direct vision, allowing the procedure to be carried out safely.

ROBOTIC-ASSISTED THORACOSCOPIC SURGERY LUNG BIOPSY

RATS has become increasingly used over the past two decades. It is considered a minimally invasive technique that uses a robot with multiple arms that operate through various small port holes and that are controlled by the thoracic surgeon.[65,66] The technique is capable of performing small wedge resections but can be used for larger procedures such as segmentectomies and even pneumonectomies. Various configurations exist allowing for slightly different functionality including two-arm, three-arm, and four-arm platforms.[67-69]

Studies have shown that RATS provides satisfactory operative outcomes comparable to those of VATS and open surgery.[70-72] Studies have also shown that RATS can improve the rate of postoperative complications as compared to VATS, particularly in older patients.[73,74] As the technique is capable of procuring larger biopsies (wedge biopsies), it is capable of providing more diagnostic material compared to bronchoscopic biopsies and may be used for diffuse parenchymal processes, infectious processes, and inflammatory conditions.

The main drawback of this technology is the cost of the equipment as well as the availability of trained operators. Advantages include quicker recovery times and ability to sample larger amounts of lung tissue. Some studies have also shown that lymph node sampling is superior to VATS with an increased rate of nodal upstaging for RATS.[75] Ultimately, RATS procedures may become more common place as technology advances, and it is adopted at more centers.

HANDLING AND PROCESSING OF THE LUNG BIOPSY

Lung biopsy samples should be placed immediately into fixative or sterile transport medium. If transport medium is not available, the material may be placed on a sterile nonstick dressing and immediately transported fresh to the laboratory for processing. Placing of a biopsy on saline-soaked gauze or mesh pads is discouraged as the biopsy material may become entrapped in the mesh, making extraction difficult with ensuing tissue damage. Exposure to air should be minimized to avoid air-drying artifacts. Procuring tissue for special techniques such as microbiologic cultures, cytogenetics, molecular studies, flow cytometry, electron microscopy (EM), or immunofluorescence always needs to be coordinated in advance with the pathology department. Tissues for microbial cultures should be sampled under sterile conditions in the operating room and submitted directly to the microbiology laboratory in a sterile container. Once the tissue has been transported to surgical pathology, the chance of contamination is great, thus compromising the results of microbiologic culture studies. If direct immunofluorescence is to be performed, a tissue sample must be frozen. Freezing to −20 °C is usually sufficient for the initial handling of the specimen. If the specimen is to be retained longer than a few weeks, freezing at −70 °C will be required. Tissues for EM need to be sampled fresh, carefully diced into 1 mm^3 cubes, and placed in a solution of 2% to 3% glutaraldehyde or other EM fixative. The vials containing the tissue must be carefully labeled, stored at 4 °C, and transferred to the EM facility. Tissues for cytogenetics or flow cytometry must be placed in an appropriate transport solution and transferred immediately to the appropriate facility for proper processing. Tissues intended for routine histopathologic examination are best placed in 10% neutral buffered formalin using a tissue to volume ratio of approximately 1:10. Alternative nonformalin fixatives such as alcohol and others may also be used, depending on the local usage at any given laboratory. PCR-based tests and NGS assays can be performed on formalin-fixed paraffin-embedded tissue fixed in 10% to 20% neutral buffered formalin or fresh, frozen, or alcohol-fixed specimens.[76,77]

With increasing use of molecular testing to guide patient management, adequate tissue sampling and optimal processing are more important than ever. Acquiring biopsy and FNA material for molecular diagnostics may pose several problems. Without intraoperative evaluation of material, tumor cellularity on small sample specimens cannot be guaranteed. Low tumor cellularity generally leads to low yields of genomic material and limits the number of ancillary tests that can be performed. Assays with higher analytic sensitivity or multiplex assay platforms than can test panels of genes are becoming increasingly available and may help when material is limited.[78] In addition, certain fixatives contain reagents that degrade nucleic acids and prevent adequate molecular testing by PCR and NGS; this is of particular concern when metastases to bone are being sampled. Pathology departments should have adequate specific protocols in place to manage the handling of metastatic bone specimens being taken with molecular testing in mind. In addition, some larger academic centers are beginning to implement so-called rapid molecular protocols in which intraoperative frozen section analysis of biopsy material is performed to ensure adequate tumor cellularity, which is then sent for immediate molecular testing. With or without intraoperative frozen section examination to ensure tumor cellularity, the procurement of several tissue cores during biopsy has been shown to increase the yield of molecular testing. Proper specimen triaging with separate cores in separate cassettes is recommended; different tissue blocks can then be used for routine and ancillary testing (Fig. 1.19).[79]

Specimens obtained through video-assisted thoracoscopy or thoracotomy may require different handling techniques than small endoscopic or core biopsy samples. In many instances, such specimens are subjected to intraoperative consultation with frozen section examination at the time of surgery. This is best accomplished by sectioning the specimen fresh with a sharp new blade avoiding unnecessary compression and distortion of the tissue. After frozen section consultation is complete, the remainder of the specimen can be routinely fixed in neutral buffered formalin or carefully injected with formalin using a 21G to 23G needle and syringe. Frozen section consultation is obtained in some instances to determine whether

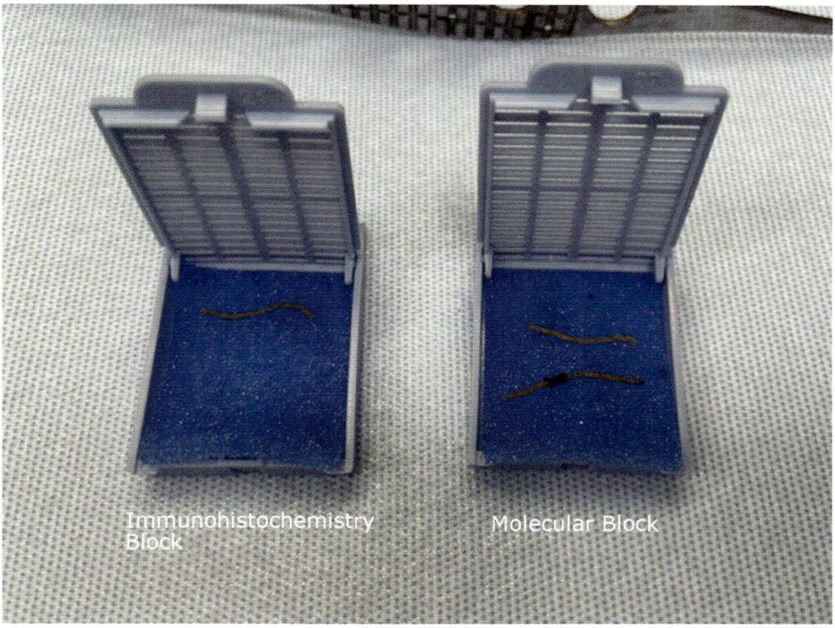

FIGURE 1.19 **Example of a lung biopsy received as three small needle cores.** The biopsy was split into two separate plastic cassettes in order to create two separate tissue blocks. Assuming that diagnostic material is available in all cores, this method preserves tissue for diagnosis, immunohistochemical testing, and downstream molecular testing as compared to placing all the biopsies into a single block.

the sample is representative for the evaluation of interstitial lung disease; however, the frozen section must be followed by an additional sample, preferably from the same site, because the frozen tissues will become distorted by the freezing artifact, rendering them useless for proper evaluation on permanent sections. Frozen section examination is not an optimal modality for evaluating interstitial lung disease and should be discouraged, unless there is a proper indication for it and additional, properly fixed, tissue will be subsequently submitted for definitive evaluation.

REFERENCES

1. Edell ES, Sanderson DR. History of bronchoscopy. In: Prakash UBS, ed. *Bronchoscopy*. Raven Press; 1994:7-11.
2. Herbut PA, Clerf LH. Bronchogenic carcinoma: diagnosis by cytological study of bronchoscopically removed secretions. *JAMA*. 1946;130:1006.
3. Ikeda S. Flexible bronchofiberscope. *Ann Otol Rhinol Laryngol*. 1970;79:916-923.
4. Kovnat DM, Rath GS, Anderson WM, et al. Maximal extent of visualization of bronchial tree by flexible fiberoptic bronchoscopy. *Am Rev Respir Dis*. 1974;110:88-90.
5. Lauver GI, Hasan FM, Morgan RB, Campbell SC. The usefulness of fiberoptic bronchoscopy in evaluating new pulmonary lesions in the compromised host. *Am J Med*. 1979;66:580-587.

6. Poletti V, Patelli M, Poggi S, Bertanti T, Spiga L, Ferracini R. Transbronchial lung biopsy and bronchoalveolar lavage in diagnosis of diffuse infiltrative lung diseases. *Respiration.* 1988;54(suppl):66-79.
7. Pue CA, Pacht ER. Complications of fiberoptic bronchoscopy at a university hospital. *Chest.* 1995;107:430-432.
8. Savage C, Morrison RJ, Zwischenberger JB. Bronchoscopic diagnosis and staging of lung cancer. *Chest Surg Clin N Am.* 2001;11:701-721.
9. Konaka C, Hirano T, Kato H, et al. Comparison of endoscopic features of early-stage squamous cell lung cancer and histological findings. *Br J Cancer.* 1999;80:1435-1439.
10. Herth FJF, Eberhardt R, Becker HD, Ernst A. Endobronchial ultrasound-guided transbronchial lung biopsy in fluoroscopically invisible solitary pulmonary nodules: a prospective trial. *Chest.* 2006;129:147-150.
11. Dursun AB, Demirag F, Bayiz H, Sertkaya D. Endobronchial metastases: a clinicopathological analysis. *Respirology.* 2005;10:510-514.
12. Poe RH, Utell MJ, Israel RH, Hall WJ, Eshleman JD. Sensitivity and specificity of the nonspecific transbronchial lung biopsy. *Am Rev Respir Dis.* 1979;119:25-32.
13. House AJS. Biopsy techniques in the investigation of diseases of the lung, mediastinum, and chest wall. *Radiol Clin North Am.* 1979;17:393-412.
14. Fraire AE, Cooper SP, Greenberg SD, Rowland LP, Langston C. Transbronchial lung biopsy. Histopathologic and morphometric assessment of diagnostic utility. *Chest.* 1992;102:748-753.
15. Shure D. Transbronchial biopsy and needle aspiration. *Chest.* 1989;95:1130-1138.
16. DiBardino DM, Yarmus LB, Semaan RW. Transthoracic needle biopsy of the lung. *J Thorac Dis.* 2015;7:S304-S316.
17. Khandhar SJ, Bowling MR, Flandes J, et al; NAVIGATE Study Investigators. Electromagnetic navigation bronchoscopy to access lung lesions in 1,000 subjects: first results of the prospective, multicenter NAVIGATE study. *BMC Pulm Med.* 2017;17:59.
18. Mondoni M, Rinaldo RF, Carlucci P, et al. Bronchoscopic sampling techniques in the era of technological bronchoscopy. *Pulmonology.* 2022;28:461-471.
19. Gal AA. Use and abuse of lung biopsy. *Adv Anat Pathol.* 2005;12:195-202.
20. Travis WD, King TE Jr, Bateman ED, et al. American Thoracic Society/European Respiratory Society international multidisciplinary consensus classification of the idiopathic interstitial pneumonias. *Am J Respir Crit Care Med.* 2002;165:277-304.
21. Wall CP, Gaensler EA, Carrington CB, Hayes JA. Comparison of transbronchial and open biopsies in chronic infiltrative lung diseases. *Am Rev Respir Dis.* 1981;123:280-285.
22. Katzenstein AL, Askin FB. Interpretation and significance of pathologic findings in transbronchial lung biopsy. *Am J Surg Pathol.* 1980;4:223-234.
23. Ferson PF, Landreneau RJ. Thoracoscopic lung biopsy or open lung biopsy for interstitial lung disease. *Chest Surg Clin N Am.* 1998;8:749-762.
24. Tiitto L, Heiskanen U, Bloigu R, Pääkkö P, Kinnula V, Kaarteenaho-Wiik R. Thoracoscopic lung biopsy is a safe procedure in diagnosing usual interstitial pneumonia. *Chest.* 2005;128:2375-2380.
25. Riley DJ, Costanzo EJ. Surgical biopsy: its appropriateness in diagnosing interstitial lung disease. *Curr Opin Pulm Med.* 2006;12:331-336.
26. Rodgers BM, Talbert JL. Clinical application of endotracheal cryotherapy. *J Pediatr Surg.* 1978;13(6D):662-668. doi:10.7196/10.1016/s0022-3468(78)80111-0
27. Esmail A, Dheda K. The cool new kid on the block: lung cryobiopsy. *Afr J Thorac Crit Care Med.* 2023;29. doi:10.7196/AJTCCM.2023.v29i3.1494
28. Segmen F, Aktaş Z, Öztürk A, et al. How many samples would be optimal for endobronchial cryobiopsy? *Surg Endosc.* 2017;31:1219-1224.

29. Simon M, Simon I, Tent PA, Todea DA, Haranguş A. Cryobiopsy in lung cancer diagnosis–a literature review. *Medicina (Kaunas)*. 2021;57:393.
30. Castro HM, Wainstein EJ, Castro Azcurra R, Seehaus A. Pneumatocele following lung cryobiopsy. *Arch Bronconeumol*. 2021;57:-600. doi:599
31. Asaoka M, Baba T, Ogura T. Pleural emphysema after transbronchial lung cryobiopsy. *Intern Med*. 2020;59:2331-2332.
32. Babiak A, Hetzel J, Krishna G, et al. Transbronchial cryobiopsy: a new tool for lung biopsies. *Respiration*. 2009;78:203-208.
33. Ankudavicius V, Miliauskas S, Poskiene L, Vajauskas D, Zemaitis M. Diagnostic yield of transbronchial cryobiopsy guided by radial endobronchial ultrasound and fluoroscopy in the radiologically suspected lung cancer: a single institution prospective study. *Cancers (Basel)*. 2022;14:1563.
34. Maldonado F, Danoff SK, Wells AU, et al. Transbronchial cryobiopsy for the diagnosis of interstitial lung diseases: CHEST guideline and Expert Panel Report. *Chest*. 2020;157:1030-1042.
35. Korevaar DA, Colella S, Fally M, et al. European Respiratory Society guidelines on transbronchial lung cryobiopsy in the diagnosis of interstitial lung diseases. *Eur Respir J*. 2022;60:2200425.
36. Rodrigues I, Estêvão Gomes R, Coutinho LM, et al. Diagnostic yield and safety of transbronchial lung cryobiopsy and surgical lung biopsy in interstitial lung diseases: a systematic review and meta-analysis. *Eur Respir Rev*. 2022;31:210280.
37. Fortin M, Liberman M, Delage A, et al. Transbronchial Lung Cryobiopsy and Surgical Lung Biopsy: A Prospective Multi-Centre Agreement Clinical Trial (CAN-ICE). *Am J Respir Crit Care Med*. 2023;207:1612-1619.
38. Montero MA, de Gracia J, Culebras Amigo M, et al. The role of transbronchial cryobiopsy in lung transplantation. *Histopathology*. 2018;73:593-600.
39. Davidsen JR, Skov IR, Louw IG, Laursen CB. Implementation of transbronchial lung cryobiopsy in a tertiary referral center for interstitial lung diseases: a cohort study on diagnostic yield, complications, and learning curves. *BMC Pulm Med*. 2021;21:67.
40. Keating DT, Taverner J. Transbronchial cryobiopsy in lung transplantation: risk, reward and relevance. *Eur Respir J*. 2023;61:2201942.
41. Loor K, Culebras M, Sansano I, et al. Lung allograft transbronchial cryobiopsy for critical ventilated patients: a randomised trial. *Eur Respir J*. 2023;61:2102354.
42. Clore F, Virapongse C, Saterfiel J. Low-risk large-needle biopsy of chest lesions. *Chest*. 1989;96:538-541.
43. Yang PC, Chang DB, Yu CJ, et al. Ultrasound-guided core biopsy of thoracic tumors. *Am Rev Respir Dis*. 1992;146:763-767.
44. Tsushima K, Sone S, Hanaoka T, Takayama F, Honda T, Kubo K. Comparison of bronchoscopic diagnosis for peripheral pulmonary nodule under fluoroscopic guidance with CT guidance. *Respir Med*. 2006;100:737-745.
45. Aviram G, Schwartz DS, Meirsdorf S, Rosen G, Greif J, Graif M. Transthoracic needle biopsy of lung masses: a survey of techniques. *Clin Radiol*. 2005;60:370-374.
46. Richardson CM, Pointon KS, Manhire AR, Macfarlane JT. Percutaneous lung biopsies: a survey of UK practice based on 5444 biopsies. *Br J Radiol*. 2002;75:731-735.
47. Yamagami T, Iida S, Kato T, Tanaka O, Nishimura T. Combining fine-needle aspiration and core biopsy under CT fluoroscopy guidance: a better way to treat patients with lung nodules? *AJR Am J Roentgenol*. 2003;180:811-815.
48. Kim HK, Shin BK, Cho SJ, et al. Transthoracic fine needle aspiration and core biopsy of pulmonary lesions. A study of 296 patients. *Acta Cytol*. 2002;46:1061-1068.
49. Li H, Chen R, Zhao J. Correlation between percutaneous transthoracic needle biopsy and recurrence in stage I lung cancer: a systematic review and meta-analysis. *BMC Pulm Med*. 2020;20:198.

50. Cheng D, Wang Z, Cui J, Liu L. Does percutaneous transthoracic needle biopsy increase the risk of pleural recurrence in patients with stage I lung cancer? *Interact Cardiovasc Thorac Surg.* 2020;30:834-838.
51. Jelitto-Gorska M, Studniarek M, Durawa A, Marjanski T, Szurowska E. Percutaneous lung needle biopsies–utility and complications in various chest lesions: a single-institution experience. *Pol J Radiol.* 2018;83:e103-e108.
52. Manhire A, Charig M, Clelland C, et al. Guidelines for radiologically guided lung biopsy. *Thorax.* 2003;58:920-936.
53. Pang JA, Tsang V, Hom BL, Metreweli C. Ultrasound-guided tissue-core biopsy of thoracic lesions with Trucut and Surecut needles. *Chest.* 1987;91:823-828.
54. Yamagami T, Iida S, Kato T, et al. Usefulness of new automated cutting needle for tissue-core biopsy of lung nodules under CT fluoroscopic guidance. *Chest.* 2003;124:147-154.
55. Zavala DC, Schoell JE. Ultrathin needle aspiration of the lung in infectious and malignant disease. *Am Rev Respir Dis.* 1981;123:125-131.
56. Greif J, Marmor S, Schwarz Y, Staroselsky AN. Percutaneous core needle biopsy vs. fine needle aspiration in diagnosing benign lung lesions. *Acta Cytol.* 1999;43:756-760.
57. Thanos L, Galani P, Mylona S, Pomoni M, Mpatakis N. Percutaneous CT-guided core needle biopsy versus fine needle aspiration in diagnosing pneumonia and mimics of pneumonia. *Cardiovasc Intervent Radiol.* 2004;27:329-334.
58. Anderson JM, Murchison J, Patel D. CT-guided lung biopsy: factors influencing diagnostic yield and complication rate. *Clin Radiol.* 2003;58:791-797.
59. Ayed AK. Video-assisted thoracoscopic lung biopsy in the diagnosis of diffuse interstitial lung disease. A prospective study. *J Cardiovasc Surg (Torino).* 2003;44:115-118.
60. Ferson PF, Landreneau RJ, Dowling RD, et al. Comparison of open versus thoracoscopic lung biopsy for diffuse infiltrative pulmonary disease. *J Thorac Cardiovasc Surg.* 1993;106:194-199.
61. Kreider ME, Hansen-Flaschen J, Ahmad NN, et al. Complications of video-assisted thoracoscopic lung biopsy in patients with interstitial lung disease. *Ann Thorac Surg.* 2007;83:1140-1145.
62. Mack MJ, Hazelrigg SR, Landreneau RJ, Acuff TE. Thoracoscopy for the diagnosis of the indeterminate solitary pulmonary nodule. *Ann Thorac Surg.* 1993;56:825-830.
63. Santambrogio L, Nosotti M, Bellaviti N, Mezzetti M. Videothoracoscopy versus thoracotomy for the diagnosis of the indeterminate solitary pulmonary nodule. *Ann Thorac Surg.* 1995;59:868-870.
64. Calhoun P, Feldman PS, Armstrong P, et al. The clinical outcome of needle aspirations of the lung when cancer is not diagnosed. *Ann Thorac Surg.* 1986;41:592-596.
65. Chen S, Geraci TC, Cerfolio RJ. Techniques for lung surgery: a review of robotic lobectomy. *Expert Rev Respir Med.* 2018;12:315-322.
66. Yamashita S, Yoshida Y, Iwasaki A. Robotic surgery for thoracic disease. *Ann Thorac Cardiovasc Surg.* 2016;22:1-5.
67. Veronesi G, Galetta D, Maisonneuve P, et al. Four-arm robotic lobectomy for the treatment of early-stage lung cancer. *J Thorac Cardiovasc Surg.* 2010;140:19-25.
68. Jang HJ, Lee HS, Park SY, Zo JI. Comparison of the early robot-assisted lobectomy experience to video-assisted thoracic surgery lobectomy for lung cancer: a single-institution case series matching study. *Innovations (Phila).* 2011;6:305-310.
69. Anderson CA, Hellan M, Falebella A, Lau CS, Grannis FW, Kernstine KH. Robotic-assisted lung resection for malignant disease. *Innovations (Phila).* 2007;2:254-258.
70. Zirafa CC, Romano G, Sicolo E, et al. Robotic versus open surgery in locally advanced non-small cell lung cancer: evaluation of surgical and oncological outcomes. *Curr Oncol.* 2023;30:9104-9115.

71. Terra RM, Bibas BJ, Haddad R, et al. Robotic thoracic surgery for non-small cell lung cancer: initial experience in Brazil. *J Bras Pneumol.* 2019;46:e20190003.
72. Ye X, Xie L, Chen G, Tang J-M, Ben X-S. Robotic thoracic surgery versus video-assisted thoracic surgery for lung cancer: a meta-analysis. *Interact Cardiovasc Thorac Surg.* 2015;21:409-414.
73. Veluswamy RR, Whittaker Brown SA, Mhango G, et al. Comparative effectiveness of robotic-assisted surgery for resectable lung cancer in older patients. *Chest.* 2020;157:1313-1321.
74. Chen DL, Kang PM, Tao SL, Wu L-C, Li Q-Y, Tan Q-Y. Comparative short-term outcomes of robotic-assisted surgery for older patients with non-small cell lung cancer: a propensity matched study. *Updates Surg.* 2022;74:1087-1096.
75. Wilson JL, Louie BE, Cerfolio RJ, et al. The prevalence of nodal upstaging during robotic lung resection in early-stage non-small cell lung cancer. *Ann Thorac Surg.* 2014;97:1901-1906; discussion 1906-1907.
76. Lindeman N, Cagle PT, Aisner DL, et al. Molecular testing guideline for the selection of lung cancer patients for treatment with targeted tyrosine kinase inhibitors: guideline from the College of American Pathologists, the International Association for the Study of Lung Cancer, and the Association for Molecular Pathology. *J Mol Diagn.* 2018;20(2):129-159.
77. Kage H, Kohsaka S, Shinozaki-Ushiku A, et al. Small lung tumor biopsy samples are feasible for high quality targeted next generation sequencing. *Cancer Sci.* 2019;110(8):2652-2657.
78. Frampton GM, Fichtenholtz A, Otto GA, et al. Development and validation of a clinical cancer genomic profiling test based on massively parallel DNA sequencing. *Nat Biotechnol.* 2013;31(11):1023-1031.
79. Beck KS, Kim TJ, Lee KY, Kim YK, Kang JH, Han DH. CT-guided coaxial biopsy of malignant lung lesions: are cores from 20-gauge needle adequate for histologic diagnosis and molecular analysis? *J Thorac Dis.* 2019;11(3):753-765.

2

INFLAMMATORY LUNG CONDITIONS

Lung injury can result from various inflammatory conditions. The changes affecting the lung parenchyma may be relatively nonspecific, and a detailed clinical history and results of imaging studies and ancillary tests will be required to arrive at a definitive or more specific diagnosis. Inflammatory conditions may lead to diverse changes ranging from acute inflammation to subacute and chronic inflammation to reparative changes characterized by fibrous scarring of lung parenchyma. It is important to understand that such changes do not constitute specific diagnoses or discrete clinicopathologic entities but merely represent patterns of tissue response to injury that are nonspecific and that may be observed in a wide variety of conditions (Table 2.1).

TABLE 2.1 **Nonspecific Patterns of Tissue Response to Injury in Lung Parenchyma**
Diffuse alveolar damage with hyaline membranes
Organizing bronchopneumonia
Bronchiolitis obliterans (peribronchial fibrosis)
Acute fibrinous and organizing pneumonia
Interstitial pneumonitis
Interstitial fibrosis
Hyperplasia of alveolar type II pneumocytes
Bronchiolar and squamous metaplasia
Respiratory bronchiolitis
Vasculitis/capillaritis
Granulomatous inflammation

ACUTE LUNG INJURY

Several conditions can result in acute lung inflammation. The acute inflammatory reaction may affect any component of the lung parenchyma, including the alveolus, the bronchial tree, the mucosa, the stroma, and bronchial vasculature.

The most common form of acute lung injury involves the alveolus and is characterized histologically by diffuse alveolar damage (DAD). The clinical counterpart of DAD has been designated over the years by different terms, including "shock lung," "postperfusion lung," and "acute respiratory distress syndrome" (ARDS). The term "ARDS" was introduced in 1967 by Ashbaugh et al[1] for patients characterized by severe respiratory distress of acute onset following different insults, with dyspnea, reduction in lung diffusing capacity, radiographic changes, and hypoxemia refractory to oxygen administration. ARDS follows a rapidly progressing clinical course and is associated with a high mortality rate, with approximately more than half of patients dying of respiratory insufficiency within days to weeks.[2,3]

Because the lung reacts to various types of injuries in a similar fashion regardless of the etiology, the histologic changes observed in acute lung injury are nonspecific and have been generically designated as "DAD." Causes of DAD in patients with ARDS include infections, drugs, radiation, ingestion or inhalation of poisons and chemicals, oxygen toxicity, shock, sepsis, collagen vascular diseases, and others (Table 2.2). ARDS can also be the result of diffuse alveolar hemorrhage or acute eosinophilic pneumonia (AEP).[4,5]

In the workup of ARDS open lung biopsy is sometimes performed for diagnosis; specifically, when (1) less invasive procedures are nondiagnostic and there is high suspicion for a curable etiology and/or (2) when trying to identify the fibrotic phase of the disease where steroid therapy can be useful.[6-8] The histologic picture in DAD can be quite variable,

TABLE 2.2 Causes of Acute Lung Injury
Infection
Drugs
Poisons, toxins
Inhalants (smoke, toxic gases, etc.)
Oxygen toxicity
Shock/sepsis
Radiation
Collagen vascular/autoimmune diseases
Surgery, trauma

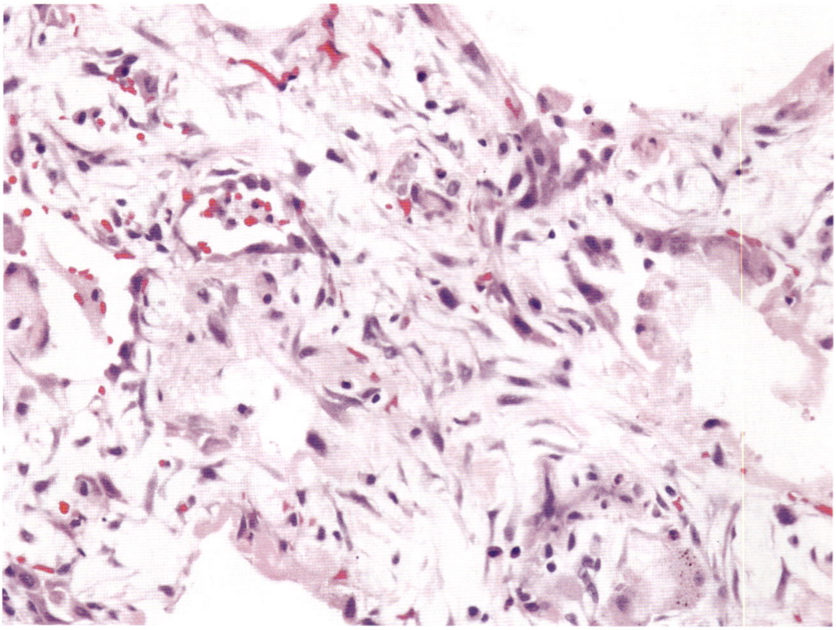

FIGURE 2.1 **Exudative phase of diffuse alveolar damage.** Notice acute endothelial and mucosal damage with abundant edema fluid in the interstitium.

depending on the stage of the process. The initial phase is characterized by acute endothelial and mucosal injury with resulting exudation of fluid and cells (so-called exudative phase) (Fig. 2.1; eFig. 2.1). The alveolar walls are characterized by interstitial and intra-alveolar edema with varying amounts of hemorrhage and fibrin deposition (eFig. 2.2). The interstitial inflammatory infiltrates comprise small lymphocytes and histiocytes. Small fibrin thrombi within the pulmonary microvasculature may also be present. The morphologic hallmark of the exudative phase is the formation of so-called hyaline membranes characterized by deposition of acellular eosinophilic proteinaceous exudates lining the alveolar walls (Fig. 2.2; eFig. 2.3). Another change that occurs toward the end of the exudative phase is hyperplasia of type II pneumocytes. The reactive type II pneumocytes may display marked cytologic atypia with enlarged, hyperchromatic nuclei and mitotic figures (Fig. 2.3). The exudative phase generally lasts from 3 to 7 days and is followed by a proliferative phase characterized by an active fibroblastic proliferation mainly involving the interstitium and eventually extending into the alveolar spaces (Fig. 2.4). The fibroblastic plugs are usually composed of loose aggregates of fibroblasts against a myxoid stroma admixed with scattered inflammatory cells and are devoid of significant collagen deposition (Fig. 2.5; eFig. 2.4). Hyperplasia of type II pneumocytes persists during this phase and may be accompanied by immature squamous metaplasia with atypia (Fig. 2.6). Hyaline membranes

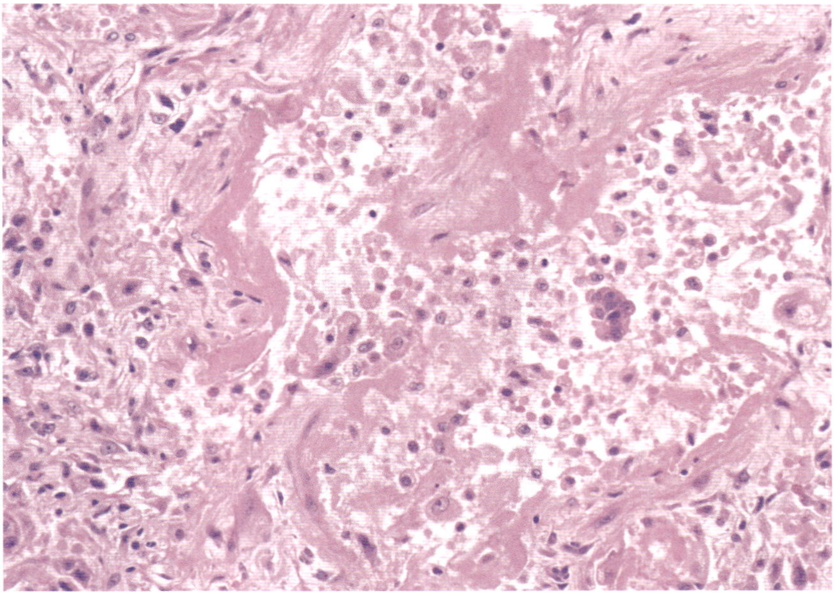

FIGURE 2.2 **Exudative phase of diffuse alveolar damage showing formation of hyaline membranes characterized by acellular eosinophilic proteinaceous material lining the surface of alveolar walls.**

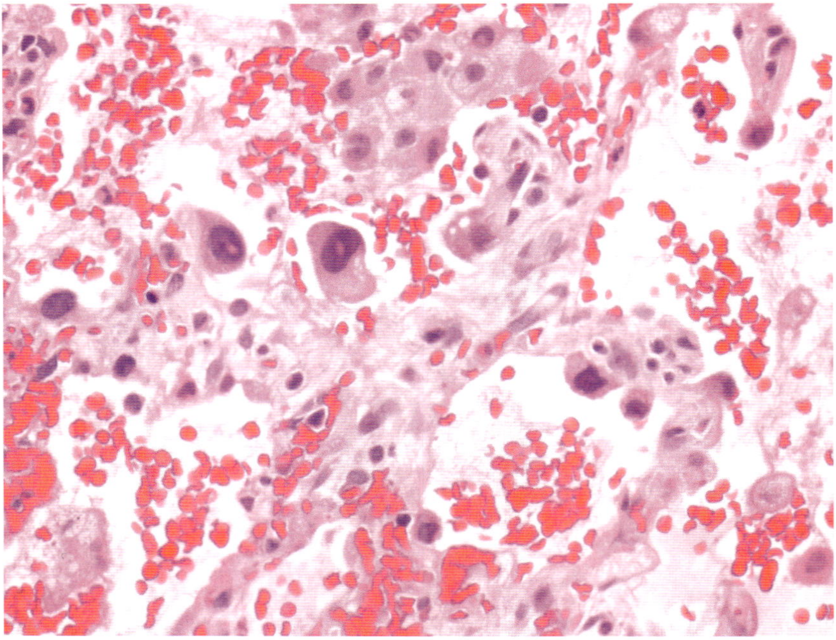

FIGURE 2.3 **Exudative phase of diffuse alveolar damage showing hyperplasia of type II alveolar pneumocytes.** Notice enlarged, atypical nuclei protruding from the alveolar walls.

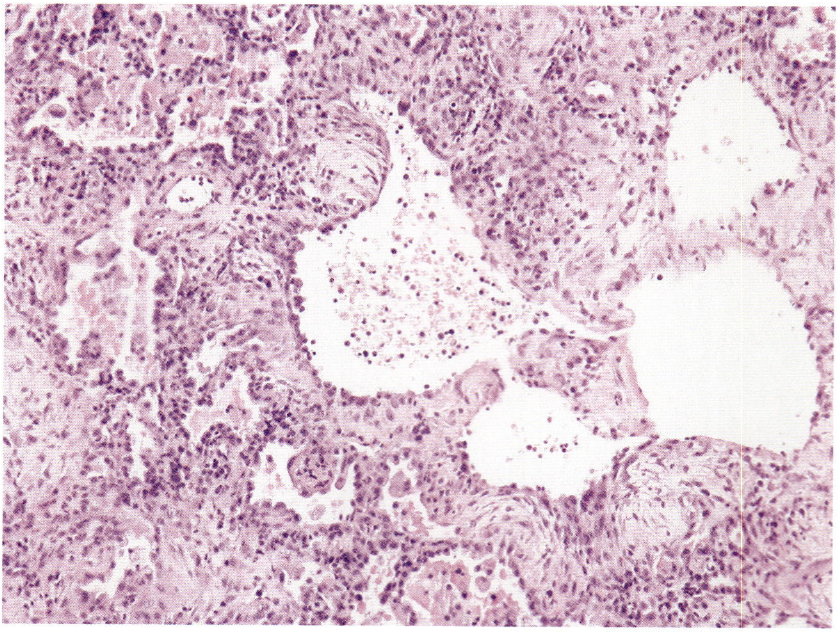

FIGURE 2.4 Proliferative phase of diffuse alveolar damage characterized by active fibroblastic proliferation involving the interstitium of the alveolar walls and extending into alveolar spaces.

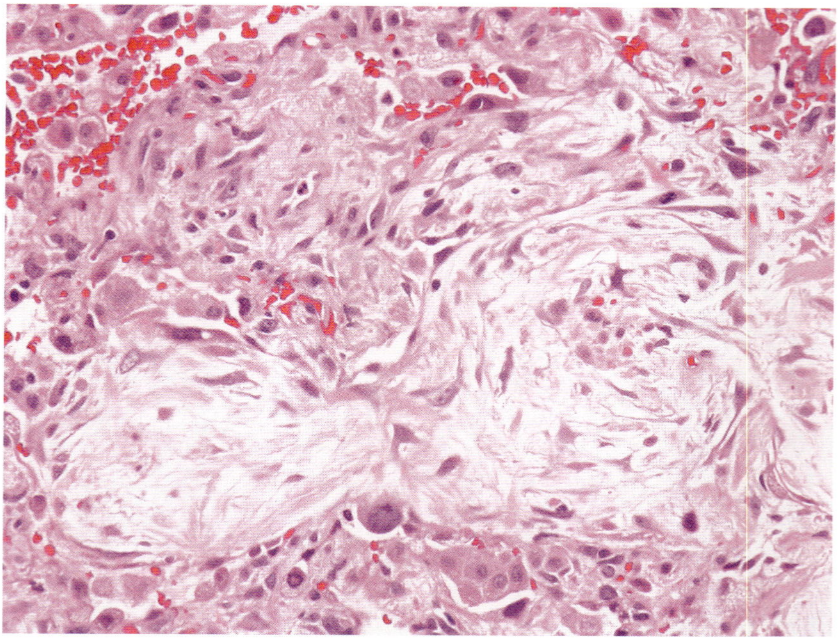

FIGURE 2.5 Proliferative phase of diffuse alveolar damage showing fibroblastic plugs within the alveolar lumens comprising aggregates of spindle fibroblasts embedded in loose myxoid matrix.

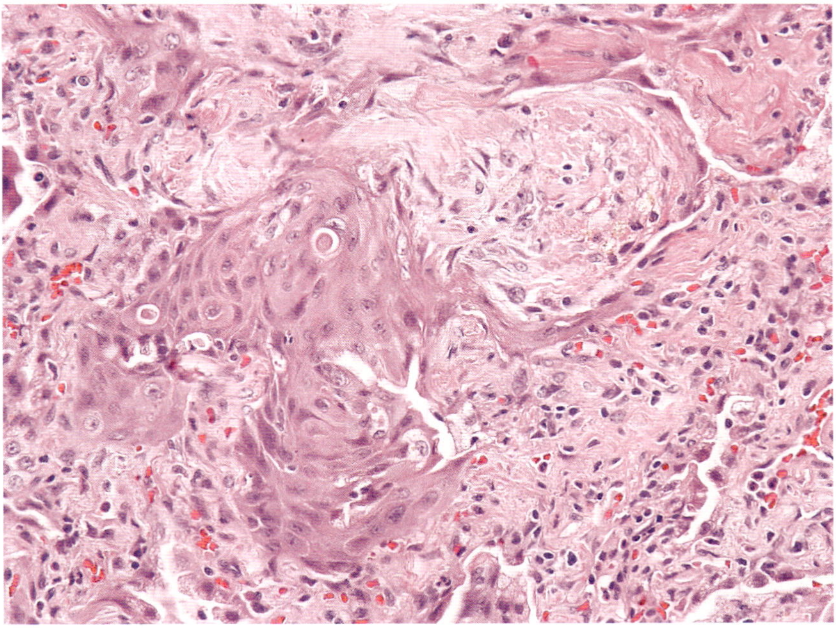

FIGURE 2.6 Proliferative phase of diffuse alveolar damage with hyperplasia of type II pneumocytes and squamous metaplasia of alveolar lining.

are usually reabsorbed by the end of the exudative phase but may persist into the proliferative phase. The natural evolution of the process at this phase may be followed by complete resolution with little residual change and complete regeneration of the alveolar lining, or it may progress to a fibrotic phase, characterized by extensive collagen deposition in and around alveolar septa, eventually resulting in extensive remodeling and honeycombing of lung parenchyma (Fig. 2.7). It should be noted that DAD in any given patient may be the result of repeated injury over a period, in which case the lung biopsy may show superimposed features of acute early exudative damage along with reparative and proliferative changes in the same biopsy specimen (eFig. 2.5). DAD will usually regress if the inciting stimulus is removed.

SPECIFIC FORMS OF ACUTE LUNG INFLAMMATION

There may be several specific etiologic causes of acute lung inflammation. Most of them result in a similar nonspecific histopathologic picture; however, in some instances, some specific features may point to a specific diagnosis, or a more specific diagnosis can be achieved with the aid of a good clinical history or results of additional clinical tests. In the absence of corroborating history or laboratory tests supporting a specific etiology for the changes observed in the lung biopsy, the pathologist's role is limited

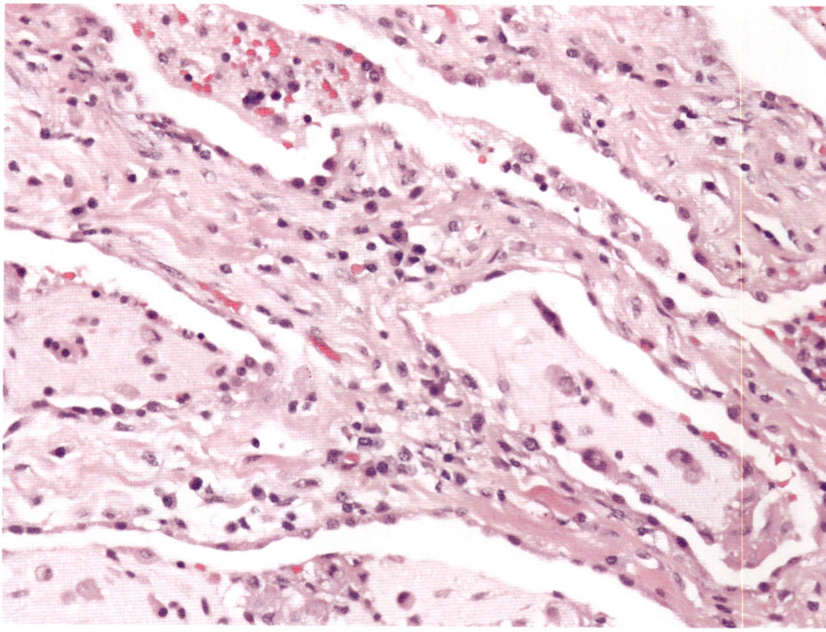

FIGURE 2.7 **Fibrotic phase of diffuse alveolar damage showing extensive collagen deposition in and around alveolar septa with remodeling of lung parenchyma.**

to making a detailed reporting of the findings of acute injury and making a generic diagnosis of DAD.

ACUTE FIBRINOUS AND ORGANIZING PNEUMONIA

Acute fibrinous and organizing pneumonia (AFOP) is a distinctive histologic manifestation of acute lung injury described as a histologic variant of DAD.[9] The clinical presentation in most cases is that of an acute or subacute process similar to but less severe than ARDS. The process may be patchy or diffuse. The histologic hallmark of AFOP is filling of the alveolar lumens with "balls" of fibrin (Fig. 2.8). A distinctive feature is the absence of neutrophils, histiocytes, or eosinophils admixed with the intra-alveolar fibrin. The alveolar septa may show mild interstitial thickening or sparse lymphoid infiltrates, but hyaline membranes are not found and inflammatory cells in the walls of the alveoli should be scarce (Fig. 2.9). Organization of the intra-alveolar fibrin such as that seen in cryptogenic organizing pneumonia (COP) is also not a feature. AFOP has been found in association with a wide variety of underlying conditions similar to those seen in DAD, although some cases is idiopathic. In the original study, patients were reported to show an association with underlying collagen vascular disease, environmental exposure to extrinsic antigens, altered immune status, ingestion of various drugs, lymphoma, and positive cultures for *Haemophilus influenzae*

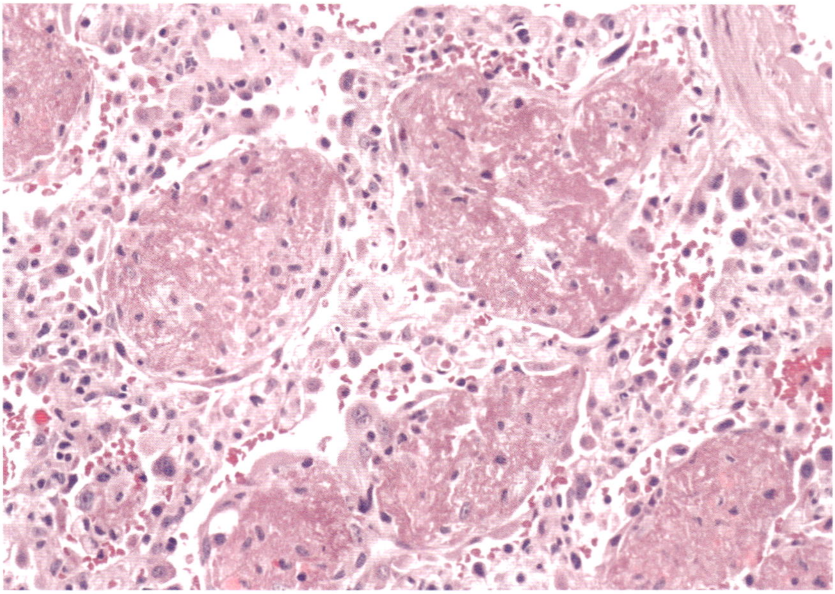

FIGURE 2.8 **Acute fibrinous and organizing pneumonia is characterized by filling of the alveolar lumens by "balls" of fibrin.**

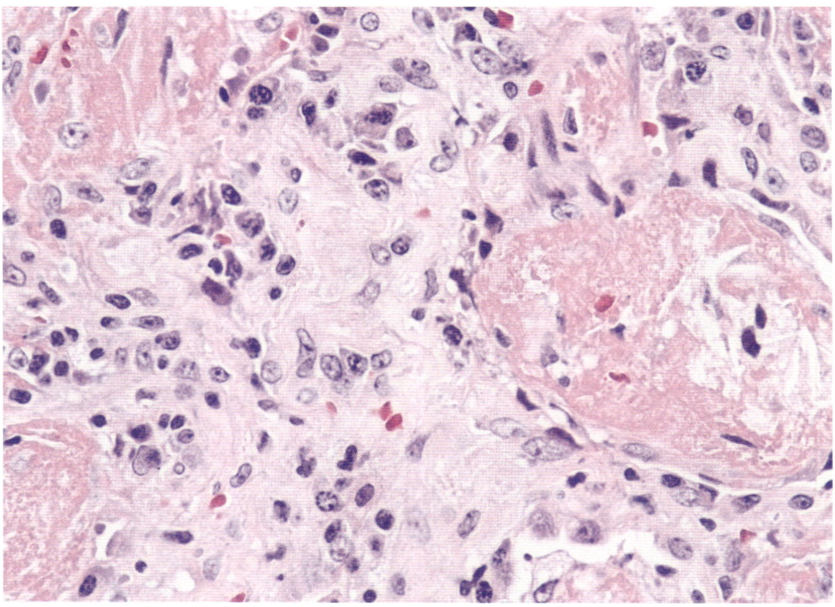

FIGURE 2.9 **Higher magnification in acute fibrinous and organizing pneumonia shows mild interstitial thickening with prominent reactive fibroblastic cells and some scattered admixed lymphocytes and plasma cells.** Notice the absence of eosinophils and neutrophils.

and *Acinetobacter baumannii*. Although most cases presented with clinical symptoms of mild ARDS, some of the patients displayed a subacute clinical course that did not require mechanical ventilation; such patients had a more favorable outcome than those requiring mechanical ventilation.

Acute Interstitial Pneumonia (Hamman-Rich Syndrome)

Acute interstitial pneumonia (AIP), previously also known as the Hamman-Rich syndrome, represents a fulminant and rapidly progressive lung condition of unknown etiology mostly affecting previously healthy young adults. It is characterized clinically by sudden onset of fever, cough, and shortness of breath with diffuse bilateral pulmonary infiltrates on chest X-rays.[10,11] Patients usually develop respiratory failure with a high mortality rate–usually within a few days to weeks.

Histologically, AIP is characterized by changes indistinguishable from DAD as seen in ARDS. Unlike ARDS in which DAD can be traced to a well-defined inciting stimulus such as infection, drugs, shock, radiation, trauma, oxygen toxicity, and noxious inhalants, the term "AIP" is reserved for cases where the etiology is unknown.[3] A thorough clinical history, serologic tests, and microbiologic studies are indicated to rule out specific causes of acute lung injury in these patients. The early changes resemble the exudative phase of DAD, with inflammation and edema of alveolar walls and formation of hyaline membranes (Fig. 2.10). This is followed by

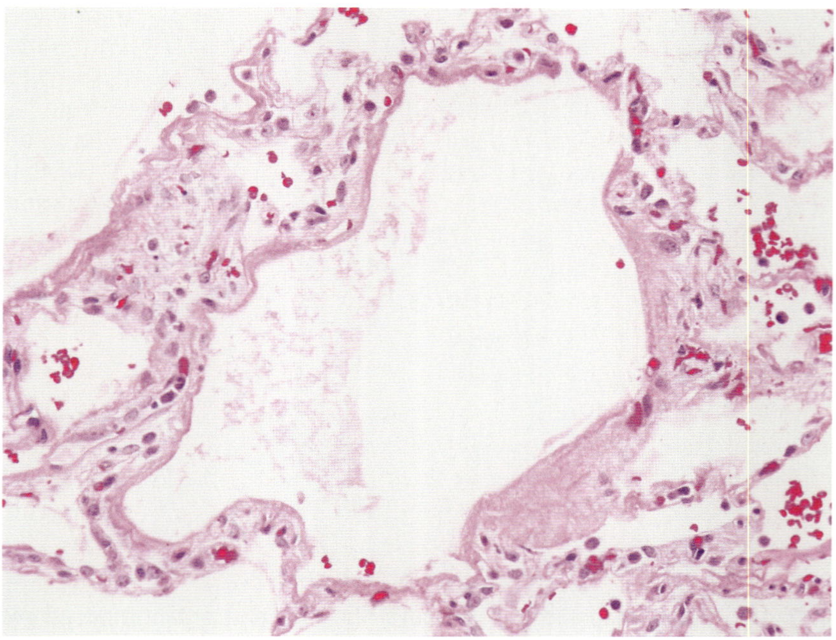

FIGURE 2.10 Formation of hyaline membrane lining the alveolar wall is seen in a patient with acute interstitial pneumonia.

an organizing phase with acute interstitial and intra-alveolar fibrosis accompanied by hyperplasia of type II pneumocytes. If the patient survives, residual scarring with severe interstitial fibrosis will ensue. AIP should also be distinguished from acute exacerbations of fibrotic pulmonary diseases where the manifestations of acute lung injury are superimposed upon an underlying fibrotic disorder such as usual interstitial pneumonia (UIP), idiopathic pulmonary fibrosis, or nonspecific interstitial pneumonia (NSIP), which usually requires close clinical and radiologic correlation to rule out underlying interstitial lung disease.[12-14]

Collagen Vascular Diseases

Lung involvement is a frequent manifestation of collagen vascular diseases. There may be several specific etiologic causes of acute lung inflammation due to collagen vascular disease. Most of them result in a similar nonspecific histopathologic picture; however, in the setting of a well-defined clinical picture and with the support of appropriate laboratory tests, a more specific diagnosis may be rendered.

Systemic Lupus Erythematosus

Patients with systemic lupus erythematosus (SLE) may present with diffuse acute or chronic inflammation of the lungs or with changes affecting primarily the pulmonary vasculature (vasculitis and thromboembolic phenomena). Acute lupus pneumonitis is a form of the disease associated with highly aggressive evolution and a high mortality rate.[15] This condition is characterized by dyspnea, tachypnea, fever, and hypoxemia. The histopathologic changes are primarily those of DAD, although acute alveolar hemorrhage with capillaritis and small vessel vasculitis can also be observed.[16,17] Diffuse fibrosis with changes indistinguishable from those of UIP will develop in 1% to 5% of patients with SLE.[18] Vascular changes are also a common manifestation of lung involvement by SLE. Capillaritis with diffuse alveolar hemorrhage, small vessel vasculitis, and pulmonary hypertension are a major cause of morbidity and mortality in patients with SLE.[19,20] Immune complex deposition, including immunoglobulin IgG, IgM, IgA, and C3, can be demonstrated by immunofluorescence in the alveolar interstitium and vessel walls.[21,22]

Rheumatoid Arthritis

Pulmonary manifestations of rheumatoid arthritis (RA) can vary from acute lung injury to the characteristic rheumatoid nodule. Acute lung injury in patients with RA takes the form of DAD, and the findings are indistinguishable from those seen in ARDS.[23,24] Correlation with serologic tests and a good clinical history are indispensable for diagnosis.

Polymyositis and Dermatomyositis

These conditions can also be associated with pulmonary manifestations, that can range from acute respiratory distress with DAD-like changes to organizing pneumonia to interstitial lung disease.[25,26]

Drug Toxicity

Many drugs can result in damage to the airways that may range from acute alveolar damage, organizing pneumonia, interstitial pneumonitis, obliterative bronchiolitis, veno-occlusive disease, granulomatous inflammation, and diffuse fibrosing pneumonitis.[27,28] The most common manifestation of acute drug toxicity is DAD.[27]

Chemotherapeutic Agents

Cytotoxic drugs are a common cause of acute lung damage. The most common agents are busulfan and bleomycin, although methotrexate and carmustine have also been implicated.[27,29] The histologic findings are characterized by nonspecific changes of DAD with extensive hyaline membrane formation. Busulfan toxicity is characterized by a combination of DAD with prominent hyperplasia of type II pneumocytes displaying markedly enlarged and pleomorphic nuclei with prominent nucleoli (Fig. 2.11).[30]

Amiodarone

The β-blocker, amiodarone, used for the control of cardiac arrhythmias is another well-recognized cause of pulmonary toxicity. The pathologic findings comprise DAD, chronic interstitial pneumonitis with fibrosis, and organizing pneumonia.[31,32] A fairly distinctive finding in amiodarone toxicity is the presence of fine cytoplasmic vacuolation of intra-alveolar macrophages and hyperplasia of type II pneumocytes (Fig. 2.12).

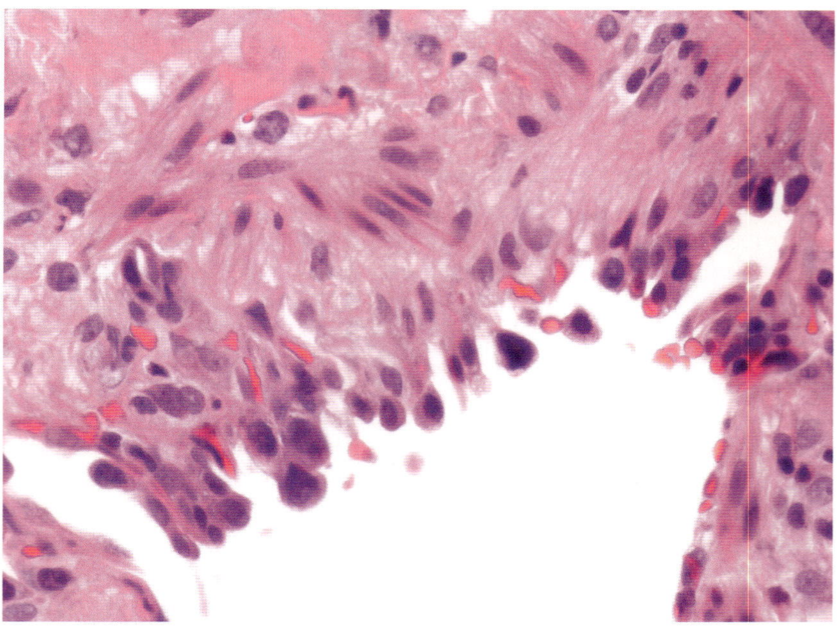

FIGURE 2.11 **Acute lung injury in a patient with drug toxicity secondary to busulfan.** Notice alveolar type II pneumocytes displaying markedly enlarged and pleomorphic nuclei with prominent nucleoli.

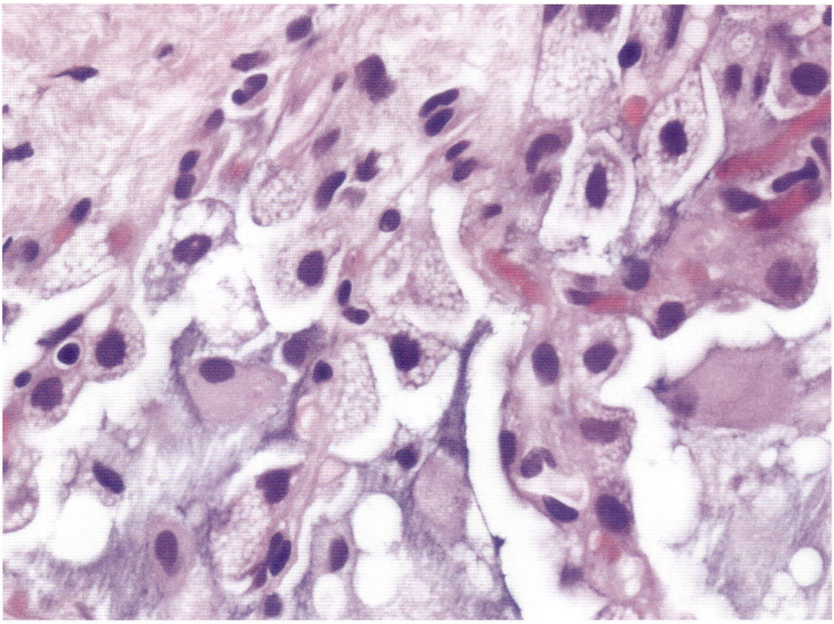

FIGURE 2.12 Acute lung injury in amiodarone toxicity characterized by prominent fine cytoplasmic vacuoles in intra-alveolar macrophages and type II alveolar pneumocytes.

Acute Eosinophilic Pneumonia

Eosinophilic pneumonia is a condition that can present clinically as acute respiratory distress or as a more chronic process, often without any identifiable underlying cause.[33] Identifiable causes of eosinophilic pneumonia include cigarette smoking, inhalational chemicals, infectious agents, and a wide variety of drugs.[34] Clinically, patients present with a typical clinical syndrome and radiographic appearance that includes fever, weight loss, cough and dyspnea with or without peripheral blood eosinophilia, and bilateral subpleural infiltrates with poorly defined margins that may disappear spontaneously only to recur later at the same sites ("migratory" infiltrates). Eosinophilic pneumonia is most often encountered as a subacute clinical process, but it can also present as an acute illness. Two distinct forms of the disease are recognized: AEP and chronic eosinophilic pneumonia; the histologic features are similar in both, and the distinction is based mostly on the duration and clinical presentation of the disease. In general, eosinophilic pneumonia is histologically characterized by alveolar septal edema admixed with macrophages and reactive atypia of alveolar type II macrophages. The distinctive feature of the process is the presence of eosinophils in varying numbers within the alveolar lumens. Hyaline membranes and intra-alveolar fibrin deposition may also be seen. It is important to recognize the eosinophils because patients respond favorably to treatment with corticosteroids.

AEP presents clinically as ARDS and is often associated with fever. Unlike the chronic form of the disease, peripheral eosinophilia is more often absent.[35] Patients may show an association with various underlying processes such as toxic inhalation, infection, cigarette smoking, and drug reactions.[36] Some cases are idiopathic.[36] A case has been reported in association with vaping.[37] Histologically, the process is characterized by fibrin deposition within alveolar lumens admixed with numerous eosinophils (Fig. 2.13). Some cases may also display hyaline membrane formation. The differential diagnosis includes AFOP and eosinophilic granulomatosis with polyangiitis, formerly known as Churg-Strauss syndrome. AEP is distinguished from AFOP by the admixture of abundant eosinophils with the intra-alveolar fibrinous exudate. It is distinguished from Churg-Strauss by the acute onset and the absence of vasculitis.

CHRONIC LUNG INJURY

Chronic lung inflammation results from long-standing lung injury that may affect alveolar walls, bronchioles, segmental bronchi, and the interstitium. The findings in subacute and chronic inflammation of the pulmonary parenchyma range from organizing pneumonia with obliterative bronchiolitis to extensive interstitial fibrosis with remodeling of lung parenchyma. These patterns are quite nonspecific and represent a common tissue

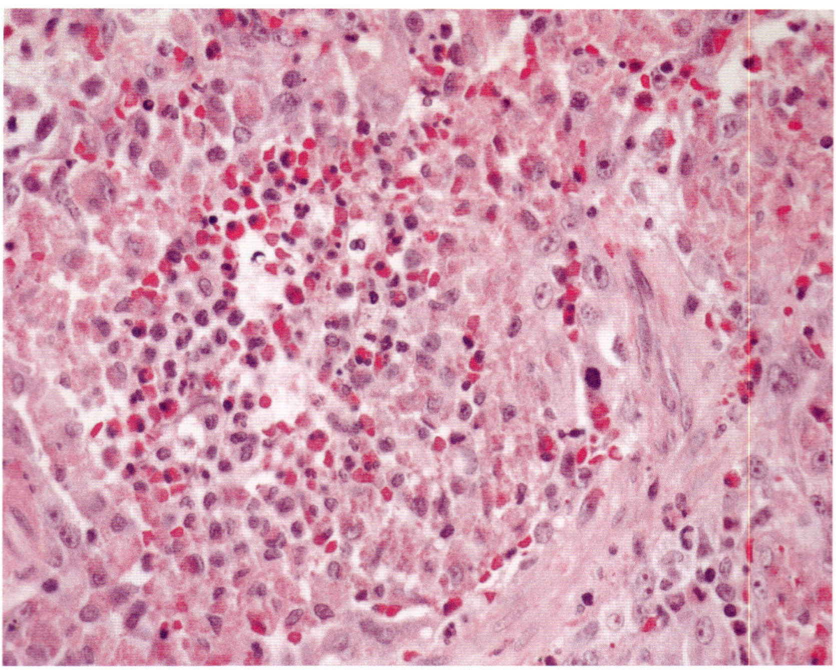

FIGURE 2.13 Acute eosinophilic pneumonia shows filling of alveolar lumens by numerous eosinophils admixed with fibrin and other inflammatory cells.

response to various injuries and stimuli. In the majority of instances, correlation with the clinical history and radiographic and laboratory test results is required for a more specific diagnosis.

The term "idiopathic bronchiolitis obliterans organizing pneumonia (BOOP)" is of historical interest and was used in the past to refer to a form of idiopathic interstitial lung disease characterized by abundance of intra-alveolar fibroblastic polyps in the terminal airways and surrounding alveoli.[38] This process is currently referred to as COP. The term "bronchiolitis obliterans" is also sometimes employed to refer to the airway injury in chronic lung transplant rejection (so-called bronchiolitis obliterans syndrome).[39,40] "BOOP" should no longer be used to define a specific "entity," and the more descriptive term of organizing pneumonia or airspace organization should be employed, as this pattern may be observed in a large number of conditions (Table 2.3).

The organizing pneumonia pattern of chronic inflammation is characterized by plugs of granulation tissue that are located within the lumen of small airways and extend into the alveolar ducts and alveoli (Fig. 2.14; eFig. 2.6). These plugs comprise inflammatory cells (neutrophils, macrophages, lymphocytes, and plasma cells) that may be admixed with small vessels and occasional fibroblasts and are embedded in a loose myxoid matrix (Fig. 2.15). The plugs may appear as polypoid masses that penetrate through the walls of the alveoli into adjacent spaces (so-called Masson bodies) or may completely fill the alveoli obliterating their lumen (Fig. 2.16). The fibrous plugs may also completely fill the alveolar ducts, adopting a branching configuration (Fig. 2.17; eFigs. 2.7 and 2.8).

TABLE 2.3 Conditions Associated With Organizing Pneumonia Pattern
In advanced stages of diffuse alveolar damage
As a complication of aspiration pneumonia
As a response to drug reactions or inhalation of toxic gases
In systemic connective tissue disorders
In the vicinity of malignant neoplasms or distal to obstructed bronchi
In association with idiopathic interstitial pneumonia (usual interstitial pneumonia)
In hypersensitivity pneumonitis
In association with other inflammatory lung diseases such as abscess, infarcts, and infections
In association with chronic obstructive bronchiolitis
In chronic lung transplant rejection
As an idiopathic process associated with mild interstitial pneumonia (cryptogenic organizing pneumonia)

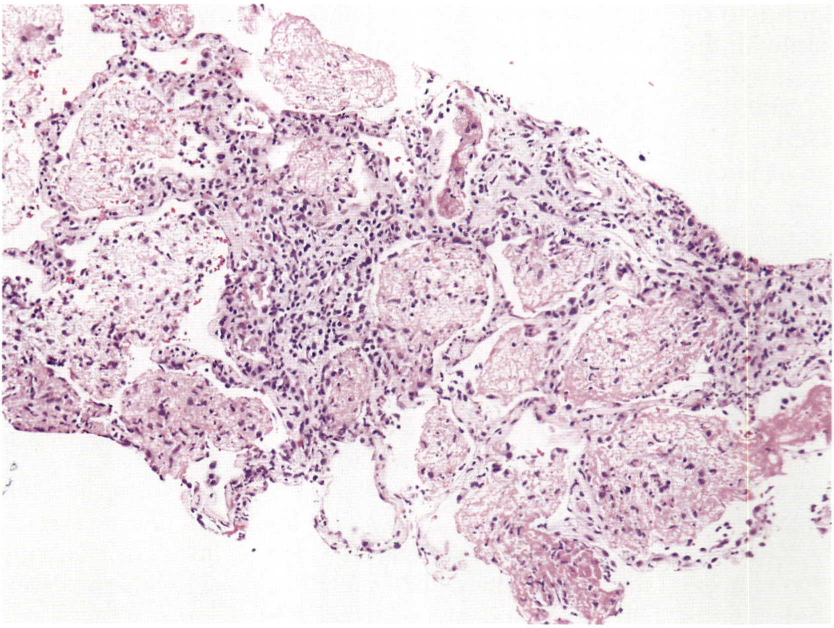

FIGURE 2.14 **Chronic lung injury tissue response pattern characterized by organizing pneumonia (formerly known as bronchiolitis obliterans organizing pneumonia).** Notice the plugs of granulation tissue located within the lumen of the small airways and extending into alveolar ducts and alveoli.

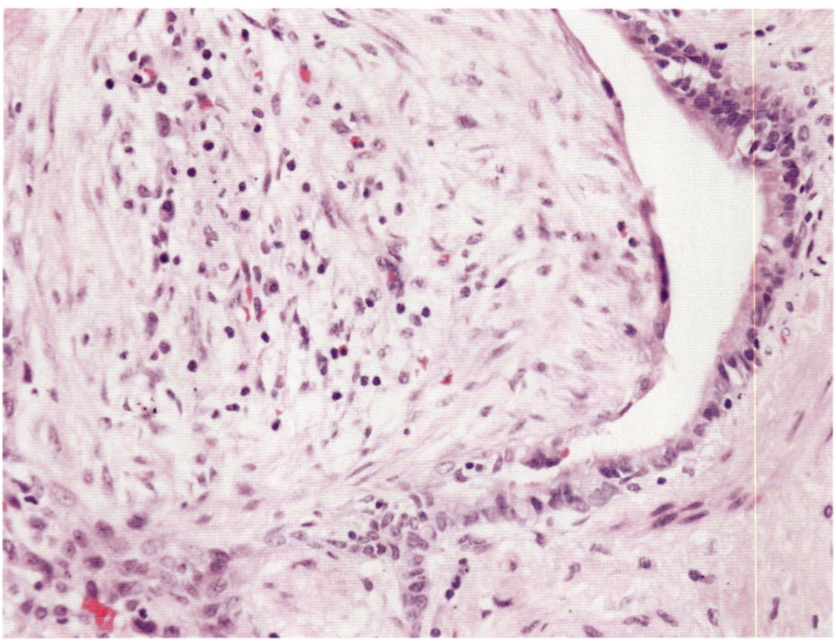

FIGURE 2.15 **Organizing pneumonia pattern showing admixture of inflammatory cells (neutrophils, plasma cells, small lymphocytes, and macrophages) with small vessels and spindled fibroblasts.**

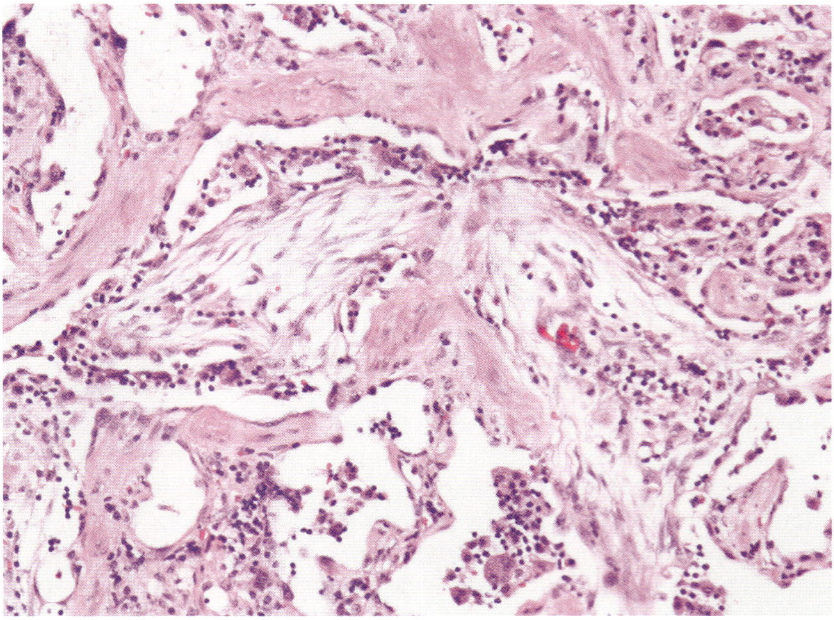

FIGURE 2.16 Polypoid masses in chronic lung injury comprising a fibroblastic proliferation with a loose myxoid matrix that fills the lumen of alveolar spaces and penetrates through the pores of Kohn into the adjacent alveoli.

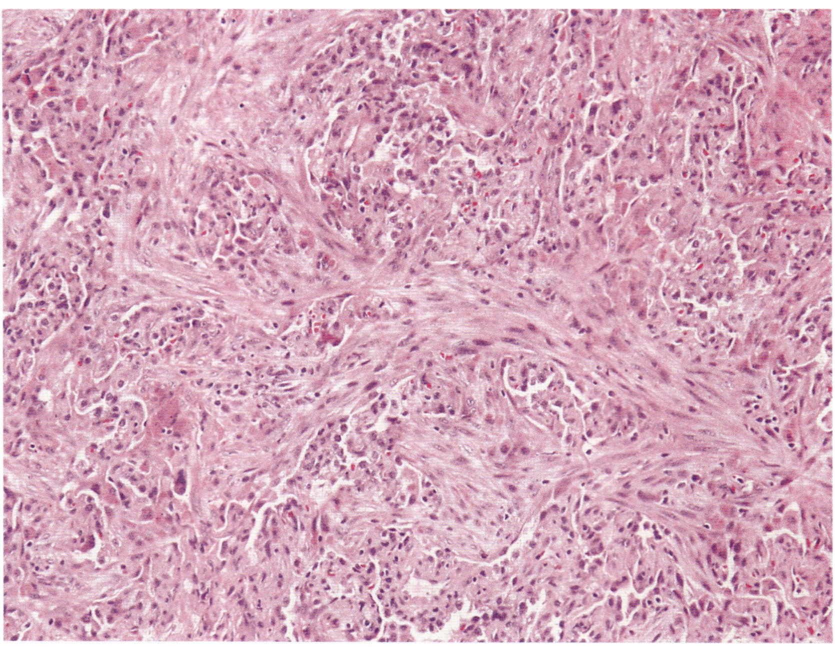

FIGURE 2.17 Chronic lung injury in which the fibrous plugs have filled multiple alveolar spaces in a branching configuration.

Another pattern of chronic inflammation that must be distinguished from the organizing pneumonia pattern is constrictive bronchiolitis (bronchiolitis obliterans). The latter is comprised of mucosal, submucosal, and peribronchiolar inflammatory infiltrates that eventually progress to peribronchiolar fibrosis and collagenization, leading to partial or total obstruction of the bronchiole (Fig. 2.18). Colloquially, this process is known as "popcorn" lung because of its association with popcorn factory workers.[41] This pattern may be observed in association with pulmonary infections such as mycoplasma or viruses, exposure to dusts, drug reactions, toxic gases, and collagen vascular disorders such as RA. It may also be seen in the posttransplant setting and in users of electronic cigarettes.[42] It can also be seen as a nonspecific response complicating DAD and other injuries to lung parenchyma.

Another nonspecific pattern that may result from long-standing chronic inflammation is interstitial fibrosis. This must be distinguished from the idiopathic interstitial fibrosing pneumonitis that will be dealt with in Chapter 9. Interstitial fibrosis is characterized by narrowing and obliteration of alveolar spaces by interstitial collagen deposition (Fig. 2.19; eFig. 2.9). When the process is advanced, it leads to dilatation and honeycombing of lung parenchyma. Interstitial fibrosis may be associated with various metaplastic processes, including bronchiolar metaplasia and squamous metaplasia. The former is characterized by replacement of the alveolar lining by columnar, ciliated bronchiolar epithelium (Fig. 2.20).

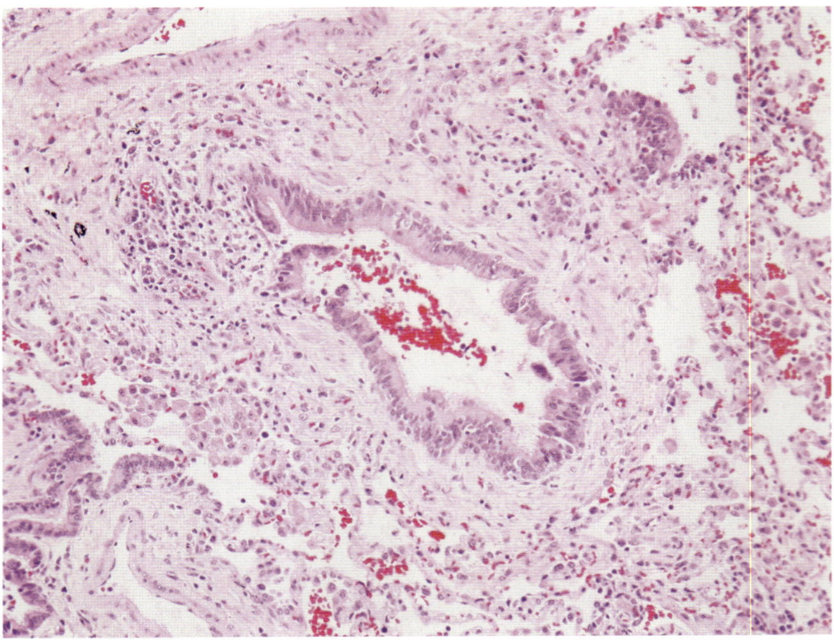

FIGURE 2.18 Early peribronchial fibrosis and collagenization with mild distortion of the bronchial lumen.

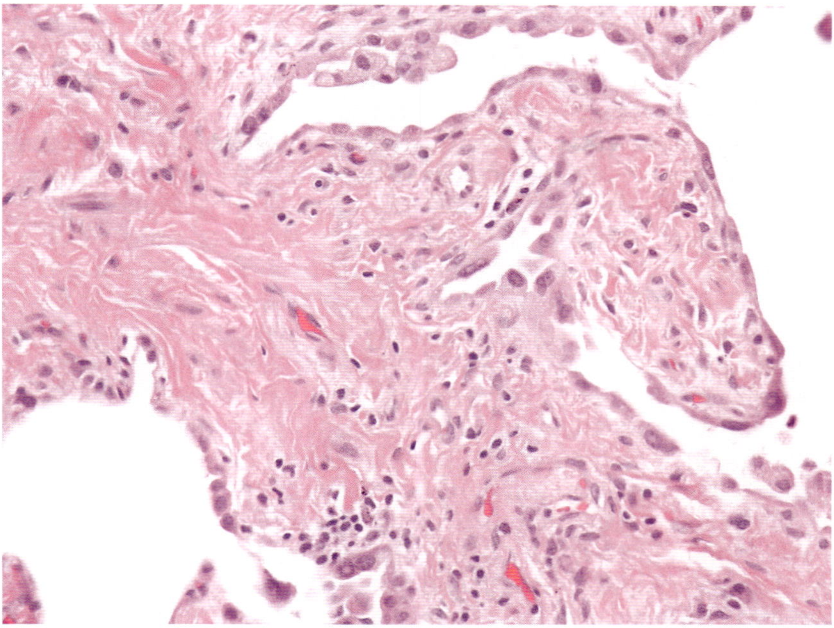

FIGURE 2.19 Nonspecific pattern of interstitial fibrosis in a patient with long-standing chronic inflammation; notice the expansion of the interstitium secondary to collagen deposition.

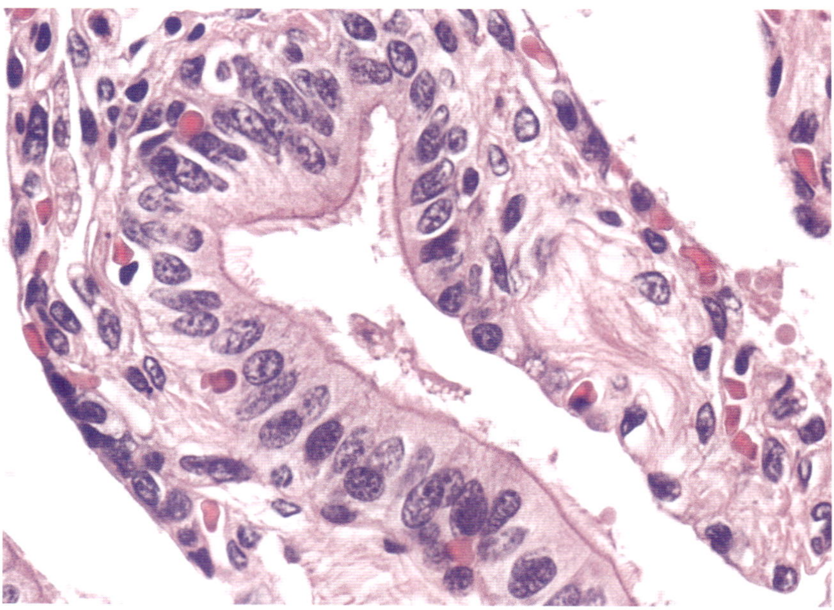

FIGURE 2.20 Bronchiolar metaplasia ("lambertosis") in chronic lung injury characterized by replacement of the alveolar lining by columnar, ciliated bronchiolar epithelium.

It has been hypothesized that the metaplastic epithelium derives from the canals of Lambert that normally connect the bronchioles with the alveoli, hence the alternate designation of "Lambertosis" for this phenomenon. Squamous metaplasia can also be observed under a wide range of circumstances and can be most striking in advanced stages of interstitial fibrosis. Another phenomenon that can be commonly observed in advanced stages of interstitial fibrosis is bronchiolar smooth muscle hyperplasia, which in advanced stages may lead to a distinctive macroscopic appearance that was termed in the old literature as "pulmonary cirrhosis" (eFig. 2.10).

Finally, another manifestation of chronic inflammation is the presence of specific types of granulomatous pneumonitis, which will be discussed separately in more detail. There is one recently described variant of organizing pneumonia, however, that has been termed granulomatous organizing pneumonia, which is unassociated with microorganisms, suggesting that the granulomas may be related to an allergic or immunologic stimulus.[43] The histology shows poorly formed granulomas in association with organizing pneumonia. It is not yet clear whether this represents a variation in the pattern of COP or corresponds to a separate and specific type of granulomatous pulmonary process. One study has found that it is more likely to present as masses or nodules than COP, suggesting it may represent a distinctive form of organizing pneumonia.[43]

SPECIFIC CAUSES OF CHRONIC LUNG INFLAMMATION

There may be several specific etiologic causes of chronic lung inflammation. Most of them result in a similar nonspecific histopathologic picture; however, in some instances, some specific features may point to a specific diagnosis, or a more specific diagnosis can be achieved with the aid of a good clinical history or results of additional clinical tests.

Collagen Vascular Diseases

Collagen vascular diseases affecting the lungs are principally characterized by a chronic inflammatory response of the pulmonary parenchyma sometimes including lymphoid aggregates with germinal center formation. Most of them result in a similar nonspecific histopathologic picture. Advanced cases can show increased fibrotic changes throughout the lung. The interstitial inflammatory infiltrates in collagen vascular diseases tend to contain more prominent plasma cells than in chronic inflammation caused by other conditions. Results of laboratory tests and a detailed clinical history are required for arriving at a more specific diagnosis.

Rheumatoid Arthritis

It has been estimated that about 14% of patients who meet the criteria for the diagnosis of RA by the American Rheumatism Association develop significant lung disease.[44] The cumulative incidence of RA-associated interstitial lung disease in the U.S. adult population has been estimated at 15.3%.[45]

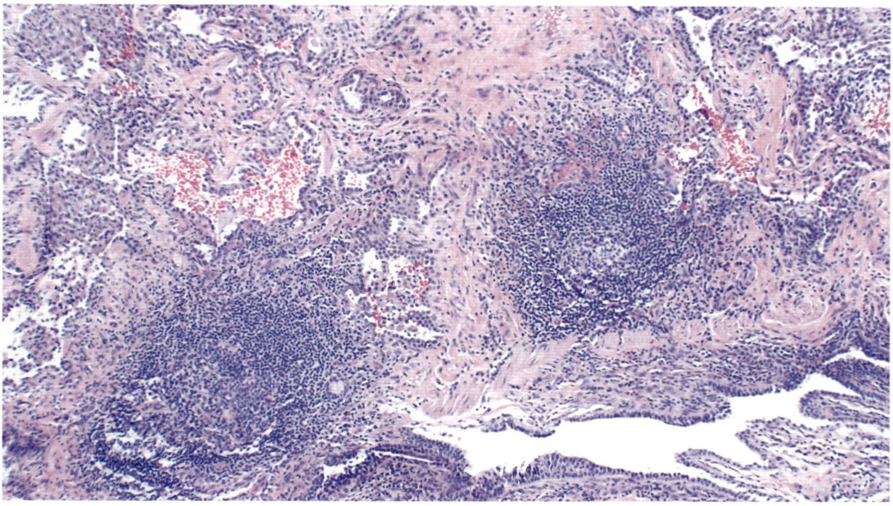

FIGURE 2.21 Prominent lymphoid follicular hyperplasia with germinal center formation is seen in a case of rheumatoid arthritis–associated interstitial lung disease.

A distinctive, but not unique, feature of lung involvement by RA is the development of multiple discrete lymphoid follicles with germinal centers (Fig. 2.21). When these lymphoid follicles aggregate around the terminal airways, the pattern is designated as "follicular bronchiolitis." A variable cellular chronic interstitial infiltrate rich in plasma cells and small lymphocytes is usually present in the vicinity of the lymphoid nodules. Another common finding is the combination of subacute and chronic inflammation manifested by hyperplasia of type II pneumocytes and interstitial pneumonia that may progress to diffuse interstitial fibrosis. The end stage of the fibrotic process will lead to the formation of the typical rheumatoid nodules, which must be distinguished from the nodules in granulomatosis with polyangiitis and of various infectious processes. It cannot be overemphasized that a specific diagnosis of RA cannot be rendered solely on the basis of biopsy material and requires strict correlation and confirmation from the clinical findings.

Systemic Lupus Erythematosus

SLE is a chronic systemic autoimmune disease that may often affect the lungs and can range from acute lupus pneumonitis to advanced fibrosis. Acute lung injury and pulmonary hemorrhage and vasculitis are more commonly associated with SLE than with other connective tissue disorders and are the more common pulmonary manifestation of the disease.[20] However, a significant number of patients will present in advanced stages with cellular interstitial pneumonia and variable degrees of interstitial fibrosis. This latter presentation is associated with a more favorable prognosis than acute lupus pneumonitis. The subacute and chronic manifestations of lupus

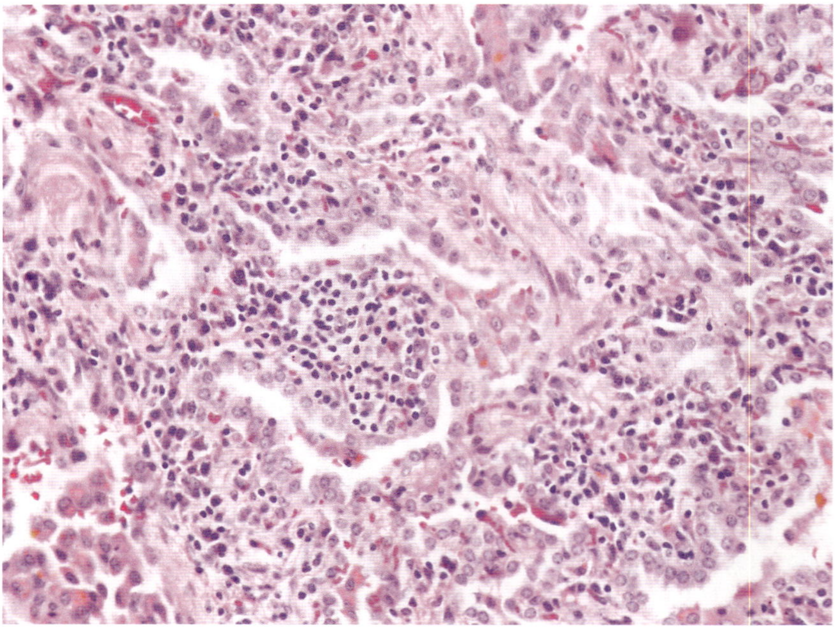

FIGURE 2.22 **Cellular interstitial pneumonia in a patient with lupus erythematosus.** Notice the dense interstitial lymphoid infiltrate expanding the alveolar walls.

pneumonitis usually present with a NSIP pattern, which is characterized by a cellular interstitial pneumonia with variable interstitial fibrosis (Fig. 2.22). More rarely, the process will progress to a more advanced pattern of interstitial fibrosis that may be indistinguishable from UIP (Fig. 2.23). Clinical correlation and laboratory findings are indispensable for correct diagnosis. Other less common chronic pulmonary manifestations of SLE include bronchiolitis obliterans and lymphocytic interstitial pneumonia.[46,47] In general, the development of interstitial lung disease in patients with SLE is considered to have an overall good prognosis but with possible risk of progression in a minority of patients.[48]

Scleroderma (Progressive Systemic Sclerosis)

Diffuse lung involvement represents the fourth most common manifestation of progressive systemic sclerosis (PSS) after skin, peripheral vascular, and esophageal involvement.[49] Patients with pulmonary involvement in scleroderma are associated with increased morbidity and mortality. A rare complication of pulmonary involvement in PSS is the development of lung carcinoma from areas of fibrosis. Lung involvement in PSS is usually characterized by diffuse interstitial fibrosis. The interstitial fibrosis is characterized by a paucicellular collagenization of the interstitium with preservation of the underlying lung architecture; however, in more advanced stages, it may closely resemble that seen in UIP (Fig. 2.24). The absence of "temporal and spatial heterogeneity" of the lesions, a distinctive feature

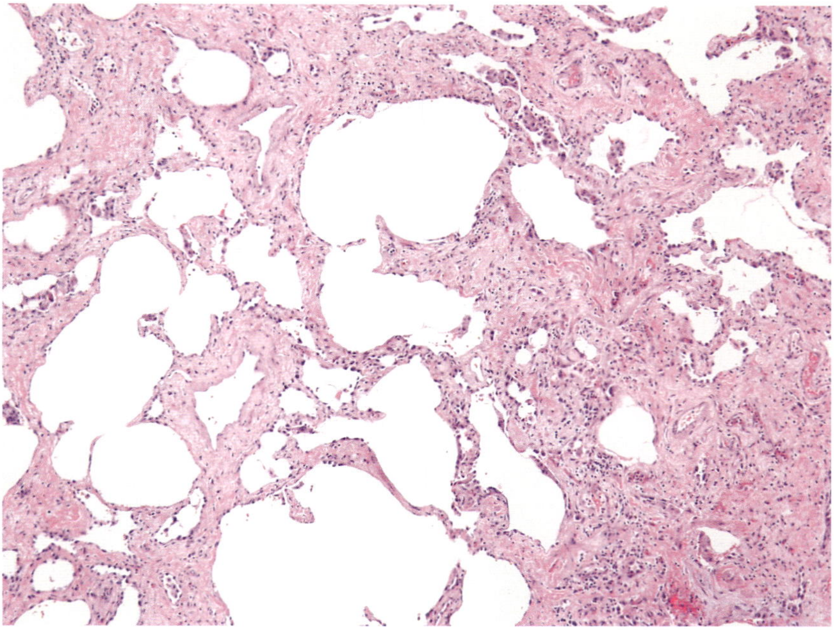

FIGURE 2.23 **Advanced stage of lupus pneumonitis showing severe interstitial fibrosis with extensive remodeling of lung parenchyma.** This picture is morphologically indistinguishable from idiopathic usual interstitial pneumonia, and a diagnosis of lupus cannot be rendered in the absence of a clinical history.

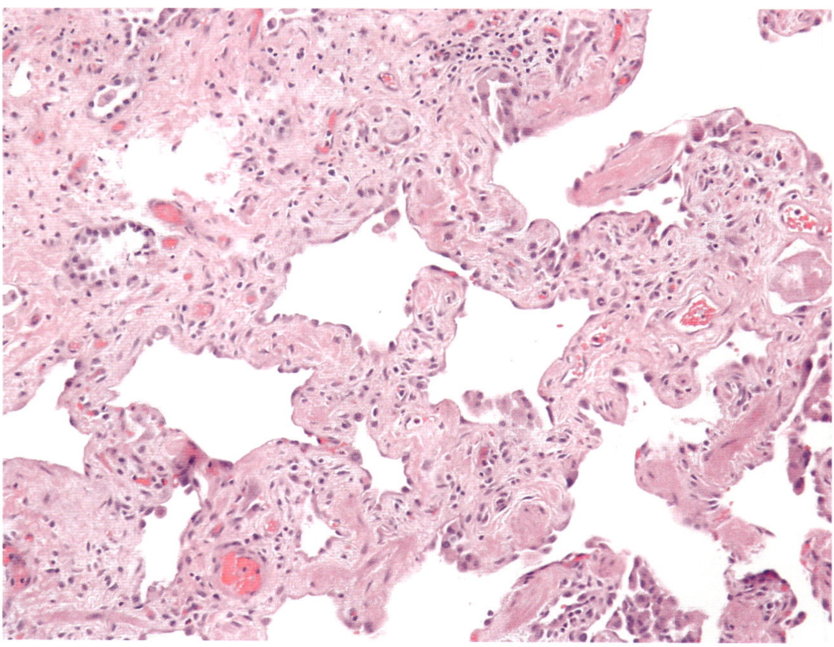

FIGURE 2.24 **Interstitial fibrosis in progressive systemic sclerosis.** This pattern of fibrosis is nonspecific and may be observed in various other disorders. Clinical correlation is required to establish the cause of the sclerosing process.

of UIP, is helpful to differentiate PSS from the latter.[50] Vascular changes secondary to pulmonary hypertension is another feature seen in the lungs of patients with PSS and represents a major cause of mortality in such patients.[51]

Polymyositis and Dermatomyositis

Pulmonary involvement in polymyositis (PM) and dermatomyositis (DM) occurs with much less frequency than in other systemic diseases and usually manifests late in the course of the process. However, in occasional cases, they may precede the clinical and serologic diagnoses of the disease.[26] As mentioned previously, PM/DM can show acute manifestations of lung injury; however, the most common manifestation of PM/DM in the lungs is chronic interstitial pneumonitis with a pattern very similar to that of NSIP. The interstitium usually shows cellular interstitial pneumonia. There is a variable degree of fibrosis, and the changes may resemble those seen in the cellular or fibrotic forms of NSIP. In more advanced stages, the fibrosis associated with PM/DM may be indistinguishable from that of idiopathic UIP (Fig. 2.25). Clinical correlation and a good history will be essential for correct interpretation. In limited biopsy samples, it may be impossible to establish a definitive diagnosis.

Sjögren Syndrome

Sjögren syndrome (SS) is an autoimmune disease characterized by dense lymphocytic infiltration of the salivary glands resulting in the clinical manifestations of dry mouth and dry eyes. The prevalence of interstitial lung disease in patients with SS has been estimated at 9.1% in one study.[52]

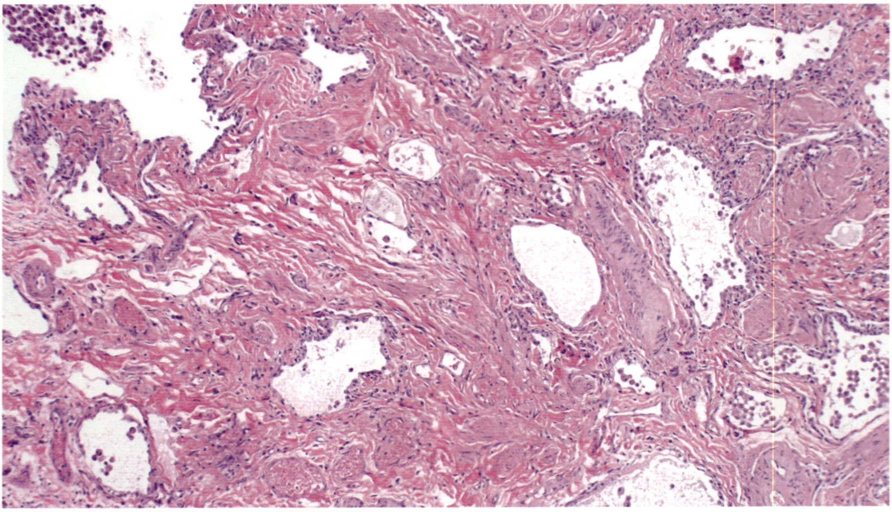

FIGURE 2.25 Advanced stage of interstitial fibrosis in dermatomyositis shows widening of the interstitium separating the alveolar septa by dense acellular collagen.

Lung involvement often occurs in SS and is characterized by a lymphocytic interstitial pneumonitis principally distributed around the airways. When the infiltrates form lymphoid follicles, they can result in a pattern of follicular bronchiolitis. The most common pattern is that of lymphoid interstitial pneumonia that may closely resemble a low-grade lymphoproliferative disorder. A common finding is the presence of small, nonnecrotizing interstitial granulomas admixed with the lymphoid cell population. It should be kept in mind that patients with SS are at increased risk for developing lymphoproliferative disorders, and proper evaluation of dense lymphoid infiltrates in SS patients with lung involvement to rule out lymphoma should always be considered.

Drug Toxicity

Many drugs, including amiodarone, bleomycin, carmustine, and methotrexate, can result in lung damage, leading to chronic inflammation and fibrosis. Most of the chronic inflammatory changes induced by drugs are nonspecific and can resemble other causes of diffuse lung injury, such as cellular interstitial pneumonia, bronchiolitis obliterans, and diffuse interstitial fibrosis.[53,54] Clinical correlation, with adequate information regarding specific types of drugs, and timing of administration in relation to the onset of symptoms are important for specific diagnosis. Cessation of symptoms or their improvement following discontinuation of the drug is also a helpful clue to verify the etiology of the pathologic findings. Chronic lung inflammation caused by drugs may manifest as diffuse interstitial fibrosis that can resemble UIP, sometimes leading to honeycombing of lung parenchyma. Tissue eosinophilia can be seen in some cases, and some drugs may be associated with the formation of small interstitial granulomas, in particular, methotrexate.[29] Clinical correlation is necessary for adequate interpretation of the pathologic findings.

Chronic Eosinophilic Pneumonia

Chronic eosinophilic pneumonia most commonly presents with a subacute clinical course but may also become protracted. The radiologic appearance has been likened to the photographic negative of pulmonary edema.[55] The disease occurs most often in middle-aged women and can be accompanied by asthma or nasal symptoms as well as peripheral eosinophilia.[56] The histologic features are very similar to those of the acute form of the disease, and the distinction is made based on the constellation of clinical findings. Usually, there is mild interstitial pneumonia with hyperplasia of type II pneumocytes and accumulation of fibrin within alveolar spaces. Macrophages are also seen within the lumen of alveolar spaces. The cytologic atypia of type II pneumocyte hyperplasia can be quite striking, sometimes simulating viral cytopathic effect. The most distinctive feature of the process, however, is the dense accumulation of eosinophils admixed with the macrophages within the alveolar lumens (Fig. 2.26).

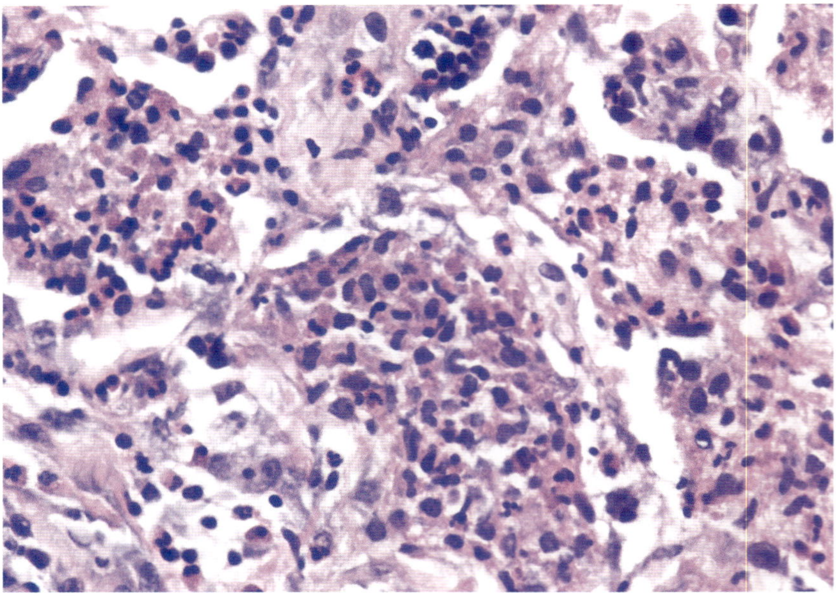

FIGURE 2.26 **Chronic eosinophilic pneumonia showing intra-alveolar accumulations of eosinophils, macrophages, and additional scattered inflammatory cells.** The histologic picture is similar to that of acute eosinophilic pneumonia.

Discrete eosinophilic microabscesses may also be present. The main differential diagnosis for this condition is with eosinophilic granulomatosis with polyangiitis, from which it is distinguished histologically by the absence of vasculitis. The condition responds well to treatment with corticosteroids.

REFERENCES

1. Ashbaugh D, Bigelow D, Petty T, Levine BE. Acute respiratory distress in adults. *Lancet*. 1967;2:319-323.
2. Tomashefsky J Jr. Pulmonary pathology of acute respiratory distress syndrome. *Clin Chest Med*. 2000;21:435-466.
3. Katzenstein A, Bloor C, Liebow A. Diffuse alveolar damage–the role of oxygen, shock and related factors. *Am J Pathol*. 1976;85:209-228.
4. De Giacomi F, Decker PA, Vassallo R, Ryu JH. Acute eosinophilic pneumonia: correlation of clinical characteristics with underlying cause. *Chest*. 2017;152(2):379-385.
5. Kao KC, Hu HC, Chang CH, et al. Diffuse alveolar damage associated mortality in selected acute respiratory distress syndrome patients with open lung biopsy. *Crit Care*. 2015;19:228.
6. Rios F, Iscar T, Cardinal-Fernandez P. What every intensivist should know about acute respiratory distress syndrome and diffuse alveolar damage. *Rev Bras Ter Intensiva*. 2017;29(3):354-363.
7. Wong A, Walkey A. Open lung biopsy among critically ill, mechanically ventilated patients. A meta-analysis. *Ann Am Thorac Soc*. 2015;12(8):1226-1230.

8. Palakshappa JA, Meyer NJ. Which patients with ARDS benefit from lung biopsy? *Chest.* 2015;148(4):1073-1082.
9. Beasley MB, Franks TJ, Galvin JR, Gochuico B, Travis WD. Acute fibrinous and organizing pneumonia. A histologic pattern of lung injury and possible variant of diffuse alveolar damage. *Arch Pathol Lab Med.* 2002;126:1064-1070.
10. Hamman L, Rich A. Acute diffuse interstitial fibrosis of the lungs. *Bull Johns Hopkins Hosp.* 1944;74:177-212.
11. Katzenstein A-L, Myers J, Mazur M. Acute interstitial pneumonia. A clinicopathologic, ultrastructural and cell kinetic study. *Am J Surg Pathol.* 1986;10:256-267.
12. Mukhopadhyay S, Parambil JG. Acute interstitial pneumonia (AIP): relationship to Hamman-Rich syndrome, diffuse alveolar damage (DAD), and acute respiratory distress syndrome (ARDS). *Semin Respir Crit Care Med.* 2012;33(5):476-485.
13. Ryerson CJ, Cottin V, Brown KK, Collard HR. Acute exacerbation of idiopathic pulmonary fibrosis: shifting the paradigm. *Eur Respir J.* 2015;46(2):512-520.
14. Miyamoto A, Sharma A, Nishino M. Expanded acceptance of acute exacerbation of nonspecific interstitial pneumonia, including 7 additional cases with detailed clinical pathologic correlation. *Pathol Int.* 2018;68(7):401-408.
15. Matthay R, Schwanz M, Petty T, et al. Pulmonary manifestations of systemic lupus erythematosus: review of twelve cases of acute lupus pneumonia. *Medicine.* 1974;54:392-409.
16. Colby T. Pulmonary pathology in patients with systemic autoimmune disease. *Clin Chest Med.* 1998;19:587-612.
17. Quismorio F Jr, Cheema G. Interstitial lung disease in systemic lupus erythematosus. *Curr Opin Pulm Med.* 2000;6:424-429.
18. Eisenberg H. The interstitial lung diseases associated with collagen-vascular disorders. *Clin Chest Med.* 1982;3:565-573.
19. Haupt HM, Moore GW, Hutchins GM. The lung in systemic lupus erythematosus: analysis of the pathologic changes in 120 patients. *Am J Med.* 1981;71:791-813.
20. Myers JL, Katzenstein AA. Microangiitis in lupus-induced pulmonary hemorrhage. *Am J Clin Pathol.* 1986;85:552-556.
21. Pertschuk LP, Moccia LF, Rosen Y, et al. Acute pulmonary complications in systemic lupus erythematosus. Immunofluorescence and light microscopic study. *Am J Clin Pathol.* 1977;68:553-559.
22. Eagen JW, Roberts H, Schwartz MM, Lewis EJ. The composition of pulmonary immune deposits in systemic lupus erythematosus. *Clin Immunol Immunopathol.* 1979;12:204-212.
23. Yousem S, Colby T, Carrington C. Lung biopsy in rheumatoid arthritis. *Am Rev Respir Dis.* 1985;131:770-777.
24. Hakala M, Paakko P, Huhti E, Tarkka M, Sutinen S. Open lung biopsy of patients with rheumatoid arthritis. *Clin Rheumatol.* 1990;9:452-460.
25. Lakhanpal S, Lie J, Conn D, Martin WJ II. Pulmonary disease in polymyositis/dermatomyositis: a clinicopathologic analysis of 65 autopsy cases. *Ann Rheum Dis.* 1987;46:23-29.
26. Tazelaar HD, Viggiano RW, Pickersgill J, Colby TV. Interstitial lung disease in polymyositis and dermatomyositis. Clinical features and prognosis as correlated with histologic findings. *Am Rev Respir Dis.* 1990;141:727-733.
27. Rossi S, Erasmus J, McAdams H, Sporn TA, Goodman PC. Pulmonary drug toxicity: radiologic and pathologic manifestations. *Radiographics.* 2000;20:1245-1259.
28. Cooper JA Jr. Drug-induced lung disease. *Adv Intern Med.* 1997;42:231-268.
29. Imokawa S, Colby TV, Leslie KO, Helmers RA. Methotrexate pneumonitis: review of the literature and histopathological findings in nine patients. *Eur Respir J.* 2000;15:373-381.

30. Littler W, Kay J, Haselton P, Heath D. Busulphan lung. *Thorax*. 1969;24:639-655.
31. Myers JL, Kennedy JI, Plumb VJ, Fulmer JD. Amiodarone pulmonary toxicity: clinical, radiologic and pathologic correlation. *Arch Intern Med*. 1987;147:50-55.
32. Myers JL, Kennedy JI, Plumb VJ. Amiodarone lung: pathologic findings in clinically toxic patients. *Hum Pathol*. 1987;18:349-354.
33. Tazelaar H, Linz L, Colby TV, Myers JL, Limper AH. Acute eosinophilic pneumonia: histopathologic findings in nine patients. *Am J Respir Crit Care Med*. 1997;155:296-302.
34. De Giacomi F, Vassallo R, Yi ES, Ryu JH. Acute eosinophilic pneumonia. Causes, diagnosis, and management. *Am J Respir Crit Care Med*. 2018;197(6):728-736.
35. Allen JN, Pacht ER, Gadek JE, Davis WB. Acute eosinophilic pneumonia as a reversible cause of noninfectious respiratory failure. *N Engl J Med*. 1989;321:569-574.
36. Philit F, Etienne-Mastroianni B, Parrot A, Guérin C, Robert D, Cordier JF. Idiopathic acute eosinophilic pneumonia: a study of 22 patients. *Am J Respir Crit Care Med*. 2002;166:1235-1239.
37. Bonnier A, Nida A, Chong WH, Saha S, Saha BK. Vaping associated acute eosinophilic pneumonia: a clinical and radiologic mimicker of COVID-19. *Prague Med Rep*. 2023;124:283-292.
38. Epler GR, Colby TV, McLoud TC, Carrington CB, Gaensler EA. Bronchiolitis obliterans organizing pneumonia. *N Engl J Med*. 1985;312:152-158.
39. Paradis I, Yousem S, Griffith B. Airway obstruction and bronchiolitis obliterans after lung transplantation. *Clin Chest Med*. 1993;14:751-763.
40. Estenne M, Maurer JR, Boehler A, et al. Bronchiolitis obliterans syndrome 2001: an update of the diagnostic criteria. *J Heart Lung Transplant*. 2002;21:297-310.
41. Kreiss K, Gomaa A, Kullman G, Fedan K, Simoes EJ, Enright PL. Clinical bronchiolitis obliterans in workers at a microwave-popcorn plant. *N Engl J Med*. 2002;347(5):330-338.
42. Todd JL, Palmer SM. Bronchiolitis obliterans syndrome: the final frontier for lung transplantation. *Chest*. 2011;140(2):502-508.
43. Feinstein MB, DeSouza SA, Moreira AL, et al. A comparison of the pathological, clinical and radiographical features of cryptogenic organizing pneumonia, acute fibrinous and organizing pneumonia and granulomatous organizing pneumonia. *J Clin Pathol*. 2015;68:441-447.
44. Gabbay E, Tarala R, Will R, et al. Interstitial lung disease in recent onset rheumatoid arthritis. *Am J Respir Crit Care Med*. 1997;156:528-535.
45. Samhouri BF, Vassallo R, Achenbach SJ, et al. Incidence, risk factors, and mortality of clinical and subclinical rheumatoid arthritis-associated interstitial lung disease: a population-based cohort. *Arthritis Care Res*. 2022;74:2042-2049.
46. Kinney WW, Angelillo VA. Bronchiolitis in systemic lupus erythematosus. *Chest*. 1982;82:646-648.
47. Yum MN, Ziegler JR, Walker PD, Ridolfo AS, Brashear RE. Pseudolymphoma of the lung in a patient with systemic lupus erythematosus. *Am J Med*. 1979;66:172-175.
48. Deneuville L, Mageau A, Debray MP, et al. Chronic interstitial lung disease associated with systemic lupus erythematosus: a multicentric study of 89 cases. *Respirology*. 2024;29:713-721.
49. Cheema GS, Quismorio FP Jr. Interstitial lung disease in systemic sclerosis. *Curr Opin Pulm Med*. 2001;7:283-290.
50. Bouros D, Wells AU, Nicholson AG, et al. Histopathologic subsets of fibrosing alveolitis in patients with systemic sclerosis and their relationship to outcome. *Am J Respir Crit Care Med*. 2002;165:1581-1586.
51. Yamane K, Ihn H, Asano Y, et al. Clinical and laboratory features of scleroderma patients with pulmonary hypertension. *Rheumatology (Oxford)*. 2000;39:1269-1271.

52. La Rocca G, Ferro F, Sambataro G, et al. Interstitial lung disease phenotypes and predictive risk factors in primary Sjogren's syndrome. *J Clin Med.* 2024;13:4963.
53. Kreisman H, Wolcove N. Pulmonary toxicity of antineoplastic therapy. *Semin Oncol.* 1992;19:508-520.
54. Zitnik RJ, Matthay RA. Drug-induced lung disease. In: Schwartz MI, King TE, eds. *Interstitial Lung Disease.* BC Decker; 1998:423-449.
55. Gaensler E, Carrington C. Peripheral opacities in chronic eosinophilic pneumonia. The photographic negative of pulmonary edema. *AJR Am J Roentgenol.* 1977;128:1-13.
56. Liebow A, Carrington C. The eosinophilic pneumonias. *Medicine (Baltimore).* 1969;48:251-285.

3

PULMONARY NONINFECTIOUS GRANULOMAS

Granulomas can occur in the lung under different circumstances, including infectious and noninfectious processes. For the most part, granulomatous pneumonitis is a relatively nonspecific reaction pattern that requires strict clinicopathologic correlation for proper interpretation. Granulomas are frequent findings in endoscopic lung biopsies; a specific diagnosis is often not attainable in most circumstances from the review of the biopsy material alone.

The most frequent cause of pulmonary granulomas is infectious diseases, and these will be discussed separately in other chapters. This chapter will deal with noninfectious granulomas and their possible etiology (Table 3.1).

TABLE 3.1 Causes of Noninfectious Granulomas in the Lung
Sarcoidosis
Berylliosis
Necrotizing sarcoid granulomatosis
Granulomatosis with polyangiitis
Bronchocentric granulomatosis
Hypersensitivity pneumonitis
Aspiration pneumonia
Less common causes of granulomas:
• Hard metal pneumoconiosis
• Autoimmune disorder (Sjögren syndrome)
• Drug reaction (methotrexate)
• Hematologic malignancies (Hodgkin lymphoma, lymphomatoid granulomatosis)
• Intravenous drug abuse
• Exogenous lipid pneumonia

SARCOIDOSIS

Sarcoidosis is a systemic disease of unknown etiology. It is currently believed that it may be caused by an inappropriate immune response to certain infectious or inorganic antigens mediated by tumor necrosis factor alpha produced by activated macrophages.[1] Pulmonary involvement is a common feature of the disease.[2,3] Pulmonary involvement by sarcoidosis is usually accompanied by cough and shortness of breath. As many as two-thirds of patients may be asymptomatic. The disease has a predilection for young adults and for African Americans. Serum angiotensin-converting enzyme can be detected in 30% to 80% of patients and may be helpful for diagnosis or monitoring active disease. In addition, serum levels of YKL-40, sIL-2R, neopterin, adenosine deaminase, and C-reactive protein have been shown to become elevated in patients with sarcoidosis.[4] However, these tests are not specific, and elevated levels can be observed in other conditions as well, including infectious granulomas, lymphomas, hepatitis, and diabetes. The Kveim test, which employs an injected antigenic serum derived from human sarcoid granuloma extracts, is relatively specific but has largely been abandoned for the use of endoscopic lung biopsy to confirm the presence of the granulomas.[3,5] On chest X-rays, the disease tends to preferentially occupy the upper lobes and is characterized by reticulonodular infiltrates with a lymphatic distribution.

The histopathologic hallmark of sarcoidosis is the formation of nonnecrotizing ("productive") epithelioid granulomas (Fig. 3.1; eFig. 3.1).

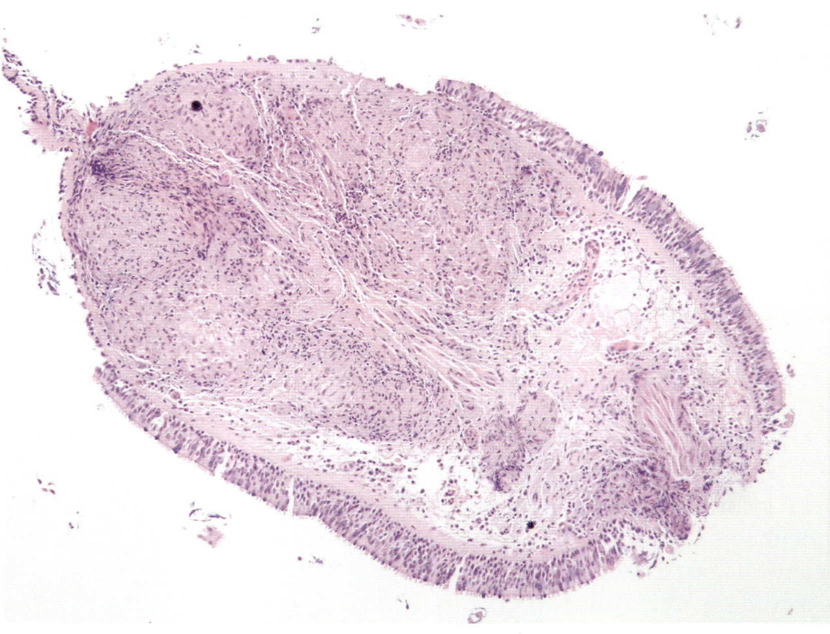

FIGURE 3.1 Endobronchial biopsy showing multiple small, confluent epithelioid granulomas in the subepithelial lamina propria in a patient with sarcoidosis.

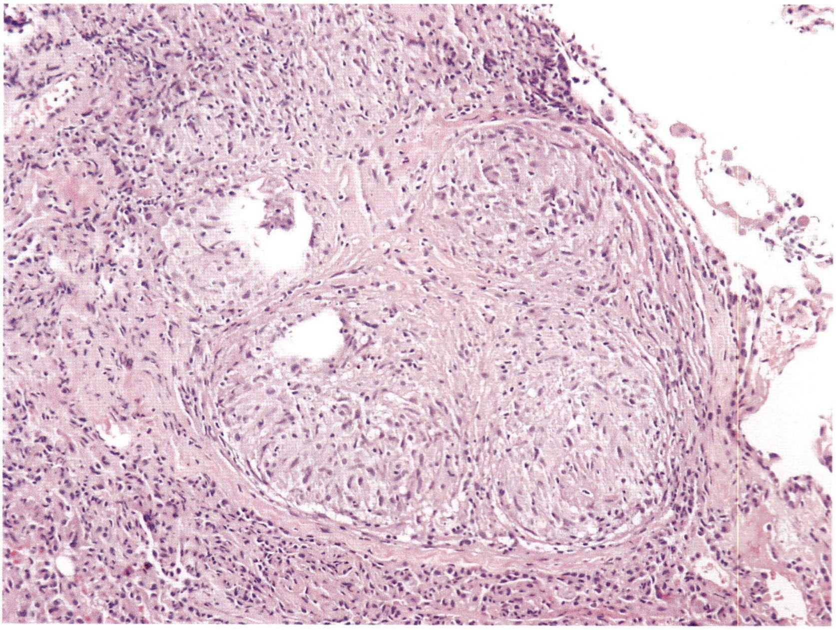

FIGURE 3.2 **Typical sarcoid granuloma characterized by nodular aggregate of epithelioid histiocytes.** Notice that the granuloma is surrounded by a thin rim of collagenous stroma that separates it from the surrounding tissues. Small scattered lymphocytes are seen in the vicinity of the granuloma.

The granulomas show a tendency to be surrounded by a rim of collagenous stroma (Fig. 3.2). They are usually small but tend to coalesce to form larger granulomas. Scattered small lymphocytes are often present in the vicinity of the granulomas. The granulomas are characteristically distributed along lymphatics and bronchovascular bundles and can often adopt a perivascular distribution (Figs. 3.3 and 3.4). The granulomas comprise collections of epithelioid histiocytes that contain abundant lightly eosinophilic cytoplasm (Fig. 3.5; eFigs. 3.2 and 3.3). The histiocytes are devoid of cytologic atypia or mitotic activity (Fig. 3.6). Multinucleated giant cells are characteristically seen within the granulomas and may contain various cytoplasmic inclusions such as Schaumann bodies and asteroid bodies. The latter are nonspecific and can be seen in various granulomatous conditions other than sarcoidosis.

Transbronchial biopsies are the preferred method for demonstrating the granulomas in sarcoidosis. The granulomas will show a tendency to occur in submucosal distribution and may sometimes be quite subtle, presenting as discrete subepithelial accumulations of epithelioid histiocytes (Figs. 3.7 and 3.8). The positive yield of the biopsy is directly proportional to the amount of tissue biopsied. It has been demonstrated that the chance of obtaining a positive biopsy in patients with sarcoidosis is increased when four biopsy specimens are obtained rather than a single biopsy.[5]

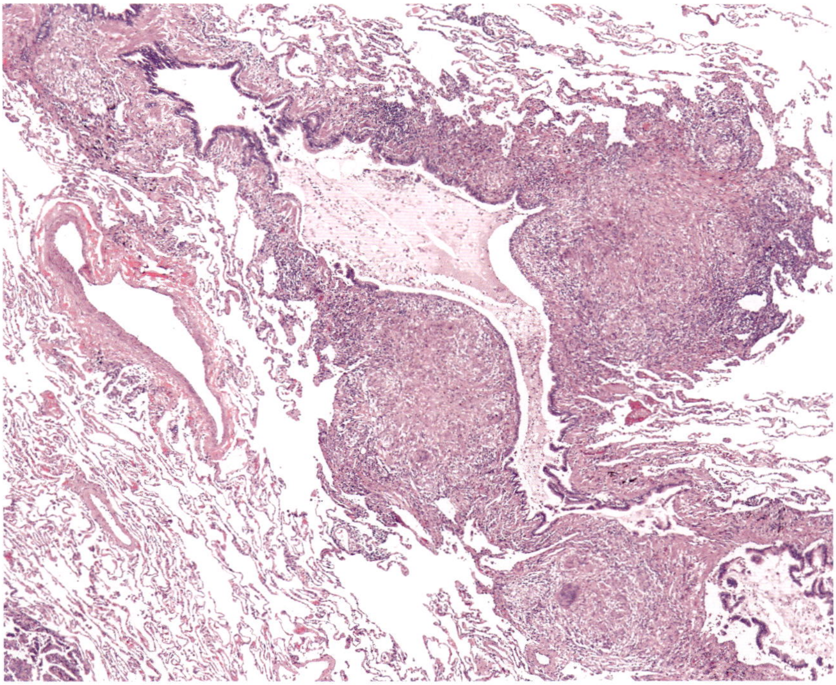

FIGURE 3.3 Characteristic distribution of sarcoid granulomas along lymphatics and bronchovascular bundles.

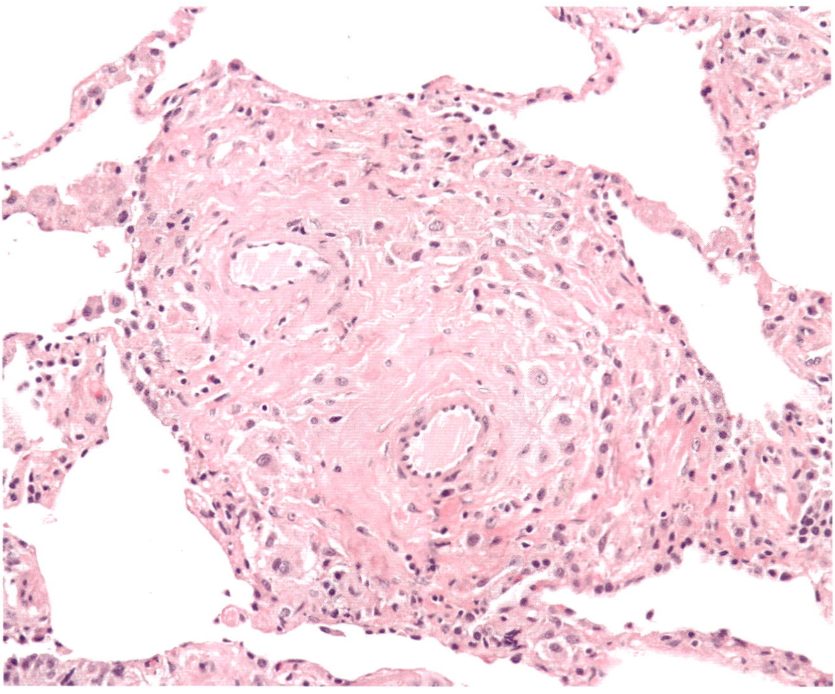

FIGURE 3.4 Perivascular distribution in sarcoid granuloma.

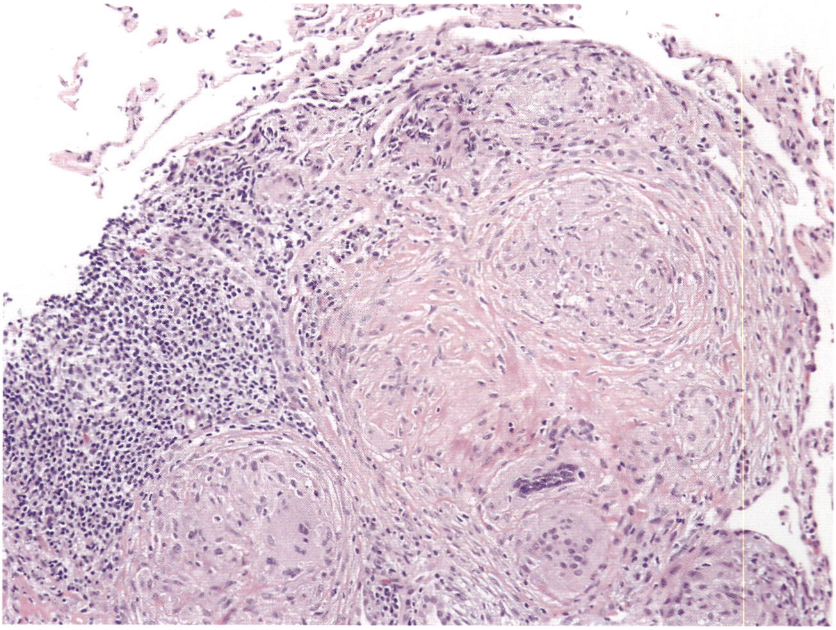

FIGURE 3.5 Sarcoid granulomas comprising collections of epithelioid histiocytes surrounded by dense collections of small lymphocytes.

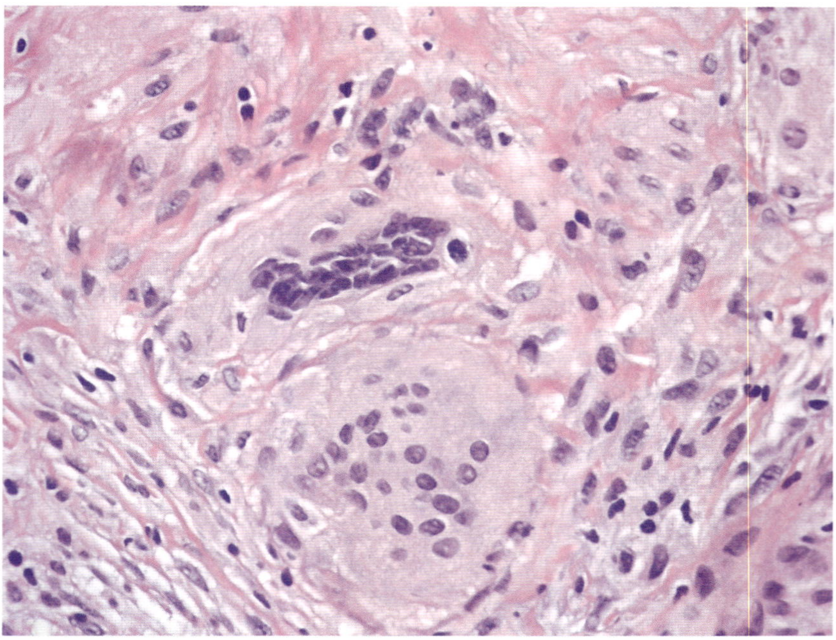

FIGURE 3.6 High magnification of sarcoid granuloma showing epithelioid histiocytes and multinucleated giant cells.

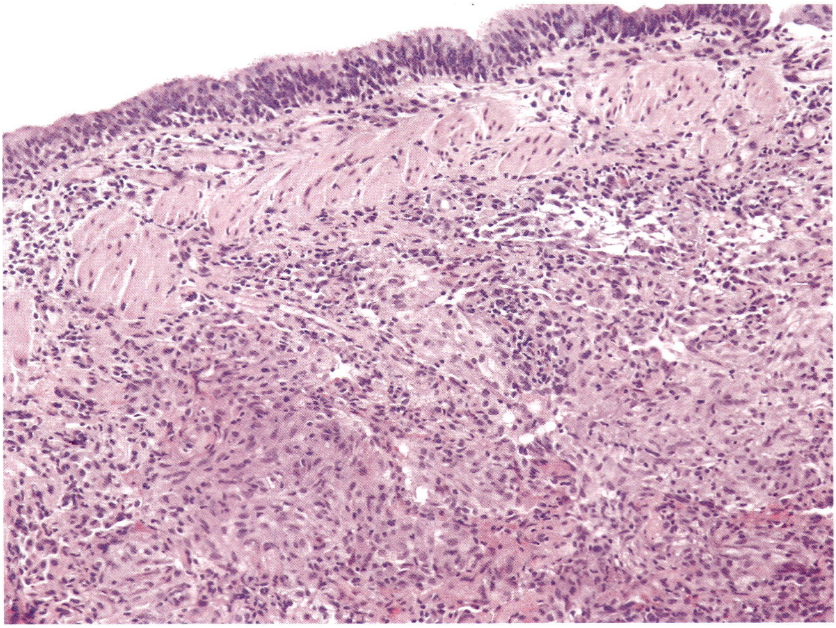

FIGURE 3.7 Discrete submucosal granulomas in bronchial biopsy in a patient with sarcoidosis.

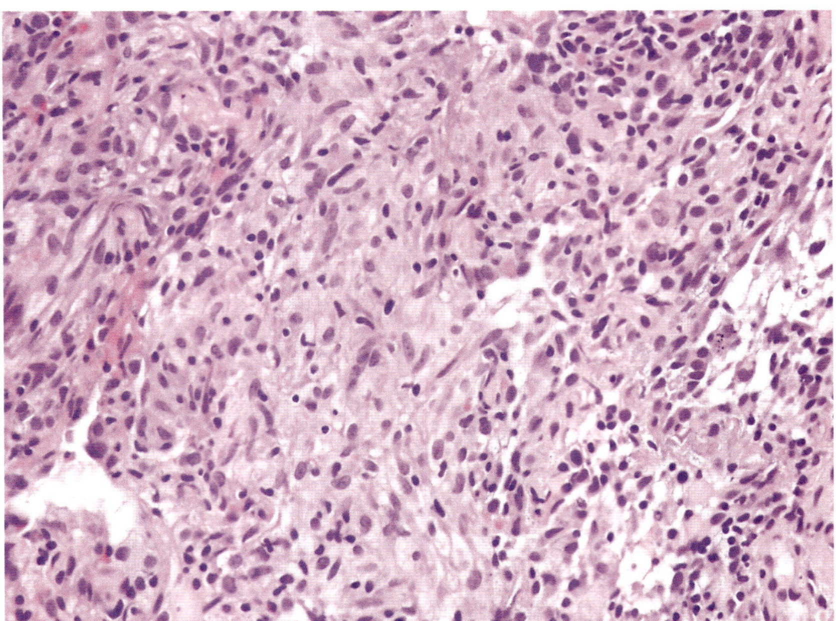

FIGURE 3.8 Higher magnification showing discrete clusters of epithelioid histiocytes gradually merging with the surrounding tissues.

The diagnosis of sarcoidosis is a diagnosis of exclusion. The pathology report on transbronchial biopsies should read only "nonnecrotizing epithelioid granulomas present" or "nonnecrotizing granulomatous pneumonitis." The pathologist can then state in a note that the findings are consistent with sarcoidosis if the clinical information provided was suggestive of the disease but should also suggest that alternate diagnostic possibilities must first be ruled out clinically. It is always a sound practice to routinely order special stains for microorganisms in cases of pulmonary granulomas to exclude infection, even in the absence of necrosis. We recommend routinely ordering acid-fast and silver stains. Submitting tissue for microbiologic cultures on cases in which clinical and radiographic findings are not highly suspicious for sarcoidosis is recommended because one study documented positive microbiologic cultures in up to 11% of biopsies of granulomas that were negative for microorganisms on special stains.[6]

More recently, cases of sarcoidosis and idiopathic pulmonary fibrosis presenting in the same patient have been described.[7] Such patients share the same clinical outcome of patients with idiopathic pulmonary fibrosis without sarcoidosis. It is postulated that such patients developed both diseases either coincidentally or have an occult genetic predisposition for both diseases.

BERYLLIOSIS

Berylliosis is a chronic occupational lung disease caused by inhalation of beryllium or its salts.[8,9] Because of its unique properties, beryllium (Be) continues to be used in many industries including ceramics, aerospace, defense, and electronics. Because chronic berylliosis can develop in patients at relatively low levels of exposure and in a minority of individuals at risk, it has been postulated that the mechanism of disease may be the result of a hypersensitivity reaction, whereby beryllium will function as a hapten binding to some large carrier molecules to form an antigen.[10] Studies have also now shown that there may be a genetic basis for sensitivity to beryllium by demonstrating increased frequency of HLA-DPGluβ69 and other human leukocyte antigen (HLA) alleles in these patient populations.[11] The histopathologic findings in chronic berylliosis are essentially indistinguishable from those of sarcoidosis and are characterized by multiple nonnecrotizing epithelioid granulomas with giant cells associated with variable degrees of fibrosis.[12] In advanced stages, the granulomas may coalesce to form large, centrally hyalinized masses that can resemble old lesions of histoplasmosis. There is also an acute form of the disease characterized by a chemical pneumonitis with diffuse alveolar damage that develops rapidly following short-term, massive exposure to soluble beryllium salts. This form of the disease has now disappeared in the United States of America (USA) owing to the air quality standards imposed in 1949 following the first cases of acute beryllium exposure reported in the USA.[13]

The diagnosis of berylliosis is dependent on the demonstration of a history of beryllium exposure and can be confirmed by demonstration of beryllium in lung tissue by wet chemical spectrometry techniques. A screening test, the beryllium lymphocyte proliferation test, which can be done on peripheral blood or bronchioloalveolar lavage lymphocytes, measures the beryllium-specific cellular immune response; this test has been shown to be useful in the surveillance of beryllium exposure, although there does appear to be variation between labs in the performance of the test.[14,15] Electron energy loss spectrometry and laser microprobe or ion microprobe mass spectrometry have also been utilized to demonstrate beryllium in tissue sections.[16] In the past, beryllium was an important component of fluorescent lights, but it is now mainly used in the aerospace industry and computer manufacturing among others, as mentioned earlier.[17] Exposure can also occur during mining and extraction of beryllium ores.

ALUMINOSIS

Aluminum is a metal utilized in a variety of industries, particularly aluminum welders, millers, refiners, and other activities requiring metal work. Exposure to airborne aluminum particles created during grinding, cutting, or welding of aluminum sheets can lead to the development of lung pathology.[18] Inhalation of aluminum particles can result in a granulomatous histiocytic response with focal interstitial accumulation of histiocytes which engulf the aluminum particles leading to the formation of discrete nodules along bronchovascular bundles (Fig. 3.9). Aluminum particles do

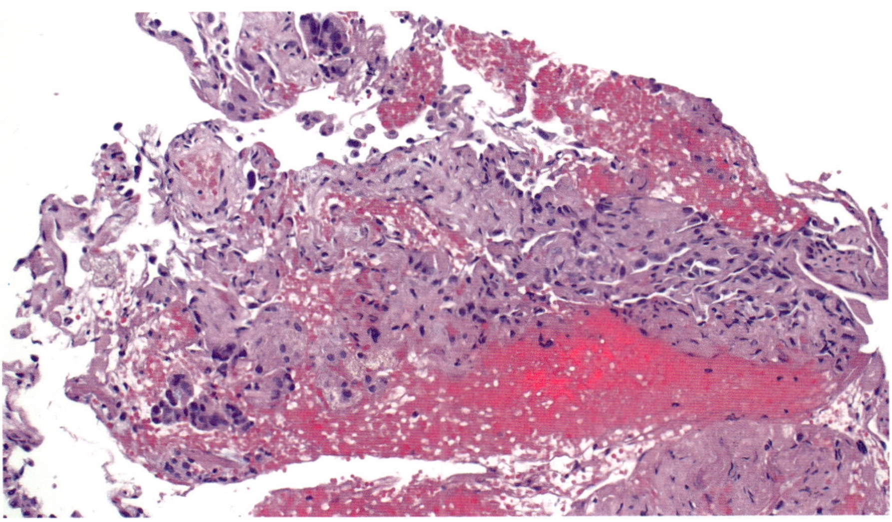

FIGURE 3.9 Endobronchial biopsy in a patient with a history of exposure to aluminum dust (arc welder) shows sheets of histiocytes with a grayish appearance in the interstitium.

not show birefringence under polarized light but may become visible if the dust exposure is admixed with silicates. The particles can be confirmed using scanning electron microscopy on tissue sections or by energy dispersive spectroscopy on particles extracted from lung tissue by digestion.[19] As with berylliosis, the diagnosis requires strict correlation with a history of exposure.

NECROTIZING SARCOID GRANULOMATOSIS

Necrotizing sarcoid granulomatosis (NSG) is a rare condition of unknown etiology characterized by nodular masses of necrotizing epithelioid granulomas involving the lung parenchyma. It is still not clear whether this condition represents a variant of sarcoidosis or whether it belongs to the family of pulmonary vasculitides.[20,21] The condition affects mostly adults older than 50 years but can also occur in adolescents or in elderly patients. There is an increased incidence in women (~1:2 male/female ratio). The disease is usually confined to the lungs and presents with cough, fever, weight loss, and chest pain. Up to 25% of patients may be asymptomatic. There has been no evidence found of systemic vasculitis, multiorgan involvement, or positive antineutrophil cytoplasmic antibodies (ANCA) in these patients.[22,23] NSG presents radiologically as bilateral, multifocal nodular opacities involving the lung parenchyma following a bronchovascular and subpleural distribution. Solitary lesions have also been reported.

Histologically, the lesions are characterized by confluent epithelioid granulomas with large areas of necrosis (Fig. 3.10). Foci of vasculitis may be present involving the media and subintimal region of small pulmonary arteries and veins. The granulomas may also circumferentially surround large arteries impinging on the adventitia. Scattered giant cells may be seen in the areas of vasculitis. The viable portions of the granulomas, however, are indistinguishable from those seen in sarcoidosis and comprise epithelioid histiocytes admixed with multinucleated giant cells. The granulomas may vary considerably in size and usually coalesce to form larger granulomas. They follow a similar lymphangitic distribution as in sarcoidosis and differ only because of the prominent areas of necrosis and the foci of vasculitis.[22-24] NSG may be very difficult to diagnose in transbronchial biopsies and may require video-assisted thoracoscopic surgery or wedge resection for adequate evaluation. Special stains for organisms are mandatory to rule out the possibility of infectious granulomas.

The differential diagnosis of NSG includes infectious granulomas, sarcoidosis, and granulomatosis with polyangiitis (GPA). Infectious granulomas may be the most difficult to exclude because they too can produce vasculitis and sarcoid-like epithelioid necrotizing granulomas. Special stains for organisms and microbiologic culture studies are the only reliable means for making this distinction. Separation from GPA may be problematic in some cases but can be accomplished by identifying the palisaded necrotizing granulomas with deeply basophilic areas of necrosis in GPA as

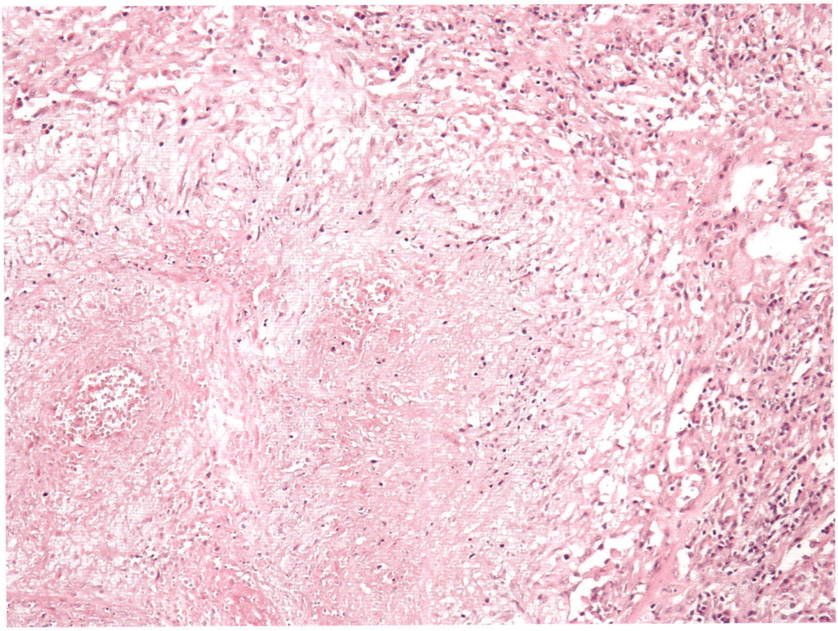

FIGURE 3.10 Necrotizing sarcoid granulomatosis showing an epithelioid granuloma with a large central area of necrosis.

opposed to the nonpalisading epithelioid granulomas of NSG and by the absence of cytoplasmic ANCA (C-ANCA) reactivity in the latter.

The prognosis for NSG is generally excellent. Most patients respond to systemic corticosteroids. A small percentage of patients will develop a relapse or have persistent disease. Death is rare and is usually the result of opportunistic infections.[22-25]

GRANULOMATOSIS WITH POLYANGIITIS

GPA represents one of the ANCA-associated pulmonary vasculitides, together with microscopic polyangiitis and eosinophilic GPA. The term "ANCA vasculitis" has been used by some to refer to this group of autoimmune disorders characterized by necrotizing vasculitis, absence or paucity of immune deposits, and predominant involvement of small vessels.[26] GPA primarily affects the upper and lower respiratory tract and the kidneys. GPA occurs in adults with a mean age of 50 years. Clinically, it presents with various symptoms that may involve the head and neck, eyes, lungs, and kidney, including sinusitis, nasal ulceration, otitis media, ear pain, oral lesions, cough, hemoptysis, pleuritic pain, conjunctivitis, eye pain, corneal ulcers, iritis, renal manifestations, and systemic manifestations including arthritis, weight loss, fever, and peripheral neuropathy.[27-30] The most important laboratory diagnostic test for GPA is the determination of serum ANCA. Two immunofluorescent patterns have been demonstrated–cytoplasmic or classical type (C-ANCA) and the perinuclear pattern (P-ANCA). The C-ANCA pattern is the one most closely associated with GPA and is present in most patients with generalized disease.[31,32] Histopathologically, the granulomas in GPA resemble more closely infectious granulomas than the granulomas of sarcoidosis owing to extensive central necrosis with peripheral palisading of macrophages (Fig. 3.11; eFig. 3.4). The basic histopathologic feature in GPA is a necrotizing vasculitis affecting small- to medium-sized arteries and veins (small/medium vessel vasculitis) (Fig. 3.12; eFig. 3.5). The vasculitis is often centered in areas of necrosis and may display granulomas involving the media and the adventitia of the vessel (Figs. 3.13 and 3.14). Fibrinoid necrosis is not a feature seen in this process. Capillaritis is another form of small vessel damage that has been observed in biopsies of patients with GPA in up to 30% of cases[33] and is discussed in Chapter 4. Small neutrophilic microabscesses are also a distinctive feature of GPA (Fig. 3.15; eFig. 3.6). They are seen within connective tissue and may contain a central area of necrosis surrounded by variable numbers of lymphocytes, plasma cells, histiocytes, and fibroblasts (Fig. 3.16). The areas of necrosis in GPA are often large and irregular with "geographic" contours. Unlike infectious granulomas,

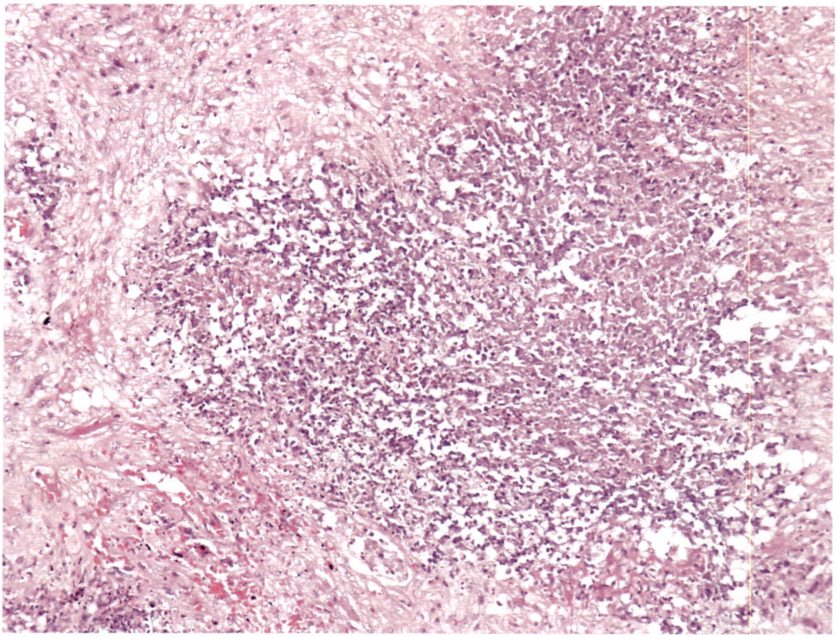

FIGURE 3.11 Granulomatosis with polyangiitis showing granuloma with characteristic area of geographic necrosis with deep basophilic appearance owing to abundant nuclear debris, surrounded by a palisaded rim of histiocytes.

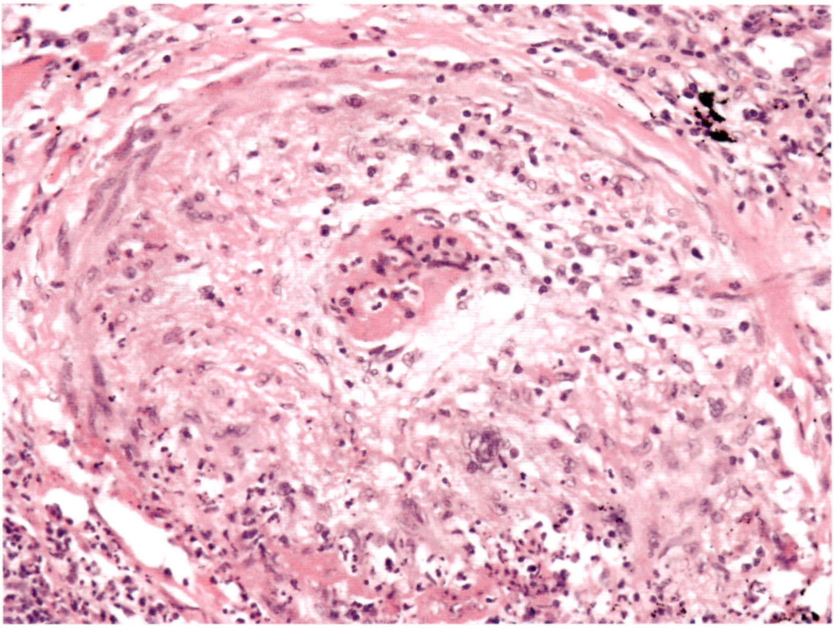

FIGURE 3.12 Granulomatosis with polyangiitis showing necrotizing vasculitis involving a small artery with small areas of necrosis in the media and adventitia of the vessels.

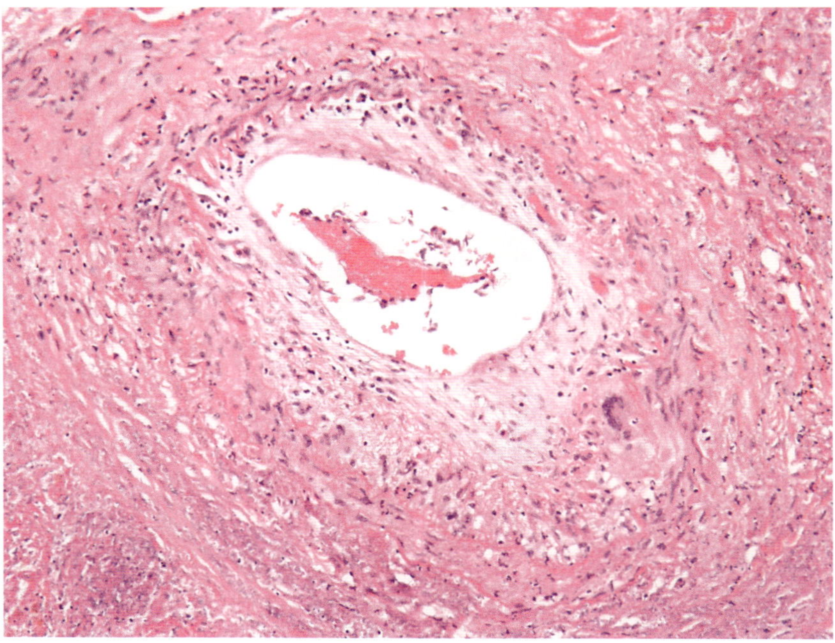

FIGURE 3.13 Medium-sized vessel in granulomatosis with polyangiitis showing involvement of the media by granulomatous inflammation.

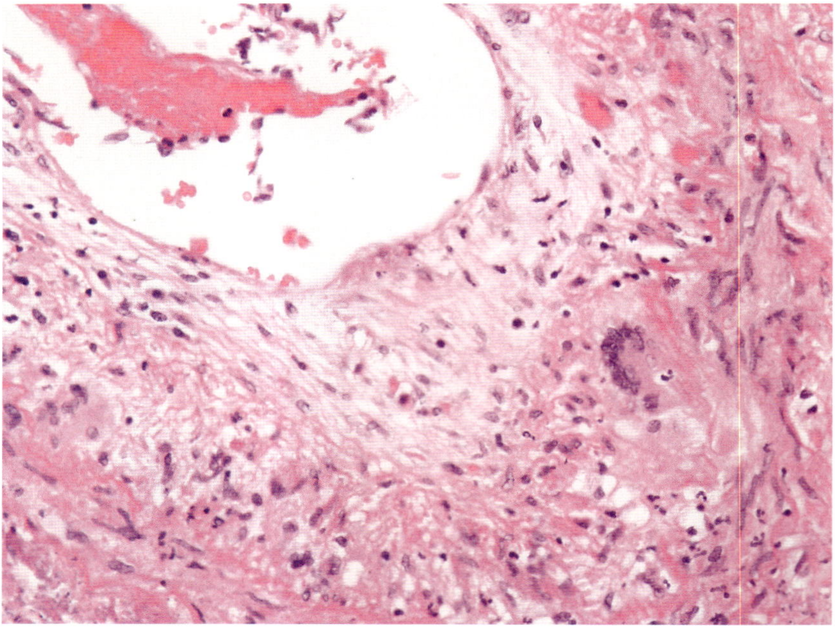

FIGURE 3.14 Higher magnification of vasculitis in granulomatosis with polyangiitis showing multinucleated giant cells and mononuclear cells within the wall of the vessel.

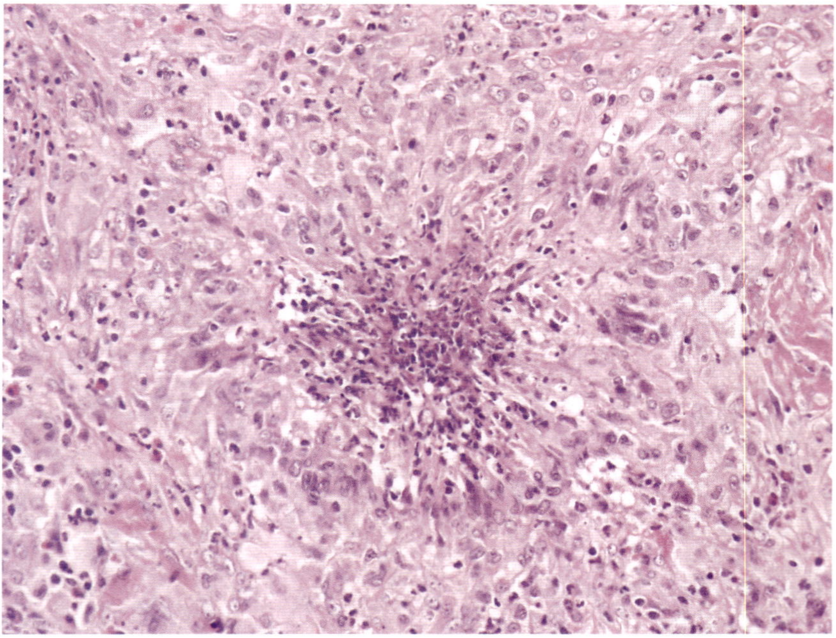

FIGURE 3.15 Small neutrophilic microabscesses in granulomatosis with polyangiitis with central area of suppuration and necrosis and numerous scattered eosinophils in the periphery of the granuloma.

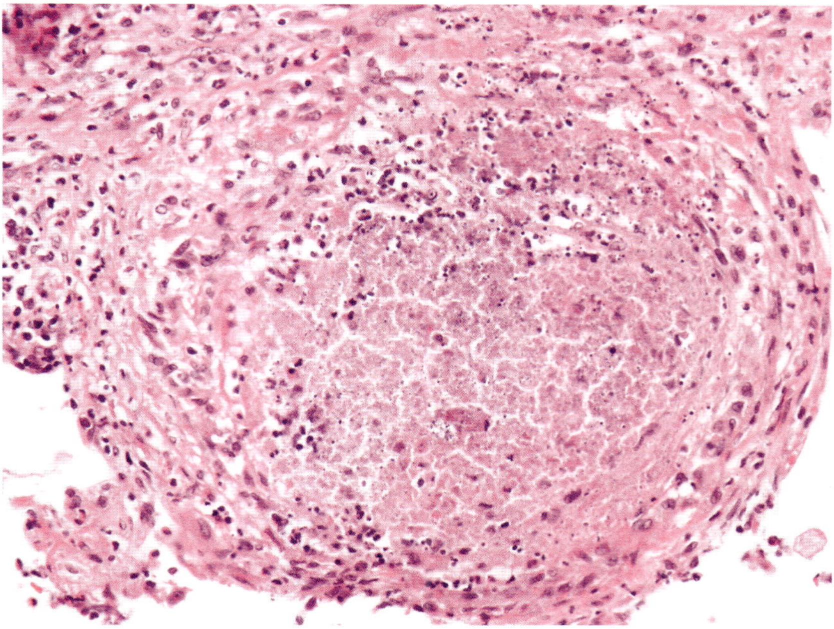

FIGURE 3.16 Another example of a small necrotizing microabscess in granulomatosis with polyangiitis showing an extensive central area of necrosis surrounded by neutrophils and nuclear debris and bounded by a peripheral rim of histiocytes.

the areas of necrosis tend to display a deeply basophilic appearance owing to the accumulation of abundant nuclear debris rather than the pink (eosinophilic) areas of necrosis seen in infectious granulomas. The areas of necrosis are characteristically surrounded by a rim of palisaded histiocytes. Multinucleated giant cells can be seen scattered singly or forming small aggregates at the edges of the areas of necrosis; however, they are not always present and may in fact be an uncommon finding in GPA. Well-formed, nonnecrotizing epithelioid granulomas are not a feature of GPA and should suggest an alternative diagnosis. Central cavitation with necrotic centers can often be seen in large granulomas. Extensive degeneration of collagen may also be appreciated surrounding the areas of necrosis. The lesions are often multiple and nodular with skip areas of uninvolved normal parenchyma. Secondary nonspecific changes that can be seen in association with GPA include an organizing pneumonia pattern, alveolar hemorrhage, interstitial fibrosis, lipid pneumonia, lymphoid hyperplasia, and acute bronchiolitis. GPA may be very difficult to diagnose on small transbronchial biopsies, but the diagnosis can be suggested when the characteristic granulomatous vasculitis is identified. Video-assisted thoracoscopic surgery or robotic-assisted thoracoscopic surgery biopsy is usually required for proper histopathologic evaluation. Clinical correlation and serologic testing are required for making a definitive diagnosis.

BRONCHOCENTRIC GRANULOMATOSIS

Bronchocentric granulomatosis (BG) is a condition characterized by necrotizing granulomatous inflammation that surrounds and replaces the bronchial wall and mucosa. The process involves the bronchi and the more distal bronchioles. BG is purely a descriptive diagnosis rather than a specific pathologic entity and may be the result of infectious and noninfectious conditions, including allergic bronchopulmonary fungal disease, bacterial or parasitic infection, rheumatoid arthritis, GPA, drugs, and necrotizing sarcoidosis. Between one-third and one-half of all cases occur in the setting of allergic bronchopulmonary aspergillosis in patients with asthma. Serum precipitin titers to *Aspergillus* or *Candida* species are elevated in about 50% of patients.[34] Cultures will grow the fungus in 20% to 50% of cases.[35] In asthmatic patients, the condition usually presents with progressive wheezing, cough, and fever with mucoid impaction. The lesions usually present as localized areas of consolidation or nodular parenchymal lesions on chest radiographs. Cavitation may be present in some of the nodules. The prognosis for patients with this condition is generally good. Asthmatic patients usually respond to corticosteroid treatment. Isolated lesions can be cured by simple surgical excision. Approximately half of the cases of BG are of noninfectious nature and may be owing to a specific etiology, such as rheumatoid arthritis or GPA, drug effect, or of unknown etiology.[36-38]

Histologically, the hallmark of the process is the destruction of the airway lumen by necrotizing palisaded granulomas (Fig. 3.17; eFig. 3.7). In some cases, the bronchial or bronchiolar wall may be partially preserved, and there will be only partial obliteration of the airway by the necrotizing granulomatous process. In cases where there is complete obliteration of the bronchial wall, identification of residual bronchial epithelium or identification of adjacent pulmonary arteries will help to confirm the bronchocentric nature of the process. In equivocal cases, elastic stains may help to identify the residual elastic lamina of the airway or to highlight the proximity to a pulmonary artery. The centers of the granulomas may contain abundant eosinophils, particularly in asthmatic patients. A foreign body giant cell reaction to the necrotic debris can also be observed in some cases. Fungal hyphae can be found in 20% to 90% of samples of patients with allergic bronchopulmonary aspergillosis.[34-36,39] The hyphae are often distorted and fragmented and are noninvasive. They are more frequently present within proximal bronchial plugs rather than in the necrotizing granulomas. Special stains for organisms should always be routinely ordered in cases of BG. Some cases of BG do not display any eosinophilia but are characterized instead by intense neutrophilia and total absence of organisms on special stains. Such cases may represent a manifestation of rheumatoid arthritis or GPA. Clinical correlation with serologic tests and identification of the other features distinctive for these conditions are necessary for correct interpretation. BG can also occur in patients with

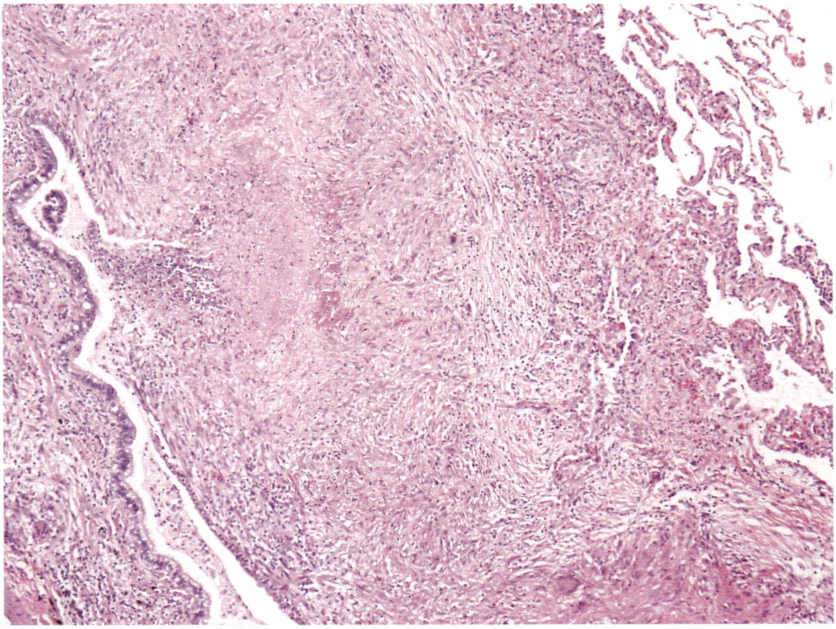

FIGURE 3.17 Necrotizing palisaded granulomas are seen causing destruction of the airway lumen in bronchocentric granulomatosis.

tuberculosis, blastomycosis, and histoplasmosis.[40,41] Transbronchial biopsies may yield limited information in cases of BG and an open lung biopsy may be preferable for more definitive interpretation. However, destruction of bronchial walls by necrotizing granulomas, especially when containing prominent eosinophils, should raise the suspicion of this condition and prompt further clinical studies and special stains to rule out organisms. It needs to be emphasized that BG is not a specific disease process but a nonspecific reaction pattern of lung airway damage to a variety of stimuli. Clinical correlation is always indicated to identify the underlying process responsible for the findings.

HYPERSENSITIVITY PNEUMONITIS

Hypersensitivity pneumonitis (HP), also known as extrinsic allergic alveolitis, represents an allergic response of the small airways and lung parenchyma to various inhaled organic antigens. The immunologic reaction in HP appears to represent a combination of immune complex–mediated (type III) and delayed-type hypersensitivity (type IV) reaction after exposure to an inciting agent.[42] Over the past several years, components of a genetic basis for HP have also been described including genetic alterations of the MUC5B promoter, telomere length, and specific HLA alleles.[43,44] The most well-known examples are farmer's lung, caused by sensitivity to thermophilic actinomycetes, and pigeon breeder or "bird fancier" lung, caused by inhalation of avian antigens. Although a similar effect can be observed with some ingested antigens, extrinsic allergic alveolitis generally refers to disease occurring as a result of inhalation exposure. These antigens include thermophilic bacteria such as actinomyces, other bacteria or bacterial products (humidifier lung, byssinosis, *Mycobacterium avium infections*), molds, amoeba, and chemicals (such as toluene diisocyanate used in plastics manufacture, or pyromellitic dianhydride used in epoxy resin).

The disease can occur as an acute or chronic process. The acute form occurs within hours of exposure to the inhaled antigen. The symptoms resemble an acute viral infection, with fever, chills, malaise, shortness of breath, and dry cough. The chronic form of the disease may be initially more subtle but will lead to progressive symptoms of shortness of breath.[45,46] Some cases can progress to end-stage diffuse interstitial fibrosis, leading to death because of respiratory compromise. Radiologic studies show diffuse ground-glass infiltrates, sometimes accompanied by reticulonodular densities. The findings mostly involve the upper half of the lung fields and generally spare the apices and bases.

The pathologic features of HP in the acute form are not well-characterized because they are seldom biopsied and most often confused for a viral-like illness. The histologic features in the subacute and chronic phases are mainly characterized by a chronic interstitial pneumonitis associated with bronchiolitis and small, poorly formed epithelioid granulomas (Fig. 3.18). The granulomas are characteristically small, ill-defined and nonnecrotizing, and they are located in the interstitium. They can be sometimes difficult to identify and will blend imperceptibly with the surrounding inflammatory cells in the alveolar septa (Fig. 3.19). The interstitial pneumonia is usually mild and causes only slight widening of the alveolar septa by small lymphocytes and occasional plasma cells. The inflammatory infiltrate is often present around the walls of terminal bronchioles. With progression of the disease, the lymphoid infiltrates can become denser and resemble a lymphoid interstitial pneumonia. In more advanced stages of chronic HP, there will be evidence of interstitial fibrosis with centrilobular accentuation that can be easily confused for usual interstitial pneumonia (UIP) and other interstitial fibrosing processes.[47] Identification of microgranulomas may be of help in suggesting a diagnosis of HP. Acute or abrupt exacerbation of chronic HP will present with extensive intra-alveolar fibrin deposition that can mimic acute fibrinous organizing pneumonia, but the underlying features of chronic HP will also be present.[48] The interstitial granulomas in HP can be very subtle and often only recognizable on higher magnification (eFig. 3.8), although we have seen examples of "hot tub" pneumonitis containing large, well-formed epithelioid granulomas (Fig. 3.20). The granulomas in such cases occur as an immunologic response to contamination with *M avium*, but the organisms are not demonstrable in the tissue. Similar features have been described with exposure to humidifiers and wind instruments. Scattered,

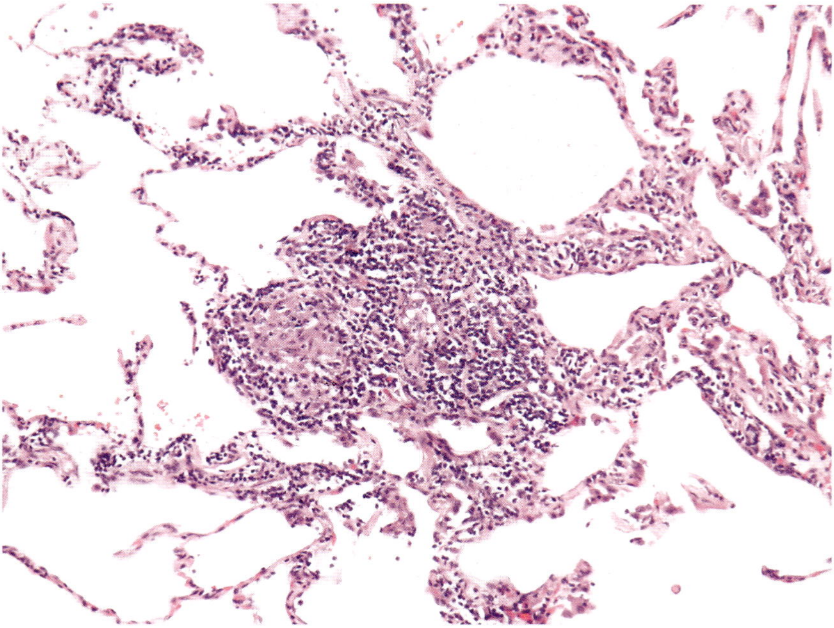

FIGURE 3.18 Chronic interstitial pneumonia in a patient with extrinsic allergic alveolitis (hypersensitivity pneumonitis) showing interstitial lymphoid infiltrates within alveolar walls and scattered small epithelioid granulomas.

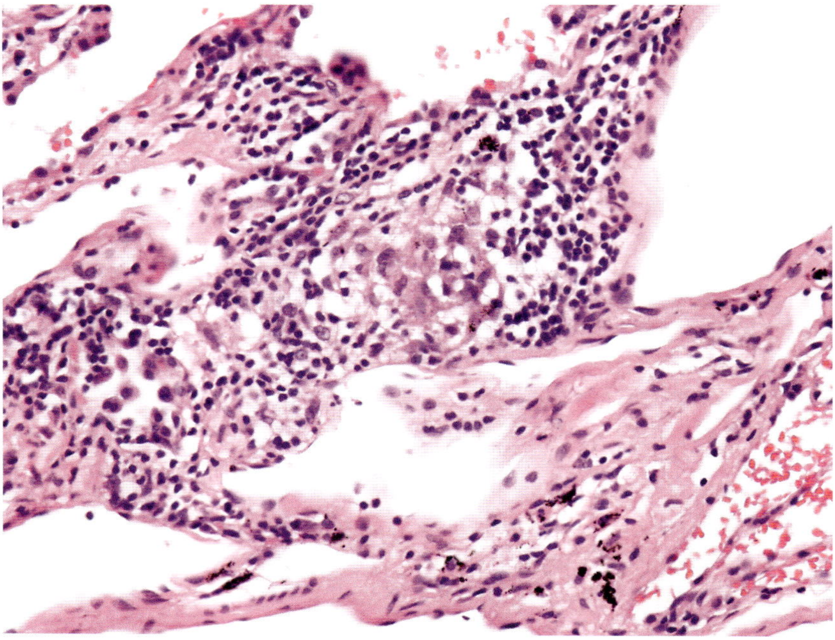

FIGURE 3.19 Higher magnification of extrinsic allergic alveolitis (hypersensitivity pneumonitis) showing ill-defined, poorly formed small epithelioid granulomas characteristic of this condition.

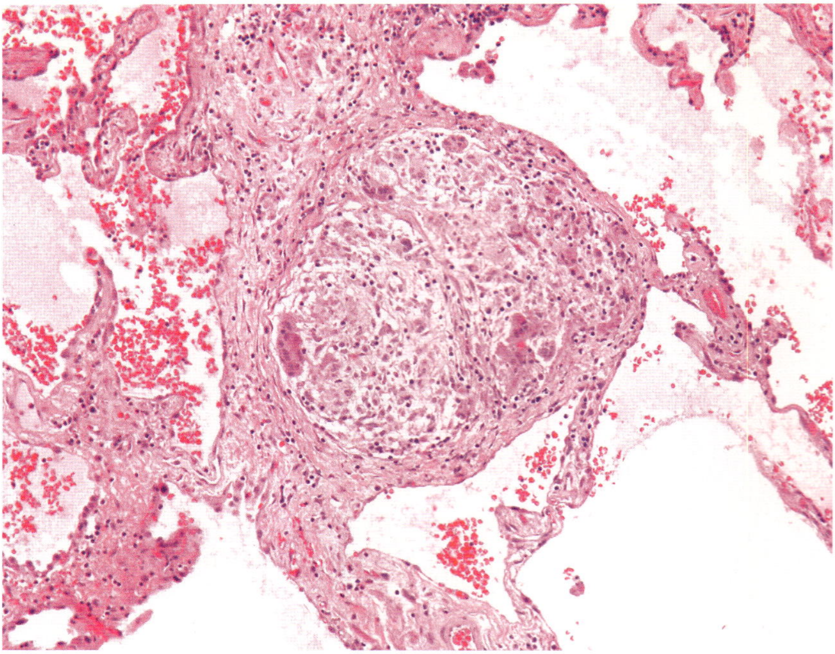

FIGURE 3.20 Large, well-formed epithelioid granulomas can be seen in "hot tub" hypersensitivity pneumonitis, reminiscent of sarcoidosis, but lacking the bronchovascular distribution of sarcoid granulomas.

isolated multinucleated giant cells may also be seen in the interstitium unassociated with the granulomas in cases of conventional HP (Fig. 3.21). Refractile oxalate crystals can be present within the giant cells and can lead to confusion with aspiration pneumonia or pneumoconiosis. Patchy airspace organization with features of organizing pneumonia can be observed in as many as 60% of cases and is characterized by discrete small foci of fibroblastic plugs within alveolar lumens. In more chronic cases of unresolved HP, prominent bronchiolization of alveolar spaces can be observed and dense fibrosis with extensive honeycombing closely resembling UIP will develop.[49-51]

The differential diagnosis for HP includes drug reactions and low-grade infections caused by atypical mycobacteria. Sarcoidosis is another differential diagnostic consideration, but the granulomas in sarcoidosis are more discrete and well defined and separated from the surrounding stroma by a rim of sclerosis. Furthermore, sarcoidosis is not usually accompanied by marked interstitial inflammation as seen in HP. Given that the histologic findings in HP are not specific and show significant overlap with many other conditions, the diagnosis requires clinicopathologic correlation. Clinical diagnostic criteria for HP have been recently proposed that stratify patients into definite, probable, and subclinical types based on a combination of exposure history, clinical and radiographic

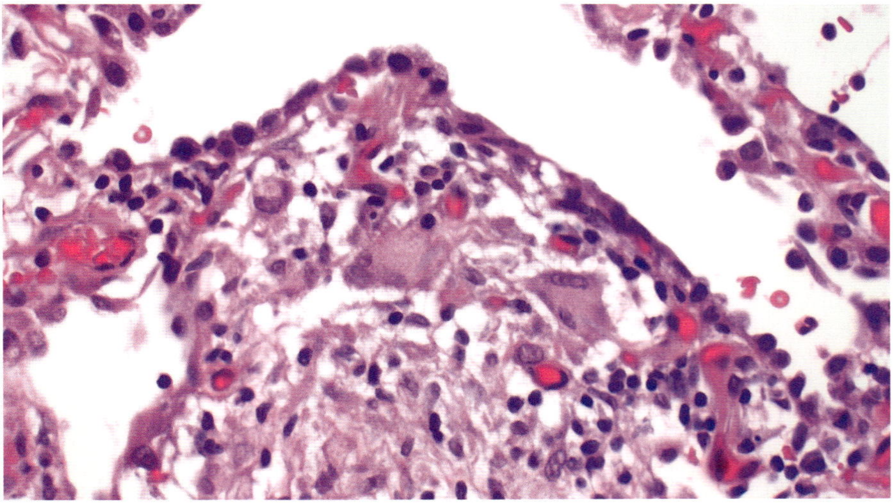

FIGURE 3.21 High power magnification of a transbronchial biopsy performed in a patient with suspected hypersensitivity pneumonitis demonstrates two multinucleated giant cells with the interstitial wall of the lung without granuloma formation.

findings, results of bronchoalveolar lavage, positive inhalational challenge test, and histopathologic features.[45,50,51] If the classical triad of interstitial pneumonitis, bronchiolitis, and ill-defined granulomas is present, the pathologist can suggest the diagnosis of HP or describe the findings as "consistent with hypersensitivity pneumonitis." Suggesting thorough clinical investigation that includes a history of exposure to antigens is indicated in the pathology report given the broad overlap of the histology with other conditions.

GRANULOMATOUS INFLAMMATION

Granulomatous Inflammation in Aspiration Pneumonia

Aspiration of particulate material is a common complication of severely debilitated patients as well as older patient populations.[52] The right lung is more often involved owing to gravitational effect and the trajectory of the right main bronchus, but the affected region can vary depending on the position of the patient at the time of aspiration. Most aspirated materials are foods and other organic materials, including seeds, meat particles, vegetable peels and pits, chicken bones, candy, and gum.[53] Aspiration pneumonia tends to be more common in older patients with individuals aged 75 or older accounting for approximately 75% of aspiration pneumonia-related deaths. It is estimated that there is approximately 17,000 deaths per year in the United States from aspiration pneumonia.[54] Complications of aspiration of particulate material can include lung abscess formation, bronchial stenosis, bronchiectasis, bronchocutaneous fistula, pneumothorax, empyema, obliterative bronchiolitis, and granulomatous inflammation. In a study of 59 patients, bilateral infiltrates or nodules were identified in 17 cases, unilateral nodules or infiltrates were found in 17 cases, and solitary nodules were seen in 13 cases. Foreign material was identified in all cases, including vegetable or food remnants in 54 cases, talc or microcrystalline cellulose in 7, crospovidone in 4, and Kayexalate in 2 patients.[55]

The histopathologic features of aspiration pneumonia include necrotizing pneumonitis with abscess formation, acute necrotizing and granulomatous bronchiolitis, and necrotizing suppurative granulomas with foreign body–type giant cell reaction to the aspirated material (Fig. 3.22). An organizing pneumonia pattern is often found distal to the obstructed bronchus or bronchioles. Hyaline membranes can develop within 48 to 72 hours and may lead to confusion with diffuse alveolar damage on endoscopic biopsies. Careful search for aspirated foreign material is necessary for a correct diagnosis. The foreign material is usually surrounded by multinucleated giant cells. The diagnosis must be suspected when multinucleated giant cells, acute bronchopneumonia or bronchiolitis, and suppurative granulomas are seen in a background of organizing pneumonia. It is important to examine the sections always under polarized microscopy to identify birefringent foreign particles. Polarized microscopy may help identify crystalline material within macrophages and multinucleated giant cells. Care must be taken,

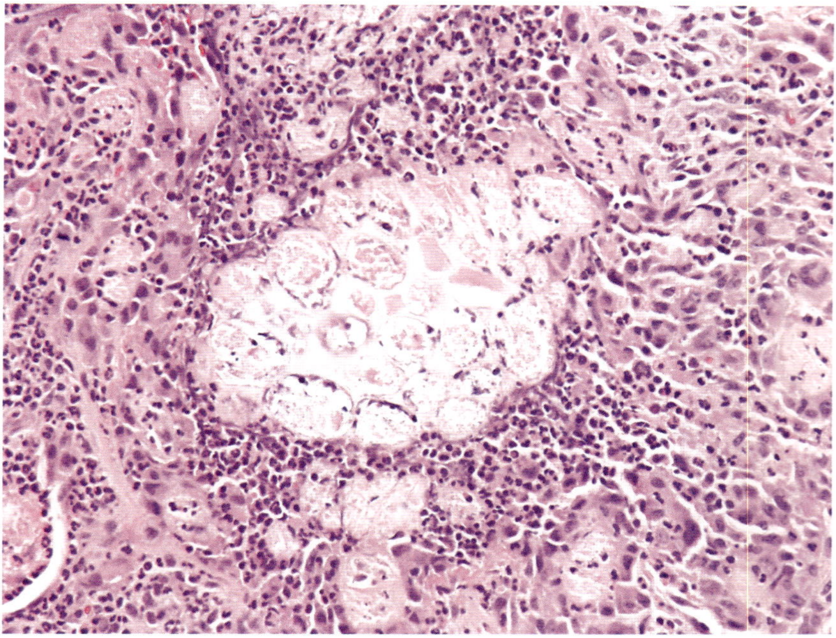

FIGURE 3.22 **Necrotizing suppurative granulomas are seen in aspiration pneumonia.** Notice the foreign body–type giant cell reaction surrounding the aspirated material.

however, not to misinterpret the presence of conchoidal calcifications or calcium oxalate crystals for evidence of aspiration, as these can occur in various inflammatory granulomatous reactions unrelated to aspiration.

Chronic aspiration of small volumes of gastric or oral contents can also lead to chronic aspiration pneumonia. Most patients have a history of gastroesophageal reflux, esophageal dysfunction, hiatal hernia, oropharyngeal dysfunction, and obstructive sleep apnea.[56] The histology is characterized by exogenous lipid pneumonia, poorly formed granulomas, and foreign body–type giant cells, with or without foreign material. The diagnosis requires clinical correlation with a careful clinical history.

Less Frequent Causes of Pulmonary Granulomatous Inflammation

Less frequent causes of pulmonary granulomatous inflammation can be seen in patients with hard metal pneumoconiosis, autoimmune disorders (particularly Sjögren syndrome [SS]), drug reactions (particularly with methotrexate), and in certain hematolymphoid neoplasms, particularly Hodgkin lymphoma and lymphomatoid granulomatosis.

Hard Metal Pneumoconiosis

Hard metal lung disease occurs as the consequence of the inhalation of hard metal dusts. Exposure can occur during the manufacture of products containing hard metals or during their use.[57-60] The two most frequent agents involved in hard metal pneumoconiosis are tungsten carbide used in the manufacture of cutting tools and drilling equipment and cobalt. Patients usually present with insidious onset of dyspnea and restrictive changes on pulmonary function tests. Radiologic studies show diffuse interstitial infiltrates with ground-glass opacities and small nodules.[61-63] The fact that a very low percentage (<1%) of exposed workers develop the disease suggests that the underlying pathogenetic mechanism may be related to a hypersensitivity reaction. Similar to other hypersensitivity-related processes, hard metal lung disease in some instances has been shown to have an association with the HLA system.[64]

The histopathologic hallmark of hard metal lung disease is the presence of abundant multinucleated giant cells within the alveolar spaces and lining the alveolar septa (Fig. 3.23; eFig. 3.9). In fact, a term applied in the past to this condition was giant cell interstitial pneumonia, which was believed to represent one of the idiopathic interstitial pneumonias.[65] The alveolar septa are usually thickened and fibrotic and lined by hyperplastic type II pneumocytes. The alveolar lumens are filled with abundant macrophages in a pattern reminiscent of desquamative interstitial pneumonia. In advanced cases, interstitial fibrosis may be very striking, leading to honeycombing of lung parenchyma and extensive bronchiolar metaplasia similar to that observed in the advanced stages of UIP. Discrete or well-formed epithelioid granulomas are *not* a feature of the disease. The metal particles can be visualized using analytic electron microscopy.[66]

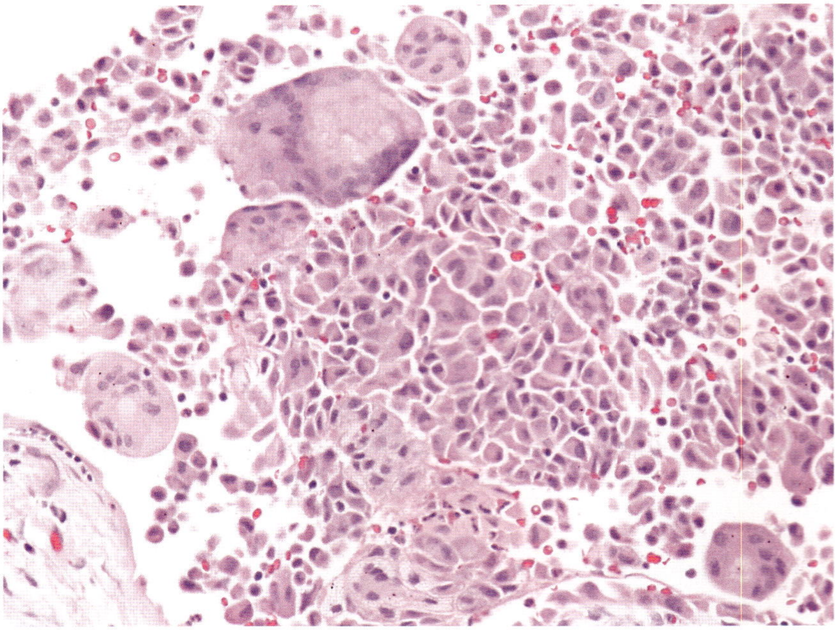

FIGURE 3.23 **Hard metal pneumoconiosis showing multinucleated giant cells admixed with macrophages within the alveolar spaces and lining the alveolar septa.**

Sjögren Syndrome

SS is an autoimmune disease characterized by a dense lymphocytic infiltration of the salivary glands, resulting in the clinical manifestations of dry mouth and dry eyes (also known as the sicca syndrome). Pulmonary involvement manifests itself in the form of interstitial pneumonia, airway disease, and sometimes with the development of hematolymphoid disease.[67-70] The principal morphologic manifestation of SS in the lungs is a lymphocytic interstitial pneumonitis principally distributed around the airways. However, a common finding is the presence of small, nonnecrotizing interstitial granulomas admixed with the lymphoid cell population.[71] For the most part, the granulomas are small and poorly formed, somewhat reminiscent of those seen in allergic extrinsic alveolitis, and are commonly admixed with the dense lymphoid interstitial infiltrate along with scattered multinucleated giant cells (Fig. 3.24). However, in some instances, the granulomas may become more numerous and diffuse, raising the possibility of an infectious process or aspiration pneumonia in the differential diagnosis. In severe cases, pulmonary involvement by SS may be complicated by bronchiectasis, bronchiolitis, interstitial fibrosis, organizing pneumonia, pleural effusion, amyloidosis, and intrapulmonary lymphoma.[72]

Methotrexate Toxicity

Methotrexate, a drug used in the treatment of various disorders, including rheumatoid arthritis and cancer, may cause interstitial inflammation with airspace organization and fibrosis. Hyperplasia of type II pneumocytes and

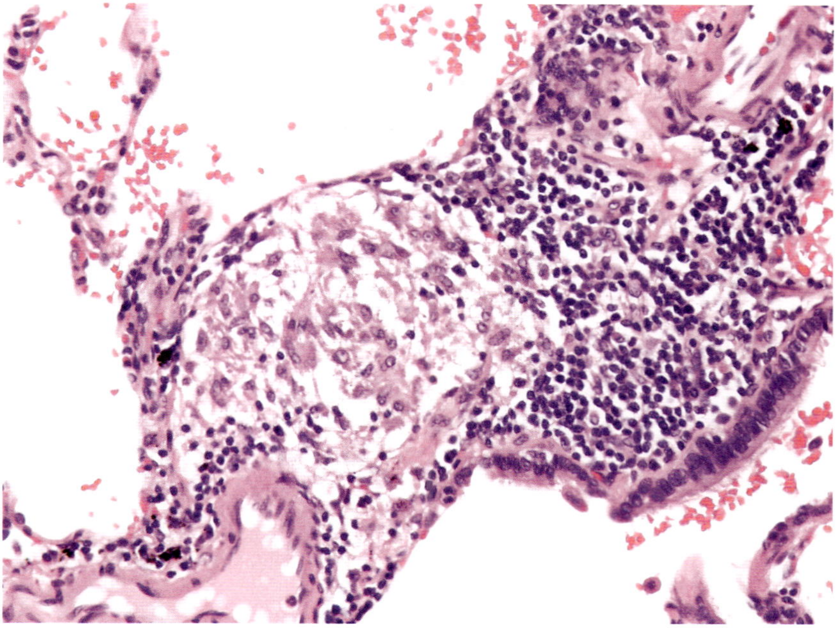

FIGURE 3.24 Small granulomas can be seen in Sjögren syndrome admixed with dense lymphoid cell infiltrates.

tissue eosinophilia can be seen in some cases. The findings are nonspecific, except for the presence of giant cells and small nonnecrotizing granulomas (Fig. 3.25), which are the only relatively specific features for this drug in comparison with other drugs causing lung toxicity.[73] In one study, it was found that the prognosis of patients with methotrexate-induced interstitial lung disease was dependent on the severity of the interstitial lung disease present.[74]

Hematolymphoid Neoplasms

Hematolymphoid neoplasms involving the lung may occasionally be accompanied by granulomas. These include Hodgkin lymphoma and lymphomatoid granulomatosis. Both will be discussed in more detail under hematolymphoid malignancies (Chapter 11).

Inflammatory Bowel Disease

Pulmonary manifestations in inflammatory bowel disease have been well documented.[75,76] These include bronchitis, bronchiectasis, obliterative bronchiolitis, organizing pneumonia, vasculitis, and granulomatous inflammation. Granulomatous pneumonitis can be observed in patients with Crohn disease and has also been reported in patients with ulcerative colitis under treatment with azathioprine.[77] In patients with Crohn disease, small, nonnecrotizing epithelioid granulomas with multinucleated giant cells tend to involve the interstitium and surrounding bronchioles. Special stains for organisms are indicated to rule out infectious agents. Clinical correlation is indispensable for correct interpretation.

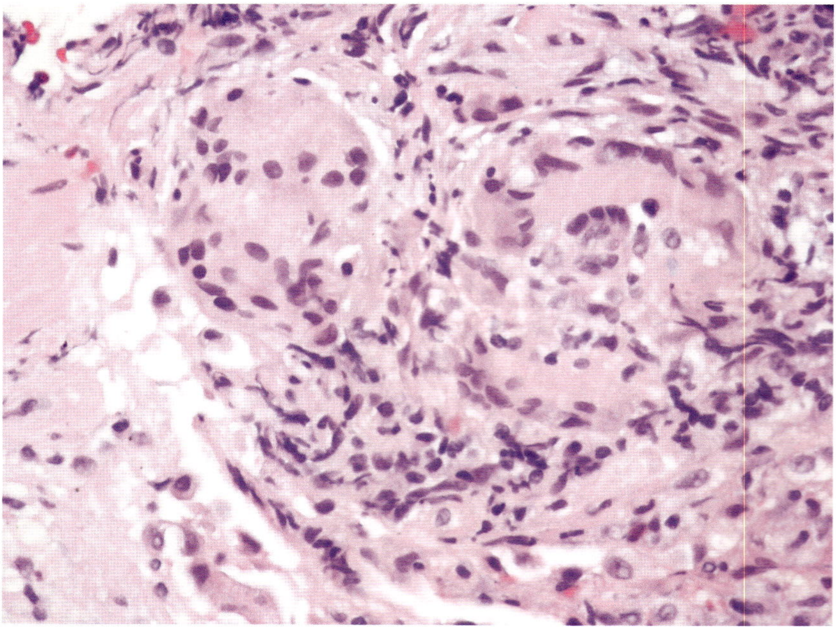

FIGURE 3.25 Small, poorly formed epithelioid granulomas similar to those observed in extrinsic allergic alveolitis can be seen in methotrexate toxicity.

Intravenous Drug Abuse

Intravenous injection of drugs that are normally intended for oral administration elicits a foreign body granulomatous reaction in the lung parenchyma secondary to the deposition of "filler" substances such as talc, starch, cellulose, and others within capillaries, arterioles, or small vessels. Talc used for "cutting" or diluting illicit drugs such as heroin can also deposit in the lung microvasculature in intravenous drug users. The granulomatous reaction can take place within the vasculature or may occur in the interstitium (Fig. 3.26). Multinucleated giant cells will usually contain polarizable crystalline foreign material. The most common types of foreign material include cornstarch, which shows a characteristic "Maltese cross" pattern of polarization, or talc, which assumes the shape of elongated plate-like crystalline material (Fig. 3.27).

Lipoid Pneumonia

Lipoid pneumonia may result from exogenous airway aspiration of mineral oils or by endogenous causes owing to breakdown of cells and release of their lipid constituents. The alveoli in exogenous lipoid pneumonia become filled with lipid-rich histiocytes containing abundant vacuolated cytoplasm (Fig. 3.28; eFig. 3.10). The vacuoles are filled with the engulfed mineral oil particles. Lipid stains, such as oil red-O, can be of help in identifying the lipid content of the vacuoles. With organization of the process, fibroblastic proliferation ensues, leading to the formation of a tumor mass (paraffinoma).[77-80]

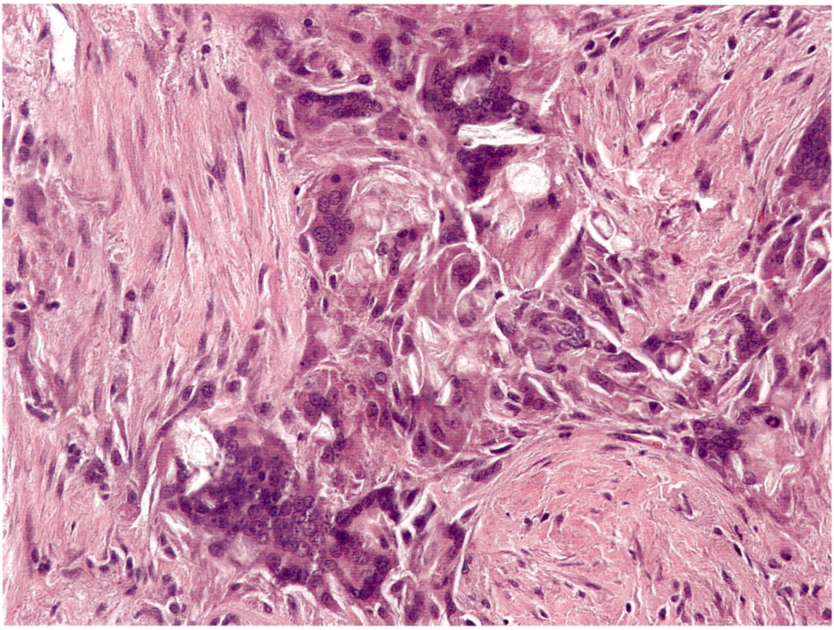

FIGURE 3.26 Small plate-like crystalline particles are seen surrounded by foreign body–type multinucleated giant cells in intravenous drug abuse.

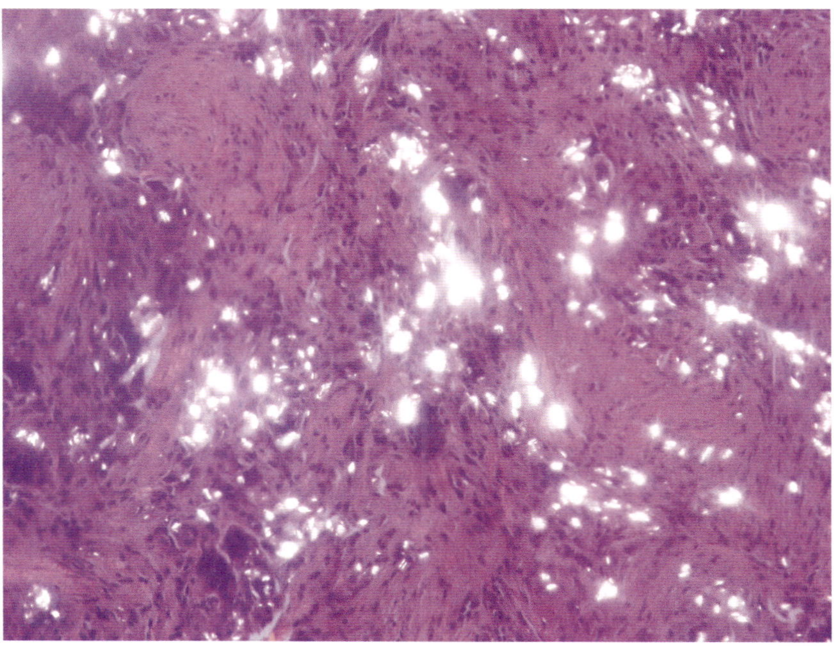

FIGURE 3.27 Intense polarization is observed under polarized light in the foreign particles in intravenous drug abuse.

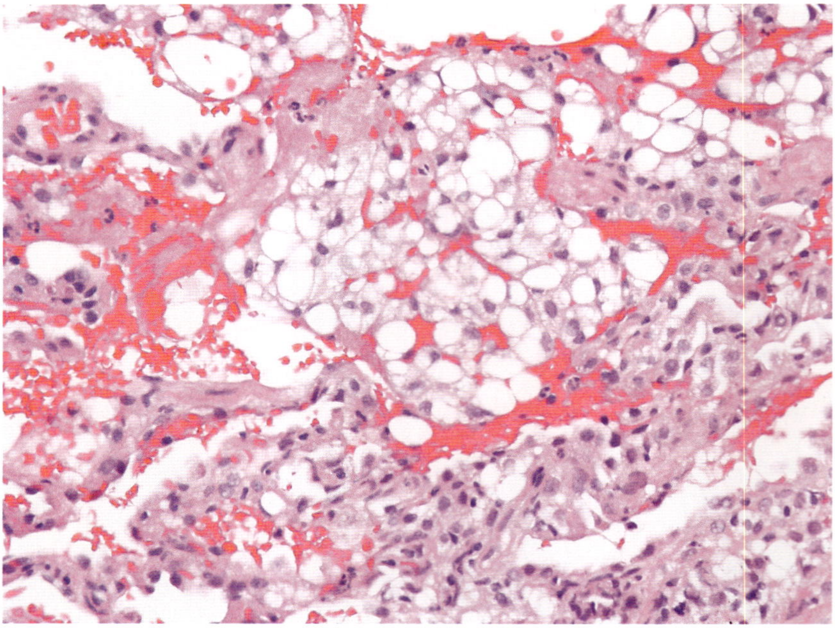

FIGURE 3.28 **Transbronchial biopsy showing vacuolated histiocytes filling the alveolar lumens in lipid pneumonia.**

REFERENCES

1. Greaves AS, Atif SM, Fontenot AP. Adaptive immunity in pulmonary sarcoidosis and chronic beryllium disease. *Front Immunol.* 2020;11:474.
2. Lynch JP III, Kazerooni EA, Gay SE. Pulmonary sarcoidosis. *Clin Chest Med.* 1997;18:755-785.
3. Hunninghake GW, Costabel U, Ando M, et al. ATS/ERS/WASOG statement on sarcoidosis. American Thoracic Society/European Respiratory Society/Word Association of Sarcoidosis and Other Granulomatous Disorders. *Sarcoidosis Vasc Diffuse Lung Dis.* 1999;16:149-173.
4. Uysal P, Durmus S, Sozer V, et al. YKL-40, soluble IL-2 receptor, angiotensin converting enzyme, and c-reactive protein: comparison of markers of sarcoidosis activity. *Biomolecules.* 2018;8(3):94.
5. Gilman MJ, Wang KP. Transbronchial lung biopsy in sarcoidosis. An approach to determine the optimal number of biopsies. *Am Rev Respir Dis.* 1980;122:721-724.
6. Hsu RM, Connors AF Jr, Tomashefski JF Jr. Histologic, microbiologic and clinical correlates of the diagnosis of sarcoidosis by transbronchial biopsy. *Arch Pathol Lab Med.* 1996;120:364-368.
7. Collins BF, McClelland RL, Ho LA, et al. Sarcoidosis and IPF in the same patient–a coincidence, an association or a phenotype? *Resp Med.* 2018;144:S20-S27.
8. Kriebel D, Brain JD, Sprince NL, Kazemi H. The pulmonary toxicity of beryllium. *Am Rev Respir Dis.* 1988;137:464-473.
9. Freiman D, Hardy H. Beryllium disease: the relation of pulmonary pathology to clinical course and prognosis based on a study of 130 cases from the U.S. Beryllium Case Registry. *Hum Pathol.* 1970;1:25-44.

10. Newman LS, Kreiss K, King TE Jr, Seay S, Campbell PA. Pathologic and immunologic alterations in early stages of beryllium disease: re-examination of disease definition and natural history. *Am Rev Respir Dis.* 1989;139:1479-1487.
11. Amicosante M, Berreta F, Rossman M, et al. Identification of HLA-DRPhebeta47 as the susceptibility marker of hypersensitivity to beryllium in individuals lacking the berylliosis-associated supratypic marker HLA-DPGlubeta69. *Respir Res.* 2005;6(1):94.
12. Balmes JR, Abraham JL, Dweik RA, et al. An official American Thoracic Society statement: diagnosis and management of beryllium sensitivity and chronic beryllium disease. *Am J Respir Crit Care Med.* 2014;190(10):e34-e59.
13. Eisenbud M. Origins of the standards for control of beryllium disease (1947–1949). *Environ Res.* 1982;27:79-85.
14. Stange AW, Furman FJ, Hillmas DE. The beryllium lymphocyte proliferation test: relevant issues in beryllium health surveillance. *Am J Ind Med.* 2004;46(5):453-462.
15. Deubner DC, Goodman M, Ianuzzi J. Variability, predictive value and uses of the beryllium blood lymphocyte proliferation test (BLPT): preliminary analysis of the ongoing workforce survey. *Appl Occup Environ Hyg.* 2001;16(5):521-526.
16. Ingram P, Shelburne JD, Roggli VL, eds. *Microprobe Analysis in Medicine.* Hemisphere; 1989.
17. Kriebel D, Sprince NL, Eisen EA, Greaves IA, Feldman HA, Greene RE. Beryllium exposure and pulmonary function: a cross-sectional study of beryllium workers. *Br J Ind Med.* 1988;45:167-173.
18. Taiwo OA. Diffuse parenchymal diseases associated with aluminum use and primary aluminum production. *J Occup Environ Med.* 2014;56(5, suppl):S71-S72.
19. Carney J, McAdams P, McCluskey J, Roggli VL. Aluminum-induced pneumoconiosis confirmed by analytical scanning electron microscopy: a case report and review of the literature. *Ultrastruct Pathol.* 2016;40:155-158.
20. Rosen Y. Four cases of necrotizing sarcoid granulomatosis: what do we know now? *Arch Pathol Lab Med.* 2015;139(2):252-262.
21. Karpathiou G, Batistatou A, Stefanou D, et al. Necrotizing sarcoid granulomatosis: a distinctive form of pulmonary granulomatous disease. *Clin Respir J.* 2018;12(4):1313-1319.
22. Churg A, Carrington C, Gupta R. Necrotizing sarcoid granulomatosis. *Chest.* 1979;76:406-413.
23. Koss M, Hochholzer L, Feigin D, Garancis JC, Ward PA. Necrotizing sarcoid-like granulomatosis: clinical, pathologic and immunopathologic findings. *Hum Pathol.* 1980;11(suppl 5):510-519.
24. Singh H, Cole S, Krause P, Conway M, Garcia L. Necrotizing sarcoid granulomatosis with extrapulmonary involvement. Clinical, pathologic, ultrastructural and immunologic features. *Am Rev Respir Dis.* 1981;124:189-192.
25. Spiteri M, Gledhill A, Campbell D, Clarke SW. Necrotizing sarcoid granulomatosis. *Br J Dis Chest.* 1987;81:70-75.
26. Alba MA, Jennette JC, Falk RJ. Pathogenesis of ANCA-associated pulmonary vasculitis. *Semin Respir Crit Care Med.* 2018;39:413-424.
27. Hoffman G, Kerr G, Leavitt R, et al. Wegener's granulomatosis: an analysis of 158 patients. *Ann Int Med.* 1992;116:488-498.
28. Cotch M, Hoffman G, Yerg D, Kaufman GI, Targonski P, Kaslow RA. The epidemiology of Wegener's granulomatosis. Estimates of the five-year period prevalence, annual mortality, and geographic disease distribution from population-based data sources. *Arthritis Rheum.* 1996;39:87-92.
29. Comarmond C, Cacoub P. Granulomatosis with polyangiitis (Wegener): clinical aspects and treatment. *Autoimmun Rev.* 2014;13(11):1121-1125.

30. Lutalo PM, D'Cruz DP. Diagnosis and classification of granulomatosis with polyangiitis (aka Wegener's granulomatosis). *J Autoimmun.* 2014;48–49:94-98.
31. Gross W, Csernok E. Immunodiagnostic and pathophysiologic aspects of antineutrophil cytoplasmic antibodies in vasculitis. *Curr Opin Rheumatol.* 1995;7:11-19.
32. Nolle B, Specks U, Ludemann J, Rohrbach MS, DeRemee RA, Gross WL. Anticytoplasmic autoantibodies: their immunodiagnostic value in Wegener's granulomatosis. *Ann Intern Med.* 1989;111:28-40.
33. Travis WD, Hoffman GS, Leavitt RY, et al. Surgical pathology of the lung in Wegener's granulomatosis. Review of 87 open lung biopsies from 67 patients. *Am J Surg Pathol.* 1991;15:315-333.
34. Katzenstein AL, Liebow A, Pass HI, Fauci AS. Bronchocentric granulomatosis, mucoid impaction, and hypersensitivity reactions to fungi. *Am Rev Respir Dis.* 1975;111:497-509.
35. Koss M, Robinson R, Hochholzer L. Bronchocentric granulomatosis. *Hum Pathol.* 1981;12:632-639.
36. Ohshimo S, Guzman J, Costabel U, Bonella F. Differential diagnosis of granulomatous lung disease: clues and pitfalls: Number 4 in the series "pathology for the clinician" edited by Peter Dorfmüller and Alberto Cavazza. *Eur Respir Rev.* 2017;26(145).
37. Pitsilka DA, Kampolis CF, Rontogianni D, Zisis C, Loukeri AA, Vlachoyiannopoulos PG. Bronchocentric granulomatosis in rheumatoid arthritis: case report and literature review. *Acta Reumatol Port.* 2020;45:214-219.
38. Hernández Pérez JM, Pérez Negrín L, López Charry CV. Bronchocentric granulomatosis as expression of pulmonary toxicity by lamotrigine. *Med Clin (Barc).* 2020;155:229-230.
39. Bosken CH, Myers JL, Greenberger PA, Katzenstein AL. Pathologic features of allergic bronchopulmonary aspergillosis. *Am J Surg Pathol.* 1988;12:216-220.
40. Maguire G, Lee M, Rosen Y, Lyons HA. Pulmonary tuberculosis and bronchocentric granulomatosis. *Chest.* 1986;89:606-609.
41. Myers J, Katzenstein AL. Granulomatous infection mimicking bronchocentric granulomatosis. *Am J Surg Pathol.* 1986;10:317-320.
42. Miller R, Allen TC, Barrios RJ, et al. Hypersensitivity pneumonitis. A perspective from members of the Pulmonary Pathology Society. *Arch Pathol Lab Med.* 2018;142:120-126.
43. Ley B, Newton CA, Arnould I, et al. The MUC5B promoter polymorphism and telomere length in patients with chronic hypersensitivity pneumonitis: an observational cohort-control study. *Lancet Respir Med.* 2017;5(8):639-647.
44. Falfán-Valencia R, Camarena A, Pineda CL. Genetic susceptibility to multicase hypersensitivity pneumonitis is associated with the TNF-238 GG genotype of the promoter region and HLA-DRB1*04 bearing HLA haplotypes. *Respir Med.* 2014;108(1):211-217.
45. Bourke SJ, Dalphin JC, Boyd G, McSharry C, Baldwin CI, Calvert JE. Hypersensitivity pneumonitis: current concepts. *Eur Respir J Suppl.* 2001;32:81s-92s.
46. Patel AM, Ryu JH, Reed CE. Hypersensitivity pneumonitis: current concepts and future questions. *J Allergy Clin Immunol.* 2001;108:661-670.
47. Larson BT, Smith ML, Elicker BM, et al. Diagnostic approach to advanced fibrotic interstitial lung disease: bridging together clinical, radiologic, and histologic clues. *Arch Pathol Lab Med.* 2017;141:901-915.
48. Hariri LP, Mino-Kenudson M, Shea B, et al. Distinct histopathology of acute onset or abrupt exacerbation of hypersensitivity pneumonitis. *Hum Pathol.* 2012;43:660-668.
49. Spagnolo P, Rossi G, Cavazza A. Hypersensitivity pneumonitis: a comprehensive review. *J Investig Allergol Clin Immunol.* 2015;25(4):237-250.
50. Churg A, Bilawich A, Wright JL. Pathology of chronic hypersensitivity pneumonitis what is it? What are the diagnostic criteria? Why do we care? *Arch Pathol Lab Med.* 2018;142(1):109-119.

51. Walters GI, Mokhlis JM, Moore VC, et al. Characteristics of hypersensitivity pneumonitis diagnosed by interstitial and occupational lung disease multi-disciplinary team consensus. *Respir Med.* 2019;155:19-25.
52. Shigemitsu H, Ashfar K. Aspiration pneumonias: under-diagnosed and under-treated. *Curr Opin Pulm Med.* 2007;13:192-198.
53. Kollef MR, Winn RE. Occult coiled drinking straw aspiration. *Heart Lung.* 1990;19:24-28.
54. Gupte T, Knack A, Cramer JD. Mortality from aspiration pneumonia: incidence, trends, and risk factors. *Dysphagia.* 2022;37:1493-1500.
55. Mukhopadhyay S, Katzenstein AL. Pulmonary disease due to aspiration of food and other particulate matter: a clinicopathologic study of 59 cases diagnosed on biopsy or resection specimens. *Am J Surg Pathol.* 2007;31:752-759.
56. Cardasis JJ, MacMahon H, Husain AN. The spectrum of lung disease due to chronic occult aspiration. *Ann Am Thorac Soc.* 2014;11:865-873.
57. Sprince NL, Oliver LC, Eisen EA, Greene RE, Chamberlin RI. Cobalt exposure and lung disease in tungsten carbide production: a cross-sectional study of current workers. *Am Rev Respir Dis.* 1988;138:1220-1226.
58. Chiba Y, Kido T, Tahara M. Hard metal lung disease with favorable response to corticosteroid treatment: a case report and literature review. *Tohoku J Exp Med.* 2019;247(1):51-58.
59. Seaman DM, Meyer CA, Kanne JP. Occupational and environmental lung disease. *Clin Chest Med.* 2015;36(2):249-269.
60. Hua JT, Cool CD, Green FHY. Pathology and mineralogy of the pneumoconioses. *Semin Respir Crit Care Med.* 2023;44:327-339.
61. Chiarchiaro J, Tomsic LR, Strock S, et al. A case series describing common radiographic and pathologic patterns of hard metal pneumoconiosis. *Respir Med Case Rep.* 2018;25:124-128.
62. Mizutani RF, Terra-Filho M, Lima E, et al. Hard metal lung disease: a case series. *J Bras Pneumol.* 2016;42(6):447-452.
63. Akira M, Suganuma N. Imaging diagnosis of pneumoconiosis with predominant nodular pattern: HRCT and pathologic findings. *Clin Imaging.* 2023;97:28-33.
64. Potolicchio I, Mosconi G, Forni A. Susceptibility to hard metal lung disease is strongly associated with the presence of glutamate 69 in HLA-DP beta chain. *Eur J Immunol.* 1997;27(10):2741-2743.
65. Ohori NP, Sciuba FC, Owens GR, Hodgson MJ, Yousem SA. Giant cell interstitial pneumonia and hard-metal pneumoconiosis: a clinicopathologic study of four cases and review of the literature. *Am J Surg Pathol.* 1989;13:581-587.
66. Stettler LE, Groth DH, Platek SF. Automated characterization of particles extracted from human lungs: three cases of tungsten carbide exposure. *Scan Electron Microsc.* 1983;1:439-448.
67. Mestre-Torres J, Solans-Laque R. Pulmonary involvement in Sjögren's syndrome. *Med Clin (Barc).* 2022;158(4):181-185. English, Spanish. doi:10.1016/j.medcli.2021.06.016. PMID: 34392987.
68. Luppi F, Sebastiani M, Silva M, et al. Interstitial lung disease in Sjögren's syndrome: a clinical review. *Clin Exp Rheumatol.* 2020;38(Suppl 126):291-300.
69. Luppi F, Sebastiani M, Sverzellati N, Cavazza A, Salvarani C, Manfredi A. Lung complications of Sjogren syndrome. *Eur Respir Rev.* 2020;29:200021.
70. Berardicurti O, Marino A, Genovali I, et al. Interstitial lung disease and pulmonary damage in primary Sjögren's syndrome: a systematic review and meta-analysis. *J Clin Med.* 2023;12:2586.
71. Deheinzelin D, Capelozzi VL, Kairalla RA, Barbas Filho JV, Saldiva PH, de Carvalho CR. Interstitial lung disease in primary Sjogren's syndrome. Clinical–pathological evaluation and response to treatment. *Am J Respir Crit Care Med.* 1996;154:794-799.

72. Chung A, Wilgus ML, Fishbein G, Lynch JP III. Pulmonary and bronchiolar involvement in Sjogren's syndrome. *Semin Respir Crit Care Med.* 2019;40:235-254.
73. Imokawa S, Colby TV, Leslie KO, Helmers RA. Methotrexate pneumonitis: review of the literature and histopathological findings in nine patients. *Eur Respir J.* 2000;15:373-381.
74. Rojas-Serrano J, Herrera-Bringas D, Perez-Roman DI, Pérez-Dorame R, Mateos-Toledo H, Mejía M. Rheumatoid arthritis-related interstitial lung disease (RA-ILD): methotrexate and the severity of lung disease are associated to prognosis. *Clin Rheumatol.* 2017;36:1493-1500.
75. Black H, Mendoza M, Murin S. Thoracic manifestations of inflammatory bowel disease. *Chest.* 2007;131:524-532.
76. Casey MB, Tazelaar HD, Myers JL, et al. Noninfectious lung pathology in patients with Crohn's disease. *Am J Surg Pathol.* 2003;27:213-219.
77. Nagy F, Molnar T, Makula E, et al. A case of interstitial pneumonitis in a patient with ulcerative colitis treated with azathioprine. *World J Gastroenterol.* 2007;13:316-319.
78. Byerley JS, Hernandez ML, Leigh MW, Antoon JW. Clinical approach to endogenous lipoid pneumonia. *Clin Respir J.* 2016;10(2):259-263.
79. Worringer E, Schroeder K, Oh E, et al. Lipoid pneumonia. *Am J Med Sci.* 2015;349(1):72.
80. Hadda V, Khilnani GC. Lipoid pneumonia: an overview. *Expert Rev Respir Med.* 2010;4(6):799-807.

4

LUNG VASCULITIS AND HEMORRHAGIC DISORDERS

The involvement of blood vessels and hemorrhage as the primary pathologic findings can affect the lung parenchyma under many conditions. Vasculitis can be the result of autoimmune-mediated disease or can be secondary to infections and other types of inflammation. Although rare, vasculitic processes in the lung can be the source of major morbidity. A diagnosis of vasculitis has serious implications as it generally requires immediate therapeutic intervention. Clinical correlation and, in many instances, ancillary serologic testing are required for a specific and definitive diagnosis.

For ease and convenience of presentation, lung vasculitis can be categorized into conditions where vasculitis is the main or major manifestation of the disease and those where it is a secondary phenomenon (Table 4.1).

TABLE 4.1 Conditions in Which Pulmonary Vasculitis Is the Principal Manifestation and Those in Which It Represents a Secondary Manifestation of the Disease

Principal Manifestation	Secondary Manifestation
Granulomatosis with polyangiitis	Necrotizing sarcoid granulomatosis
Microscopic polyangiitis	Classical sarcoid
Eosinophilic granulomatosis with polyangiitis	Collagen vascular disease
Polyarteritis nodosa	Inflammatory bowel disease
Small vessel vasculitis (capillaritis)	Malignancy
Takayasu syndrome	Pulmonary infection
Henoch-Schönlein purpura	Bronchocentric granulomatosis
Behçet syndrome	Sequestration
Cryoglobulinemia	Drug or toxic substances
Giant cell arteritis	Transplantation
	Radiation
	Malignant lymphoma

The majority of vasculitic syndromes affecting the lung belong to the category of idiopathic vasculitides. The most common ones affecting the lungs are granulomatosis with polyangiitis (GPA) and microscopic polyangiitis (MP). Other idiopathic vasculitides that affect the lung parenchyma less commonly include eosinophilic granulomatosis with polyangiitis (EGPA; Churg-Strauss syndrome), polyarteritis nodosa, small vessel vasculitis, Takayasu syndrome, Henoch-Schönlein purpura (HSP), Behçet syndrome, cryoglobulinemia, and giant cell arteritis. The diagnosis of these conditions is often fraught with difficulties and relies heavily on a good clinical history and correlation with the radiology and the results of specialized laboratory tests.

GRANULOMATOSIS WITH POLYANGIITIS

This condition, formerly classified by Liebow under the category of "pulmonary angiitis and granulomatosis,"[1] represents a vasculitic process with predominant involvement of the lungs and sometimes a prominent granulomatous component. The disease can occur at all extremes of age but is most common in middle-aged adults. The classic presentation of the disease is the triad of upper respiratory tract, lung involvement, and glomerulonephritis. Other organs, including skin, eyes, joints, and nervous system, can also be affected. Less than 20% of patients present initially with renal disease but at least 75% eventually develop a focal segmental necrotizing glomerulonephritis. However, the disease can be limited to the lungs (ie, limited or localized form of GPA); such patients are usually associated with a better prognosis.[2-4] The main clinical symptoms of GPA include cough, chest pain, hemoptysis, nasal ulceration, sinus pain, fever, malaise, and weight loss. Other symptoms include hematuria, renal failure, otitis, arthralgia, myalgia, neurologic abnormalities, and skin lesions. Some patients may develop other presentations including cavitary lesions, isolated lung lesions mimicking malignancy, lung abscesses, and massive life-threatening hemoptysis.[5-9] It is interesting to note that some patients may be relatively asymptomatic despite having numerous necrotic nodules involving the lungs.[10,11] As indicated previously, the most reliable diagnostic laboratory abnormality is the presence of antineutrophil cytoplasmic antibodies (ANCA) in the serum. ANCA are autoantibodies to components of neutrophil and monocyte granules (specifically proteinase 3 and myeloperoxidase) that can be detected by indirect immunofluorescence or by enzyme-linked immunosorbent assay techniques. Of the two immunofluorescent patterns observed (cytoplasmic ANCA or C-ANCA and perinuclear ANCA or P-ANCA), the one characterized by diffuse cytoplasmic immunofluorescence staining (C-ANCA) appears to be highly specific for GPA and can be found in more than 90% of systemic cases and in about 60% of localized cases.[12,13] False-positive results, however, can also be observed under various circumstances. Imaging features of GPA are relatively nonspecific and may mimic a large number of diseases including tumors, infections, and other inflammatory disease.[14] Lung biopsies are usually indicated for definitive diagnosis.

The granulomatous features of GPA have been explained in detail in Chapter 3. In this chapter, we will detail the vascular changes that characterize the disease. The vascular changes in GPA can be of various types, including capillaritis, acute necrotizing vasculitis affecting small arteries and veins, and granulomatous vasculitis. *Capillaritis* is a distinctive feature of GPA and normally involves alveolar septal capillaries and venules. It is frequently present within the parenchyma surrounding areas of necrosis. Transbronchial lung biopsy can be highly useful in identifying capillaritis in GPA. The process is characterized by acute neutrophilic inflammation that expands and destroys alveolar septa (Figs. 4.1 and 4.2; eFigs. 4.1 and 4.2). When extensive destruction of alveolar walls ensues, the capillaritis can only be inferred from the distribution of the acute inflammation, which will outline preexisting alveolar septa (Fig. 4.3; eFig. 4.3). A distinctive histologic presentation of GPA is characterized by the absence of granulomas and necrosis

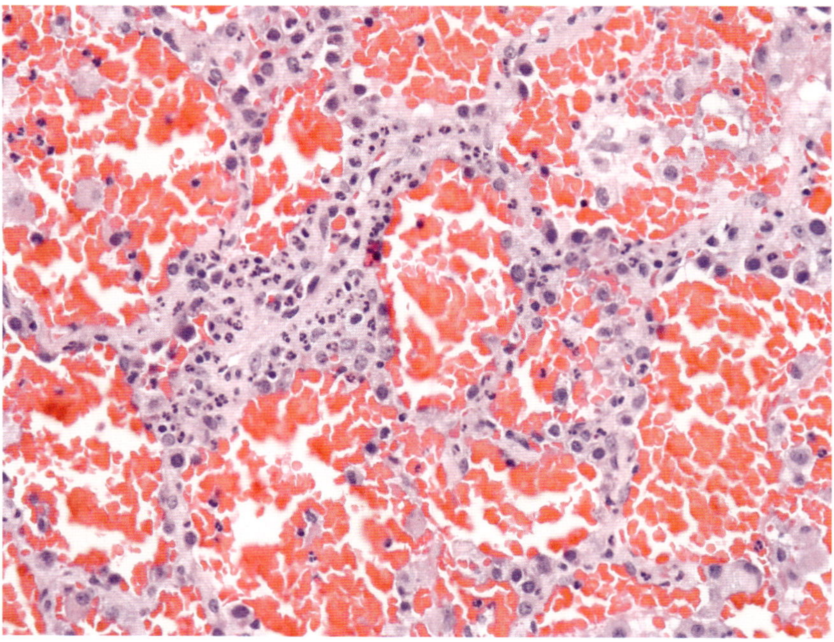

FIGURE 4.1 Capillaritis in granulomatosis with polyangiitis characterized by acute neutrophilic infiltration that expands the alveolar septa.

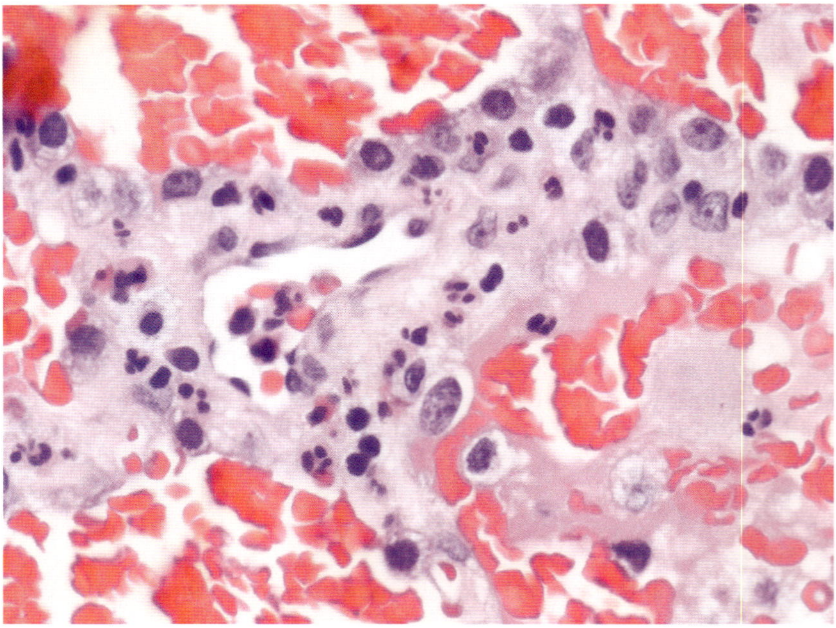

FIGURE 4.2 **Higher magnification of capillaritis in granulomatosis with polyangiitis.** Notice the expansion of the alveolar septa by abundant neutrophils.

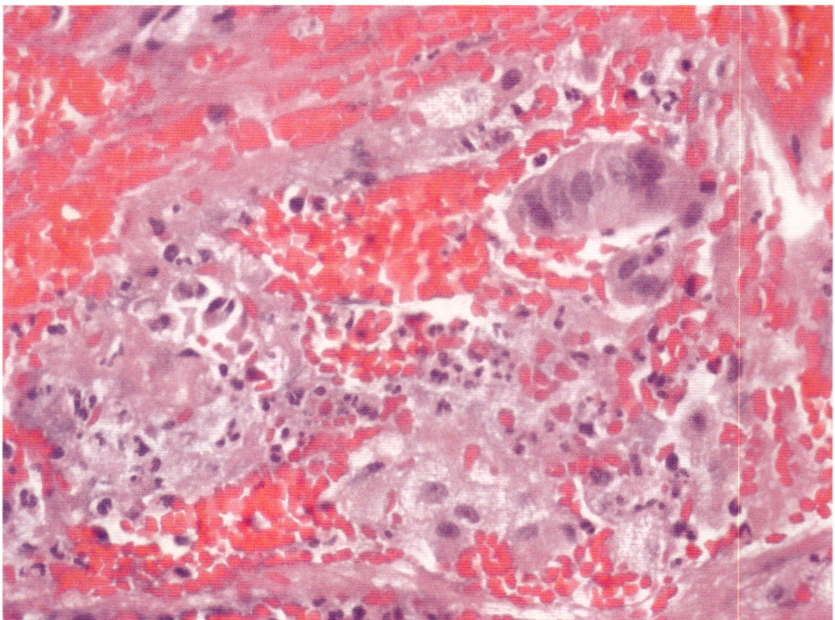

FIGURE 4.3 **Necrotizing capillaritis in granulomatosis with polyangiitis.** The process has already destroyed the alveolar septa and only their outline can be discerned by tracing the distribution of the neutrophils.

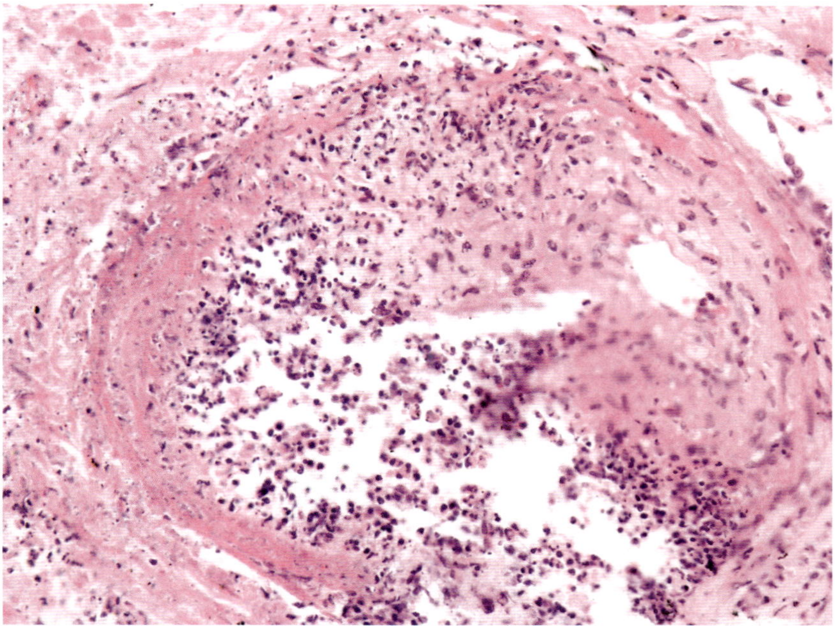

FIGURE 4.4 Necrotizing vasculitis in granulomatosis with polyangiitis shows destruction of vessel walls by neutrophilic infiltrate admixed with fibrinoid exudates.

and by prominent alveolar hemorrhage and capillaritis. Clinically, such patients usually present with hemoptysis and diffuse pulmonary infiltrates and follow a fulminant clinical course. The biopsy will show extensive intra-alveolar hemorrhage and capillaritis characterized by focal expansion of alveolar septa by neutrophils admixed with nuclear debris. *Necrotizing vasculitis* is a constant feature of most cases of GPA characterized by infiltration and destruction of vessel walls by a neutrophilic infiltrate, sometimes accompanied by fibrinoid necrosis (Fig. 4.4). The vasculitis can be seen involving only a portion of the vessel wall leading to an "eccentric" or partial distribution. Circumferential and transmural involvement by acute and chronic inflammatory infiltrate, accompanied by necrosis and destruction of the vessel wall, however, is the more common manifestation. Elastic tissue stains can help demonstrate the destruction of the internal elastic lamina (Fig. 4.5). The necrotizing vasculitis may lead to complete destruction of the vessel walls (Fig. 4.6). *Granulomatous vasculitis* was covered in detail in Chapter 3 on granulomatous pneumonitis and is characterized by necrotizing granulomas and multinucleated giant cells involving the adventitia and media of small and middle-sized vessels (Fig. 4.7; eFigs. 4.4-4.6).

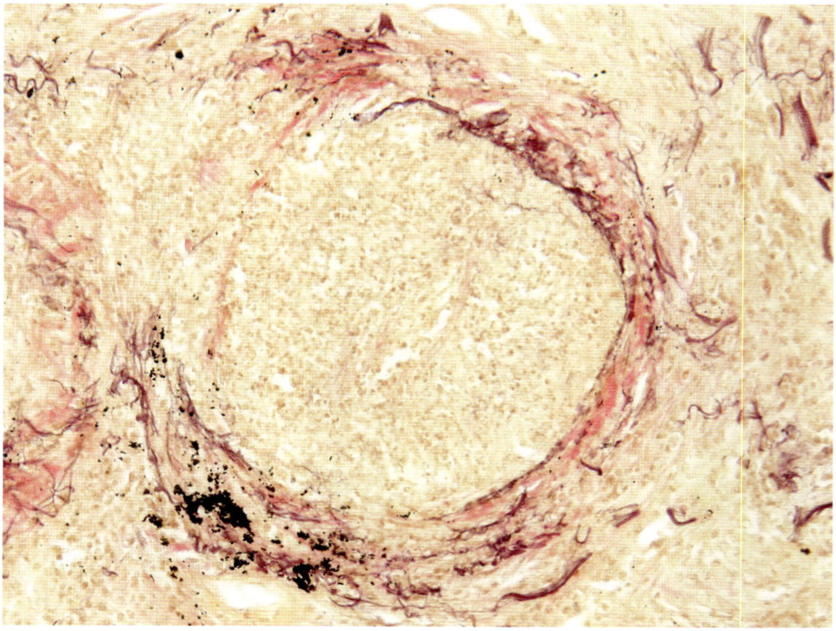

FIGURE 4.5 Verhoeff Van Gieson stain in granulomatosis with polyangiitis shows almost complete destruction of internal elastic lamina.

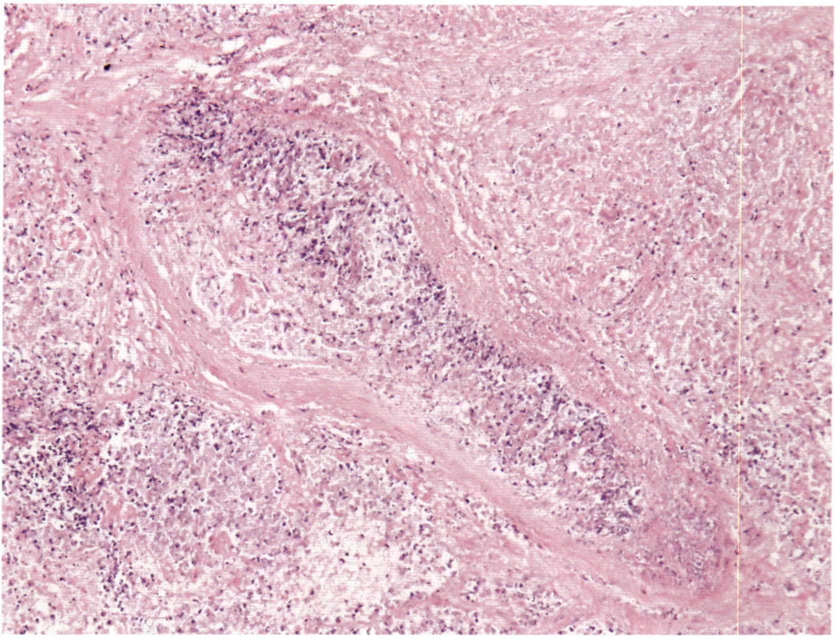

FIGURE 4.6 Necrotizing vasculitis in granulomatosis with polyangiitis showing complete destruction of vessel wall with fibrinoid necrosis.

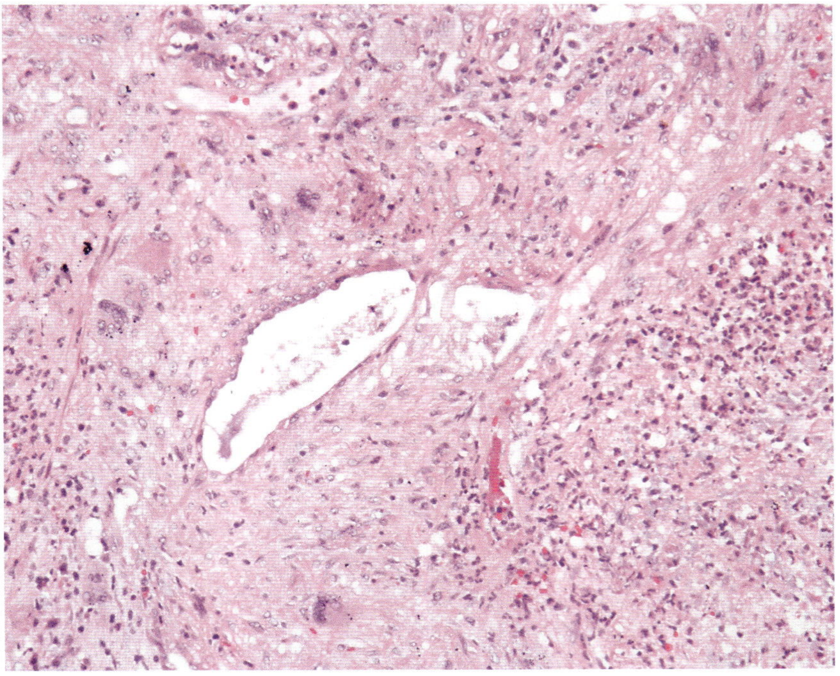

FIGURE 4.7 Granulomatous vasculitis in granulomatosis with polyangiitis shows necrotizing granulomas and multinucleated giant cells involving the adventitia and the media of a mid-sized artery.

The histologic features of GPA can be quite distinctive in fully developed lesions that are sampled on open lung or video-assisted thoracoscopic surgery biopsies. Lesions may be more difficult to appreciate on smaller biopsies; however, in rare instances, findings consistent with GPA, such as obvious evidence of vasculitis with surrounding necrosis, may be identified (Figs. 4.8-4.12).[15] A descriptive diagnosis should be rendered by the pathologist under such circumstances. In some instances, when both the clinical and histopathologic findings are highly consistent with GPA, the diagnosis can be strongly considered even in the absence of C-ANCA positivity.[16] A definitive diagnosis, however, should be rendered only after a strict correlation of the histopathologic findings with the clinical picture and serologic studies for C-ANCA are done.[17]

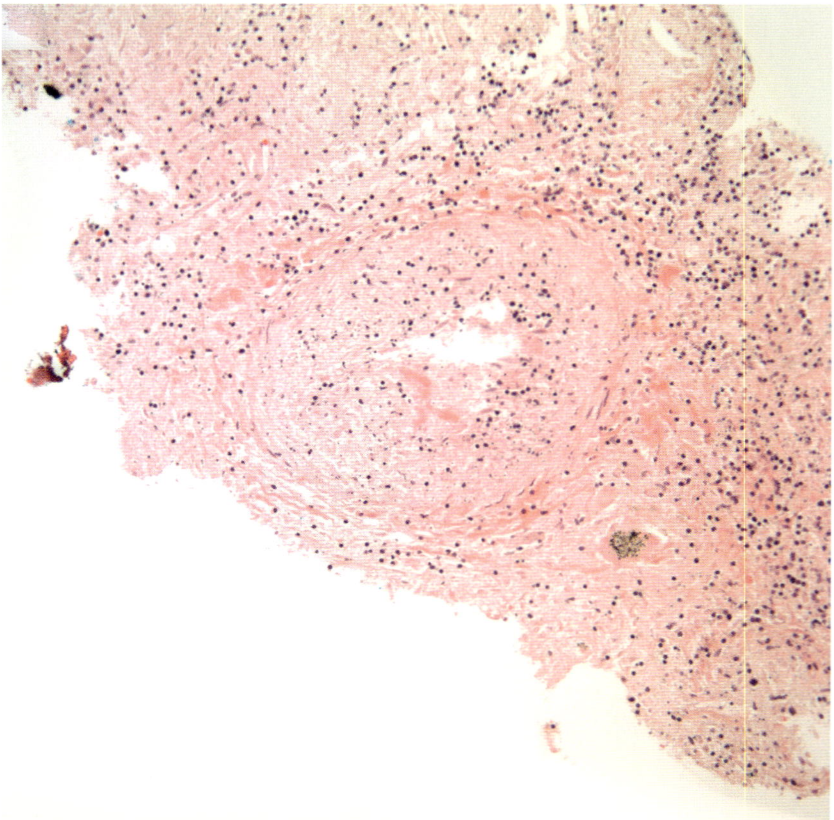

FIGURE 4.8 **Percutaneous core needle biopsy performed in a patient with suspected granulomatosis with polyangiitis vasculitis and a peripheral lung nodule.** The biopsy demonstrates a small- to medium-sized vessel with an inflammatory cell infiltrate and destruction of the vessel wall.

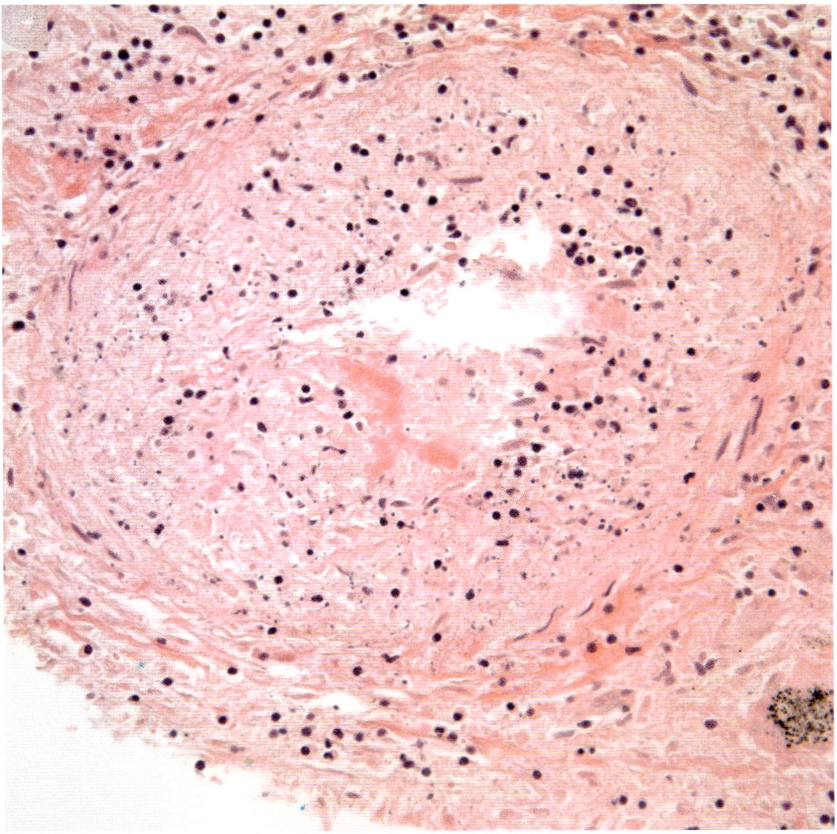

FIGURE 4.9 Higher-power magnification shows multiple mononuclear inflammatory cells and karyorrhectic debris within the wall of the blood vessel.

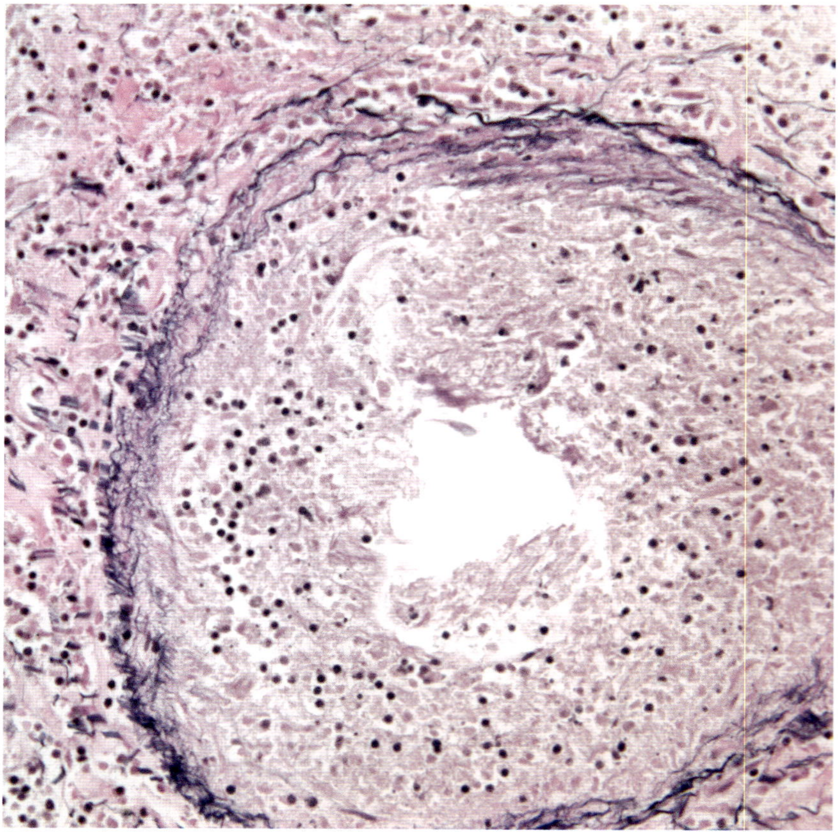

FIGURE 4.10 Elastic special stain (Verhoeff Van Gieson) highlights the destroyed remnants of the internal elastic lamina that should normally show a crisp intact circumferential layer of elastic.

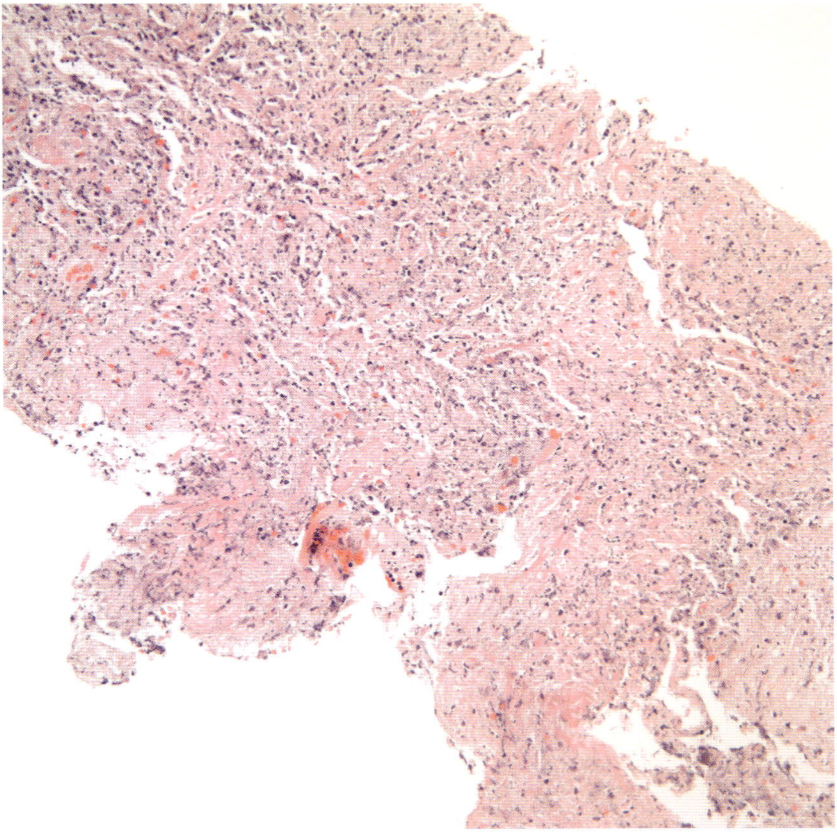

FIGURE 4.11 Adjacent portion of the same biopsy demonstrating necrotic lung parenchyma with a blueish-purple tinge due to the high degree of karyorrhectic debris.

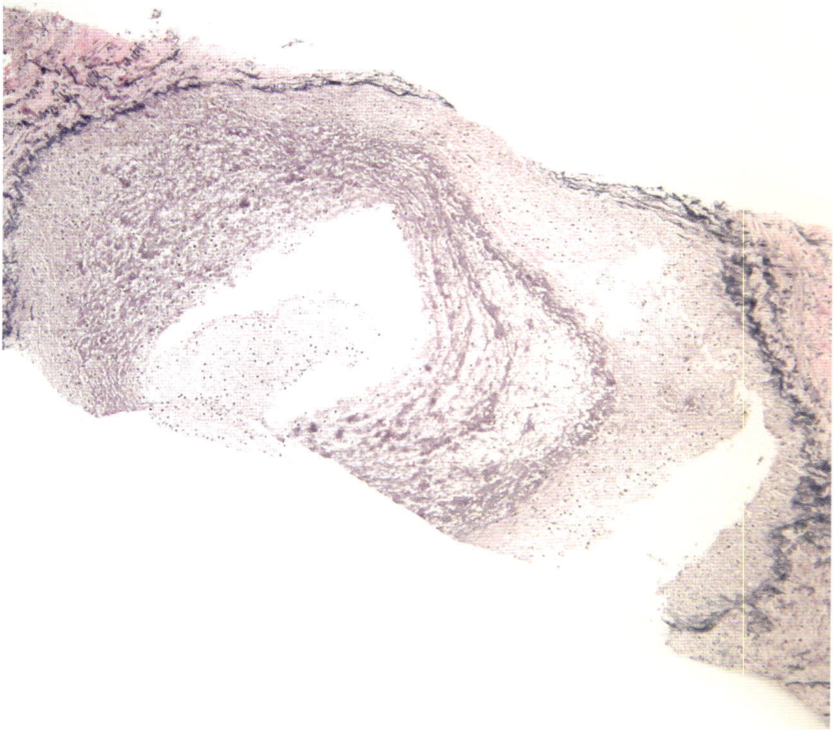

FIGURE 4.12 **Elastic special stain (Verhoeff Van Gieson) highlights another area of the same biopsy with a medium-sized vessel.** Notice the elastic lamina at the edges of the vessel is completely destroyed with only a residual smear of staining remaining. The lumen of the vessel is filled with necrotic debris. In this scenario, a diagnosis of granulomatosis with polyangiitis could be suggested despite the limited tissue sampling.

MICROSCOPIC POLYANGIITIS

MP is a term that encompasses conditions that were designated in the past as leukocytoclastic vasculitis, systemic necrotizing vasculitis, and hypersensitivity vasculitis.[18] It represents the second most common type of small vessel vasculitis affecting the lungs. An International Consensus Conference has defined MP as a vasculitis restricted to arterioles, venules, and capillaries.[19] The American College of Rheumatology and European Alliance of Associations for Rheumatology recently released classification criteria for diagnosis of patients with suspected MP. The criteria assign a score for P-ANCA or antimyeloperoxidase-ANCA positivity, pauci-immune glomerulonephritis, lung fibrosis or interstitial lung disease, sinonasal symptoms or signs, C-ANCA or antiproteinase 3 ANCA positivity, and eosinophil count $\geq 1 \times 10^9/L$.[20] If an overall score of greater than or equal 5 points is reached, a patient with a small or medium vessel vasculitis could be definitely diagnosed as having MP greater than 90% of the time. MP is a systemic disease that involves the lungs in approximately 50% of cases. Other symptoms include necrotizing glomerulonephritis, fever, myalgia, arthralgia, otitis, rhinitis, and skin involvement.[21,22] More than 80% of patients have positive ANCA, especially P-ANCA.[21]

The typical presentation of the disease is with pulmonary hemorrhage. Bilateral lung infiltrates are present in chest X-rays, and CT will usually demonstrate ground-glass attenuation, particularly involving the lower zones of the lungs. The treatment of choice is immunosuppressive agents, although supportive treatment with steroids, plasmapheresis, dialysis, and mechanical ventilation may also be needed.[23] The disease has a high mortality rate, although complete recovery was observed in up to 69% of patients in one study.[23,24]

The principal histologic manifestation of MP is alveolar hemorrhage with capillaritis (Fig. 4.13).[25] The capillaritis may appear on cursory examination as foci of increased alveolar wall cellularity against a background of alveolar hemorrhage, but on higher magnification, the alveolar walls show neutrophilic infiltration, which sometimes spills out onto the alveolar lumens simulating acute bronchopneumonia (Fig. 4.14). The intra-alveolar hemorrhage is often admixed with fibrin and hemosiderin-laden macrophages. In the healing phase, the alveolar hemorrhage can become organized, resulting in an organizing pneumonialike pattern mixed with an obliterative bronchiolitislike pattern. The lungs in MP may also be involved by fibrosis, sometimes with a pattern reminiscent of idiopathic pulmonary fibrosis (Fig. 4.15).[26-28] When present, fibrosis represents a poor prognostic indicator.[29]

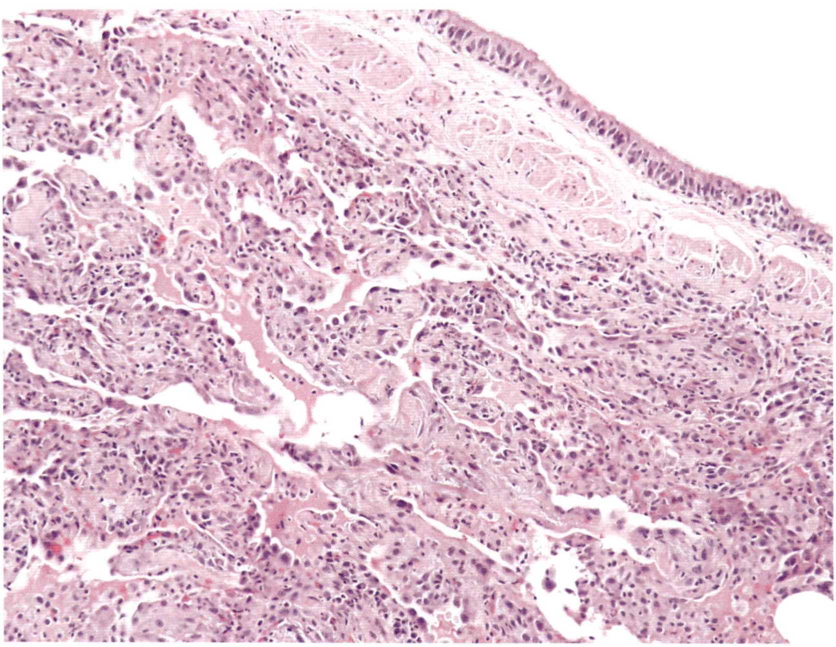

FIGURE 4.13 Transbronchial biopsy in a patient with microscopic polyangiitis showing widening of alveolar septa by cellular infiltrate.

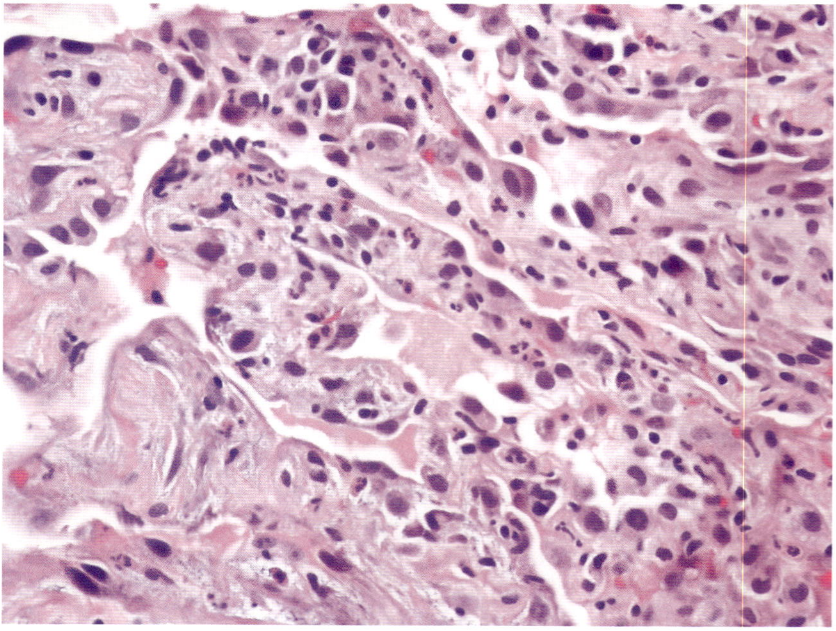

FIGURE 4.14 **Higher magnification of capillaritis in a patient with microscopic polyangiitis.** Notice the neutrophilic infiltration of alveolar walls.

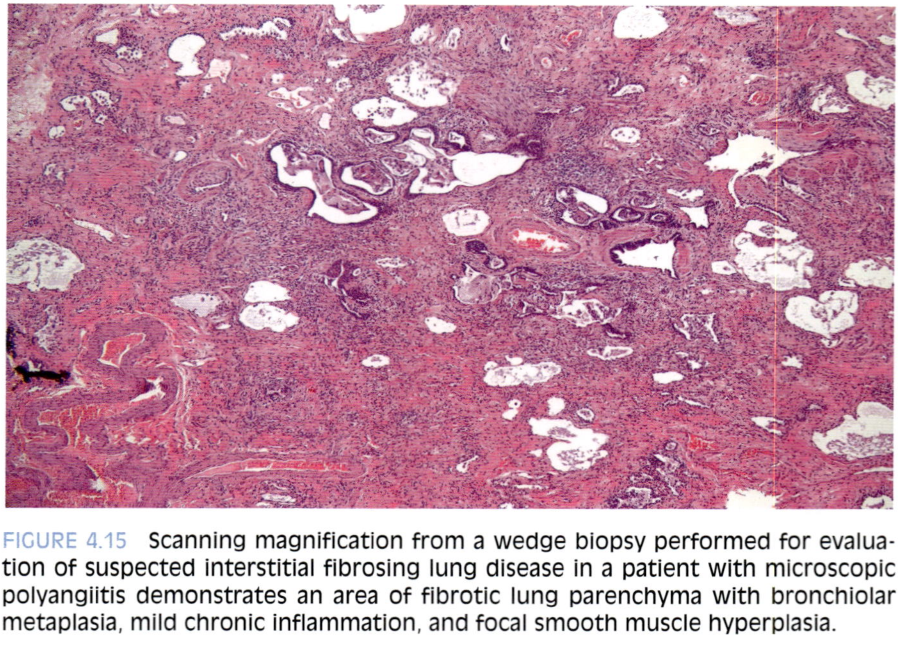

FIGURE 4.15 **Scanning magnification from a wedge biopsy performed for evaluation of suspected interstitial fibrosing lung disease in a patient with microscopic polyangiitis demonstrates an area of fibrotic lung parenchyma with bronchiolar metaplasia, mild chronic inflammation, and focal smooth muscle hyperplasia.**

The differential diagnosis includes infections, GPA, Goodpasture syndrome, and other small vessel vasculitides (eFig. 4.7). When fibrosis is present, consideration should be given to fibrosing lung diseases as well. The histologic variant of GPA characterized by alveolar hemorrhage and capillaritis in the absence of granulomas and necrosis may be impossible to distinguish from MP on histologic grounds.

EOSINOPHILIC GRANULOMATOSIS WITH POLYANGIITIS (CHURG-STRAUSS SYNDROME)

EGPA, formerly known as Churg-Strauss syndrome,[30] is a condition of unknown etiology that affects mainly the respiratory tract and is characterized by the association of vasculitis with eosinophilia. The classical triad in EGPA is asthma, peripheral blood eosinophilia, and small/medium vessel vasculitis.[31-33] Other manifestations include neuropathy, sinus abnormalities, pulmonary infiltrates, arthritis, arthralgias, serositis, skin manifestations (urticaria), central nervous system abnormalities, gastrointestinal bleeding, and renal failure.[34] EGPA is currently regarded as a clinical syndrome that requires meeting certain criteria for diagnosis as established by the American College of Rheumatology.[35] The diagnosis is no longer predicated on the results of lung biopsy but on the fulfillment of the clinical criteria. The traditional approach is based on the identification of six main criteria, including asthma, greater than 10% eosinophilia in peripheral blood, mono- or polyneuropathy, nonfixed radiographic pulmonary infiltrates, paranasal sinus abnormalities, and a biopsy containing a blood vessel with extravascular eosinophils. A fairly specific diagnosis can generally be established when four of the six criteria are met.[35] An alternate method for reaching the diagnosis involves identifying three major criteria: asthma, eosinophilia greater than 10%, and a history of allergy, although patients without asthma but with a history of allergic disease can also develop EGPA. The latter method is more sensitive but less specific.[35]

The process can affect patients at any age but shows a predilection for adults between 30 and 50 years of age. EGPA can involve the upper respiratory tract, lungs, skin, peripheral nerves, heart, and kidneys. The disease generally progresses through three stages: the prodromal phase is characterized by asthma, rhinitis, and peripheral eosinophilia. The asthma may be present over a period of years before the onset of vasculitis.[31,36,37] This is followed by the vasculitic phase during which the patients develop signs and symptoms of vasculitis and will test positive for P-ANCA. The damage sustained during this phase is usually permanent. Approximately half of the patients with EGPA develop cardiac disease, including pericarditis, hypertension, acute myocardial infarction, and heart failure.[31,38] Other common manifestations include peripheral neuritis, cutaneous leukocytoclastic vasculitis, and sinonasal compromise. Renal, gastrointestinal, and central nervous system manifestations owing to vasculitis may also occur but are rarer. The final phase, or postvasculitic phase, is characterized by persistent asthma and allergic rhinitis as well as neuropathy and hypertension.[34] There are no specific laboratory tests for EGPA. The most characteristic finding is peripheral blood eosinophilia. Bronchoalveolar lavage will also demonstrate increased eosinophilia. The radiographic abnormalities include multifocal lung infiltrates that are nonfixed (ie, they change in location and distribution over time). High-resolution computerized tomography scans will usually show parenchymal opacifications or ground-glass attenuation. The treatment of choice consists of systemic corticosteroids. Immunosuppressive agents, interferon, and high doses of immune globulin have also been used in patients with severe or fulminant symptoms. More recently, targeted therapy with monoclonal antibodies such as mepolizumab or benralizumab has shown utility in the treatment of relapsing or refractory EGPA.[39,40] Patients most often die of cardiac complications, including congestive heart failure and acute myocardial infarct.

The pathologic findings of EGPA on lung biopsy in patients with the full-blown syndrome include vasculitis, eosinophilic pneumonia, and granulomas. The lesion may extend along the pleura and interlobular septa. The most consistent finding is eosinophilic pneumonia, characterized by accumulation of eosinophils in the airspaces as well as within the interstitium. The vasculitis can affect small arteries, veins, or capillaries and is composed mainly of neutrophils admixed with eosinophils, small lymphocytes, and, sometimes, multinucleated giant cells (Figs. 4.16 and 4.17; eFig. 4.8).[41] Vasculitis can also

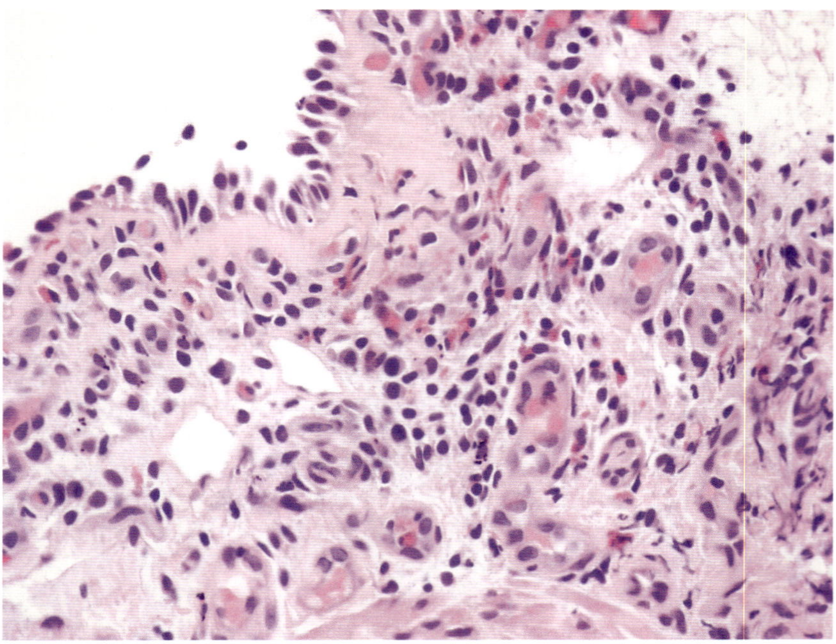

FIGURE 4.16 Endobronchial biopsy in a patient with eosinophilic granulomatosis with polyangiitis shows dense lymphoid infiltrates admixed with eosinophils surrounding the vessel walls in the submucosa.

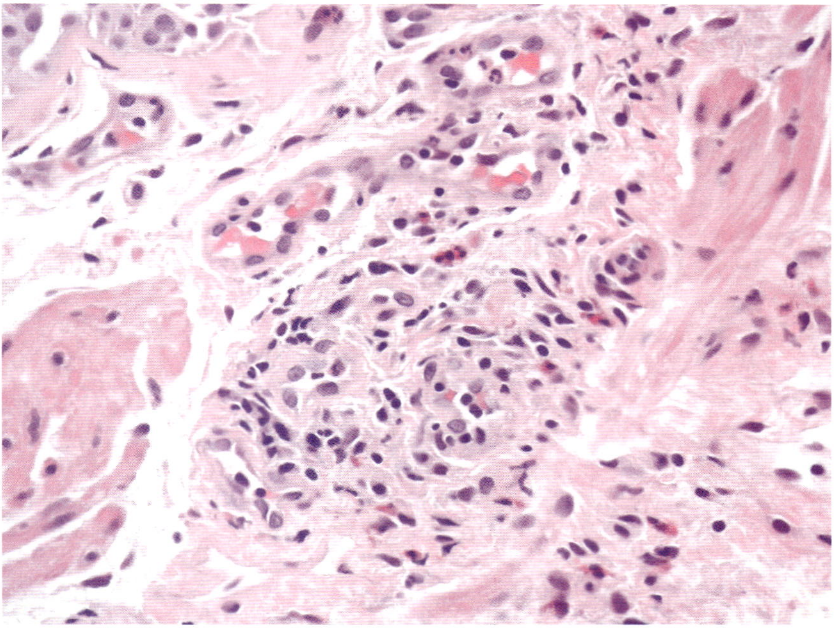

FIGURE 4.17 Higher magnification of vasculitis in eosinophilic granulomatosis with polyangiitis shows infiltration of vessel walls by neutrophils admixed with eosinophils.

manifest as capillaritis with diffuse pulmonary hemorrhage.[42] The granulomas in EGPA are usually small, with central fibrinoid necrosis and peripheral palisading of histiocytes. They can contain multinucleated giant cells.

UNCOMMON FORMS OF LUNG VASCULITIS

Various uncommon forms of vasculitis, including giant cell (temporal) arteritis, polyarteritis nodosa, Takayasu arteritis, Behçet syndrome, HSP, and the vasculitis associated with necrotizing sarcoid granulomatosis, may affect the lung.

Giant Cell (Temporal) Arteritis

Temporal arteritis is a disorder that involves primarily the temporal arteries in older adults. The disease is associated with upper respiratory tract symptoms and lower respiratory tract involvement only in a minority of cases; however, interstitial lung disease has been reported as the initial manifestation of giant cell arteritis.[43,44] Pulmonary involvement is usually bilateral, resulting in interstitial opacities or small nodules.[45,46] In rare cases, the pulmonary involvement may be unilateral and present as a mass lesion.[47] Giant cell arteritis confined exclusively to the lungs has also been described.[48] The disease involves principally the large and medium pulmonary arteries. The damage is centered principally in the elastic lamina of the vessel, which is destroyed by chronic inflammation admixed with multinucleated giant cells. On bronchoscopic biopsies, the main finding is the destruction of the media of pulmonary arteries by granulomatous inflammation with fragmentation of elastic fibers.[49] Unlike other types of granulomatous vasculitis, such as GPA, giant cell temporal arteritis is distinguished by the lesions being confined to the vessel wall without involvement of the surrounding lung parenchyma. Temporal arteritis is also distinguished from GPA by the younger age of the patients and by the involvement of the temporal arteries. Treatment usually involves steroids, though some antibody therapy has been tried as well.[50]

Takayasu Arteritis

Takayasu arteritis is a nonspecific inflammatory vasculitis that principally affects the aorta in women under the age of 40.[51] It is categorized as a disease affecting medium- to large-sized arteries.[52] In addition to the aorta, pulmonary arteries may be involved, and this may rarely be the initial manifestation of the disease. Patients with pulmonary involvement may present with pulmonary hypertension, cough, chest pain, pneumonia, and dyspnea.[52-55] Imaging findings are nonspecific and include nodules, patchy opacities, ground-glass opacities, mosaic attenuation, bronchiectasis, and others.[56] The histologic pulmonary manifestations are similar to those of systemic vasculitis and will show inflammatory infiltrates with disruption of the arterial wall.[52] Owing to the multisystem compromise and primary involvement of large caliber arteries such as the aorta and pulmonary artery, the diagnosis is generally established by angiography in the correct clinical setting.

Behçet Syndrome

Behçet syndrome is a systemic inflammatory disorder of unknown etiology that involves primarily the skin, eyes (uveitis), mouth, and genitalia (aphthous ulcers). The disease has a marked geographic distribution and predominantly affects young or middle-aged individuals of Middle Eastern, Japanese, and Mediterranean origin.[57,58] The most common clinical feature of the disease is recurrent and painful oral or genital ulcers. Symptoms of pulmonary involvement may be present and include cough, chest pain, dyspnea, and hemoptysis.[58,59] Pulmonary involvement has been reported to be as high as 70% in some populations.[60] The lesions are characterized by a necrotizing vasculitis that involves the arteries, veins, and capillaries (Fig. 4.18). The inflammatory infiltrate involving the vessel walls in Behçet syndrome comprises small lymphocytes. Resolving lesions may show recanalized thrombi and perivascular adventitial fibrosis. Hemorrhage with severe hemoptysis may result as a complication of the necrotizing vasculitis. Other secondary complications resulting from the vasculitis include pulmonary artery aneurysms, arterial and venous thrombosis, and pulmonary infarcts.[61-64] Rare reported complications include recurrent endobronchial

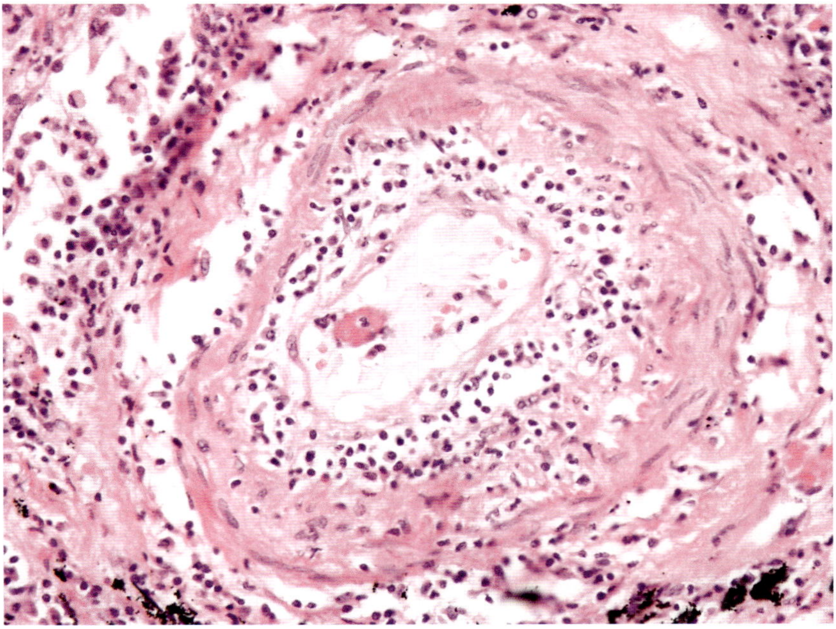

FIGURE 4.18 **Necrotizing vasculitis in Behçet disease.** The lesions are characterized by infiltration of small vessel walls by small lymphocytes.

stenosis and aortobronchial fistula formation.[65] The diagnosis is made by fulfilling the clinical requirements, including oral aphthous ulcers occurring more than three times in 1 year and at least two of the following clinical manifestations: recurrent genital aphthous ulcers, uveitis, synovitis, cutaneous vasculitis, and meningoencephalitis.[66] In addition, there should be an absence of inflammatory bowel disease or other collagen vascular disorder. Circulating immune complexes have been demonstrated in patients with active pulmonary disease, suggesting that they may play a role in the pathogenesis of the pulmonary manifestations.[59,67]

Henoch-Schönlein Purpura

HSP is a rare form of pulmonary hemorrhagic vasculitis that most often affects children. Pulmonary manifestations are quite rare, and the disease most often affects the skin, kidneys, and joints. Pulmonary involvement in HSP most commonly presents as diffuse alveolar hemorrhage.[68] Other reported pulmonary complications include pulmonary embolus, pulmonary-renal syndrome, and an unusual association with mycobacterial infections.[69-74] The pathologic findings in the lung are characterized by intra-alveolar hemorrhage, organizing pneumonia, and neutrophilic capillaritis (Fig. 4.19). The capillaritis may be subtle and masked by the capillary congestion (Fig. 4.20; eFig. 4.9). The findings are nonspecific and must be correlated with the clinical history and laboratory studies.[75]

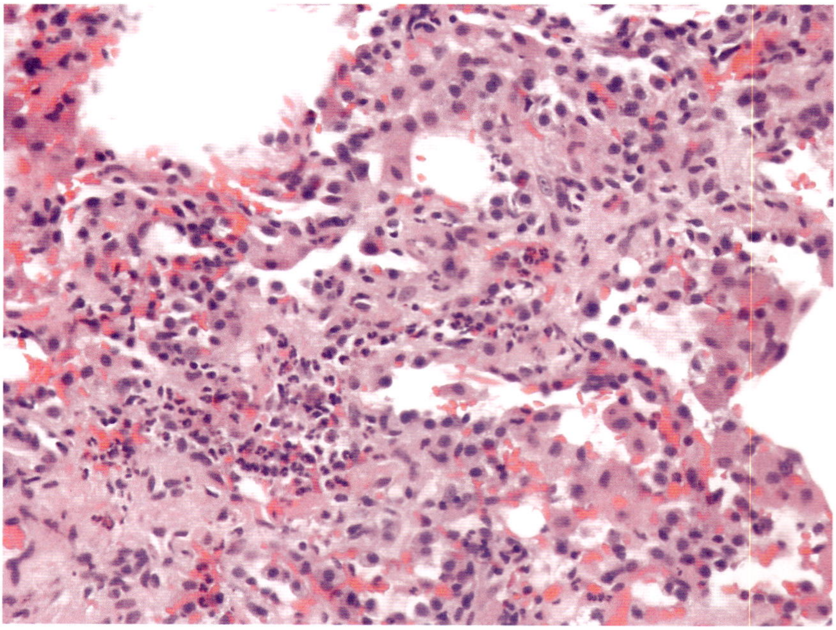

FIGURE 4.19 **Intra-alveolar hemorrhage and capillaritis in a patient with Henoch-Schönlein purpura.** Notice the thickening of alveolar septa by a cellular infiltrate.

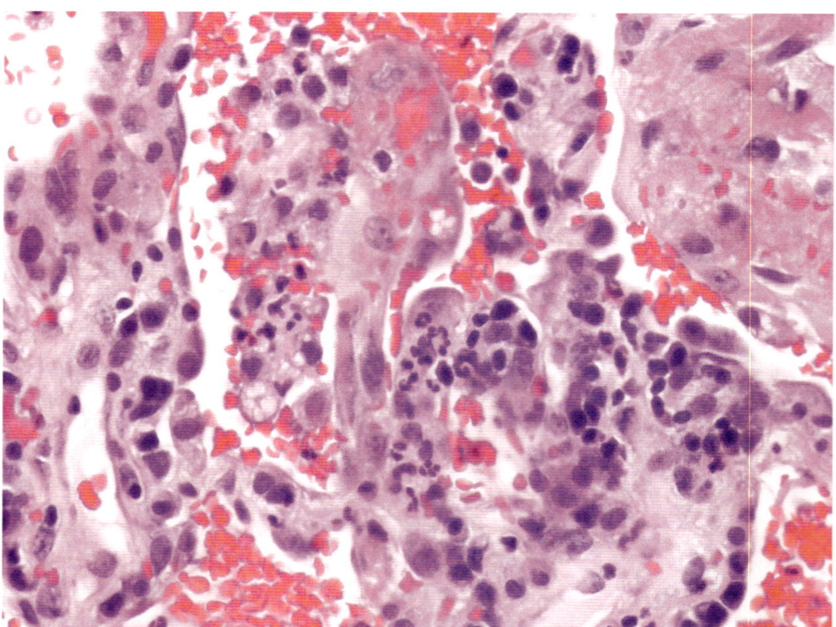

FIGURE 4.20 **Higher magnification of capillaritis in Henoch-Schönlein purpura shows congestion of alveolar wall capillaries admixed with neutrophilic infiltrates.**

Necrotizing Sarcoid Granulomatosis

Systemic vasculitis is seldom observed in patients with sarcoidosis. The pathologic findings comprise sarcoid-like granulomas involving pulmonary vessels, sometimes showing foci of necrosis. The granulomatous necrotizing vasculitis may be systemic and also involve the skin, lymph nodes, bone, synovium, liver, trachea, and bone marrow.[76] In rare instances, classical sarcoid may also show a nonnecrotizing granulomatous vasculitis as an incidental finding in lung biopsies. The lesions will display typical nonnecrotizing epithelioid granulomas with giant cells involving the walls of blood vessels.[77]

PULMONARY HEMORRHAGE

Pulmonary hemorrhage can be caused by various mechanisms. The main clinical symptom is hemoptysis, followed by cough, fever, and dyspnea. The cause can be a localized event, such as thromboembolus, hemorrhage secondary to bleeding from tumor, abscess, or bronchiectasis. Otherwise, it may be diffuse, such as in Goodpasture syndrome, vasculitis, and collagen vascular disease (eFig. 4.10). The localized form presents clinically and radiologically as a localized airspace infiltrate. Bronchoscopy in such instances can localize the source of the bleeding and determine the underlying cause. The diffuse form is characterized clinically by diffuse and often bilateral airspace infiltrates on chest X-ray and computerized tomography scans. Hemoptysis may be absent at the time of initial presentation in one-third of the patients with pulmonary hemorrhage. The radiologic features of diffuse alveolar hemorrhage comprise patchy or diffuse bilateral areas of lung consolidation, particularly in the lower lobes and perihilar regions.[78-80]

Conventional transbronchial biopsy is, in general, of very limited value in confirming a specific diagnosis. It may serve to confirm only the clinical impression of intra-alveolar hemorrhage or help to rule out other conditions. The histopathologic evaluation of intra-alveolar hemorrhage should take into consideration the clinical context for proper interpretation.[81] Some degree of extravasation of red blood cells can be observed in routine lung biopsies as a result of trauma caused by the biopsy procedure itself. The presence of fresh blood in the lumen of the alveoli per se is not an indication that the patient is suffering from clinically significant intra-alveolar hemorrhage. In such instances, the presence of red blood cells in the absence of fibrin, hemosiderin-laden macrophages, or reactive changes in the surrounding alveolar walls should suggest the possibility of artifactual hemorrhage rather than pathologic hemorrhage. When hemorrhage is accompanied by fibrin deposition and coarse granules of hemosiderin within macrophages, as well as supportive radiologic imaging demonstrating a diffuse alveolar infiltrate, the process corresponds to one of the diffuse alveolar hemorrhage syndromes (Fig. 4.21). Intra-alveolar hemorrhage should also be distinguished on small endoscopic biopsies from hemosiderin-laden macrophages seen in smoker's lungs.

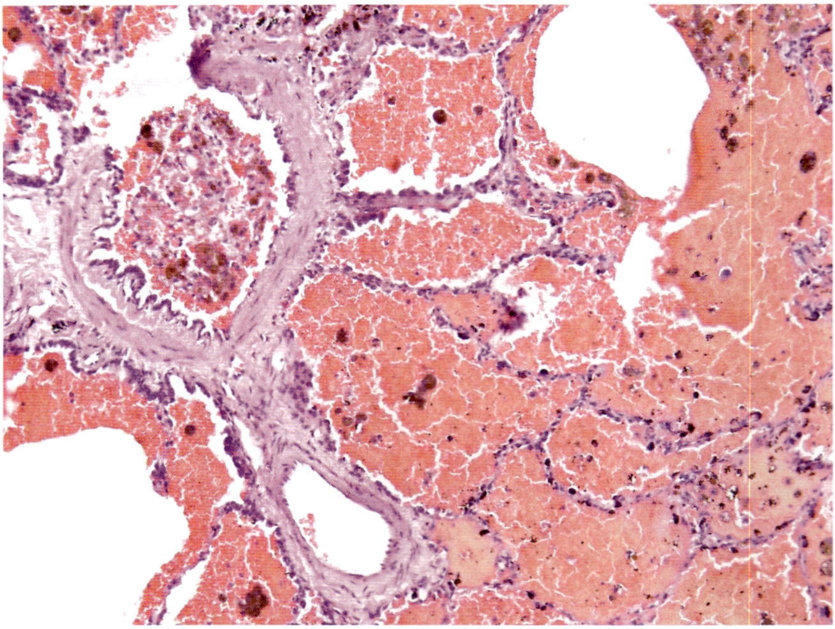

FIGURE 4.21 **Diffuse alveolar hemorrhage in a patient with Goodpasture syndrome.** The diagnosis cannot be rendered based on the biopsy findings alone. Correlation with clinical and laboratory findings and immunofluorescence studies is necessary for arriving at a definitive diagnosis.

In the latter, the macrophages filling the alveolar lumens and within the bronchioles contain very fine, dusty hemosiderin pigment, as opposed to the darkly staining, heavily pigmented macrophages seen in hemorrhagic syndromes, in which the hemosiderin granules are coarser and more abundant.

A distinctive form of diffuse alveolar hemorrhage is *idiopathic pulmonary hemosiderosis*. The condition is of unknown etiology and affects children more frequently than adults. Proposed mechanisms include immune complex mediated as well as hemorrhage being driven by histamine, vascular endothelial growth factor, and eosinophilic cationic protein inducing vascular endothelial damage leading to extravasation of red blood cells.[82] It presents clinically with hemoptysis, iron deficiency anemia, cough, and dyspnea. The condition is localized to the lungs and shows no systemic involvement or distinctive laboratory abnormalities. The episodes of pulmonary hemorrhage are recurrent and intermittent. Up to 25% of patients die because of massive hemorrhage; 50% develop chronic disease with supervening interstitial fibrosis.[83] Patients usually show variable response to corticosteroid therapy. The histology shows alveolar hemorrhage with abundant pigmented macrophages containing coarse hemosiderin granules (Fig. 4.22). The diagnosis is made in the appropriate clinical

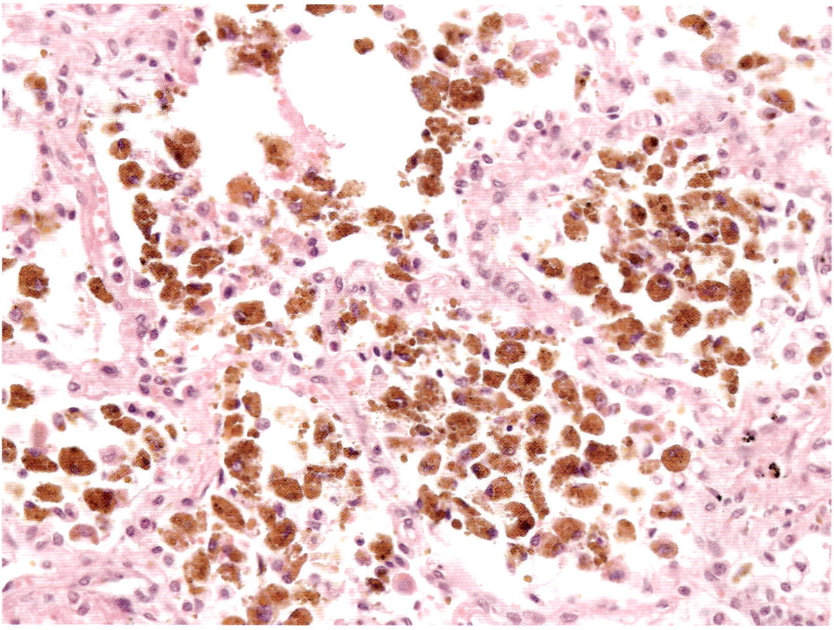

FIGURE 4.22 **Alveolar hemorrhage in idiopathic pulmonary hemosiderosis.** Notice the abundance of hemosiderin-laden macrophages admixed with red blood cells, characteristic of this disorder.

context.[84] A specific diagnosis of diffuse alveolar hemorrhage cannot be rendered in the absence of adequate clinical and laboratory data.

The various causes of diffuse alveolar hemorrhage are listed in Table 4.2. Most causes are immunologically mediated.[85] Some of these conditions display specific patterns of immunoglobulin deposition that can be demonstrated by immunofluorescence on adequately prepared tissue sections from the lung biopsy. Coordination between the clinician and the pathologist before the biopsy is carried out is therefore critical to obtain adequately processed samples for immunofluorescence microscopy if a hemorrhagic pulmonary disorder is suspected clinically. A more convenient substitute for immunofluorescent studies currently is the use of serologic tests that are widely available and reasonably specific for the various subtypes of diffuse alveolar hemorrhage.

Diffuse alveolar hemorrhage can also present histologically in association with capillaritis or without evidence of capillaritis. This particular histologic finding is of importance because specific entities are associated with capillaritis, whereas others are not (Table 4.3).

Correlation of the pathologic findings with clinical and laboratory findings is of importance for arriving at a more specific diagnosis (Table 4.4), as the histopathologic findings are generally nonspecific in the majority of cases of diffuse alveolar hemorrhage.

TABLE 4.2 Causes of Diffuse Alveolar Hemorrhage

Immunologic Conditions	Infectious Diseases
• Granulomatosis with polyangiitis • Eosinophilic granulomatosis with polyangiitis • Systemic lupus erythematosus • Microscopic polyangiitis • Goodpasture syndrome • Henoch-Schönlein purpura • Connective tissue diseases	• Bacterial (lung abscess, tuberculosis, bacterial pneumonia, etc.) • Viral • Fungal • Parasites (paragonimus westermani, leptospirosis)
Drugs and Toxins	**Neoplasia**
• Anticoagulants • Streptokinase • Cocaine • Solvents • Amiodarone	• Lung cancer • Kaposi sarcoma/angiosarcoma • Metastasis to the lung/bronchus
Bleeding Disorders	**Cardiac Causes**
• Coagulopathies • Thrombocytopenia	• Pulmonary thromboembolism • Left ventricular failure • Mitral stenosis • Aneurysms
Trauma	**Other Causes**
• Ruptured bronchus (bronchoscopy, Swan-Ganz catheter, lung biopsy, Hickman catheter) • Lung contusion • Aortic tear, others	• Idiopathic pulmonary hemosiderosis • Aspiration of foreign body • Intralobar sequestration • Endometriosis • Broncholithiasis • Lymphangioleiomyomatosis

TABLE 4.3 Causes of Diffuse Alveolar Hemorrhage Associated or Not Associated With Capillaritis

Alveolar Hemorrhage With Capillaritis	Alveolar Hemorrhage Without Capillaritis
Granulomatosis with polyangiitis	Idiopathic pulmonary hemosiderosis
Microscopic polyangiitis	Systemic lupus erythematosus
Goodpasture syndrome	Goodpasture syndrome
Henoch-Schönlein purpura	Diffuse alveolar damage
Mixed cryoglobulinemia	Coagulation disorders
Behçet syndrome	Pulmonary veno-occlusive disease
Connective tissue diseases	Mitral stenosis
Drug-induced	Neoplasms

TABLE 4.4 Clinical and Pathologic Findings in the Main Causes of Diffuse Alveolar Hemorrhage

Condition	Pathologic Findings	Laboratory Findings	Clinical Findings
Goodpasture syndrome	Nonspecific, can be associated with mild capillaritis and hyaline membranes	Antiglomerular basement membrane antibody 1	Young male smokers Also involves kidneys
Granulomatosis with polyangiitis	Diffuse alveolar hemorrhage with prominent capillaritis	C-ANCA 1	Multiorgan involvement, including kidneys, nasal passage, and others
Idiopathic pulmonary hemosiderosis	Alveolar hemorrhage unassociated with capillaritis, with abundant hemosiderin-laden macrophages	No immunologic mechanism identified	Children with recurrent bouts of hemoptysis and anemia

(continued)

TABLE 4.4 Clinical and Pathologic Findings in the Main Causes of Diffuse Alveolar Hemorrhage (*continued*)

Condition	Pathologic Findings	Laboratory Findings	Clinical Findings
Microscopic polyangiitis	Diffuse alveolar hemorrhage with prominent capillaritis	P-ANCA 1	Frequent multiorgan involvement
Systemic lupus erythematosus	Diffuse alveolar hemorrhage with prominent capillaritis	Antinuclear antibodies 1	Shows all the typical features of the disease. Patients with lupus nephritis are at increased risk for developing alveolar hemorrhage

C-ANCA, cytoplasmic antineutrophil cytoplasmic antibodies; P-ANCA, perinuclear antineutrophil cytoplasmic antibodies.

REFERENCES

1. Liebow AA. The J. Burns Amberson lecture: pulmonary angiitis and granulomatosis. *Am Rev Respir Dis.* 1973;108:1-18.
2. Katzenstein AL, Locke WK. Solitary lung lesions in Wegener's granulomatosis. Pathologic findings and clinical significance in 25 cases. *Am J Surg Pathol.* 1995;19:545-552.
3. Comarmond C, Cacoub P. Granulomatosis with polyangiitis (Wegener): clinical aspects and treatment. *Autoimmun Rev.* 2014;13(11):1121-1125.
4. Carrington C, Liebow A. Limited forms of angiitis and granulomatosis of Wegener's type. *Am J Med.* 1966;41:497-527.
5. Bernal-Bello D, Morales-Ortega A, Duarte-Millán MÁ, Tardío JC, Frutos-Pérez B. Lung cavitation in granulomatosis with polyangiitis: clinical implications. *Clin Rheumatol.* 2022;41:2915-2916.
6. Begum S, Srinivasan S, Kathirvelu S, Vaithy A. Limited granulomatosis with polyangiitis presenting as an isolated lung lesion. *Indian J Pathol Microbiol.* 2020;63:611-614.
7. Capdevila-Reniu A, Rodríguez-Garcia SC, Grafia I, et al. Localised granulomatosis with polyangiitis in an older patient with rheumatoid arthritis. *Age Ageing.* 2019;49:146-148.
8. Coviello E, Puma F, Pourmolkara D, Mandarano M, Napolitano AG. Massive, life-threatening hemoptysis due to localized granulomatosis with polyangiitis. *J Cardiothorac Surg.* 2023;18:239.
9. Chippa V, Gujarathi R, Chenna S, Candula N. Limited granulomatosis with polyangiitis presenting as recurrent lung abscess without pneumonia. *Cureus.* 2022;14:e29858.
10. Talarico R, Barsotti S, Elefante E, Baldini C, Tani C, Mosca M. Systemic vasculitis and the lung. *Curr Opin Rheumatol.* 2017;29(1):45-50.
11. Feragalli B, Mantini C, Sperandeo M, et al. The lung in systemic vasculitis: radiological patterns and differential diagnosis. *Br J Radiol.* 2016;89(1061):20150992.

12. Gal AA, Salinas FF, Staton GW Jr. The clinical and pathological spectrum of antineutrophil cytoplasmic autoantibody-related pulmonary disease. A comparison between perinuclear and cytoplasmic antineutrophil cytoplasmic autoantibodies. *Arch Pathol Lab Med.* 1994;118:1209-1214.
13. Rao JK, Weinberger M, Oddone EZ, Allen NB, Landsman P, Feussner JR. The role of antineutrophil cytoplasmic antibody (c-ANCA) testing in the diagnosis of Wegener granulomatosis. A literature review and meta-analysis. *Ann Intern Med.* 1995;123:925-932.
14. Guneyli S, Ceylan N, Bayraktaroglu S, et al. Imaging findings of pulmonary granulomatosis with polyangiitis (Wegener's granulomatosis): lesions invading the pulmonary fissure, pleura or diaphragm mimicking malignancy. *Wien Klin Wochenschr.* 2016;128:809-815.
15. Sendo S, Tsuji G, Umeda R, Ichise Y, Kumagai S, Suzuki Y. Granulomatosis with polyangiitis (Wegener's granulomatosis) diagnosed by transbronchial biopsy from stenotic portion of mainstem bronchus. *Mod Rheumatol.* 2015;25:649-652.
16. Jennings CR, Jones NS, Dugar J, Powell RJ, Lowe J. Wegener's granulomatosis–a review of diagnosis and treatment in 53 subjects. *Rhinology.* 1998;36:188-191.
17. Kubaisi B, Abu SK, Foster CS. Granulomatosis with polyangiitis (Wegener's disease): an updated review of ocular disease manifestations. *Intractable Rare Dis Res.* 2016;5(2):61-69.
18. Churg J. Nomenclature of vasculitic syndromes: a historical perspective. *Am J Kidney Dis.* 1991;18:148-153.
19. Jennette JC, Falk RJ, Andrassy K, et al. Nomenclature of systemic vasculitides. Proposal of an international consensus conference. *Arthritis Rheum.* 1994;37:187-192.
20. Suppiah R, Robson JC, Grayson PC, et al. 2022 American College of Rheumatology/European Alliance of Associations for Rheumatology classification criteria for microscopic polyangiitis. *Ann Rheum Dis.* 2022;81:321-326.
21. Jennette JC, Falk RJ. Small-vessel vasculitis. *N Engl J Med.* 1997;337:1512-1523.
22. Chung SA, Seo P. Microscopic polyangiitis. *Rheum Dis Clin North Am.* 2010;36(3):545-558.
23. Lauque D, Cadranel J, Lazor R, et al. Microscopic polyangiitis with alveolar hemorrhage. A study of 29 cases and review of the literature. *Medicine (Baltimore).* 2000;79:222-233.
24. Takakuwa Y, Yamasaki Y, Matsushita H, et al. Long-term survival, causes of death, and prognostic factors for mortality in patients with microscopic polyangiitis and those with anti-neutrophil cytoplasmic antibody-positive interstitial lung disease: a single-center retrospective study. *Int J Rheum Dis.* 2023;26:446-453.
25. Tashiro H, Takahashi K, Tanaka M, et al. Characteristics and prognosis of microscopic polyangiitis with bronchiectasis. *J Thorac Dis.* 2017;9(2):303-309.
26. Wurmann P, Sabugo F, Elgueta F, et al. Interstitial lung disease and microscopic polyangiitis in chilean patients. *Sarcoidosis Vasc Diffuse Lung Dis.* 2020;37:37-42.
27. Kim MJ, Shin K. Interstitial lung disease and diffuse alveolar hemorrhage, the two key pulmonary manifestations in microscopic polyangiitis. *Tuberc Respir Dis (Seoul).* 2021;84:255-262.
28. Manfredi A, Cassone G, Izzo R, et al; Study Group of the Italian Society for Rheumatology (SIR). Interstitial lung disease in microscopic polyangiitis and granulomatosis with polyangiitis: demographic, clinical, serological and radiological features of an Italian cohort from the Italian Society for Rheumatology. *Clin Exp Rheumatol.* 2023;41:821-828.
29. Kim MJ, Lee D, Choe J, Song JW. Long-term clinical course and outcomes of patients with microscopic polyangiitis-associated interstitial lung disease. *Front Pharmacol.* 2023;14:1064307.
30. Mouthon L, Dunogue B, Guillevin L. Diagnosis and classification of eosinophilic granulomatosis with polyangiitis (formerly named Churg-Strauss syndrome). *J Autoimmun.* 2014;48-49:99-103.

31. Lanham JG, Elkon KB, Pusey CD, Hughes GR. Systemic vasculitis with asthma and eosinophilia: a clinical approach to the Churg–Strauss syndrome. *Medicine (Baltimore).* 1984;63:65-81.
32. Guillevin L, Cohen P, Gayraud M, Lhote F, Jarrousse B, Casassus P. Churg-Strauss syndrome. Clinical study and long-term follow-up of 96 patients. *Medicine (Baltimore).* 1999;78:26-37.
33. Greco A, Rizzo MI, De Virgilio A, et al. Churg-Strauss syndrome. *Autoimmun Rev.* 2015;14(4):341-348.
34. Lanham JG, Churg J. Churg–Strauss syndrome. In: Churg A, Churg J, eds. *Systemic Vasculitides.* Igaku-Shoin; 1991:101-120.
35. Masi A, Hunder GG, Lie JT, et al. The American College of Rheumatology 1990 criteria for the classification of Churg–Strauss syndrome (allergic granulomatosis and angiitis). *Arthritis Rheum.* 1990;33:1094-1100.
36. Chumbley LC, Harrison EG Jr, DeRemee R. Allergic granulomatosis and angiitis (Churg–Strauss syndrome). Report and analysis of 30 cases. *Mayo Clin Proc.* 1977;52:477-484.
37. Specks U, DeRemee RA. Granulomatous vasculitis. Wegener's granulomatosis and Churg–Strauss syndrome. *Rheum Dis Clin North Am.* 1990;16:377-397.
38. Churg J, Strauss L. Allergic granulomatosis, allergic angiitis, and periarteritis nodosa. *Am J Pathol.* 1951;27:277-301.
39. Faverio P, Bonaiti G, Bini F, Vaghi A, Pesci A. Mepolizumab as the first targeted treatment for eosinophilic granulomatosis with polyangiitis: a review of current evidence and potential place in therapy. *Ther Clin Risk Manag.* 2018;14:2385-2396.
40. Bettiol A, Urban ML, Padoan R, et al. Benralizumab for eosinophilic granulomatosis with polyangiitis: a retrospective, multicentre, cohort study. *Lancet Rheumatol.* 2023;5:e707-e715.
41. Scapa JV, Fishbein GA, Wallace WD, Fishbein MC. Diffuse alveolar hemorrhage and pulmonary vasculitides: histopathologic findings. *Semin Respir Crit Care Med.* 2018;39(4):425-433.
42. Lai RS, Lin SL, Lai NS, Lee PC. Churg–Strauss syndrome presenting with pulmonary capillaritis and diffuse alveolar damage. *Scand J Rheumatol.* 1998;27:230-232.
43. Larson TS, Hall S, Hepper NG, Hunder GG. Respiratory tract symptoms as a clue to giant cell arteritis. *Ann Intern Med.* 1984;101:594-597.
44. Konishi C, Nakagawa K, Nakai E, et al. Interstitial lung disease as an initial manifestation of giant cell arteritis. *Intern Med.* 2017;56(19):2633-2637.
45. Bradley JD, Pinals RS, Blumenfeld HB, Poston WM. Giant cell arteritis with pulmonary nodules. *Am J Med.* 1984;77:135-140.
46. Karam GH, Fulmer JD. Giant cell arteritis presenting as interstitial lung disease. *Chest.* 1982;82:781-784.
47. Yoshimoto R, Tanaka K, Kawahata T, et al. Unusual manifestations of giant cell arteritis and granulomatosis with polyangiitis. *Immunol Med.* 2019;42:94-98. doi:10.1080/25785826.2019.1657377
48. Wagenaar SS, van den Bosch JM, Westermann CJ, Bosman HG, Lie JT. Isolated granulomatous giant cell vasculitis of the pulmonary elastic arteries. *Arch Pathol Lab Med.* 1986;110:962-964.
49. Ladanyi M, Fraser RS. Pulmonary involvement in giant cell arteritis. *Arch Pathol Lab Med.* 1987;111:1178-1180.
50. Ohta R, Nishikura N, Ikeda H, Sano C. Giant cell arteritis with chronic bronchitis successfully treated with tocilizumab. *Cureus.* 2023;15:e40146.
51. Arend WP, Michel BA, Bloch DA, et al. The American College of Rheumatology 1990 criteria for the classification of Takayasu arteritis. *Arthritis Rheum.* 1990;33:1129-1134.
52. Nakajima N. Takayasu arteritis: consideration of pulmonary involvement. *Ann Vasc Dis.* 2008;1(1):7-10.

53. Shimada Y, Shibata A, Ishikawa H, et al. Organizing pneumonia as the first presentation in a patient with Takayasu arteritis: a report of rare complication. *Intern Med.* 2021;60:1887-1891.
54. Wang J, Lei K, Li J, et al. Analysis of clinical features and prognostic factors in Takayasu arteritis involving pulmonary hypertension: a retrospective study. *Medicine (Baltimore).* 2024;103:e37992.
55. Mukoyama H, Shirakashi M, Tanaka N, et al. The clinical features of pulmonary artery involvement in Takayasu arteritis and its relationship with ischemic heart diseases and infection. *Arthritis Res Ther.* 2021;23:293.
56. Kong X, Zhang J, Lin J, et al. Pulmonary findings on high-resolution computed tomography in Takayasu arteritis. *Rheumatology (Oxford).* 2021;60:5659-5667.
57. Fairley C, Wilson JW, Barraclough D. Pulmonary involvement in Behcet's syndrome. *Chest.* 1989;96:1428-1429.
58. Raz I, Okon E, Chajek-Shaul T. Pulmonary manifestations in Behcet's syndrome. *Chest.* 1989;95:585-589.
59. Efthimiou J, Johnston C, Spiro SG, Turner-Warwick M. Pulmonary disease in Behcet's syndrome. *Q J Med.* 1986;58:259-280.
60. Edrees A, Naguib S, El Menyawi M, Ismail I, Nagah H. Pulmonary manifestations in a group of patients with Behcet's disease. *Int J Rheum Dis.* 2017;20(2):269-275.
61. Slavin RE, de Groot WJ. Pathology of the lung in Behcet's disease. Case report and review of the literature. *Am J Surg Pathol.* 1981;5:779-788.
62. Lakhanpal S, Tani K, Lie JT, Katoh K, Ishigatsubo Y, Ohokubo T. Pathologic features of Behcet's syndrome: a review of Japanese autopsy registry data. *Hum Pathol.* 1985;16:790-795.
63. Giannessi C, Smorchkova O, Cozzi D, et al. Behçet's disease: a radiological review of vascular and parenchymal pulmonary involvement. *Diagnostics (Basel).* 2022;12:2868.
64. Armağan B, Okşul M, Şener YZ, et al. Pulmonary hypertension in Behçet's disease: echocardiographic screening and multidisciplinary approach. *Turk J Med Sci.* 2023;53:563-571.
65. Rahman N, Senanayake E, Mascaro J, Situnayake D, Bishay ES, Patel AJ. Recurrent endobronchial occlusion and aorto-bronchial fistula formation in Behcet's disease. *J Cardiothorac Surg.* 2023;18:22.
66. Davatchi F. Behcet's disease. *Int J Rheum Dis.* 2014;17(4):355-357.
67. Gamble CN, Wiesner KB, Shapiro RF, Boyer WJ. The immune complex pathogenesis of glomerulonephritis and pulmonary vasculitis in Behcet's disease. *Am J Med.* 1979;66:1031-1039.
68. Maria Di Pietro G, Castellazzi ML, Mastrangelo A, Montini G, Marchisio P, Tagliabue C. Henoch-Schönlein purpura in children: not only kidney but also lung. *Pediatr Rheumatol Online J.* 2019;17:75.
69. Bender ST, Mertens PR, Gross C. Pulmonary-renal syndrome in IgA vasculitis. *Kidney Int.* 2023;103(4):800. doi:10.1016/j.kint.2022.12.010. PMID: 36948773.
70. Mosalem O, Hernandez Garcilazo N, Saleh Y, Rous FA. Pulmonary embolism as the primary presentation of IgA vasculitis. *BMJ Case Rep.* 2020;13:e235884.
71. Li J, Wang XZ, Wang RC, Yang J, Hao H-L, Xue L-Y. Pulmonary tuberculosis presenting as Henoch-Schönlein purpura: case report and literature review. *Medicine (Baltimore).* 2020;99:e22583.
72. Kiani AN, Nunez SE, O'Sullivan F, Muruganandum M, Emil NS. The coexistence of pulmonary tuberculosis and adult-onset Henoch-Schönlein purpura. *Rheumatol Adv Pract.* 2020;4:rkaa039.
73. Saliba J, Grall M, Saliba C. A rare case of Henoch-Schönlein purpura and *Mycobacterium xenopi* pulmonary infection. *Cureus.* 2021;13:e13533.

74. Yıldırım R, Üsküdar Cansu D, Uludoğan BCE, Dinler M, Tekin E, Korkmaz C. The coexistence of IgA vasculitis and tuberculosis: a case-based review. *Rheumatol Int.* 2021;41:1683-1689.
75. Rajagopala S, Parameswaran S, Ajmera JS, Ganesh RN, Katrevula A. Diffuse alveolar hemorrhage in IgA nephropathy: case series and systematic review of the literature. *Int J Rheum Dis.* 2017;20(1):109-121.
76. Fernandes SR, Singsen BH, Hoffman GS. Sarcoidosis and systemic vasculitis. *Semin Arthritis Rheum.* 2000;30:33-46.
77. Takemura T, Matsui Y, Saiki S, Mikami R. Pulmonary vascular involvement in sarcoidosis: a report of 40 autopsy cases. *Hum Pathol.* 1992;23:1216-1223.
78. Parrot A, Fartoukh M, Cadranel J. Alveolar hemorrhage [in French]. *Rev Mal Respir.* 2015;32(4):394-412.
79. Martínez-Martínez MU, Oostdam DAH, Abud-Mendoza C. Diffuse alveolar hemorrhage in autoimmune diseases. *Curr Rheumatol Rep.* 2017;19(5):27.
80. Lara AR, Schwarz MI. Diffuse alveolar hemorrhage. *Chest.* 2010;137(5):1164-1171.
81. Colby TV, Fukuoka J, Ewaskow SP, Helmers R, Leslie KO. Pathologic approach to pulmonary hemorrhage. *Ann Diagn Pathol.* 2001;5:309-319.
82. Saha BK, Chong WH, Saha S, Aiman A, Bonnier A. Proposed pathogenesis of diffuse alveolar hemorrhage in idiopathic pulmonary hemosiderosis. *Lung.* 2022;200:205-215.
83. Saha BK. Idiopathic pulmonary hemosiderosis: a state of the art review. *Respir Med.* 2021;176:106234.
84. Zhang Y, Luo F, Wang N, Song Y, Tao Y. Clinical characteristics and prognosis of idiopathic pulmonary hemosiderosis in pediatric patients. *J Int Med Res.* 2019;47:293-302.
85. Lynch J, Leatherman J. Alveolar hemorrhage syndromes. In: Fishman A, ed. *Fishman's Pulmonary Diseases and Disorders.* McGraw-Hill; 1998:1193-1210.

5

BACTERIAL LUNG INFECTIONS

Bacterial infections are a common cause of lung morbidity and mortality. Transbronchial biopsies are often used as an effective means for making a specific diagnosis, particularly in immunosuppressed and transplant patients. Various clinical settings besides immunosuppression can be associated with bacterial pneumonia, including alcoholism, aspiration, intravenous drug use, various immune deficiency syndromes, viral infections, cystic fibrosis, and chronic obstructive pulmonary disease.[1-3] Common bacterial pneumonias are found in various clinical settings, both nosocomial and community acquired. Two major types are recognized: lobar pneumonia, in which consolidation of an entire lobe of lung results from diffuse and uniform inflammation of the pulmonary parenchyma, and patchy bronchopneumonia, in which multiple foci of inflammation are present involving the terminal airways.[4] The most common causative organisms are gram-positive cocci, including *Staphylococcus aureus* and *Streptococcus pneumoniae*, and gram-negative pathogens, including *Klebsiella pneumoniae*, *Haemophilus influenzae*, *Escherichia coli*, *Acinetobacter baumannii*, *Stenotrophomonas maltophilia*, and *Pseudomonas aeruginosa* (eFigs. 5.1 and 5.2). In recent years, clinicians have faced a growing number of infections caused by multidrug-resistant pathogens. These infections can cause increased morbidity and mortality if not identified appropriately or treated early enough.[5] These types of pneumonia are generally diagnosed by cultures of sputum or other respiratory secretions and do not generally require a biopsy unless specific culture and sensitivity assays are unsuccessful on sputum samples.[6] The histologic hallmark of the process is the presence of acute inflammatory exudate filling the alveolar spaces admixed with fibrin and often with necrosis of alveolar walls (Fig. 5.1). Tissue Gram stains will usually highlight the organisms. Molecular testing for pathogens has also shown some efficacy. Next-generation sequencing to identify pathogenic organisms can be performed on formalin-fixed paraffin-embedded biopsy material or on cytologic specimens such as sputum and alveolar lavages with reasonable sensitivity, though culture remains the gold standard.[7,8]

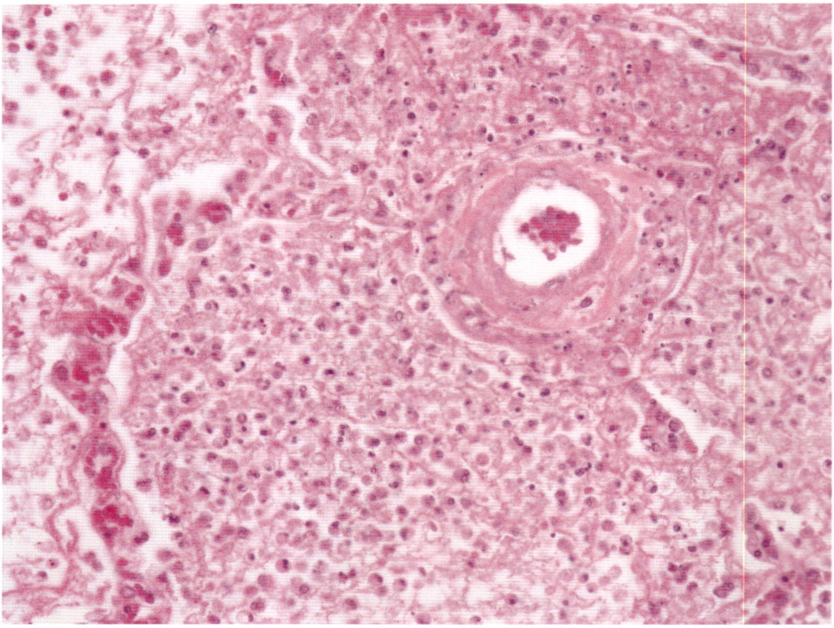

FIGURE 5.1 Acute bronchopneumonia owing to *Klebsiella pneumoniae* shows filling of alveolar spaces with abundant neutrophils.

UNCOMMON BACTERIAL PNEUMONIAS

Several uncommon bacterial pneumonias are seen in clinical practice that may be amenable to specific diagnosis by transbronchial biopsy, including *Legionella* pneumonia, botryomycosis, *Nocardia*, *Actinomyces*, tularemia, malakoplakia, bacillary angiomatosis, mycobacterial pneumonias, and others (Table 5.1).

Legionella Pneumonia

Legionella pneumonia, also known as Pontiac fever or Legionnaires' disease (when in its more severe form), is a pulmonary infection caused by the gram-negative bacteria, *Legionella pneumophila*. The disease was first described in 1977 after several members of the American Legion suffered an outbreak of severe pneumonia at the American Legion Convention held in 1976 in Philadelphia in the United States of America. Rare cases of infections caused by *Legionella longbeachae* have also been reported in Australia and New Zealand.[9] The organism is not normally transmitted by direct contact; human infection results from inhalation of aerosolized droplets from soil or from contaminated air-handling equipment, such as evaporator pans, air conditioners, humidifiers, respiratory therapy equipment, and so on. This microorganism can cause nosocomial outbreaks as well as sporadic infection.[10-12] Patients present with constitutional

TABLE 5.1 Uncommon Bacterial Pneumonias

Infection	Organisms	Histology	Stains	Clinical Features
Legionella	*Legionella pneumophila* (gram-negative bacteria)	Neutrophilic pneumonia admixed with fibrin and nuclear debris	Silver stains (Dieterle, Warthin-Starry, Steiner) Immunofluorescence staining, DNA in situ hybridization	Inhalation of aerosolized droplets in air-handling equipment
Nocardia	*Nocardia asteroides* (gram-positive, long beaded and branching filamentous bacteria)	Necrotizing neutrophilic pneumonia	GMS, B&B, and Fite-Faraco stain (weakly acid-fast)	Adult men, immunocompromised
Actinomyces	*Actinomyces israelii* (anaerobic, thin filamentous bacteria)	Suppurative inflammation with abscess formation and “sulfur granules”	GMS and B&B (filamentous branching bacteria) Negative acid-fast	Secondary to aspiration in debilitated patients
Tularemia	*Francisella tularensis* (gram-negative coccobacillus)	Acute fibrinous and necrotizing pneumonia	Immunofluorescent antibody testing	Zoonosis–bite of deer tick or deer fly
Yersinia	*Yersinia pestis* (gram-negative rod)	Necrotizing and hemorrhagic pneumonia with abundant organisms	Silver stains (Warthin-Starry, Dieterle, Steiner) Direct immunofluorescence	Zoonosis–bite of rodent tick
Melioidosis	*Burkholderia pseudomallei* (gram-negative bacteria)	Acute necrotizing bronchopneumonia with abscess formation	Bacteria, cultures	Endemic in tropic regions in Southeast Asia

(*continued*)

TABLE 5.1 **Uncommon Bacterial Pneumonias (*continued*)**

Infection	Organisms	Histology	Stains	Clinical Features
Malakoplakia	*Rhodococcus equi* (gram-positive coccobacillus)	Dense histiocytic infiltrate with scattered concentric calcifications (Michaelis-Gutmann bodies)	Bacteria stain with B&B, Fite-Faraco Michaelis-Gutmann bodies stain with Von Kossa and Alizarin red stains	Organism found in soil and feces of animals, especially horses
Whipple disease	*Tropheryma whipplei*	Sheets of macrophages with abundant clear, PAS-positive foamy cytoplasm	GMS, Warthin-Starry	Multisystem disorder associated with malabsorption, diarrhea, weight loss, and lymphadenopathy
Bacillary angiomatosis	*Bartonella henselae* (small coccobacillus)	Vascular proliferation lined by large epithelioid endothelial cells with acute inflammatory infiltrates	Modified Warthin-Starry at pH 3.2 Immunohistochemistry	Immunocompromised patients; transmitted through cats by fleas
Botryomycosis	*Staphylococcus aureus* and other bacteria	Neutrophilic pneumonia with "sulfur granules"	B&B ("grapelike" cultures composed of nonfilamentous, nonbranching bacteria)	Immunosuppressed patients

B&B, Brown and Brenn; GMS, Gomori methenamine silver; PCR, polymerase chain reaction.

symptoms including headache, fever, and myalgia. Cough, shortness of breath, and pleuritic pain are present in about half of the patients, and one-third may present with hemoptysis.[9] Chest radiographs show patchy peripheral areas of consolidation that may rapidly progress to extensive lobar involvement.[13] The organism may be difficult to culture, and microbiologic studies have yielded only up to 60% sensitivity.[14] Histologically, transbronchial biopsies will show extensive neutrophilic infiltration of alveolar spaces admixed with fibrin (Fig. 5.2; eFig. 5.3). In one-third of patients, the infiltrate may comprise monocytes and macrophages, or an admixture of neutrophils and monocytic cells. Often, there is abundant nuclear debris owing to karyorrhexis of neutrophils imparting the biopsy with a distinctive "dusty" appearance. Diffuse alveolar damage and organizing pneumonia may be seen in adjacent areas (Fig. 5.3), and secondary vasculitis can also be observed in some cases. In more advanced stages, the lung biopsy may show a desquamative interstitial pneumonia–like pattern (Fig. 5.4). The organisms can be visualized within macrophages by use of special stains.[15] The best stains for *Legionella* are silver stains, including Steiner, Warthin-Starry, and Dieterle. The organisms will present as small, short singly scattered bacilli (Fig. 5.5). Immunoperoxidase and immunofluorescent staining can also be used with specific antibodies on deparaffinized, formalin-fixed tissue samples.[16] The use of molecular

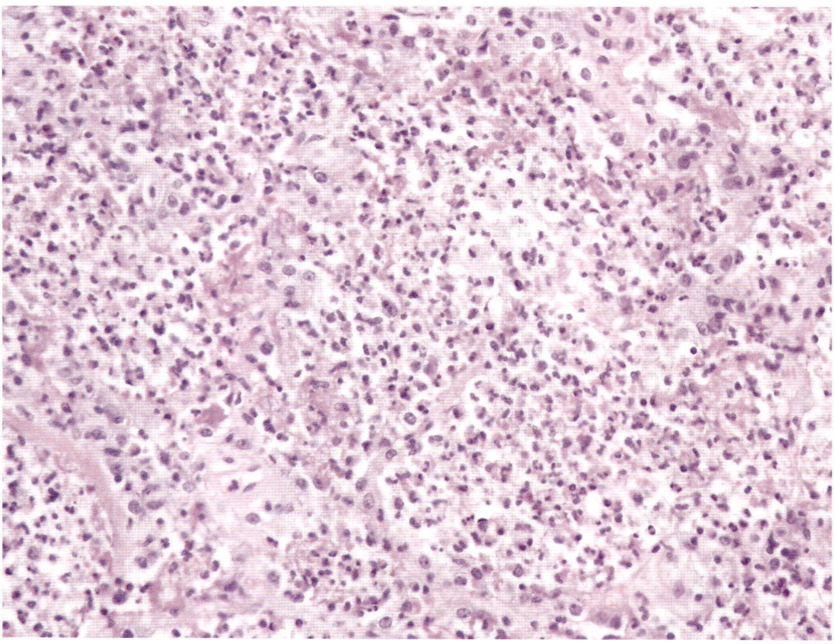

FIGURE 5.2 Transbronchial biopsy in a patient with Legionnaire disease showing massive neutrophilic infiltration of alveolar spaces admixed with fibrin and nuclear debris imparting the biopsy with a characteristic "dusty" appearance.

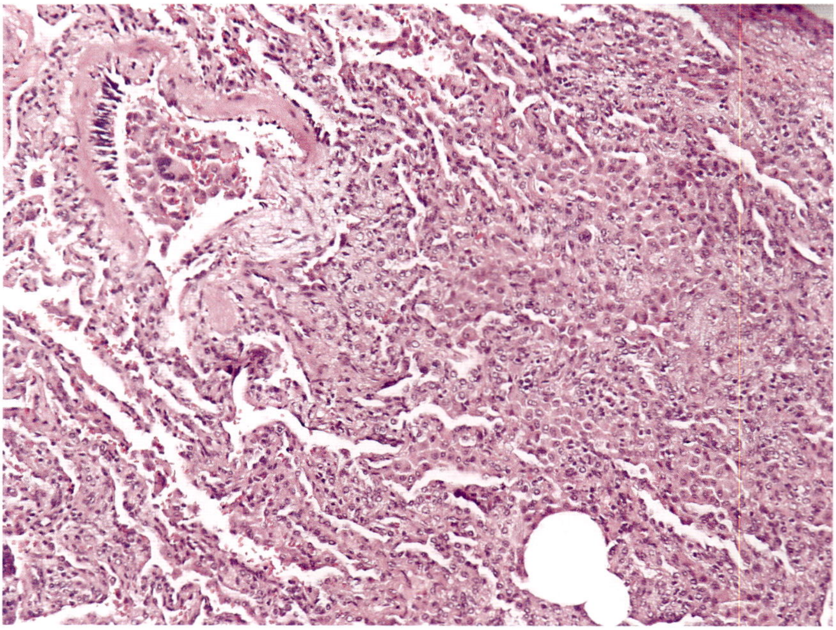

FIGURE 5.3 *Legionella* pneumonia showing a focal organizing pneumonia pattern.

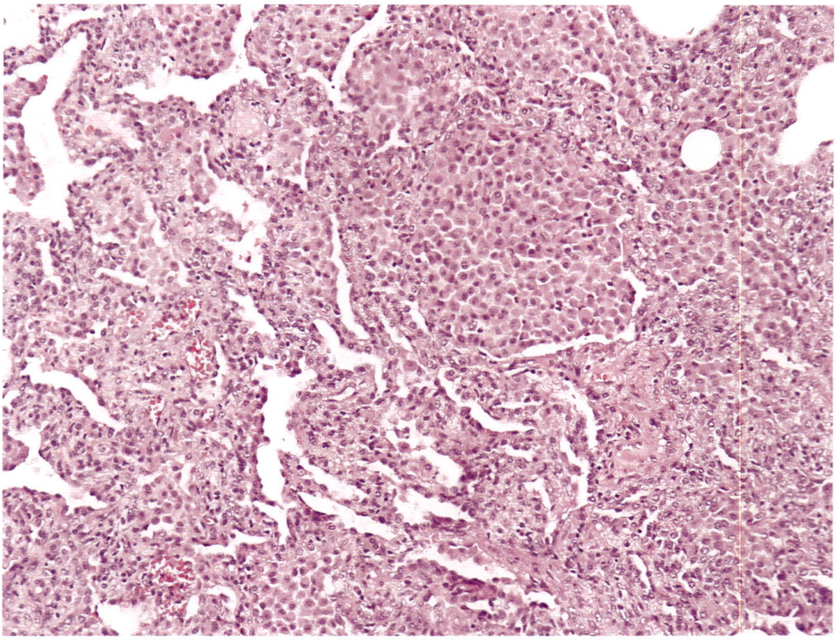

FIGURE 5.4 Desquamative interstitial pneumonia pattern in *Legionella* pneumonia.

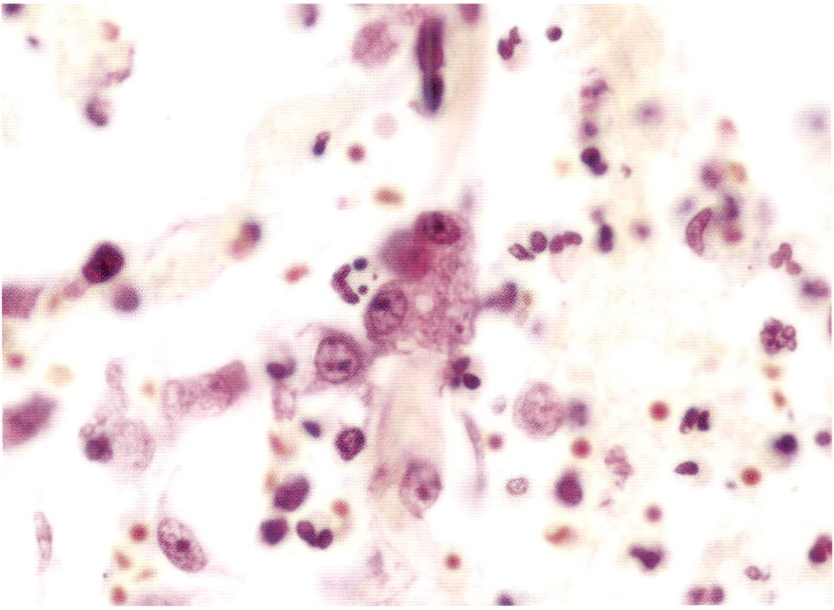

FIGURE 5.5 Steiner silver stain showing *Legionella* organisms within alveolar macrophages.

techniques such as DNA in situ hybridization, polymerase chain reaction (PCR), and next-generation sequencing studies to detect these agents has been reported as a more sensitive and rapid method for diagnosis.[17-19]

Nocardia

Nocardia is a filamentous, gram-positive bacteria with a characteristically beaded histology. Pulmonary infection occurs from inhalation of saprophytic organisms in the soil or in decaying vegetable matter.[4] There are multiple species of *Nocardia*, but lung infection most often is caused by *Nocardia asteroides*. The process most often affects adult men, particularly among immunocompromised patients, as well as patients with chronic diseases such as chronic obstructive pulmonary disease, asthma, chronic sarcoidosis, malignancy, chronic alcoholism, and human immunodeficiency virus (HIV).[20] Infections present as indolent or subacute disease with cough, thick purulent sputum, fever, weight loss, and malaise.[20] Cavitation is a common complication of nocardiosis, and pleural effusions, fistulas, and empyema can also supervene. The lesions may sometimes be reminiscent of a malignant tumor.[21] Histologically, nocardia is characterized by a necrotizing pneumonia with extensive acute inflammation and large areas of necrosis (Figs. 5.6 and 5.7). The organisms display long, thin, beaded filamentous bacteria that branch at right angles. They are not easily visualized on routine hematoxylin and eosin (H&E) tissue sections, and special stains are required for their identification. *Nocardia* stains

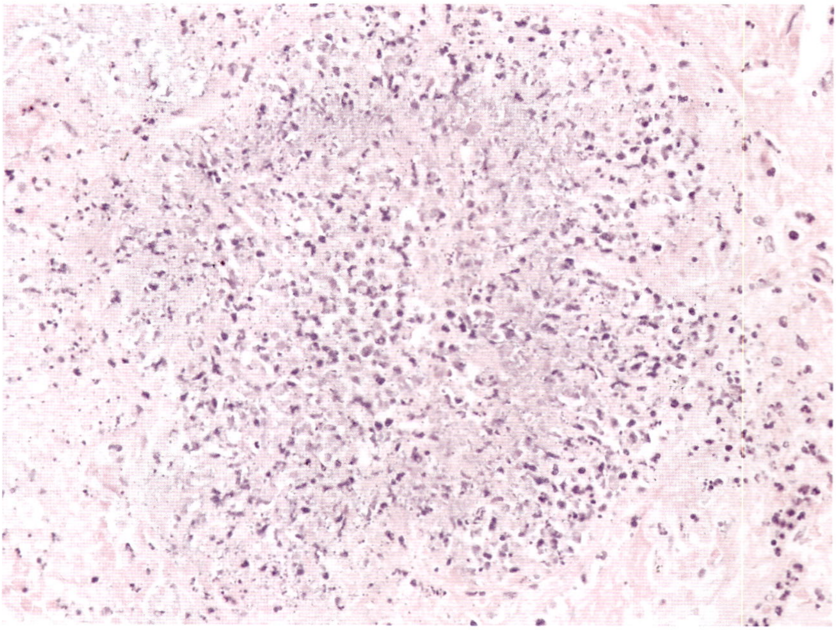

FIGURE 5.6 **Lung biopsy showing focus of necrosis owing to *Nocardia*.** The organisms are not easily visualized on routine hematoxylin and eosin stains.

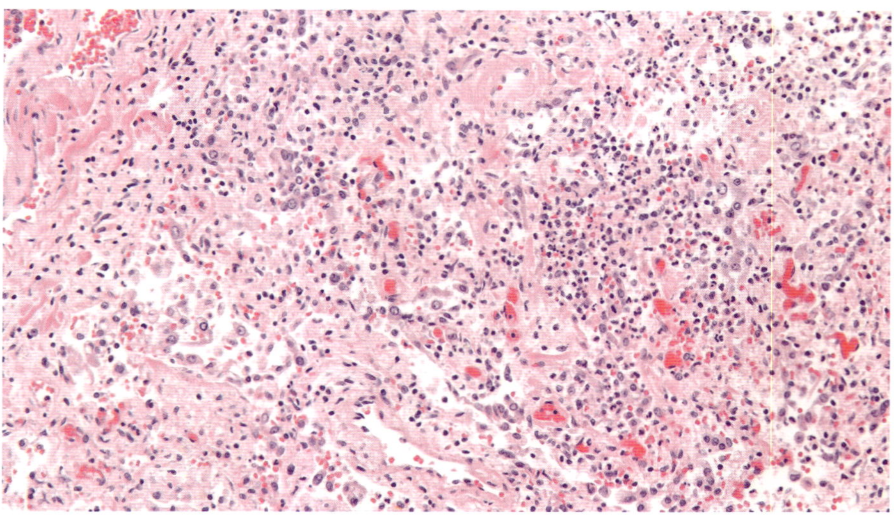

FIGURE 5.7 **Representative image from a wedge resection biopsy shows disrupted lung parenchyma with small pockets of neutrophilic microabscess and reactive pneumocyte atypia.**

with Gomori methenamine silver (GMS) and with tissue Gram stains such as Brown and Brenn and Brown and Hopps (Figs. 5.8 and 5.9). *Nocardia* is also weakly acid-fast and will be positive for the Fite-Faraco stain. However, the organisms can be difficult to detect and may be easily

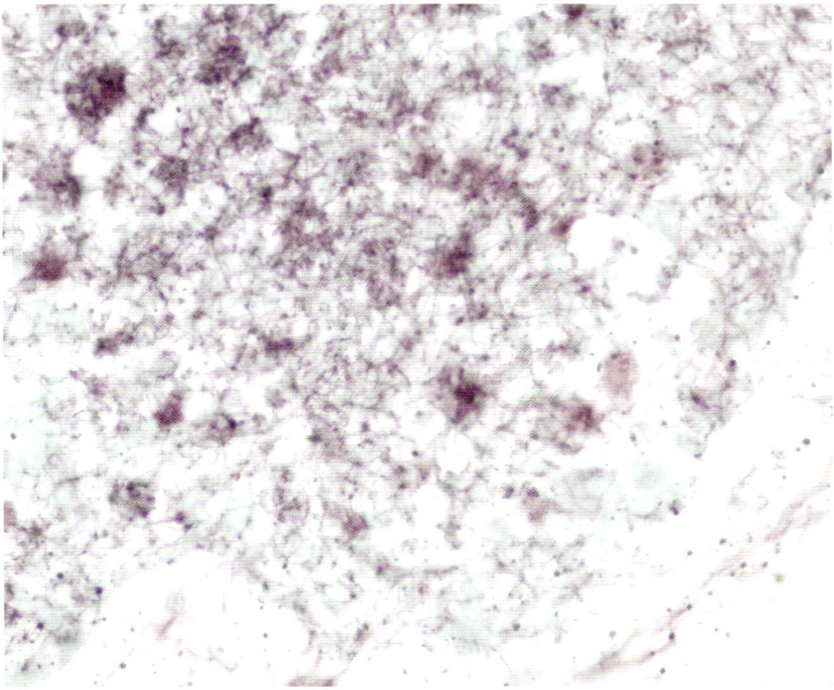

FIGURE 5.8 Thin, beaded filamentous bacteria that branch at right angles characteristic for *Nocardia* (Gomori methenamine silver stain).

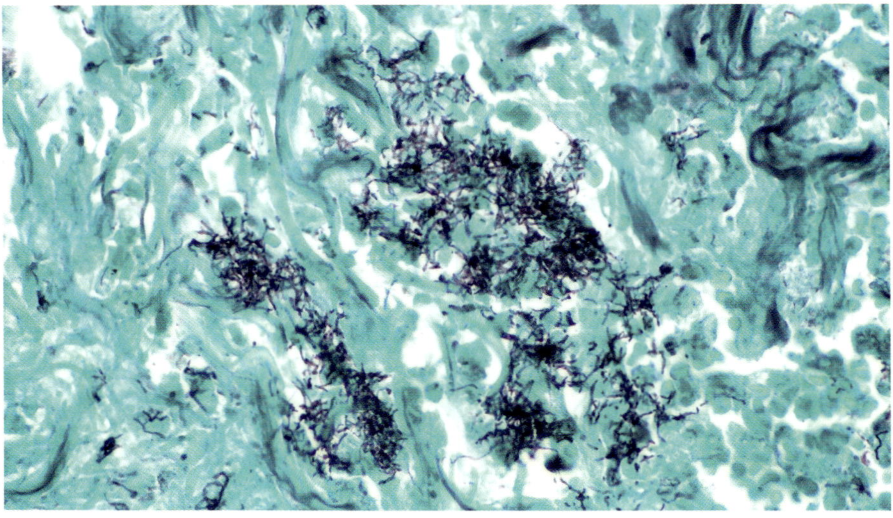

FIGURE 5.9 A small pocket of *Nocardia* is identified within the lung parenchyma. Note the tangled appearance of the mass of filamentous organisms (Gomori methenamine silver stain).

overlooked unless one pays attention to the peculiar complex branching appearance of the filamentous bacteria. Periodic acid-Schiff (PAS) stain for the fungus is usually negative. Definitive diagnosis is established by culture of lung biopsy tissue or bronchoalveolar lavage fluid. Molecular testing may sometimes help clinch the diagnosis in equivocal cases.[22] Because cultures usually require 1 to 2 weeks, a more rapid diagnosis may be obtained from a transbronchial biopsy. Identification of *Nocardia* species on biopsy material requires a high degree of suspicion and use of the appropriate special stains such as the Brown and Brenn, GMS, or Fite-Faraco acid-fast stain. *Nocardia* is distinguished from *Actinomyces* by its weak acid-fast positivity.

Actinomyces

Actinomyces is an anaerobic filamentous bacterium that commonly inhabits the mouth and nasal passages. There are several species, but the most common pathogen in the lungs is *Actinomyces israelii*. Lung infection is usually the result of aspiration of oropharyngeal contents.[23] Chest X-rays usually show unilateral patchy lower lobe areas of consolidation that may cause multifocal and nodular opacities. The process may extend to the pleura and chest wall and produce sinus tracts with bronchopleural and cutaneous fistulas. Lesions may sometimes be localized and be confused for malignancy or other tumors.[24-27] Actinomycosis is characterized by suppurative inflammation, abscess formation, and the formation of so-called sulfur granules (eFig. 5.4).[28] The latter correspond to focalized masses of organisms that seem to radiate from the center of the structure. When these structures develop an eosinophilic, amorphous layer around the periphery of the granules, the process is referred to as the "Splendore-Hoeppli" phenomenon (Fig. 5.10). The lesions often tend to cavitate and form abscesses that may be surrounded by a prominent histiocytic reaction. The organisms are thin, gram-positive, beaded filamentous bacteria that show branching at right angles. At the periphery of the sulfur granules, the organisms often show a radial orientation with club-shaped swellings at the periphery. The organisms are positive for GMS and the Brown and Brenn tissue Gram stain (Fig. 5.11). The differential diagnosis includes other organisms that can form sulfur granules with the Splendore-Hoeppli phenomenon, such as botryomycosis. *Nocardia* can closely resemble actinomycosis but is weakly acid-fast positive with the Fite-Faraco and other acid-fast stains, and it does not form sulfur granules.

Tularemia

Tularemic pneumonia is caused by a small, gram-negative coccobacillus, *Francisella tularensis* (formerly known as *Pasteurella tularensis*). The disease is transmitted through the bite of an infected deer tick or fly, handling of animal carcasses, inhalation of particles, or consumption

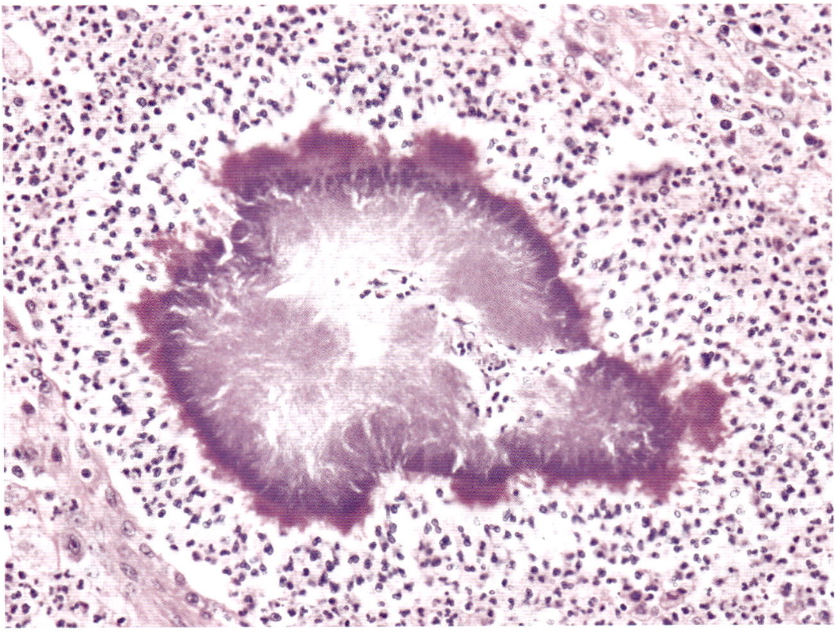

FIGURE 5.10 "Sulfur granules" in actinomycosis showing filamentous structures that radiate from the center toward the periphery and show an amorphous peripheral eosinophilic layer of proteinaceous material (so-called Splendore-Hoeppli phenomenon).

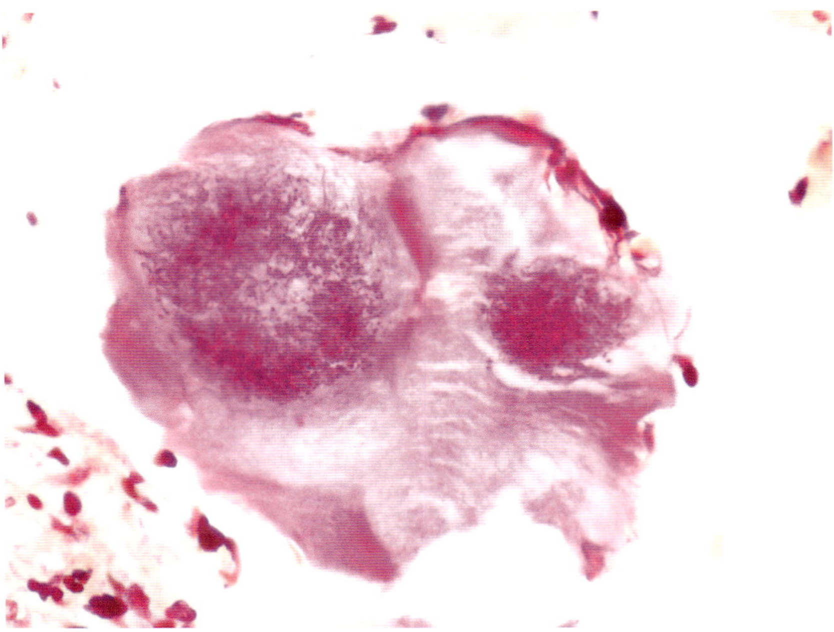

FIGURE 5.11 Positive staining of *Actinomyces* with tissue Gram stain (Brown and Brenn).

of infected food and water.[29-31] The disease also affects the skin, lymph nodes, eyes, and orophraynx.[32] Patients with pulmonary involvement often present with cough and may demonstrate parenchymal or pleural lesions on imaging studies.[33] Pneumonic tularemia is characterized by an acute fibrinous and necrotizing pneumonia with extensive necrosis of alveolar walls. The organisms may be demonstrated by immunofluorescent antibody staining.

Yersinia pestis

Yersinia pestis (formerly *Pasteurella pestis*) is a short, nonmotile gram-negative rod, best known as the causative organism of the bubonic plague. The plague is a zoonosis that is transmitted by the bite of a flea whose natural hosts are small animals, in particular rodents (especially rats). Plague was responsible for the death of millions of persons during the Middle Ages through to the 18th century, but it is very uncommon nowadays and is restricted to small rural areas in the southwest of the United States and certain parts of Africa, South America, and the Far East.[4] Pneumonia is one of the major manifestations of the disease.[34] Lung involvement is characterized by a necrotizing and hemorrhagic pneumonia with extensive necrosis of alveolar walls. The terminal airways are filled with neutrophils, but fibrin is conspicuously absent. Large numbers of organisms are seen in the alveolar lumens and can be demonstrated with silver stains such as Steiner, Warthin-Starry and Dieterle, or with the Brown and Hopps stain. The bacteria are bipolar and exhibit a “safety pin” configuration, a feature best seen on touch imprints stained with the Gram stain. The organisms can be demonstrated by direct immunofluorescence on formalin-fixed deparaffinized sections.[35,36]

Melioidosis

Melioidosis is an infection caused by a gram-negative bacterium, *Burkholderia pseudomallei* (*Pseudomonas pseudomallei*). The disease occurs exclusively in tropical regions and is endemic to Southeast Asia.[37] The disease presents with skin abscesses, necrotizing pneumonia, and sepsis, but the main target organ is the lung.[38] When lung involvement is present, it has been shown to predict an unfavorable outcome.[39] The pneumonia may be acute, subacute, or chronic. The infection causes acute necrotizing bronchopneumonia with focal abscess formation.[40] The necrotizing pneumonia contains abundant neutrophils and macrophages. Some cases may display a mixture of acute inflammation and granulomatous inflammation manifested by a rim of palisaded histiocytes and giant cells at the edges of the necrotizing neutrophilic abscesses. The giant cells and macrophages usually contain dense clusters of bacilli called globi. Most of the organisms are intracellular and can sometimes be recognized in H&E tissue sections, but the diagnosis is best established based on bacterial cultures.

Malakoplakia

Malakoplakia is a distinctive inflammatory process that results from infection with various organisms, including *Rhodococcus equi*, *E coli*, and *Acinetobacter*.[41,42] In the lungs, it is most commonly associated with *R equi* infection. The infection has a predilection for immunocompromised patients, particularly acquired immunodeficiency syndrome (AIDS) patients and transplant patients.[43-45] *R equi* is a gram-positive coccobacillus found in soil and in the feces of some animals, particularly horses. Infection is acquired through inhalation of contaminated aerosols. Lung infection generally results in areas of consolidation that may show focal cavitation. Rare, reported presentations include focalized masses and pulmonary cysts.[46-48] Histologically, the lesions are characterized by a dense histiocytic infiltrate with scattered plasma cells (Figs. 5.12 and 5.13). The hallmark of the lesion is the presence of scattered small, concentric calcifications known as Michaelis-Gutmann bodies measuring from 2 to 10 µm in diameter.[49] These structures can be found within the cytoplasm of the histiocytes or within the interstitium (Fig. 5.14). On transbronchial biopsies, these structures may be few and difficult to find. Histochemical stains for calcium such as the von Kossa or Alizarin red stain will highlight them (Fig. 5.15). The bacteria can be identified in tissue sections with a tissue Gram stain such as Brown and Brenn, and they are also weakly acid-fast and can be demonstrated with modified acid-fast stains such as the Fite-Faraco.

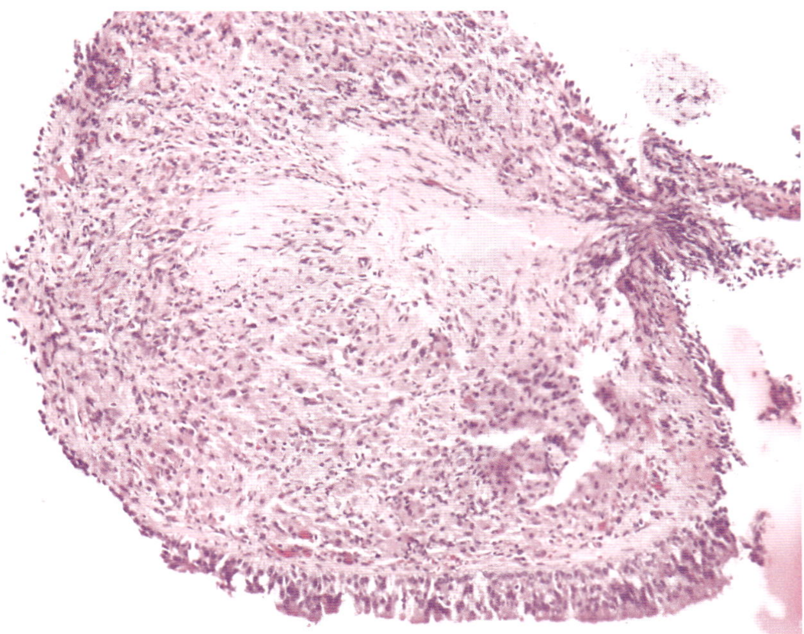

FIGURE 5.12 Transbronchial biopsy in a patient with malakoplakia shows dense histiocytic infiltrate in the submucosa.

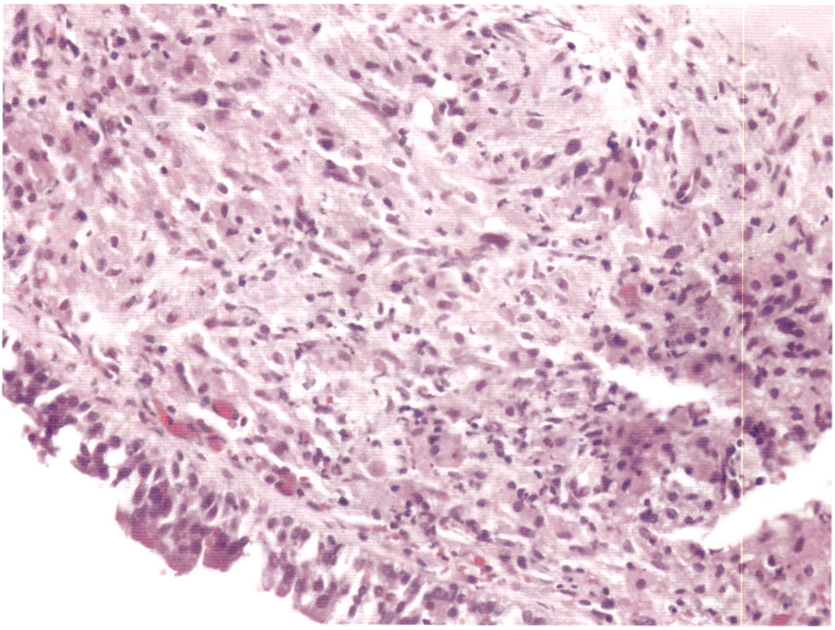

FIGURE 5.13 Higher magnification of the biopsy in a patient with pulmonary involvement with malakoplakia shows abundant epithelioid histiocytes admixed with a few small lymphocytes and plasma cells.

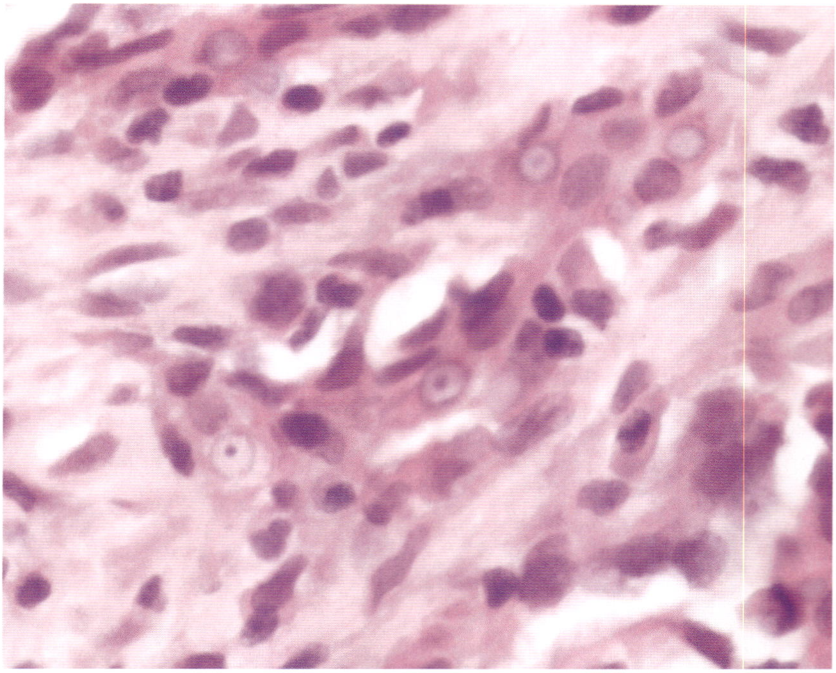

FIGURE 5.14 Small round concentric structures with central foci of calcification adopting a "targetoid" appearance characterize the Michaelis-Gutmann bodies in malakoplakia.

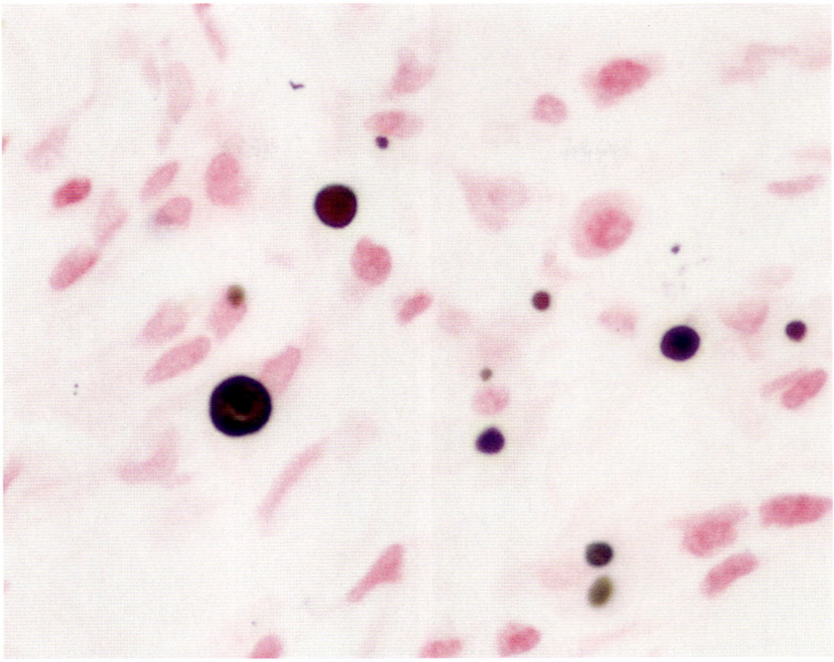

FIGURE 5.15 Von Kossa stain for calcium highlights the Michaelis-Gutmann bodies in pulmonary malakoplakia.

Whipple Disease

Whipple disease is a rare disorder caused by infection with the bacteria *Tropheryma whipplei*. The disease involves multiple organs, in particular the gastrointestinal tract, and usually presents with malabsorption, diarrhea, weight loss, and lymphadenopathy. Pulmonary involvement is uncommon but may be present in up to 30% of cases.[50-55] Histologically, the disease is characterized by sheets of macrophages with abundant clear, foamy cytoplasm (Fig. 5.16). The macrophages are filled with bacteria that stain positive with silver stains such as Warthin-Starry and GMS. The cytoplasm of the histiocytes is strongly positive for PAS (Fig. 5.17). Peribronchiolar and submucosal infiltration by histiocytes is often seen. The histiocytic infiltrate in Whipple disease can be easily confused for infection with *Mycobacterium avium-intracellulare* (MAI). Strong cytoplasmic positivity of the macrophages for PAS and negative staining of the organisms for modified acid-fast stains will help distinguish between the two. Confirmation of the diagnosis requires demonstration of the organism by PCR or other molecular techniques.[56]

Bacillary Angiomatosis

Bacillary angiomatosis is a tissue reaction pattern comprising primarily an epithelioid vascular proliferation in response to an infection caused by a small coccobacillus, *Bartonella henselae,* and *Bartonella quintana* (formerly *Rochalimaea*). Cats are the most common hosts for the

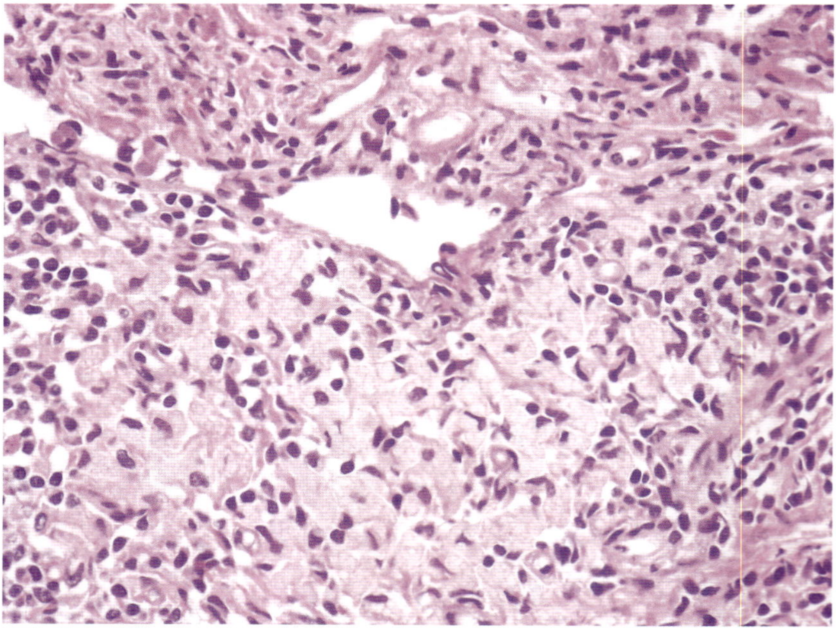

FIGURE 5.16 Sheets of vacuolated macrophages with a bubbly cytoplasm are seen in Whipple disease involving the lung.

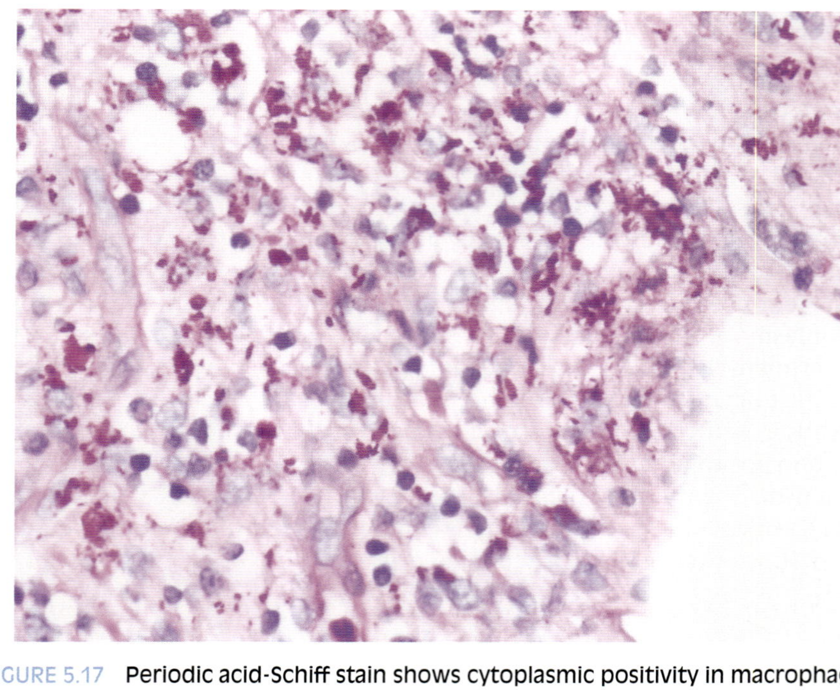

FIGURE 5.17 Periodic acid-Schiff stain shows cytoplasmic positivity in macrophages within the interstitium in Whipple's disease involving the lung

organisms, and transmission is through the cat flea. Immunocompromised patients are particularly prone to this infection. Bacillary angiomatosis most commonly affects the skin but can occur in almost all organs. Lung involvement has been reported in AIDS patients who presented with interstitial pneumonitis, lymphadenopathy, and polypoid endobronchial lesions.[57,58] Histologically, the lesions are characterized by a dense proliferation of small vessels lined by plump endothelial cells with abundant epithelioid cytoplasm (Fig. 5.18). Scattered inflammatory cells, particularly neutrophils and small lymphocytes, are often present forming discrete microabscesses (Fig. 5.19). The organisms can sometimes be visualized on H&E stains; they show a tendency to cluster within the cytoplasm of the histiocyte, imparting the lesions with a "dirty," purple appearance (eFigs. 5.5 and 5.6). The organisms are best visualized with a modified Warthin-Starry silver stain at a pH of 3.2. The organisms are negative for PAS and acid-fast stains. Both immunohistochemistry utilizing specific antibodies against *B henselae* or detection by PCR can be used to confirm the diagnosis.[59,60]

Botryomycosis

Botryomycosis is an infection caused by nonfilamentous bacteria that form "sulfur granules" similar to those seen in actinomycosis. The disease

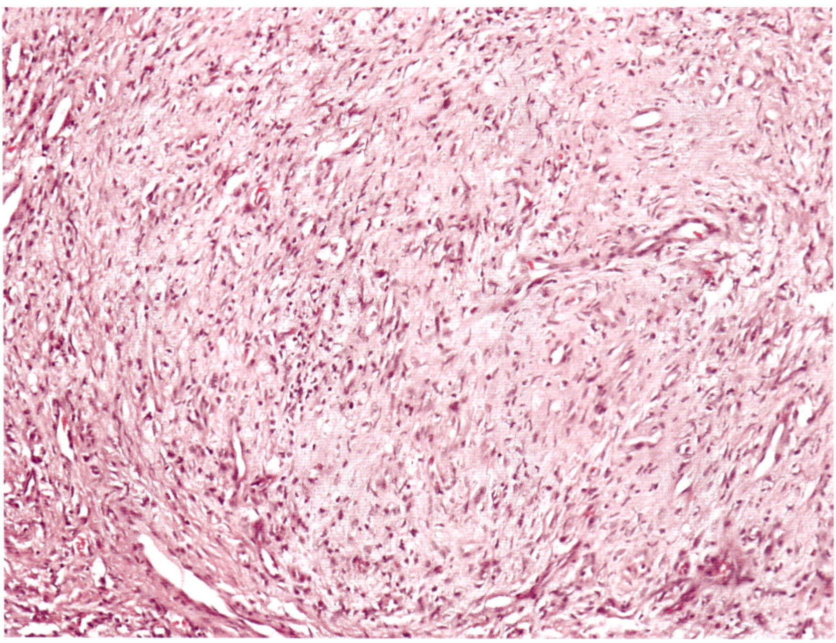

FIGURE 5.18 Proliferation of small vessels lined by plump epithelioid cells and admixed with inflammatory cells is seen in bacillary angiomatosis involving the lung.

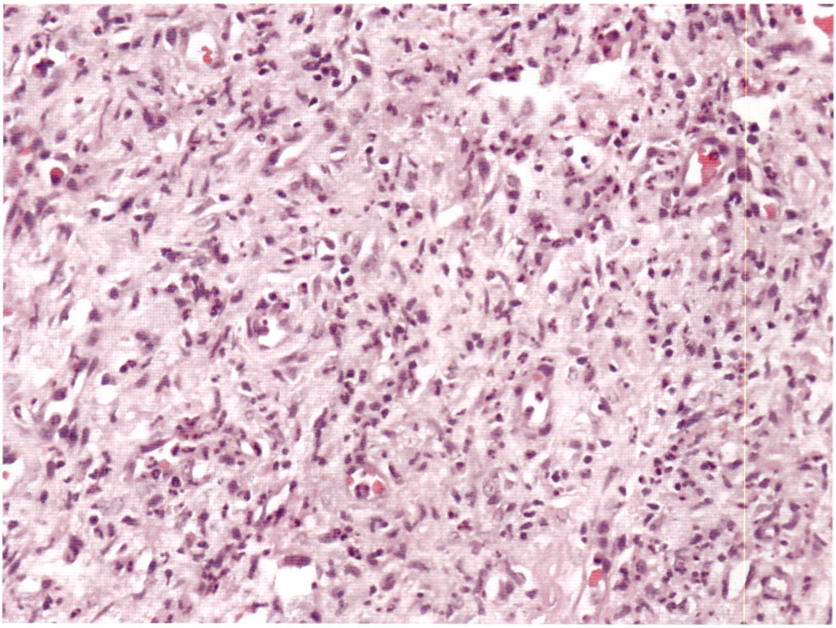

FIGURE 5.19 **Higher magnification of bacillary angiomatosis showing a population of neutrophils and small lymphocytes surrounding the small vessels.** The surrounding histiocytes have a "dirty" appearance and contain abundant organisms that are best appreciated with special stains.

can affect almost any organ. The most common organism associated with botryomycosis is *S aureus*, although other organisms can also result in the same lesions, including *P aeruginosa*, *E coli*, *Proteus*, *Streptococcus*, and others. Lung involvement is rare and can occur as bronchial infection complicating bronchiectasis, as focalized tumor-like lesions, or as diffuse bronchopneumonia.[28,61-66] The disease often presents in the setting of immunosuppression. The diagnosis is made when the distinctive "granules" measuring up to 2 mm in diameter are identified in tissue sections. These granules comprise nonfilamentous bacterial organisms, such as gram-positive cocci or gram-negative bacilli, and are typically located within areas of suppuration and necrosis (Fig. 5.20). The granules often display the Splendore-Hoeppli phenomenon, with a layer of eosinophilic amorphous material deposited at the periphery of the bacterial colonies. The organisms are visualized on tissue Gram stains and characteristically grow forming grapelike cultures, hence the designation of "botryomycosis." The main differential diagnosis is with actinomycosis, but the organisms in botryomycosis do not show the filamentous branching seen in actinomycosis.

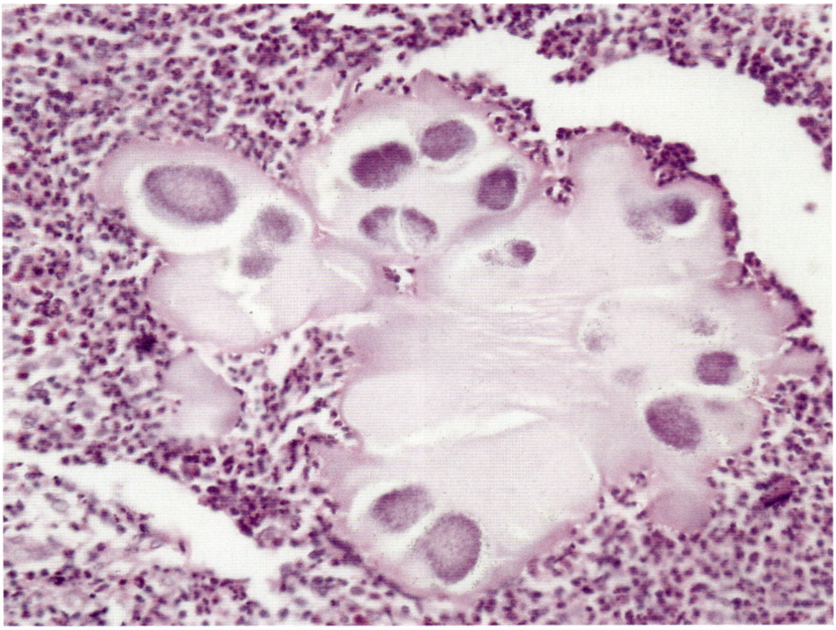

FIGURE 5.20 "Sulfur granule" comprising masses of nonfilamentous bacteria are seen in a case of botryomycosis involving the lung (tissue Gram stain; Brown and Brenn).

MYCOBACTERIAL PNEUMONIAS

Mycobacterial infection can be a frequent finding in the lungs of debilitated and immunosuppressed patients. The two main causative agents are *Mycobacterium tuberculosis* and the MAI complex, though various other mycobacterial species such as *Mycobacterium abscessus* are also implicated in pulmonary disease.[67] Although the incidence of infection with *M tuberculosis* has decreased dramatically worldwide in developed countries owing to the use of antituberculous drugs, tuberculosis (TB) remains one of the most common infectious causes of death in underdeveloped countries. In addition, the incidence of nontuberculous pulmonary disease has been rising globally.[68-71] In the United States and globally, the development of drug-resistant strains and the AIDS epidemic as well as the COVID-19 pandemic saw a resurgence in TB.[72] All mycobacteria share in common their acid-fast staining property caused by the high lipid content of the bacilli, a useful diagnostic feature.

Mycobacterium tuberculosis

The lung is one of the main targets of TB and is characterized by chronic, recurrent infection that is transmitted through inhalation of aerosolized droplets containing the tubercle bacillus. TB is often associated with various underlying diseases such as diabetes, HIV infection, alcoholism, cancer, chronic renal failure, and drug abuse. It is clinically divided into primary and secondary (reactivation TB) infections. In primary TB, the initial response to the infection is a neutrophilic reaction followed by macrophages that engulf the organisms. The macrophages can spread to the regional lymph nodes, but they usually stay in the lungs and become localized to the upper half of the upper lobes ("Simon foci"). When the infection resolves, it undergoes fibrosis and calcification ("Ghon complex"). More than 90% of primary TB will heal spontaneously without progression. The patients will most often be asymptomatic, and the infection can be demonstrated only by a positive tuberculin skin test. Ten percent of patients will develop progressive disease characterized by hematogenous spread within the lungs to form a military pattern of involvement or foci of consolidation with tuberculous bronchopneumonia. Secondary TB occurs when a dormant focus of infection is reactivated causing reinfection. This will usually result in the characteristic cavitary lesions that can affect one or both upper lobes. This is the most common form of TB in adults.[73]

The pathologic findings in TB are mainly related to the destructive tissue reaction at the sites of infection. The most common reaction pattern is characterized by large, confluent necrotizing granulomas that show peripheral palisading of histiocytes, epithelioid histiocytes, and frequent Langhans-type multinucleated giant cells (Figs. 5.21 and 5.22; eFigs. 5.7 and 5.8). A miliary pattern characterized by multiple small epithelioid granulomas can also be observed (Fig. 5.23). The lesions can sometimes be characterized by scattered microscopic granulomas and isolated Langhans giant cells distributed in peribronchial location (Fig. 5.24). The lesions

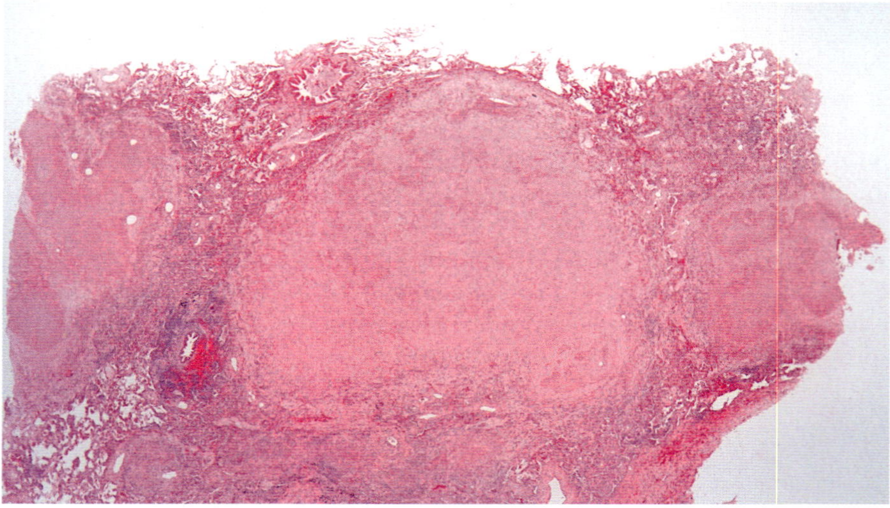

FIGURE 5.21 Low-power magnification from a wedge resection of a patient with cavitary lesions (*Mycobacterium tuberculosis*) demonstrates multiple large granulomas with geographic necrosis.

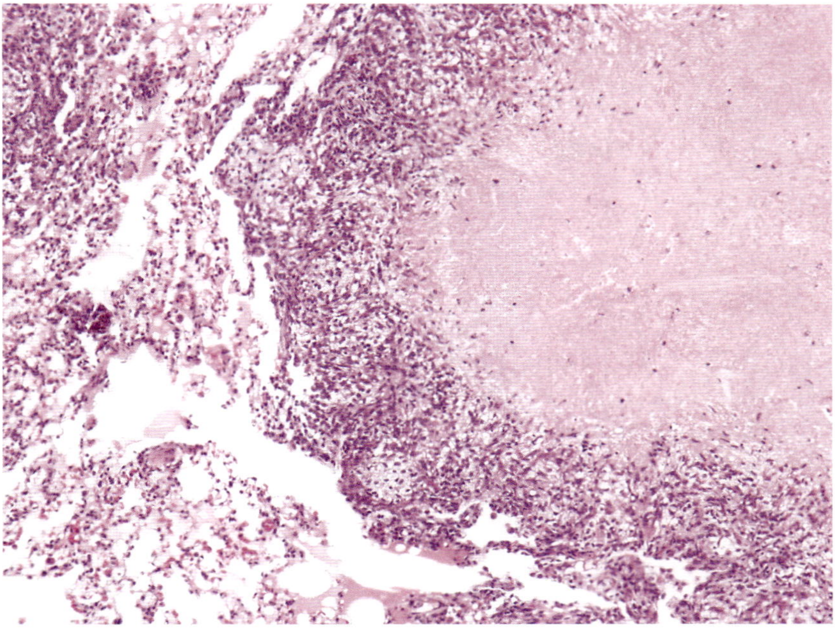

FIGURE 5.22 **Necrotizing granuloma in lung infection with *Mycobacterium tuberculosis*.** Notice peripheral palisading of histiocytes admixed with Langhans-type multinucleated giant cells surrounding the necrotic center.

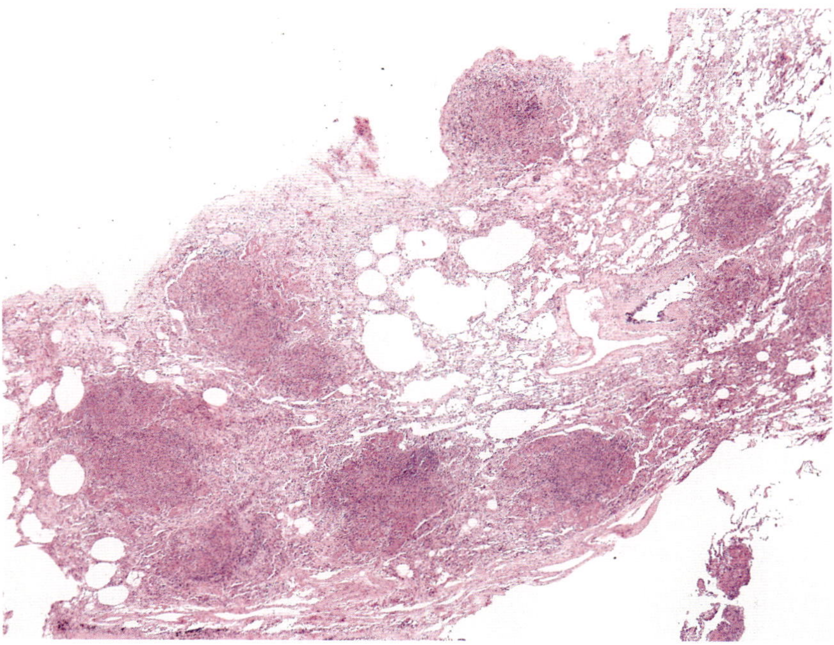

FIGURE 5.23 **Miliary pattern in transbronchial lung biopsy in a patient with tuberculosis.**

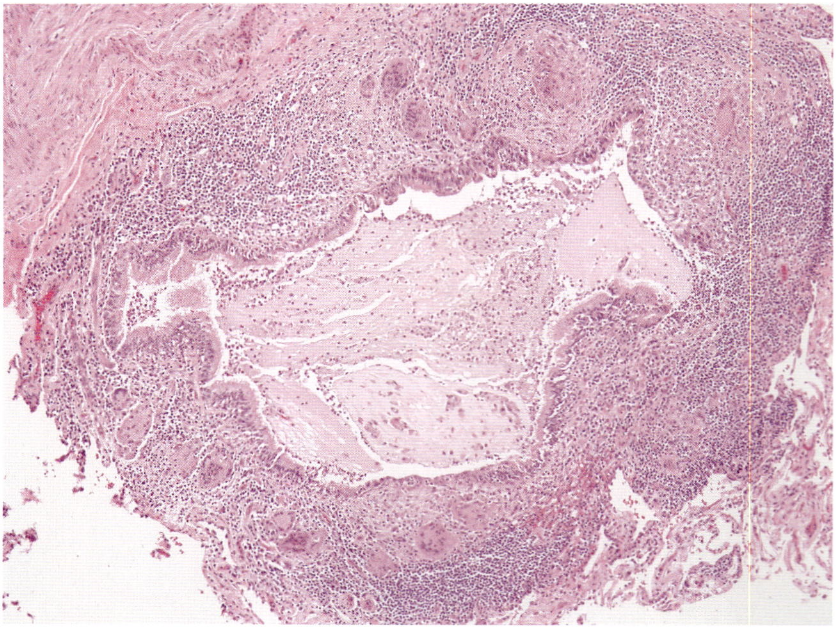

FIGURE 5.24 **Granulomatous peribronchiolitis is seen in a patient with tuberculosis.** Notice small granulomas and scattered multinucleated giant cells surrounded by abundant lymphoid infiltrates.

contain bacilli mostly in the necrotic center, but they can also be identified within epithelioid histiocytes and multinucleated giant cells.[74] The bacilli are often few and difficult to identify and will require a diligent search, best done under 60× "high-dry" magnification or oil immersion. The organisms are best identified on acid-fast stains; Ziehl-Neelsen will stain the small, beaded, and thin bacilli bright red (Fig. 5.25). Fluorescent staining, immunoperoxidase, and molecular methods can also be used to demonstrate the organism in tissues.[75,76] Long-standing lesions will tend to undergo fibrosis and calcification. Endobronchial spread occurs through lymphatic spread of organisms through the bronchial mucosa. The infection can also involve the pleura and regional lymph nodes. A rise in the incidence of TB was observed in the past three decades, mainly related to the onset of the AIDS epidemic.[77] More recently there have been some positive trends in reduction and prevalence of the disease; however, the number of drug-resistant mycobacterial cases has begun to steadily increase as well.[78]

Atypical Mycobacteria

Atypical, nontuberculous mycobacteria constitute a group of organisms that are found in soil, plants, fresh and salt water, and animals that cause infection directly from the environment rather than through human transmission. Atypical mycobacteria do not follow the same pattern of primary

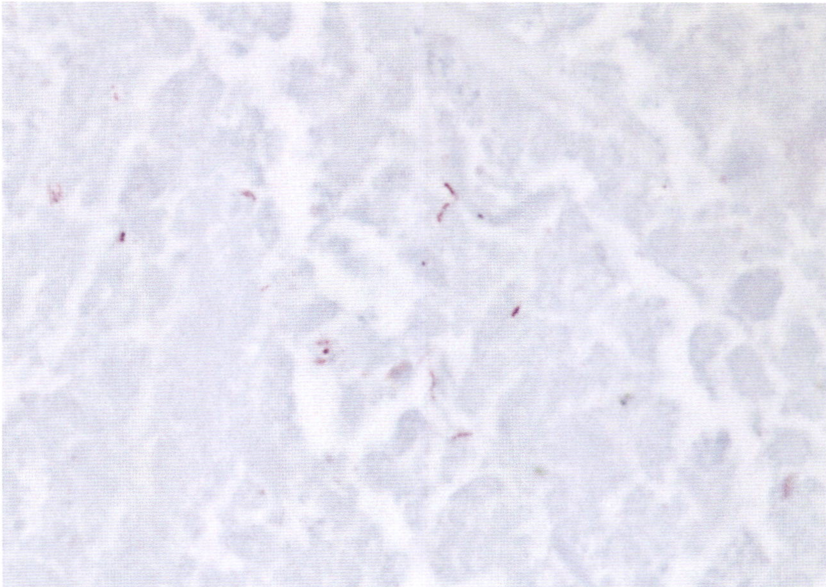

FIGURE 5.25 Few acid-fast bacilli are identified in areas of caseating necrosis within the granulomas of pulmonary tuberculosis (Ziehl-Neelsen stain).

and secondary (reactivation) infections observed in TB. Primary infection of the lungs with atypical mycobacteria usually causes cavitary lung disease. In HIV-positive patients, the lung is considered to be the initial route of infection where the organisms lie dormant until the immunosuppression activates the organisms and dissemination takes place.[79] The organisms are closely related and are often grouped together and referred to as the *M avium* complex (MAC) or MAI. The MAC is the most important atypical mycobacterial agent of human infection, with a high incidence in patients with AIDS.[80] *Mycobacterium kansasii* is another important cause of nontuberculous mycobacteriosis.[81] Although rarer, other types of atypical mycobacteria can be the source of infection in the lungs, including *M abscessus*, *Mycobacterium fortuitum*, and *Mycobacterium chelonae*.[69-71]

The histopathologic hallmark of atypical mycobacterial infection in the lung is the presence of nonnecrotizing epithelioid granulomas.[82-84] MAI also causes upper lobe cavitary lung lesions. The noncaseating granulomas can resemble those seen in sarcoidosis. Transbronchial biopsies are quite helpful in diagnosing the condition (Figs. 5.26 and 5.27). The interstitium separating the alveolar septa shows sheets of large epithelioid cells (Fig. 5.28); formation of well-defined granulomas may not always be present (eFig. 5.9). Higher magnification will show sheets of epithelioid histiocytes displaying a finely granular, "dirty" or cloudy cytoplasmic appearance (so-called pseudo-Gaucher cell) owing to the massive number of bacilli distending the cytoplasm (Fig. 5.29; eFig. 5.10). The bacilli are

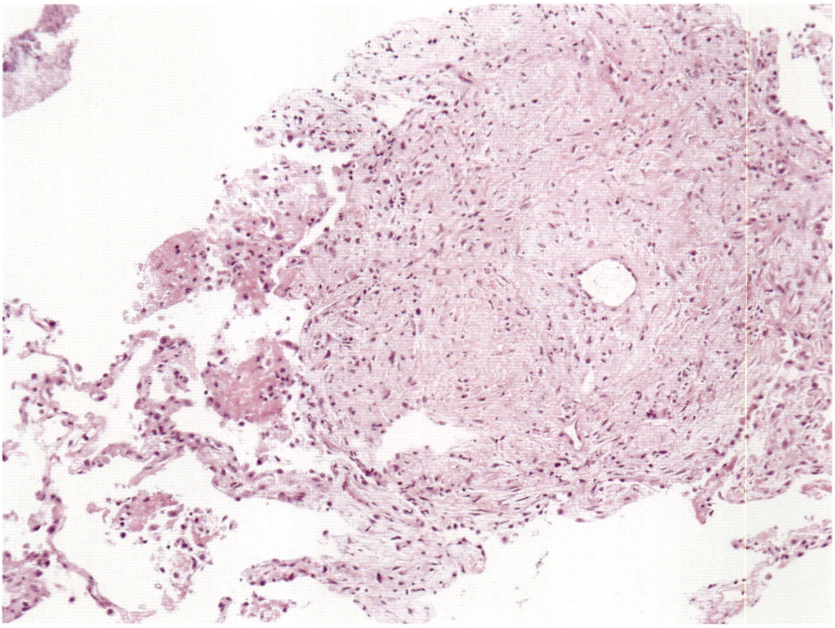

FIGURE 5.26 Transbronchial biopsy in immunosuppressed patient with *Mycobacterium avium–intracellulare* shows sheets of epithelioid histiocytes.

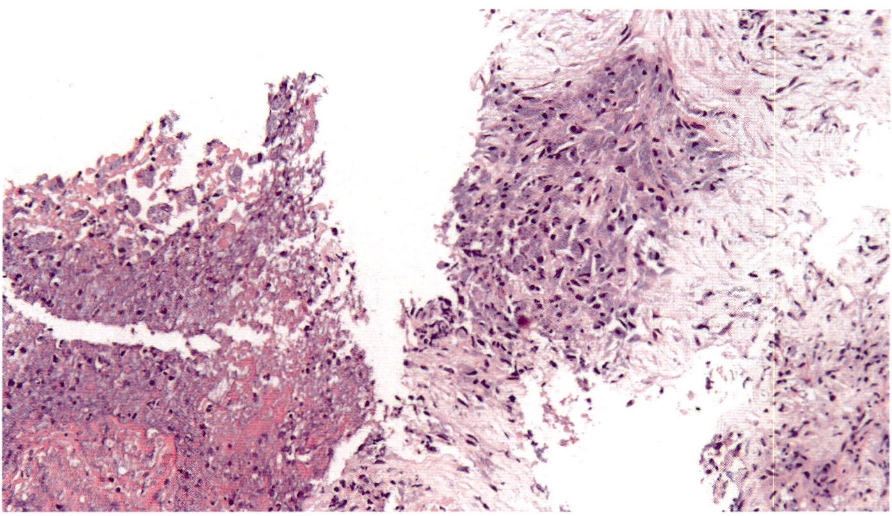

FIGURE 5.27 Transbronchial biopsy shows a small aggregate of dusty appearing epithelioid histiocytes with an associated area of necrosis adjacent to it.

easily visualized on Ziehl-Neelsen stains and are usually more slender and more abundant than in TB, particularly in AIDS patients.[79,85] The organisms can also be seen with PAS and GMS stains and modified acid-fast stains such as Fite-Faraco, which will stain them intensely (Fig. 5.30).

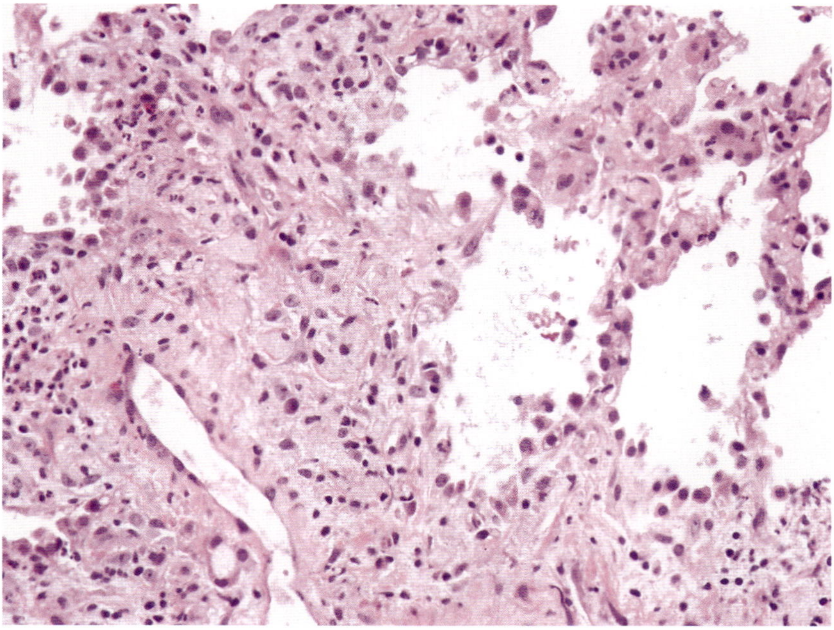

FIGURE 5.28 Lung involvement in *Mycobacterium avium–intracellulare* shows abundant epithelioid histiocytes admixed with other inflammatory elements in the interstitium.

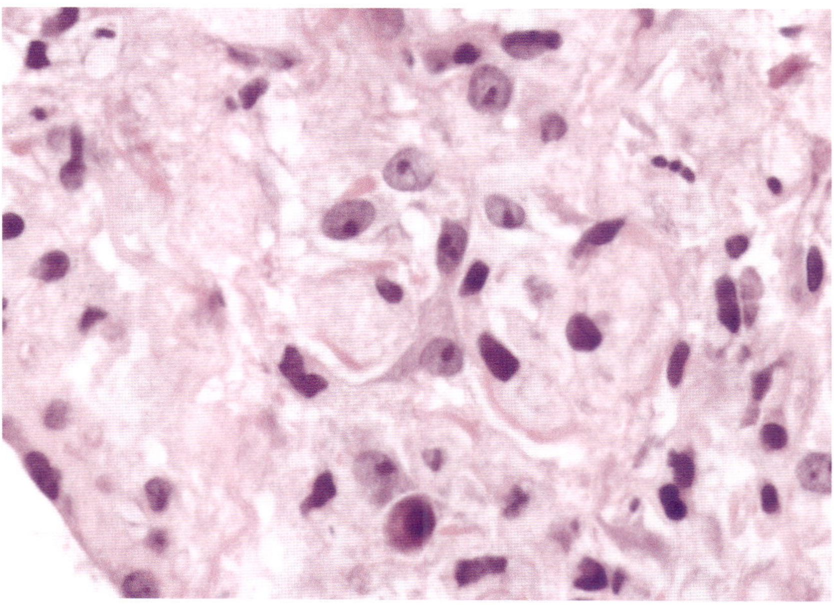

FIGURE 5.29 Higher magnification from preceding picture showing sheets of large, epithelioid histiocytes with "dirty" granular cytoplasm.

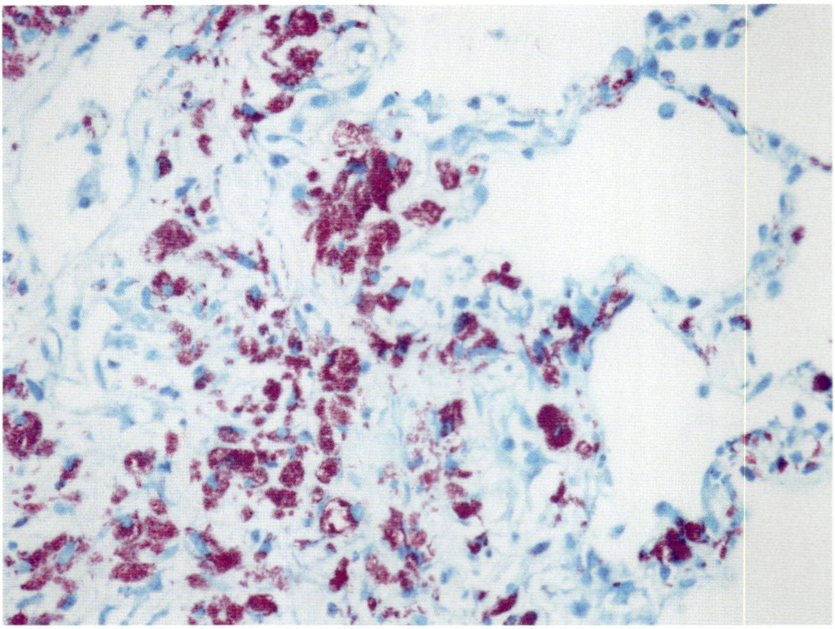

FIGURE 5.30 **Modified acid-fast stain (Fite-Faraco) intensely stains the organisms in *Mycobacterium avium–intracellulare*.** Notice the abundance of organisms and the larger size compared with those of *Mycobacterium tuberculosis*.

An unusual appearance that can be rarely encountered with MAC is the so-called mycobacterial spindle cell pseudotumor, a condition in which the histiocytes will adopt a spindled appearance with a fascicular growth pattern resembling a mesenchymal spindle cell proliferation.[86,87] Many of the spindled histiocytes, however, will display abundant "dirty" granular cytoplasm owing to the intracytoplasmic bacilli, which are easily highlighted by acid-fast stains.

REFERENCES

1. Prasso JE, Deng JC. Postviral complications: bacterial pneumonia. *Clin Chest Med.* 2017;38(1):127-138.
2. Ciofu O, Hansen CR, Høiby N. Respiratory bacterial infections in cystic fibrosis. *Curr Opin Pulm Med*. 2013;19(3):251-258.
3. Martin-Loeches I, van Someren GF, Schultz MJ. Bacterial pneumonia as an influenza complication. *Curr Opin Infect Dis*. 2017;30(2):201-207.
4. Goetz MB, Finegold SM. Pyogenic bacterial pneumonia, lung abscess and empyema. In: Murray JF, Nadel JA, Mason RJ, Boushey H, eds. *Textbook of Respiratory Medicine*. 3rd ed. WB Saunders; 2000:985-1041.
5. Wunderink RG, Matsunaga Y, Ariyasu M, et al. Cefiderocol versus high-dose, extended-infusion meropenem for the treatment of Gram-negative nosocomial pneumonia (APEKS-NP): a randomised, double-blind, phase 3, non-inferiority trial. *Lancet Infect Dis*. 2021;21:213-225.

6. Chandler F. Approaches to the pathologic diagnosis of infectious diseases. In: Connor D, Chandler FW, Schwartz DA, et al., eds. *Pathology of Infectious Disease*. Appleton & Lange; 1997:3-7.
7. Deng Z, Li C, Wang Y, et al. Targeted next-generation sequencing for pulmonary infection diagnosis in patients unsuitable for bronchoalveolar lavage. *Front Med (Lausanne)*. 2023;10:1321515.
8. Wu D, Wang W, Xun Q, et al. Metagenomic next-generation sequencing indicates more precise pathogens in patients with pulmonary infection: a retrospective study. *Front Cell Infect Microbiol*. 2022;12:977591.
9. Viasus D, Gaia V, Manzur-Barbur C, Carratalà J. Legionnaires' disease: update on diagnosis and treatment. *Infect Dis Ther*. 2022;11:973-986.
10. Weisenburger DD, Helms CM, Renner ED. Sporadic Legionnaires' disease. A pathologic study of 23 fatal cases. *Arch Pathol Lab Med*. 1981;105:130-137.
11. Chahin A, Opal SM. Severe pneumonia caused by *Legionella pneumophila*: differential diagnosis and therapeutic considerations. *Infect Dis Clin N Am*. 2017;31(1):111-121.
12. Mondino S, Schmidt S, Rolando M, et al. Legionnaires' disease: state of the art knowledge of pathogenesis mechanisms of *Legionella*. *Annu Rev Pathol*. 2020;15:439-466.
13. Poirier R, Rodrigue J, Villeneuve J, Lacasse Y. Early radiographic and tomographic manifestations of Legionnaires' disease. *Can Assoc Radiol J*. 2017;68(3):328-333.
14. Fields BS, Benson RF, Besser RE. *Legionella* and Legionnaires' disease: 25 years of investigation. *Clin Microbiol Rev*. 2002;15:506-526.
15. Winn WC Jr, Myerowitz RL. The pathology of the *Legionella pneumonias*. A review of 74 cases and the literature. *Hum Pathol*. 1981;12:401-422.
16. Veza PR, Lack EE, Chandler FW. Legionellosis. In: Connor DH, Chandler FW, Manz HJ, et al., eds. *Pathology of Infectious Diseases*. Appelton & Lange; 1997:597-604.
17. Hayden RT, Uhl JR, Qian X, et al. Direct detection of *Legionella* species from bronchoalveolar lavage and open lung biopsy specimens: comparison of light cycler PCR, in-situ hybridization, direct fluorescence, antigen detection and culture. *J Clin Microbiol*. 2001;39:2618-2626.
18. Niu S, Zhao L. Metagenomic next-generation sequencing clinches the diagnosis of Legionella pneumonia in a patient with acute myeloid leukemia: a case report and literature review. *Front Cell Infect Microbiol*. 2022;12:924597.
19. Wang Y, Dai Y, Lu H, et al. Case report: metagenomic next-generation sequencing in diagnosis of *Legionella pneumophila* pneumonia in a patient after umbilical cord blood stem cell transplantation. *Front Med (Lausanne)*. 2021;8:643473.
20. Brown-Elliott BA, Brown JM, Conville PS, Wallace RJ Jr. Clinical and laboratory features of the *Nocardia* spp. Based on current molecular taxonomy. *Clin Microbiol Rev*. 2006;19(2):259-282.
21. Lopes K, Montenegro C, Vìlchez J, Camachoa ME, Marquesa HG. IMAGES: *Nocardia* pneumonia: a surprising and rare pulmonary infection mimicking lung cancer. *Pulmonology*. 2022;28:415-417.
22. Ye J, Li Y, Hao J, et al. Rare occurrence of pulmonary coinfection involving *Aspergillus fumigatus* and *Nocardia cyriacigeorgica* in immunocompetent patients based on NGS: a case report and literature review. *Medicine (Baltimore)*. 2023;102:e36692.
23. Eschapasse E, Hussenet C, Bergeron A, Lebeaux D. Respiratory infections caused by slow-growing bacteria: *Nocardia*, *Actinomyces*. *Rhodococcus Rev Mal Respir*. 2017;34(6):661-671.
24. Aydin Y, Arslan R, Filik M. Pulmonary actinomycosis mimicks lung cancer. *Rev Soc Bras Med Trop*. 2022;55:e0195.
25. Rouis H, Moussa C, Ayadi A, et al. Pulmonary actinomycosis mimicking lung malignancy: about two cases. *Heliyon*. 2023;9:e20070.

26. Zheng M, Wei Y, Borkar NA, et al. Pulmonary actinomycosis masquerading as lung cancer. *Respir Med Case Rep*. 2024;51:102050.
27. Baykal H, Ulger AF, Çelik D, Tanrikulu FB, Tatci E. Clinical and radiological characteristics of pulmonary actinomycosis mimicking lung malignancy. *Rev Assoc Med Bras*. 1992;2022(68):372-376.
28. De Montpreville VT, Nashashibi N, Dulmet EM. Actinomycosis and other bronchopulmonary infections with bacterial granules. *Ann Diagn Pathol*. 1999;3:67-74.
29. Evans ME, Gregory DW, Schaffner W, McGee ZA. Tularemia: a 30-year experience with 88 cases. *Medicine (Baltimore)*. 1985;64:251-269.
30. Thomas LD, Schaffner W. Tularemia pneumonia. *Infect Dis Clin N Am*. 2010; 24(1):43-55.
31. Plymoth M, Lundqvist R, Nystedt A, Sjöstedt A, Gustafsson TN. Targeting tularemia: clinical, laboratory, and treatment outcomes from an 11-year retrospective observational cohort in Northern Sweden. *Clin Infect Dis*. 2024;78:1222-1231.
32. Miller RP, Bates JH. Pleuropulmonary tularemia. A review of 29 patients. *Am Rev Respir Dis*. 1969;99:31-41.
33. Martinet P, Khatchatourian L, Saidani N, et al. Hypermetabolic pulmonary lesions on FDG-PET/CT: tularemia or neoplasia? *Infect Dis Now*. 2021;51:607-613.
34. Venugopal G, Pechous RD. *Yersinia pestis* and pneumonic plague: insight into how a lethal pathogen interfaces with innate immune populations in the lung to cause severe disease. *Cell Immunol*. 2024;403-404:104856.
35. Johnson CC, Finegold SM. Pyogenic bacterial pneumonia, lung abscess and empyema. In: Murray JF, Nadel JA, eds. *Textbook of Respiratory Medicine*. 2nd ed. WB Saunders; 1994:1036-1093.
36. Smith JH, Reisner BS. Plague. In: Connor DH, Chandler FW, Manz HJ, et al., eds. *Pathology of Infectious Diseases*. Appelton & Lange; 1997:729-738.
37. Mohapatra PR, Mishra B. Burden of melioidosis in India and South Asia: challenges and ways forward. *Lancet Reg Health Southeast Asia*. 2022;2:100004.
38. Ip M, Osterberg LG, Chau PY, Raffin TA. Pulmonary melioidosis. *Chest*. 1995;108:1420-1424.
39. Khiangte HL, Vimala LR, Veeraraghavan B, Yesudhason BL, Karuppusami R. Can the imaging manifestations of melioidosis prognosticate the clinical outcome? A 6-year retrospective study. *Insights Imaging*. 2019;10(1):17.
40. Greenwald KA, Nash G, Foley FD. Acute systemic melioidosis. Autopsy findings in four patients. *Am J Clin Pathol*. 1969;52:188-198.
41. Colby TV, Hunt S, Pelzmann K, Carrington CB. Malakoplakia of the lung: a report of two cases. *Respiration*. 1980;39:295-299.
42. Crouch E, White V, Wright J, et al. Malakoplakia mimicking carcinoma metastatic to the lung. *Am J Surg Pathol*. 1984;8:151-156.
43. Verville TD, Huycke MM, Greenfield RA, Fine DP, Kuhls TL, Slater LN. *Rhodococcus equi* infections of humans. Twelve cases and a review of the literature. *Medicine (Baltimore)*. 1994;73:119-132.
44. Köksal D, Ozcan A, Demira F, et al. Pulmonary malakoplakia: a case report and review of the literature. *Tuberk Toraks*. 2014;62(3):248-252.
45. Lane RJ, Kradin R, Xia D, et al. Malakoplakia in thoracic transplant recipients. *Transplant Proc*. 2019;51(3):871-874.
46. Corrêa LF, da Silva TKB, Camargo SM, Furian BC. Pulmonary malakoplakia associated with peripheral cysts in an immunocompetent patient: a case report. *J Chest Surg*. 2022;55:422-424.
47. Grewal HS, Virk RK, Carroll ME, et al. Malakoplakia presenting as a lung mass in a lung transplant recipient: case report. *Transplant Proc*. 2022;54:173-175.

48. Narwani P, Rajendran I, Lewington A, Eltayeb A, Ganjifrockwala A, Annamalaisamy R. Malakoplakia presenting as pleuropulmonary masses: a rare clinical, radiological and histopathological diagnosis. *Radiol Case Rep*. 2021;16:3859-3863.

49. Yousef M, Naghibi B. Malakoplakia outside the urinary tract. *Arch Pathol Lab Med*. 2007;131:297-300.

50. Duss FR, Jaton K, Vollenweider P, Troillet N, Greub G. Whipple disease: a 15-year retrospective study on 36 patients with positive polymerase chain reaction for *Tropheryma whipplei*. *Clin Microbiol Infect*. 2021;27:910.e9-910.e13.

51. Kelly CA, Egan M, Rawlinson J. Whipple's disease presenting with lung involvement. *Thorax*. 1996;51:343-344.

52. Pollock JJ. Pleuropulmonary Whipple's disease. *South Med J*. 1985;78:216-217.

53. Winberg CD, Rose ME, Rappaport H. Whipple's disease of the lung. *Am J Med*. 1978;65:873-880.

54. Urbanski G, Rivereau P, Artru L, Fenollar F, Raoult D, Puéchal X. Whipple disease revealed by lung involvement: a case report and literature review. *Chest*. 2012;141(6):1595-1598.

55. Ladna M, George J, Forsmark CE. Whipple's disease presenting with a chief complaint of dyspnea and cough from pulmonary invasion without evidence of gastrointestinal involvement. *Cureus*. 2024;16:e54554.

56. Misbah SA, Mapstone NP. Whipple's disease revisited. *J Clin Pathol*. 2000;53:750-755.

57. Foltzer MA, Guiney WB Jr, Wager CC, Alpern HD. Bronchopulmonary bacillary angiomatosis. *Chest*. 1993;104:973-975.

58. Slater LN, Min KW. Polypoid endobronchial lesions. A manifestation of bacillary angiomatosis. *Chest*. 1992;102:972-974.

59. Caponetti GC, Pantanowitz L, Marconi S, Havens JM, Lamps LW, Otis CN. Evaluation of immunohistochemistry in identifying *Bartonella henselae* in cat-scratch disease. *Am J Clin Pathol*. 2009;131(2):250-256.

60. Oteo JA, Maggi R, Portillo A, et al. Prevalence of *Bartonella* spp. by culture, PCR and serology, in veterinary personnel from Spain. *Parasit Vectors*. 2017;10(1):553.

61. Bersoff-Matcha SJ, Roper CC, Liapis H, Little JR. Primary pulmonary botryomycosis: case report and review. *Clin Infect Dis*. 1998;26:620-624.

62. Katapadi K, Pujol F, Vuletin JC, Katapadi M, Pachter BR. Pulmonary botryomycosis in a patient with AIDS. *Chest*. 1996;109:276-278.

63. Speir WA Jr, Mitchener JW, Galloway RF. Primary pulmonary botryomycosis. *Chest*. 1971;60:92-93.

64. Bender-Saebelkampf S, Franke I, Alter M, Tueting T, Gaffal E. Cutaneous and pulmonary botryomycosis. *Lancet Infect Dis*. 2019;19(6):670.

65. Ariza-Prota MA, Pando-Sandoval A, García-Clemente M, Jiménez H, Álvarez-Álvarez C, Clara PC. Primary pulmonary botryomycosis: a bacterial lung infection mimicking lung cancer. *Int J Tuberc Lung Dis*. 2013;17(7):992-994.

66. Benavides-Huerto MA, Mier-Briseño A, Lagunas-Rangel FA. Primary pulmonary botryomycosis. Report of a case and literature review. *Lung India*. 2023;40:457-461.

67. Kumar K, Daley CL, Griffith DE, Loebinger MR. Management of *Mycobacterium avium* complex and *Mycobacterium abscessus* pulmonary disease: therapeutic advances and emerging treatments. *Eur Respir Rev*. 2022;31:210212.

68. Lange C, Böttger EC, Cambau E, et al; Expert panel group for management recommendations in non-tuberculous mycobacterial pulmonary diseases. Consensus management recommendations for less common non-tuberculous mycobacterial pulmonary diseases. *Lancet Infect Dis*. 2022;22:e178-e190.

69. Blakney RA, Ricotta EE, Frankland TB, et al. Incidence of nontuberculous mycobacterial pulmonary infection, by ethnic group, Hawaii, USA, 2005-2019. *Emerg Infect Dis*. 2022;28:1543-1550.

70. Kumar K, Loebinger MR. Nontuberculous mycobacterial pulmonary disease: clinical epidemiologic features, risk factors, and diagnosis: the nontuberculous mycobacterial series. *Chest*. 2022;161:637-646.

71. Prevots DR, Marshall JE, Wagner D, Morimoto K. Global epidemiology of nontuberculous mycobacterial pulmonary disease: a review. *Clin Chest Med*. 2023;44:675-721.

72. Dheda K, Perumal T, Moultrie H, et al. The intersecting pandemics of tuberculosis and COVID-19: population-level and patient-level impact, clinical presentation, and corrective interventions. *Lancet Respir Med*. 2022;10:603-622.

73. Hruban RH, Hutchin GM. Mycobacterial infections. In: Dail DH, Hammar SP, eds. *Pulmonary Pathology*. Springer-Verlag; 1994:331-350.

74. El Zammar OA, Katzenstein AL. Pathological diagnosis of granulomatous lung disease: a review. *Histopathology*. 2007;50:289-310.

75. Barbolini G, Bisetti A, Colizzi V, Damiani G, Migaldi M, Vismara D. Immunohistologic analysis of mycobacterial antigens by monoclonal antibodies in tuberculosis and mycobacteriosis. *Hum Pathol*. 1989;20:1078-1089.

76. Salian NV, Rish JA, Eisenach KD, Cave MD, Bates JH. Polymerase chain reaction detection of Mycobacterium tuberculosis in formalin-fixed tissue. *Am J Respir Crit Care Med*. 1996;153:1419-1423.

77. Chaisson RE, Schecter GF, Theuer CP, Rutherford GW, Echenberg DF, Hopewell PC. Tuberculosis in patients with the acquired immunodeficiency syndrome. Clinical features, response to therapy, and survival. *Am Rev Respir Dis*. 1987;136:570-584.

78. Wejse C, Lillebæk T, Kirk O, Ravn P, Johansen IS, Andersen AB. The current global tuberculosis state. *Ugeskr Laeger*. 2017;179(20):V12160866.

79. Hopewell PC, Bloom BR. Tuberculosis and other mycobacterial diseases. In: Murray JF, Nadel JA, Mason RJ, Boushay H, eds. *Textbook of Respiratory Medicine*. 3rd ed. WB Saunders; 2000:1043-1105.

80. Wallace JM, Hannah JB. *Mycobacterium avium* complex infection in patients with the acquired immunodeficiency syndrome. A clinicopathologic study. *Chest*. 1988;93:926-932.

81. Christensen E, Dietz GW, Ahn C, et al. Initial roentgenographic manifestations of pulmonary *Mycobacterium tuberculosis*, *M. kansasii*, and *M. intracellulare* infections. *Chest*. 1981;80:132-147.

82. Contreras MA, Cheung OT, Sanders GE, Goldstein RS. Pulmonary infection with nontuberculous mycobacteria. *Am Rev Respir Dis*. 1988;137:149-156.

83. Farhi DC, Mason UG III, Horsburg CR Jr. Pathologic findings in disseminated *Mycobacterium avium-intracellulare* infection. A report of 11 cases. *Am J Clin Pathol*. 1986;85:67-71.

84. Marchevsky A, Damsker B, Gribetz A, Tepper S, Geller SA. The spectrum of pathology of nontuberculous mycobacterial infections in open-lung biopsy specimens. *Am J Clin Pathol*. 1982;78:695-700.

85. Zakowski P, Fligiel S, Berlin GW, Johnson L Jr. Disseminated *Mycobacterium avium-intracellulare* infection in homosexual men dying of acquired immunodeficiency. *JAMA*. 1982;248:2980-2982.

86. Sekosan M, Cleto M, Senseng G, Farolan SJ. Spindle cell pseudotumors in the lungs due to *Mycobacterium tuberculosis* in a transplant patient. *Am J Surg Pathol*. 1994;18:1065-1068.

87. Boylan KE, Larsen BT, Young BA, et al. Pulmonary mycobacterial spindle cell pseudotumor: a report of 3 cases including a practical approach to histopathologic recognition of this unusual entity. *Int J Surg Pathol*. 2018;26(7):629-634.

6

FUNGAL LUNG INFECTIONS

Fungal infections are a common complication in immunocompromised patients. Transbronchial biopsies can be useful in the diagnosis of many fungal infections. Under certain circumstances, this may be the most rapid and effective method to diagnose fungal infection in an acutely ill patient in whom opportunistic infection is clinically suspected.[1] In rare cases, wedge resections may be performed to remove larger cavitary lesions. Histologic examination will often permit a rapid diagnosis and will allow the pathologist to assign the organism to a group or genus. Definitive speciation can be obtained later and confirmed by culture. Although some fungi are visible on hematoxylin and eosin (H&E), special stains such as periodic acid-Schiff (PAS), and silver stains such as Gomori methenamine silver (GMS) or Grocott stains are usually needed to highlight the organisms.

Although more than 100 fungi have been identified in the lungs, only a small number are implicated as the source of human infection.[2] Fungi may be seen in the lungs as yeast (round spherules), hyphae (long tubular structures), and pseudohyphae (long tubular structures with regularly spaced constrictions). Fungal infections can cause several patterns of tissue damage in the lung, including necrotizing and nonnecrotizing granulomas, cavitary lesions, acute bronchopneumonia, and airway disease. The morphology of the organism can be a helpful clue for diagnosis; that is, septate mycelia with branching at 45° angles are typical of *Aspergillus* species, and large spherules with endospores are characteristic of *Coccidioides immitis*. It must be kept in mind, however, that atypical forms of many organisms may be encountered, and definitive speciation may require culture or other special techniques.[3-7]

For ease of study, fungal diseases of the lung can be divided according to their morphologic appearances into fungi characterized by round yeast forms and fungi characterized by elongated hyphal or pseudohyphal forms, acknowledging the fact that an admixture of the two may be present in certain types of organisms.

FUNGI CHARACTERIZED BY ROUND YEAST FORMS

Histoplasmosis

Histoplasmosis is the most common fungal infection worldwide and is endemic to the Ohio and Mississippi River Valleys in North America. It is also the most common opportunistic fungal infection in acquired immunodeficiency syndrome (AIDS) patients.[8-10] It also represents a source of posttransplant lung infections.[11,12] Histoplasmosis is caused by a dimorphic fungus *Histoplasma capsulatum* and can present as an asymptomatic, self-limited process that will pass clinically undetected, as an acute infection causing respiratory distress,[13] a chronic process that may become progressive and disseminated, or may result in the formation of an asymptomatic, calcified pulmonary nodule.[14] The organisms may also cause chronic cavitary disease.[15] In its later stages, it may involve mediastinal lymph nodes and eventually progress to mediastinal fibrosis and sclerosing mediastinitis. The fungus lives in the soil and is contracted by inhalation of dust infected with bird droppings. Histologically, *H capsulatum* infection results in necrotizing and nonnecrotizing granulomas that can present as large, solitary lesions, miliary nodules, or cavitary lesions (Figs. 6.1 and 6.2; eFigs. 6.1-6.3). In immunocompromised patients, intra-alveolar collections of foamy macrophages filled with organisms are seen. The process can progress to a life-threatening disseminated phase with fibrinopurulent exudates

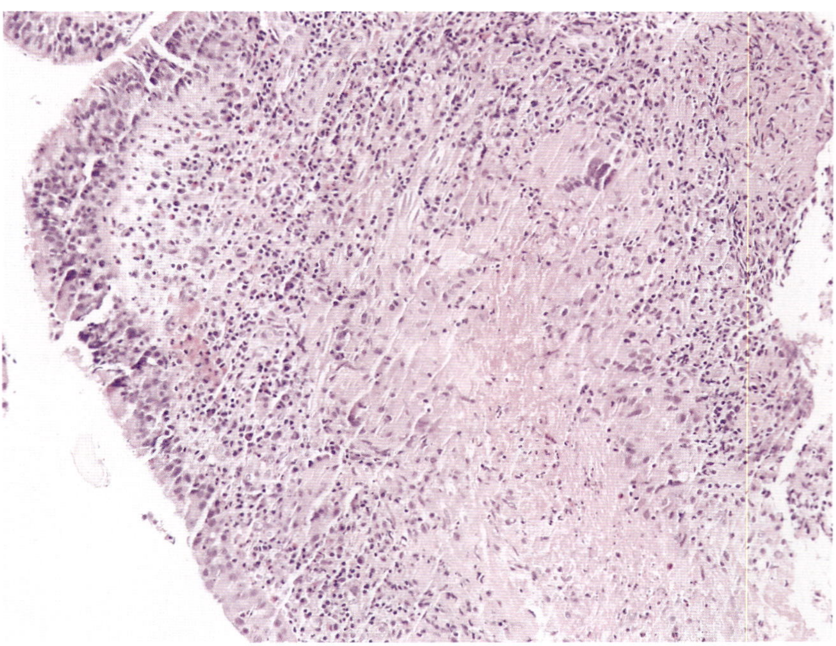

FIGURE 6.1 Bronchial biopsy showing *Histoplasma* granuloma with peripheral palisading of epithelioid histiocytes.

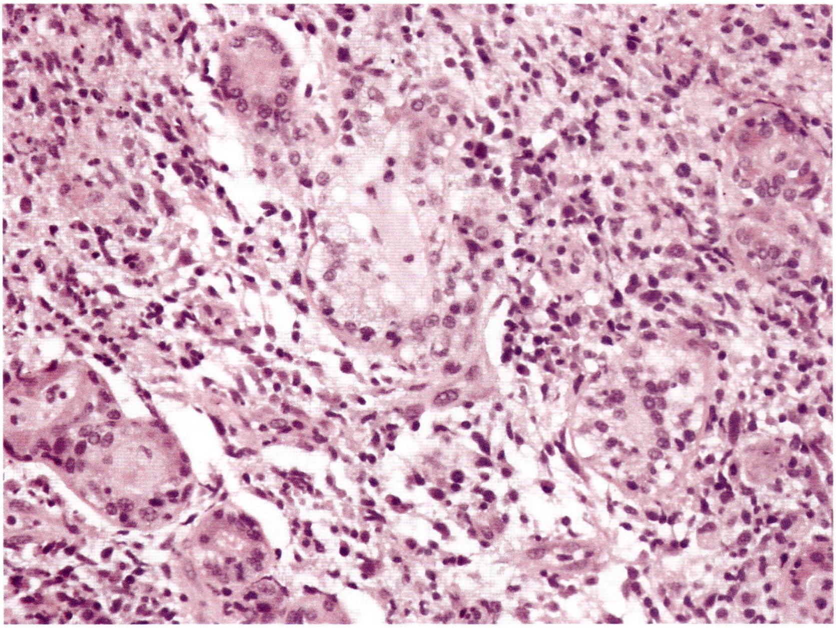

FIGURE 6.2 Higher magnification of *Histoplasma* granuloma showing round to oval, refractive structures within the cytoplasm of multinucleated giant cells.

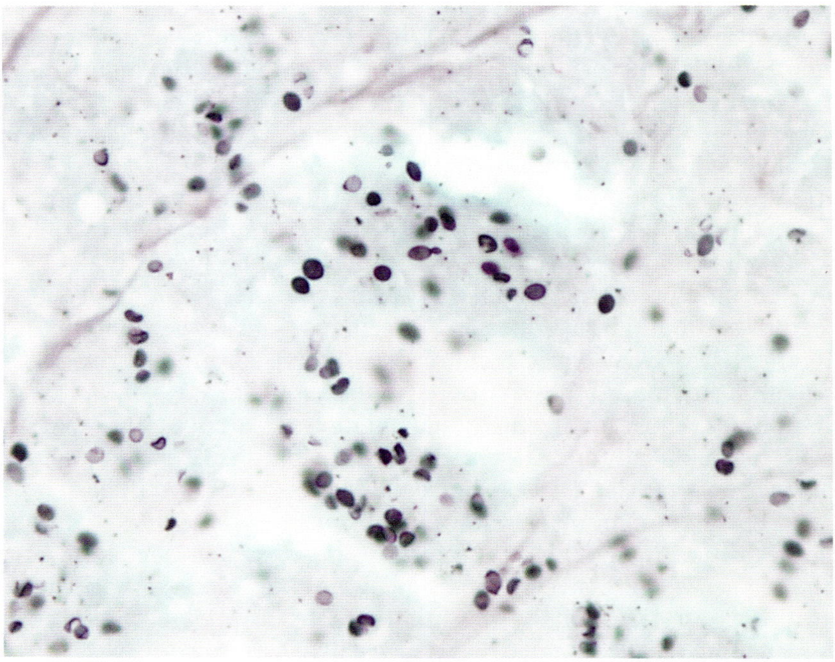

FIGURE 6.3 Gomori methenamine silver highlights the organisms in pulmonary histoplasmosis.

resembling a lobar pneumonia.[16] Chronic infection occurs most commonly in nonimmunosuppressed adults and resembles reinfection tuberculosis with cavitary lesions.

Morphologic diagnosis is based on the identification of the yeast form of *H capsulatum* in tissue sections. The organisms are characterized by small round to oval yeasts (2-4 µm), with narrow-based budding.[6] When numerous, they can be seen on H&E stains as small refractive ovoid structures within macrophages; however, they are most often very difficult to visualize on routine staining and will require the use of silver stains (ie, GMS) for identification (Fig. 6.3). Some of the organisms can show centrally placed, dotlike dark staining foci similar to those seen in *Pneumocystis jirovecii.* The diagnosis can also be established by direct immunofluorescence on histologic sections, polymerase chain reaction assays, and the use of more advanced molecular techniques such as Sanger sequencing or massively parallel sequencing assays.[17-20] The number of organisms may vary widely depending on the stage of the lesion. Early lesions can contain abundant organisms, whereas in late stage, in calcified or calcifying granulomas, the organisms may be very few or altogether absent. The small yeast of *H capsulatum* needs to be distinguished from *Pneumocystis*, capsule-deficient *Cryptococcus*, *Candida*, *Penicillium marneffei*, and *Blastomyces dermatitidis* (Table 6.1).

Blastomycosis

Blastomycosis is a fungal infection caused most commonly by *B dermatitidis* and *B gilchristii*; Dimorphic fungi is found in the soil, most commonly in North America in the Mississippi, Missouri, and Ohio River Valleys. In 2023, one of the largest documented outbreaks occurred at a paper mill in Michigan with 131 documented cases; 16 patients required hospitalization and one patient died from infection.[21] Additional clusters have also been recently identified in Minnesota.[22] The infection may be clinically asymptomatic or can be present as an acute pneumonia or chronic process.[23] The disease primarily affects the lungs but may spread to extrapulmonary sites, in particular to the skin and bone. In the lung, the disease may cause focal or diffuse lung infiltrates primarily distributed in the upper lobes, diffuse alveolar damage, and solitary or multiple nodules. Focal involvement may manifest as a pulmonary mass that can be radiologically indistinguishable from lung cancer.[24,25] Cavitation occurs in up to 20% of cases, but calcification seldom ensues. The disease is not as common in immunocompromised patients as compared to some of the other fungal lung infections but, when occurring in this setting, is more aggressive.[26] The clinical manifestations in patients with acute infection are similar to an acute bacterial pneumonia, and they can sometimes lead to acute respiratory distress syndrome.[27,28] Chronic infection is more common and is characterized by necrotizing and nonnecrotizing granulomas.

TABLE 6.1 Differential Diagnosis of Common Lung Infections Caused by Round Yeastlike Fungi

Organism	Size	Shape	Lesions	Distinguishing Features
Histoplasma capsulatum	2-4 µm	Round to oval yeast Narrow-based budding Occasional dark staining foci Intracellular location within histiocytes	Histiocytic infiltrates filled with organisms (acute form) Necrotizing and nonnecrotizing granulomas (chronic form)	Uniform small yeast with narrow-based buds Positive for periodic acid-Schiff and silver stains; negative for mucicarmine and Gram stains
Blastomyces dermatitidis	2-4 and 8-15 µm	Round to oval yeast surrounded by thick, refractile walls Broad-based buds	Suppurative inflammation (acute) Necrotizing and nonnecrotizing granulomas (chronic)	Slightly larger yeast with broad-based buds and thick, refractile walls admixed with smaller yeast
Cryptococcus neoformans	2-20 µm	Round to oval yeast surrounded by thick halo Narrow-based buds Capsule-deficient forms	Necrotizing palisading granulomas or granulomatous pneumonia (in immunocompetent patients) Histiocytic and mucoid infiltrates devoid of inflammation (in immunocompromised patients)	Positivity for mucicarmine More variable size (2-20 µm) Absence of inflammatory reaction Capsule-deficient forms may be more difficult to diagnose
Candida albicans	2-6 µm	Round to oval yeast admixed with pseudohyphae (elongated branching structures without septae)	Suppurative, necrotizing inflammation No granulomas or foamy histiocytes	Presence of pseudohyphae without septae admixed with smaller yeast forms Positive for tissue Gram stain Extracellular location

(continued)

TABLE 6.1 Differential Diagnosis of Common Lung Infections Caused by Round Yeastlike Fungi (*continued*)

Organism	Size	Shape	Lesions	Distinguishing Features
Pneumocystis jirovecii	5-7 µm cysts	Round to oval cysts with grooves and folds, and dark staining foci in the center of the cysts	Lymphocytic and fibrosing interstitial pneumonitis with foamy intra-alveolar exudates containing abundant organisms	Intra-alveolar location Foamy exudates Absence of budding walls Positive for Gomori methenamine silver and with monoclonal antibodies by immunohistochemistry
Penicillium marneffei	2.5-5 µm	Round to oval yeast with transverse septum	Abundant macrophages filled with organisms	No budding forms Also shows short hyphae and elongated, oval, and curved forms with rounded ends History of travel to Southeast Asia
Coccidioides immitis	30-100 µm	Large, round spherules with or without endospores	Necrotizing granulomas Fungus balls	Large round spherules with numerous endospores Spherules without endospores may be confused for large *Blastomyces* organisms
Paracoccidioides brasiliensis	4-60 µm	Round yeast with multiple buds	Necrotizing granulomas	Distinguished from *Cryptococcus* by the multiple buds and lack of mucicarmine staining

The histologic appearance of *B dermatitidis* is that of round to oval yeast (8-15 μm), surrounded by thick, refractile walls with double contours (Fig. 6.4). The yeasts often show buds that are single and broad-based. Occasionally, the organisms may be much smaller (2-4 μm) resembling *H capsulatum*. Larger forms (up to 30 μm) can be seen that can mimic the spherules in *Coccidioides*.[29] Organisms are highlighted by PAS and GMS stains (Fig. 6.5). Culture is the most definitive way to establish the diagnosis, but direct immunofluorescence on deparaffinized sections, immunohistochemistry, and molecular techniques can also be helpful.[18,30]

Cryptococcosis

Cryptococcosis is caused by the inhalation of spores of *Cryptococcus neoformans*, a yeast found worldwide in soil contaminated with pigeon droppings. In recent years, cases attributed to *Cryptococcus gattii* have also been identified.[31-33] There are two major clinical forms: pulmonary infection and leptomeningeal infection secondary to hematogenous spread from the lungs. Immunosuppressed patients are at higher risk for acquiring the infection. Primary lung infection is usually asymptomatic. Lung manifestations of the disease may be focal, including a nodule or mass lesion with ill-defined borders, multifocal peripheral pulmonary nodules or masses, or unilateral or bilateral parenchymal consolidation.[34]

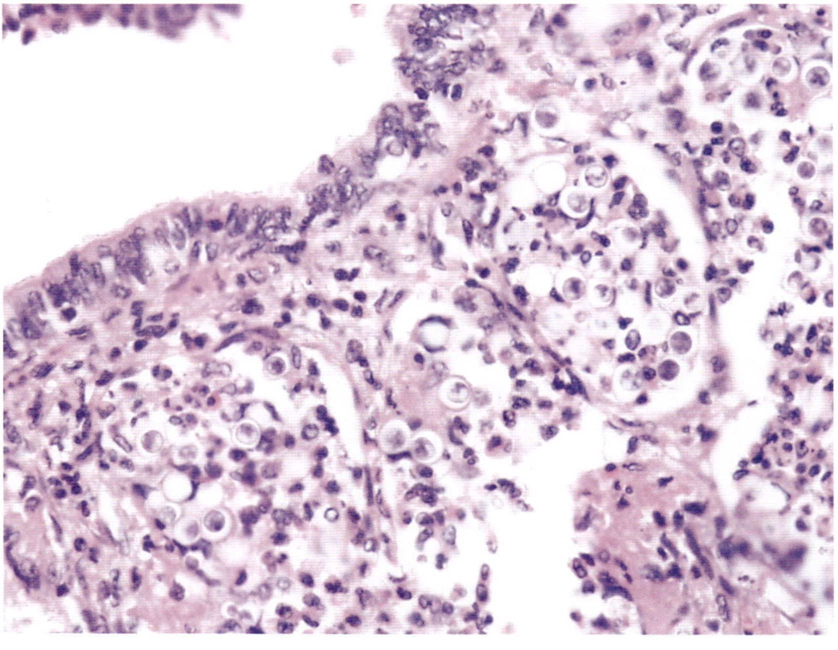

FIGURE 6.4 Endobronchial biopsy in *Blastomyces dermatitidis* pneumonia shows round yeast surrounded by a thick refractile wall with double contours and occasional single, broad-based buds.

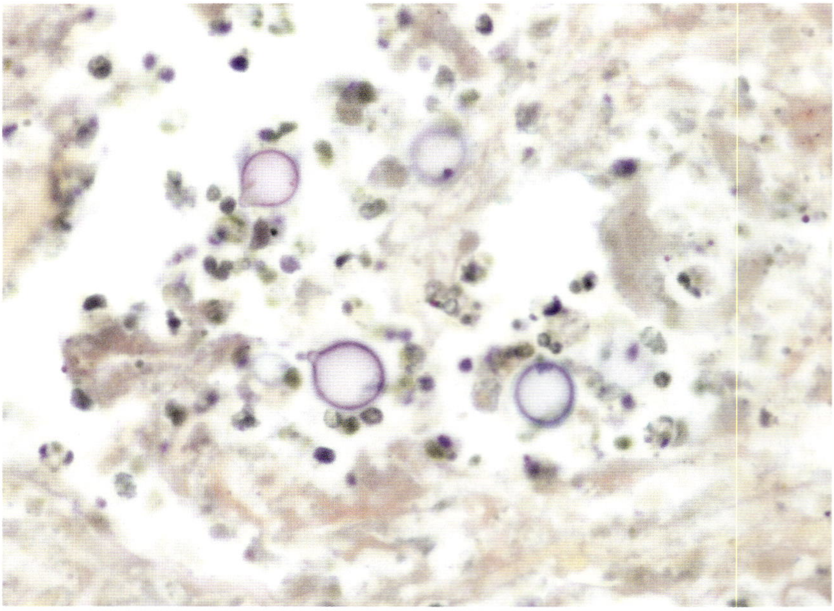

FIGURE 6.5 Periodic acid-Schiff stain in blastomycosis shows round to oval yeast surrounded by a thick refractile wall with small, broad-based single buds.

Immunocompromised patients most often exhibit disseminated disease with diffuse, bilateral interstitial infiltrates or miliary involvement that may progress to diffuse parenchymal consolidation and cavitation.[35] In immunocompetent patients, the lesions most often manifest as necrotizing palisading granulomas or as granulomatous pneumonia (Fig. 6.6); in immunocompromised patients, the infiltrates are often histiocytic and mucoid and devoid of inflammation (Fig. 6.7). In rare cases, the lesions may become fibrotic and microscopically demonstrate scattered granulomas embedded with a fibrotic stroma (Figs. 6.8-6.10).

On histology, the organisms are small, round to oval yeasts (usually 4-6 μm) that may occasionally attain larger sizes (up to 20 μm) (eFig. 6.4). Single budding with a narrow base is a characteristic feature (Fig. 6.11). The organisms are best highlighted by silver stains (Fig. 6.12; eFig. 6.5).[36] The cells appear to be surrounded by a thin halo, which actually corresponds to a mucinous capsule. This capsule is highlighted with mucin stains such as mucicarmine, a discriminating feature for diagnosis (Fig. 6.13; eFig. 6.6). The organisms can also be highlighted with PAS and Fontana-Masson. A capsule-deficient form of *C neoformans* has also been described and is typically found in immunocompetent patients. These forms may present a challenge for histologic diagnosis as they will be negative or react only weakly with the mucicarmine stain. As with other fungal diseases, definitive speciation and identification may require culture, immunohistochemistry, or advanced molecular assays such as metagenomic next-generation sequencing to establish a definitive diagnosis.[4,37]

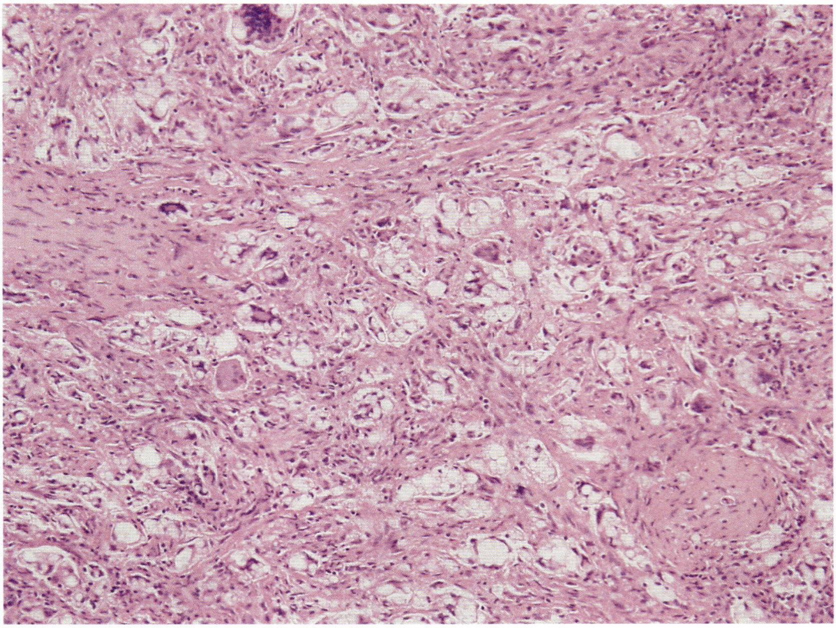

FIGURE 6.6 **Granulomatous pneumonia in an immunocompetent patient with cryptococcal infection.**

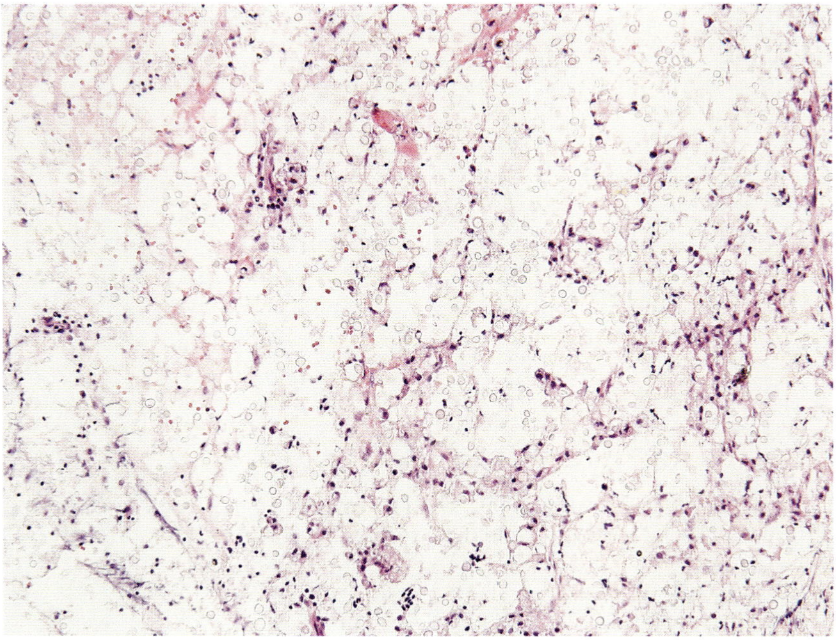

FIGURE 6.7 **Immunocompromised patient with cryptococcal pneumonia.** Notice the absence of inflammatory infiltrates and the abundance of organisms.

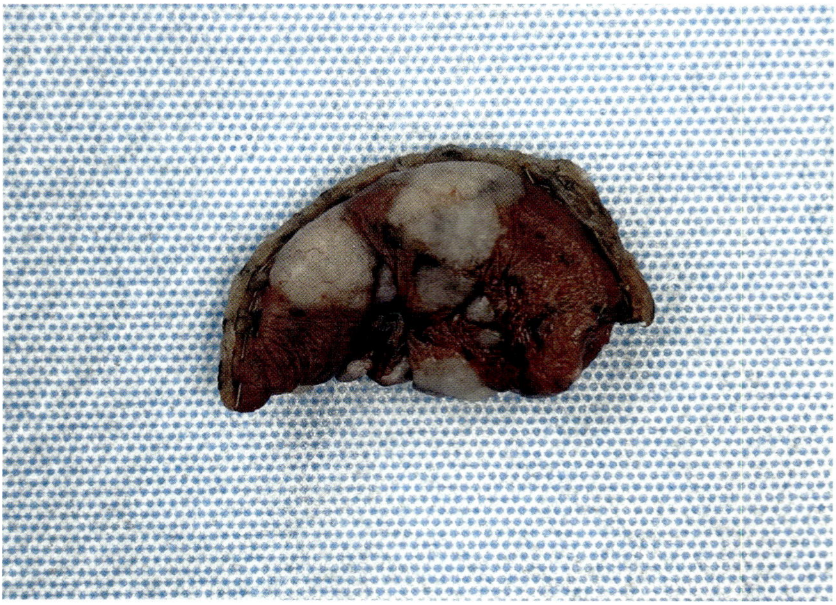

FIGURE 6.8 **Lung wedge resection in an unusual case of pulmonary *Cryptococcus* infection shows multiple small pleural based nodules.**

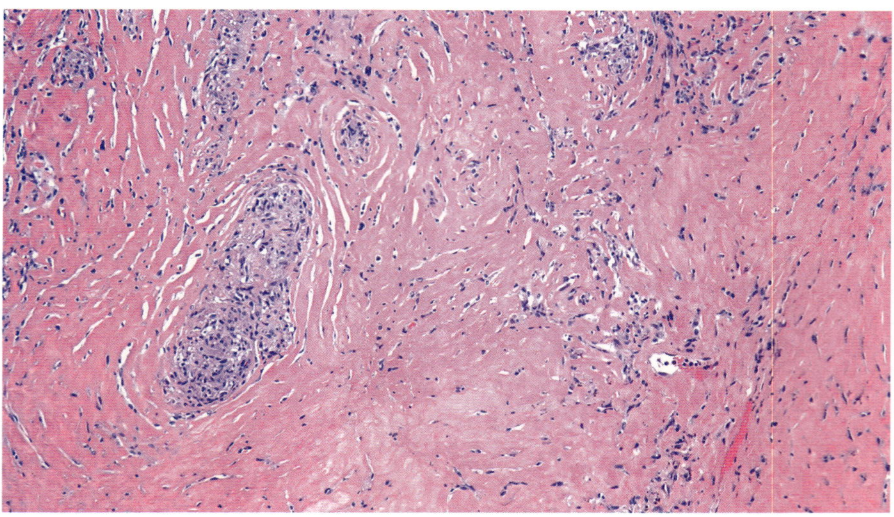

FIGURE 6.9 **Histologic examination shows areas of dense fibrotic/collagenized stroma with rare scattered granulomas.** Note that organisms are not immediately apparent.

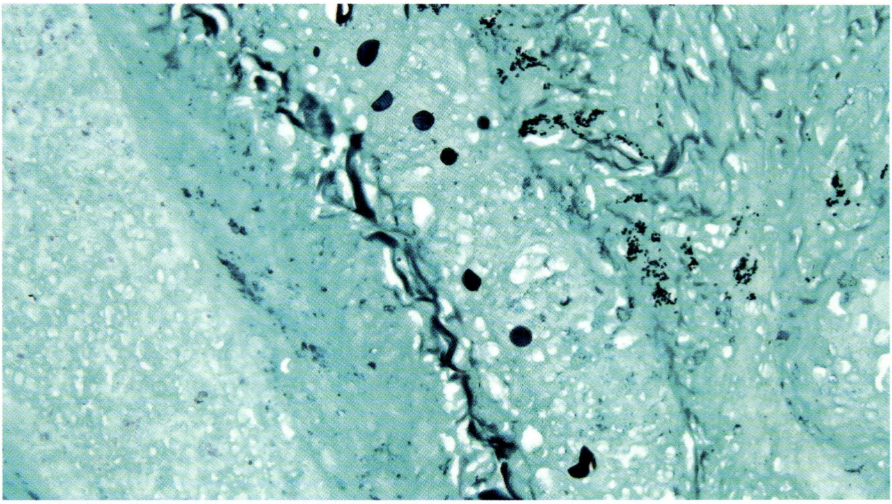

FIGURE 6.10 Sliver staining performed in multiple tissue sections identified very rare fungal yeast forms without obvious budding, but cultures of lavage fluid confirmed *Cryptococcus* spp. infection.

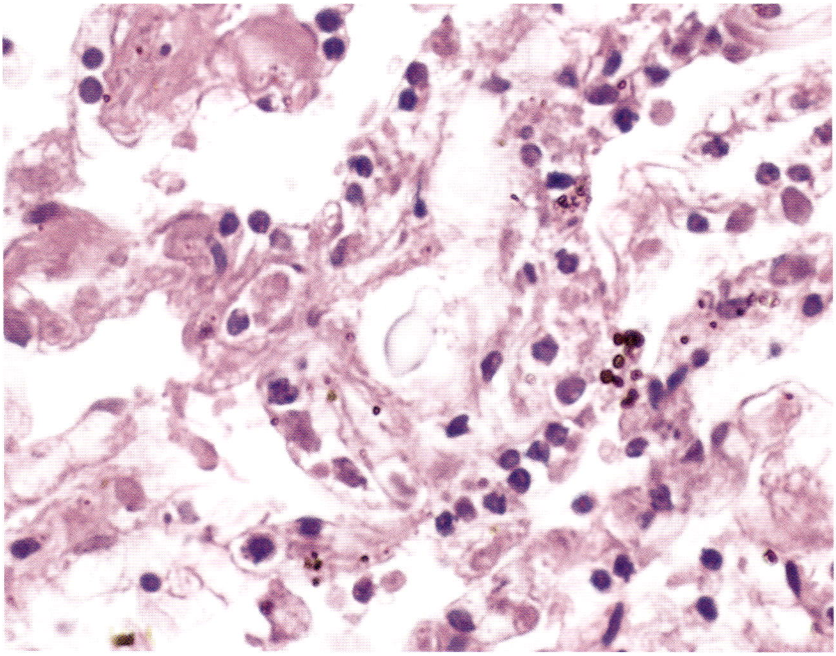

FIGURE 6.11 Lung biopsy in cryptococcal pneumonia showing an oval yeast with narrow-based single budding.

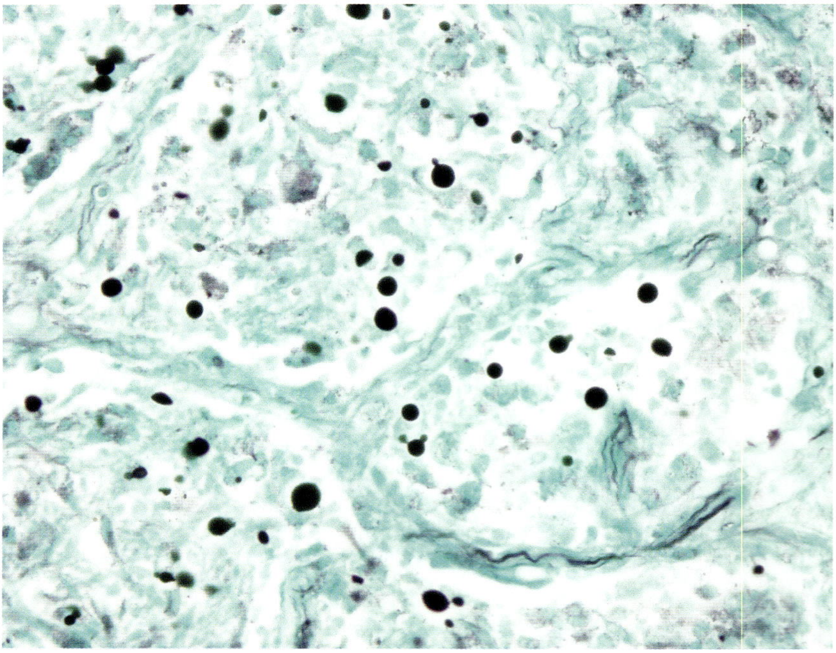

FIGURE 6.12 Methenamine silver stain in cryptococcal pneumonia shows numerous round to oval yeast with occasional single budding within alveolar spaces.

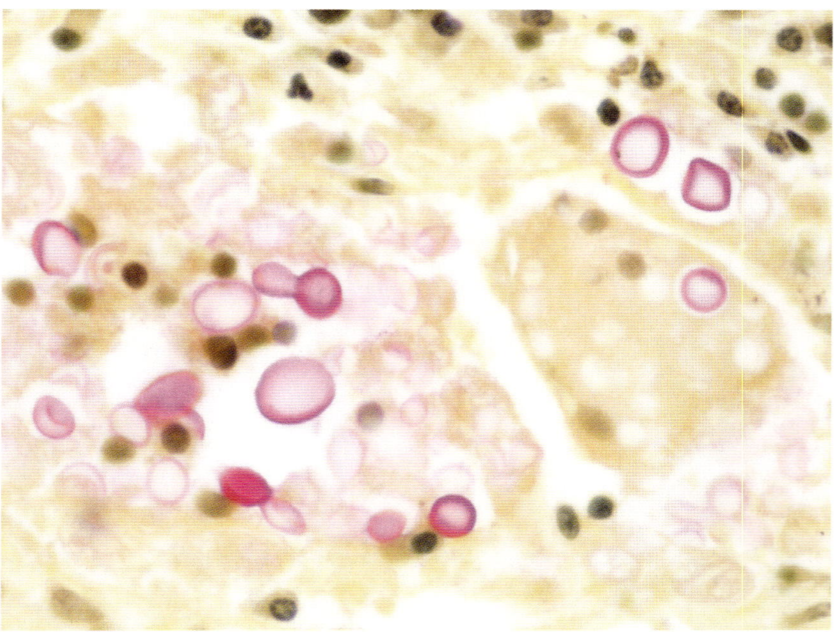

FIGURE 6.13 Mucicarmine stain in cryptococcal pneumonia shows round to oval yeast surrounded by a thick mucinous capsule and showing a few budding forms.

Candidiasis

Candidiasis is caused by yeast that is a normal commensal organism in the respiratory, gastrointestinal, and genitourinary tracts of normal individuals. In immunocompromised states, these organisms become pathogenic and invade into the tissues.[38] The most common pathogenic organism in humans is *Candida albicans*. *Candida glabrata* (formerly *Torulopsis glabrata*) is also becoming increasingly recognized as a human pathogen.[6] Pulmonary candidiasis usually manifests with unilateral or bilateral consolidation, resulting in lobar, segmental, or patchy pneumonia.[39]

Candida species are small oval yeasts (2-6 μm) that show budding and are accompanied by pseudohyphae and occasionally true hyphae. The pseudohyphae are elongated structures that often tend to line up in chains and show irregular branching at acute angles (Fig. 6.14). The pseudohyphae show constrictions at the points of attachment with other pseudohyphae but, unlike true hyphae, are not septated. The organisms are highlighted by PAS, GMS, and Gram stains. *C glabrata* is characterized only by the yeast form and does not form hyphae or pseudohyphae. Histologically, *Candida* infection is characterized by necrotic and hemorrhagic nodules containing colonies of organisms admixed with fibrinopurulent exudate. Infarcts may occur secondary

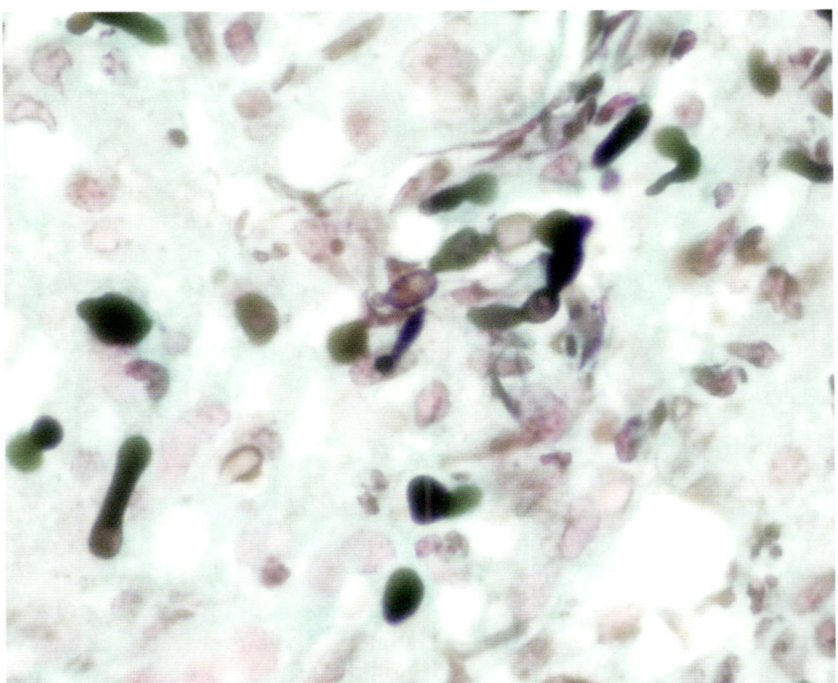

FIGURE 6.14 Silver stain in a patient with *Candida* pneumonia shows small round to oval yeast admixed with pseudohyphae.

to vascular occlusion by organisms (eFigs. 6.7 and 6.8). *Candida* may show very few pseudohyphae or present only in the yeast form, closely resembling *Histoplasma* in some cases. Unlike the organisms in histoplasmosis, *Candida* organisms will stain positive with the tissue Gram stain. Furthermore, *H capsulatum* characteristically shows an intracellular location within histiocytes, whereas *Candida* is always extracellular.

Pneumocystosis

Pneumocystosis is an important cause of opportunistic pneumonia in immunosuppressed patients.[40] Although formerly classified as a protozoan (*P carinii*), the organism is now classified as a fungus and thought to be related to the *Saccharomyces*. The species infecting humans has been renamed as *P jirovecii*.[41,42] The organism is most likely acquired through airborne inhalation of respiratory secretions. Initial exposure causes subclinical infection followed by a latent state that develops into opportunistic infection when the patient becomes immunosuppressed. Pneumocystosis can be reliably diagnosed by transbronchial lung biopsy, although equally effective approaches include cytologic examination of bronchoalveolar lavage fluid, bronchial washings, or sputum specimens.[43,44] Clinically, patients present with bilateral fine infiltrates in the perihilar region that progress to diffuse bilateral airspace consolidation involving mainly the lower lobes. AIDS patients may develop thin-walled bilateral cysts in the upper lobes in subpleural distribution.[45]

Histologically, the typical lesion of *P jirovecii* pneumonia comprises intra-alveolar foamy eosinophilic exudates containing the small organisms.[46] The frothy appearance of the eosinophilic exudate is caused by the accumulation of organisms (Figs. 6.15 and 6.16). The cysts of *Pneumocystis* are 5 to 7 μm in diameter and are round to oval. Small round, centrally placed dark staining dots are often present within the cysts. Another distinctive feature is the presence of slender grooves or longitudinal folds in the cysts owing to collapse of the cyst wall. This appearance has been likened to "crushed ping pong balls." The alveolar walls usually show mild thickening of the interstitium owing to inflammation and fibrosis, with prominence of alveolar type II pneumocytes. Fibroblastic foci with intra-alveolar plugs comprising fibromyxoid tissue may result in an organized pneumonia pattern. The best stain for demonstrating the cysts is a GMS stain (Figs. 6.17 and 6.18). Immunohistochemistry and in situ hybridization can also be performed in formalin-fixed paraffin-embedded tissue sections (Fig. 6.19).[47,48] Molecular techniques can also be used to aid in the diagnosis, including the use of next-generation sequencing assays.[49-52]

A few unusual manifestations of *Pneumocystis* pneumonia are worth underscoring. Absence of the characteristic foamy exudate may occur in up to 47% of non-HIV patients and in up to 19% of HIV-infected patients.[53,54] Granulomatous inflammation can be seen in lung biopsies in a small percentage of HIV-positive patients with *Pneumocystis* pneumonia.[55,56] The granulomas comprise clusters of small epithelioid histiocytes

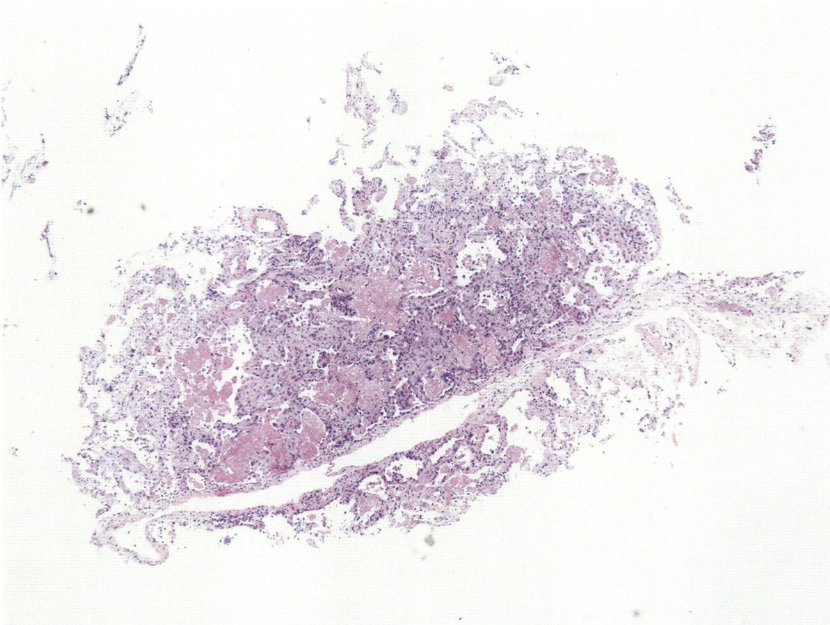

FIGURE 6.15 **Transbronchial biopsy in an AIDS patient with *Pneumocystis jirovecii* pneumonia.** Notice eosinophilic exudates within alveolar lumens.

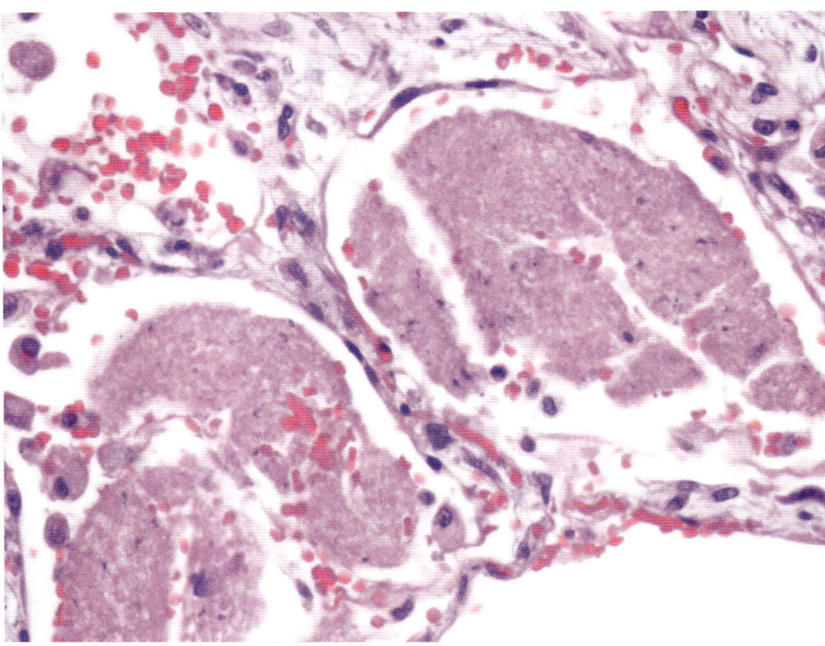

FIGURE 6.16 **Higher magnification of lung biopsy with *Pneumocystis jirovecii* pneumonia showing granular eosinophilic exudates filling the alveolar lumens.**

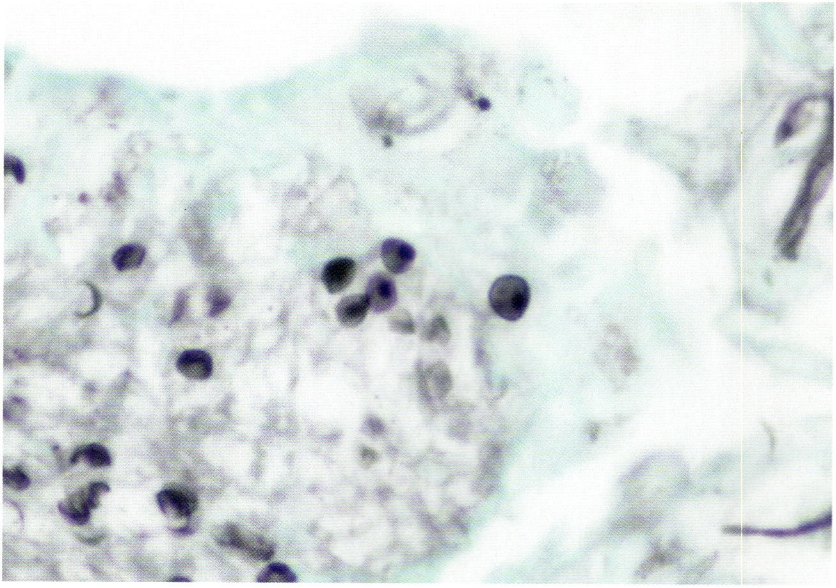

FIGURE 6.17 **Gomori methenamine silver stain highlights the organisms of *Pneumocystis jirovecii* within the intra-alveolar exudates.** The cysts are round to oval with centrally placed dark staining dots but may also show collapsed or crescent-shaped forms.

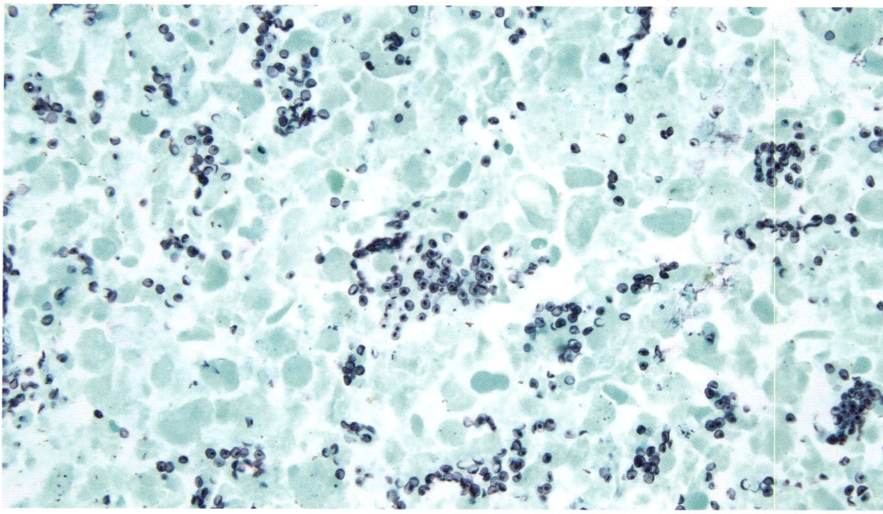

FIGURE 6.18 **Gomori methenamine silver stain highlights the organisms of *Pneumocystis jirovecii*.** Notice the prominent centrally placed dark staining dots reminiscent of large nucleoli.

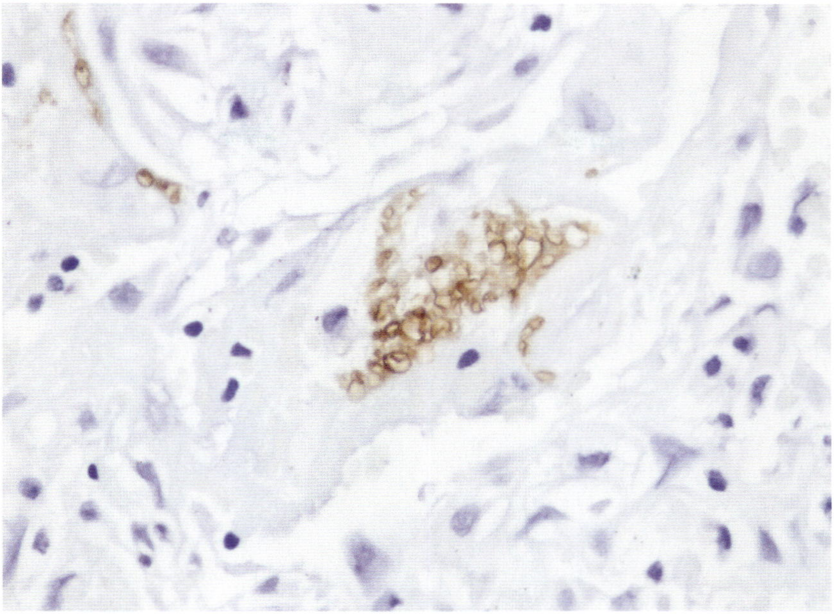

FIGURE 6.19 Immunoperoxidase stain with antibodies against *Pneumocystis jirovecii* shows positive-staining round organisms within the lumen of an alveolus.

with or without multinucleated giant cells, admixed with the characteristic frothy exudates (Fig. 6.20). In malnourished infants, the interstitium may contain a very dense lymphocytic infiltrate that can mask the intra-alveolar exudates.[57] Calcifications are another unusual occurrence in lung biopsies where alveolar exudates are absent or inconspicuous. In fact, calcifications in lymph nodes, liver, spleen, or kidney in a HIV-positive patient is highly suggestive of disseminated extrapulmonary *Pneumocystis* infection.[58,59]

Penicilliosis

Penicilliosis is caused by a dimorphic fungus that is endemic to Southeast Asia, where it represents one of the most common opportunistic infections in AIDS patients. It is seldom seen in the United States, except in immunocompromised patients who have traveled to endemic areas.[60,61] Lung infection is caused by inhalation of contaminated air. The organisms cause acute necrotizing pneumonia. Asymptomatic cases and rare cases clinically confused for malignancy have been reported.[62,63] The airspaces are stuffed with alveolar macrophages containing abundant organisms (Fig. 6.21). The organisms are round or oval yeast (2.5-5 μm) characterized by a single transverse septum. Short hyphal forms and elongated, curved sausage-shaped forms may also be seen in necrotic and cavitary lesions.

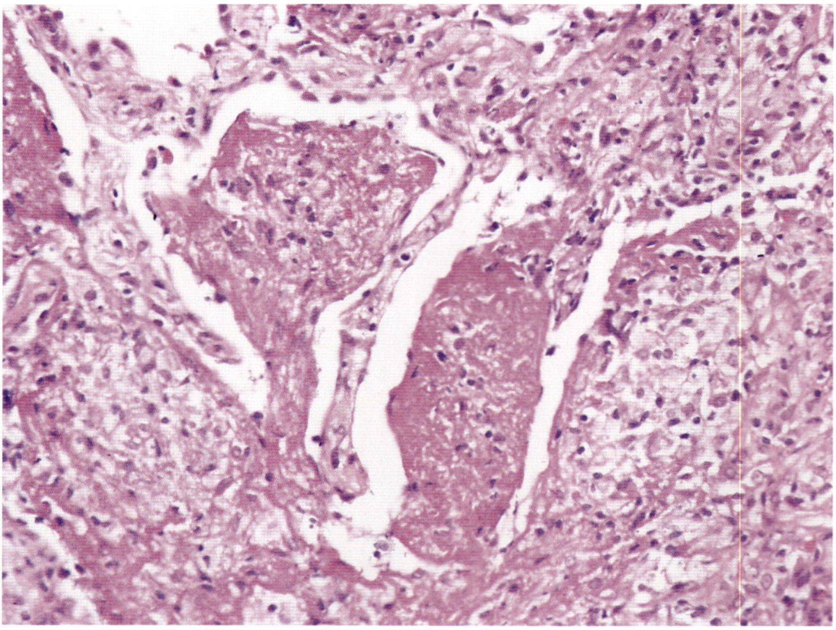

FIGURE 6.20 **Granulomatous *Pneumocystis jirovecii* lung infection characterized by clusters of epithelioid histiocytes surrounding the frothy exudates.** A high level of clinical suspicion and use of silver stains should lead to the correct diagnosis in such cases.

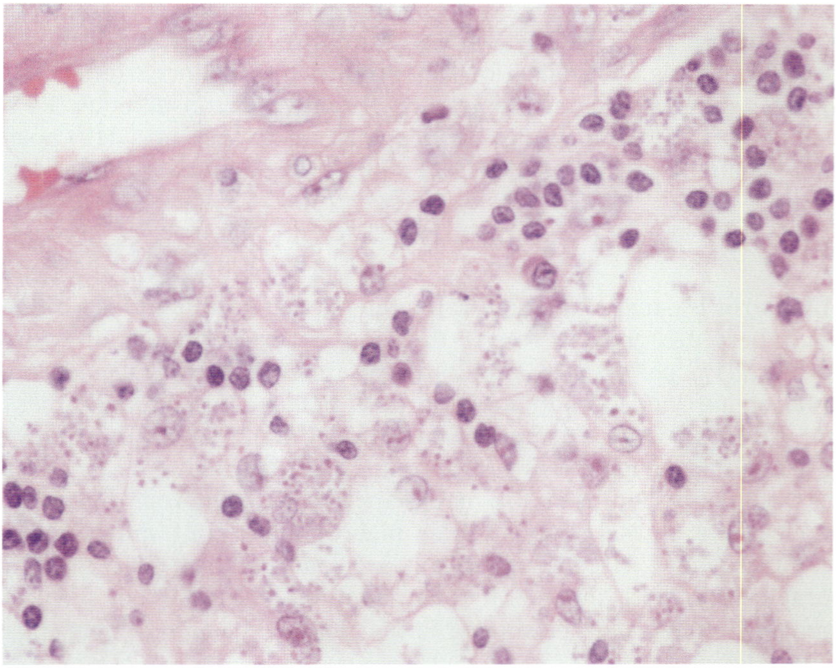

FIGURE 6.21 **Numerous small, round or oval yeast are present within alveolar macrophages in a patient with pulmonary penicilliosis.**

Coccidioidomycosis

Coccidioidomycosis is a fungal disease endemic to the southwestern United States (where it is also known as San Joaquin Valley fever) caused by a soil fungus *Coccidioides immitis* and *Coccidioides posadasii*.[64] The fungus thrives in hot, dry climates and desert soil.[65,66] The disease shows a wide spectrum of morphologic manifestations in the lungs, including asymptomatic primary infection, solitary parenchymal nodules, acute bronchopneumonia, eosinophilic pneumonia, chronic progressive disease with miliary and cavitary lesions, and systemic dissemination.[6,67,68] Histologically, the hallmark of the infection is the production of necrotizing and nonnecrotizing granulomas (Fig. 6.22). In some cases, there can be a perigranulomatous inflammatory reaction consisting of lymphocyte aggregates.[69] Mycetomas (fungus balls) may occur within cavitary lesions.[70,71] In tissue sections, *Coccidioides* is seen as mature or immature spherules and endospores (eFig. 6.9). The spherules are large (30-100 µm), round to oval, and contain multiple endospores that measure from 2 to 5 µm (Fig. 6.23). The diagnosis of the disease requires the identification of the endosporulating organism. Immature spherules lack endospores. The mature spherules have a thick refractile wall. When mature spherules rupture, they spill their endospores into the surrounding tissues; the endospores stain with GMS and PAS stains (Fig. 6.24). Vegetative forms may also be seen in tissue sections and comprise 2- to 4-µm-thick septate hyphae that produce chains of barrel-shaped arthroconidia. The latter are usually present in cavitary lesions and in fungus balls and may cause problems distinguishing them from other hyphae-producing fungi (Table 6.2).

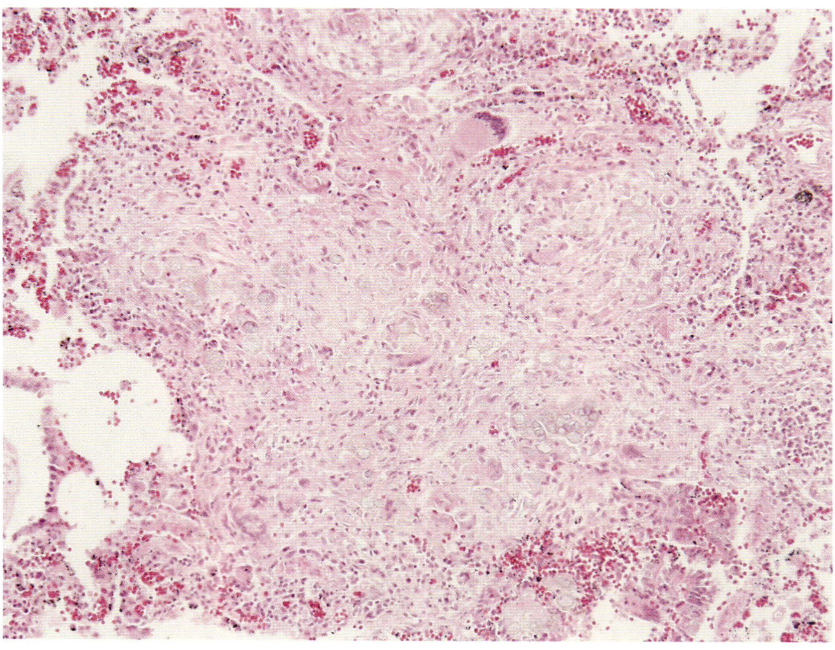

FIGURE 6.22 **Granulomatous pneumonitis in coccidioidomycosis.** Notice the epithelioid granulomas containing numerous fungal organisms within multinucleated giant cells.

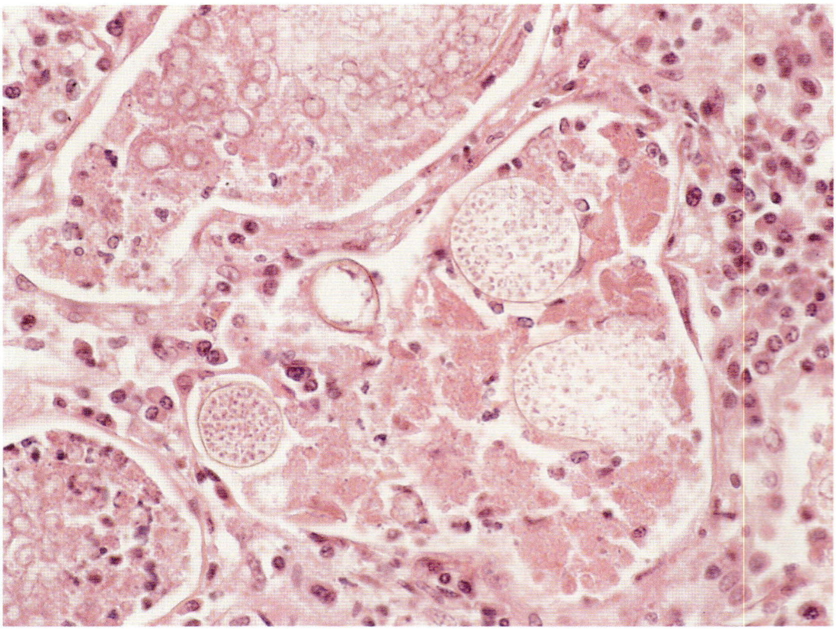

FIGURE 6.23 **Higher magnification of lung infection with *Coccidioides immitis* shows abundant spherules within multinucleated giant cells.** Some of the spherules are large and contain multiple endospores.

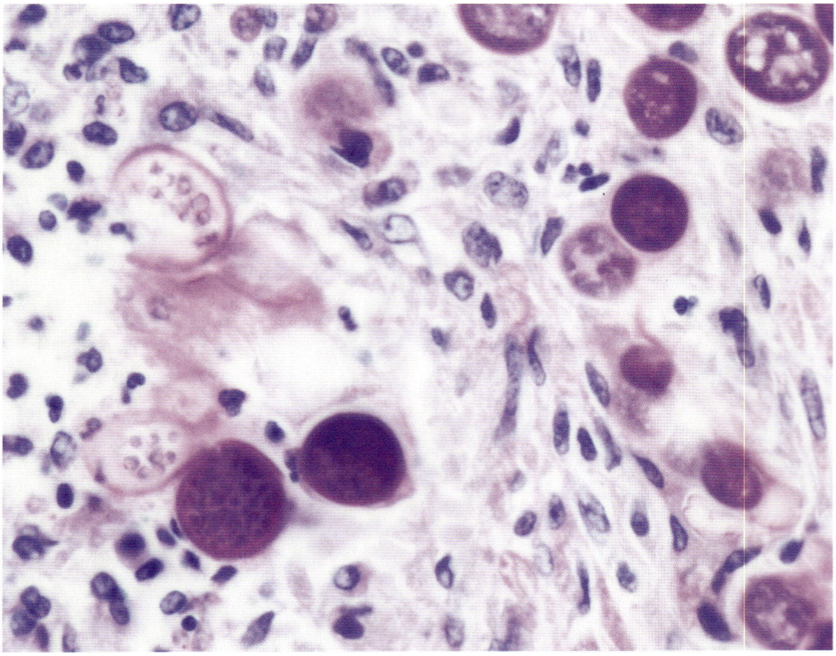

FIGURE 6.24 **Periodic acid-Schiff stain highlights the spherules in coccidioidomycosis.** Notice that some of the spherules contain abundant small endospores.

TABLE 6.2 Differential Diagnosis of Common Lung Infections Caused by Elongated Hyphal Organisms

Organism	Size	Shape	Lesions	Distinguishing Features
Candida albicans	2-6 μm width	Round to oval yeast admixed with pseudohyphae (elongated branching structures without septae)	Suppurative, necrotizing inflammation No granulomas or foamy histiocytes	Pseudohyphae without septae admixed with smaller yeast forms Gram positive Extracellular location
Aspergillus	3-6 μm width	Elongated septate hyphae with dichotomous branching Fruiting bodies and conidial heads	Necrotizing inflammation with angioinvasion	Septate hyphae with regular branching at acute angles May show swelling of hyphae resembling zygomycosis PAS and GMS positive
Zygomycetes	5-25 μm width	Broad, thin-walled hyphae with few septae and irregular branching at wide angles	Necrotizing inflammation with angioinvasion	Thick hyphae with irregular branching at wide angles GMS positive
Vegetative forms of *Coccidioides*	2-4 μm width	Septate hyphae and chains of barrel-shaped arthroconidia	Necrotizing inflammation in cavitary lesions	Need to find large spherules with endospores for definitive diagnosis

PAS, periodic acid-Schiff; GMS, Gomori methenamine silver.

When endospores cannot be identified in the spherules, definitive diagnosis may require culture, serologic testing, immunofluorescence, and molecular testing.[30,72,73]

Paracoccidioidomycosis

Paracoccidioidomycosis, also known as South American blastomycosis, is a fungal infection caused by *Paracoccidioides brasiliensis*. The disease is endemic to tropical regions of South America and is caused by inhalation of the organisms.[74,75] The lungs are the primary site of infection, but in more than 60% of patients, the disease becomes systemic. Pulmonary infection may be acute or chronic and can mimic tuberculosis and sarcoidosis. The main histologic manifestation is that of necrotizing granulomas. The histologic hallmark of the disease is the presence of yeasts (blastoconidia) with multiple buds. The organisms are large round yeast of varying sizes (4-60 µm) surrounded by a thick wall. Multiple buds are seen in the periphery of the yeast, imparting them with the distinctive "mariner's wheel" or "ship's wheel" appearance (Fig. 6.25). In tissues, the organisms are best demonstrated with GMS stains. Molecular assays are now available as well, which may aid in establishing the diagnosis.[76]

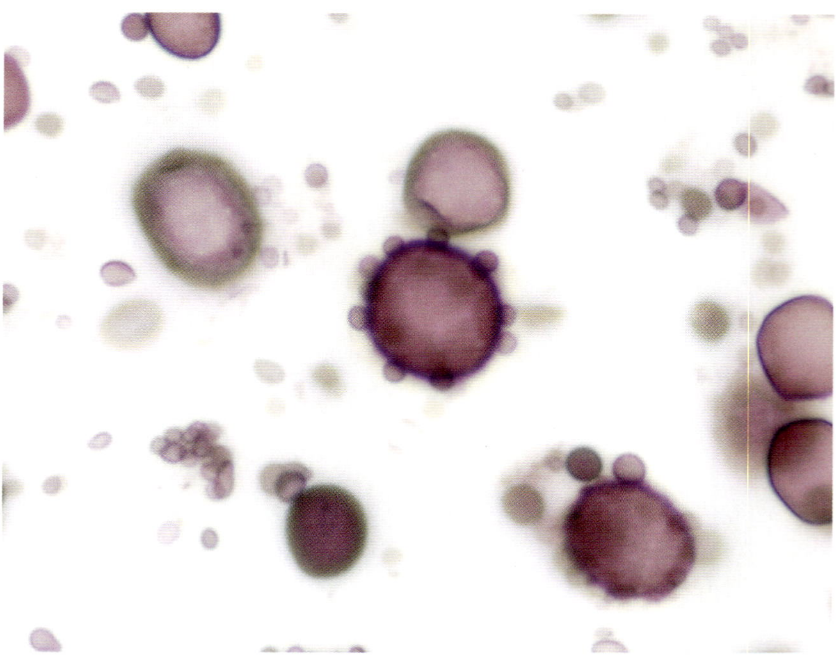

FIGURE 6.25 Pulmonary infection by *Paracoccidioides brasiliensis* shows large yeast with multiple buds resembling a mariner's wheel (Gomori methenamine silver stain).

FUNGI CHARACTERIZED BY ELONGATED HYPHAL FORMS

Aspergillosis

Aspergillosis is an infection caused by a mold, *Aspergillus*, of ubiquitous distribution. The most common types are *Aspergillus fumigatus*, *Aspergillus flavus*, and *Aspergillus niger*.[6,77] The molds are inhaled into the respiratory tract, leading to various patterns of lung injury, including colonization of the airways or preexisting cavities (fungus ball), hypersensitivity reactions, and invasive aspergillosis. Fungus balls ("aspergilloma") usually result from colonization of preexisting cavitary lesions, such as those of tuberculosis, bronchiectasis, chronic lung abscess, histoplasmosis, and cancer.[78] Hypersensitivity reactions can present in the lung in two forms: allergic bronchopulmonary aspergillosis and hypersensitivity pneumonitis. Acute invasive aspergillosis is a life-threatening condition that usually occurs in immunocompromised patients. Patients present with clinical features that resemble acute bacterial pneumonia. It can be difficult to make a correct diagnosis because sputum cultures are often negative; endoscopic or open lung biopsy may be very helpful for definitive diagnosis. Chronic necrotizing aspergillosis, the chronic form of the disease, is characterized by necrotizing granulomatous pneumonia, granulomatous bronchiectatic cavities, or bronchocentric granulomatosis.[79] In the latter, the lesions develop around bronchioles surrounded by granulomatous inflammation and contain mucus, necrotic debris, and hyphal fragments of *Aspergillus*.[79,80] The bronchioles may undergo extensive squamous metaplasia owing to the chronic irritation by the organisms (Fig. 6.26).

Aspergillus species is characterized in tissue sections by elongated, septate, and branching hyphae that are 3 to 6 µm in width. The hyphae tend to grow in an orderly, parallel fashion and show septa at regular intervals without constrictions at the points of septation. The branches of the hyphae are dichotomous, that is, the size of the branches are the same as the parent hyphae, and they are usually seen at acute angles (45°) (Fig. 6.27).[6] The hyphae may show degenerative changes such as swelling of hyphal segments, making it difficult to distinguish them from that of other fungi such as mucormycosis. The organisms are easily visualized on H&E stains but are better highlighted with PAS or GMS stains (Fig. 6.28). An anti-*Aspergillus* antibody is also available; however, the majority of diagnoses only require conventional GMS stains.[81] In allergic bronchopulmonary aspergillosis, there is usually scant hyphae with admixed mucous material harboring mixed inflammatory cells, Charcot-Leyden crystals, and Curschmann spirals. *A. niger* is associated with deposits of calcium oxalate crystals.[6] When the organisms are found in cavities exposed to air, they can develop fruiting bodies and conidial heads, which consist of a central vesicle surrounded by sterigmata and chains of conidia resembling a flower in bloom (Figs. 6.29 and 6.30). In chronic granulomatous lesions, the hyphae may be surrounded by the Splendore-Hoeppli phenomenon comprising radiating eosinophilic material at the periphery of the fungal

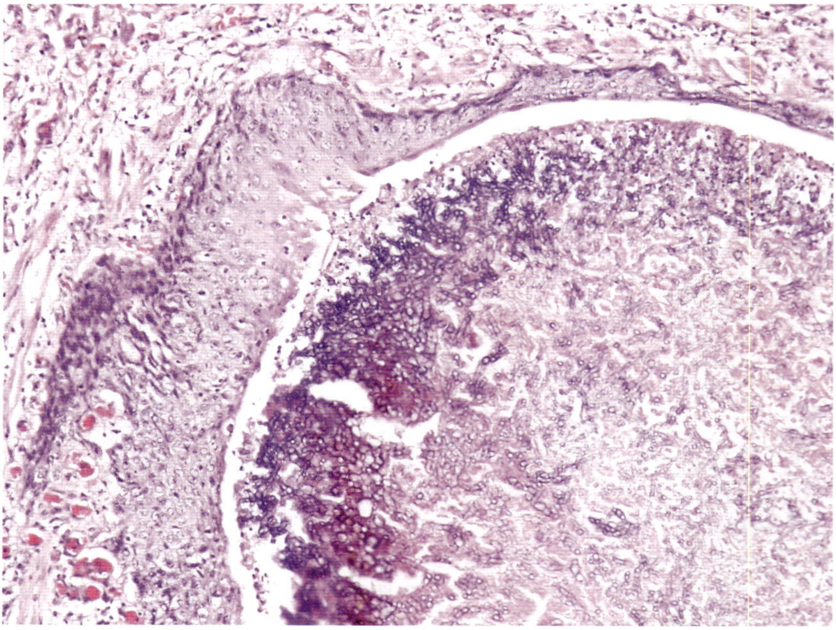

FIGURE 6.26 **Extensive squamous metaplasia of a bronchiole is observed in this biopsy.** The lumen of the bronchiole is filled with septate, branching hyphae of *Aspergillus*.

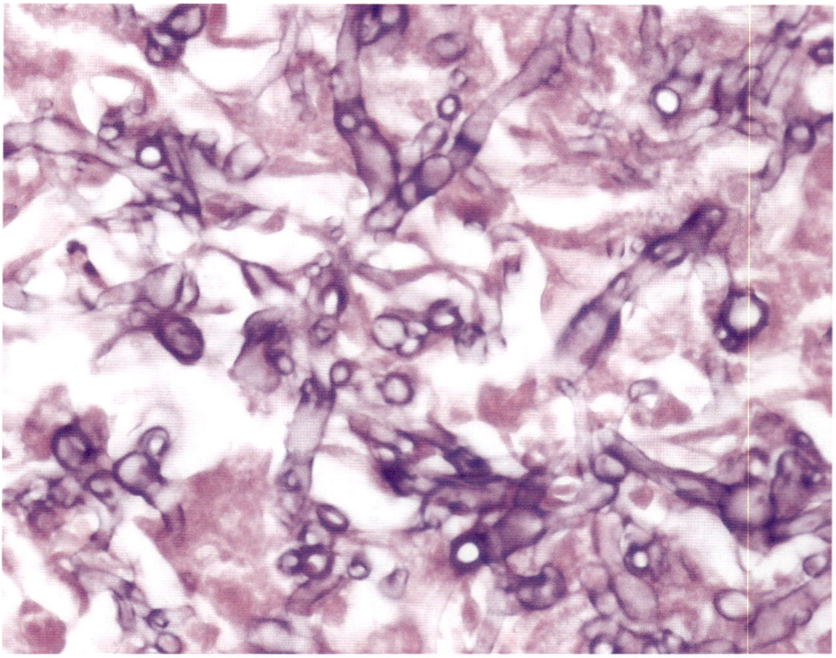

FIGURE 6.27 **Higher magnification showing the characteristic septate hyphae of *Aspergillus* sp. showing branching at acute angles.**

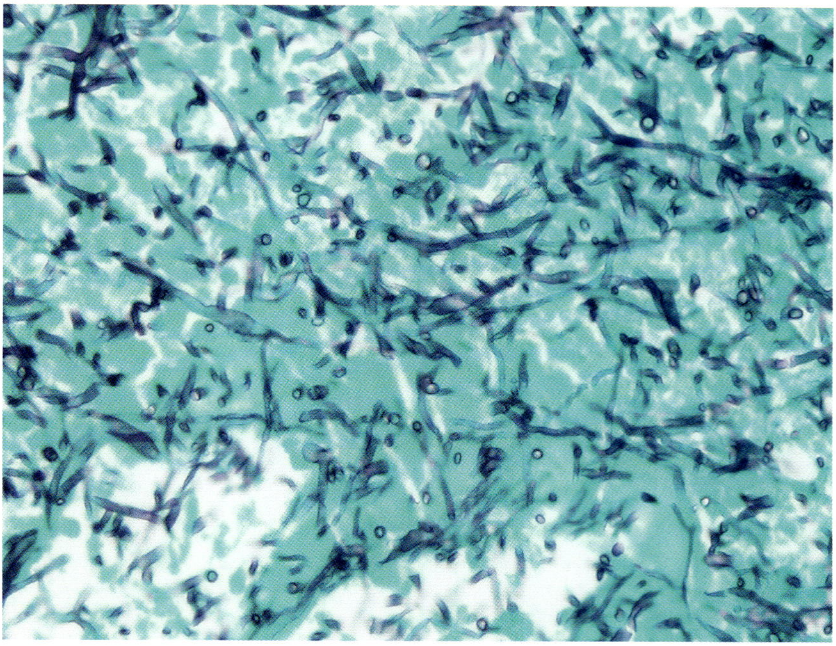

FIGURE 6.28 **Gomori methenamine silver stain highlights the organisms in invasive aspergillosis.** Notice branching septate hyphae.

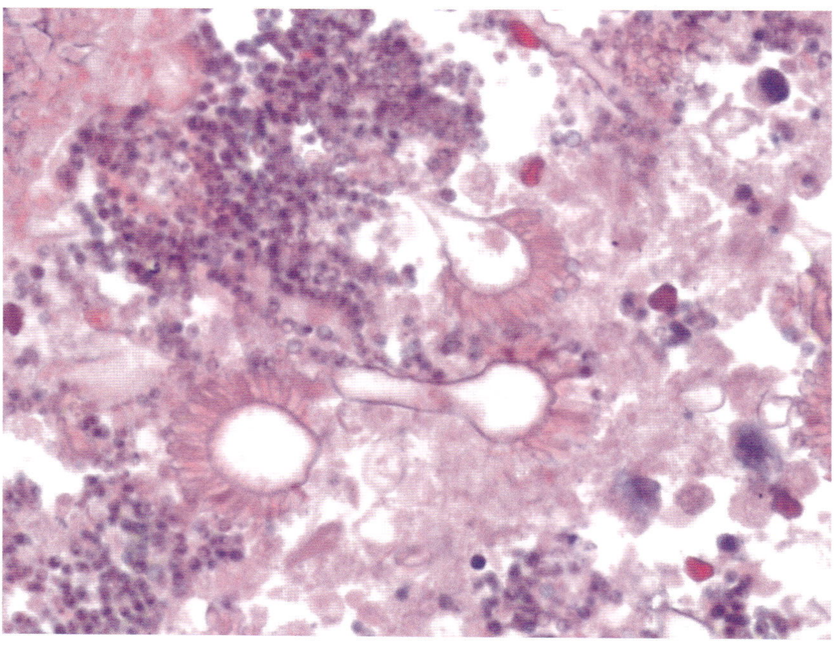

FIGURE 6.29 **Fruiting bodies and conidial heads are seen in pulmonary aspergilloma.** Notice central vesicles surrounded by multiple sterigmata resembling the petals of a flower.

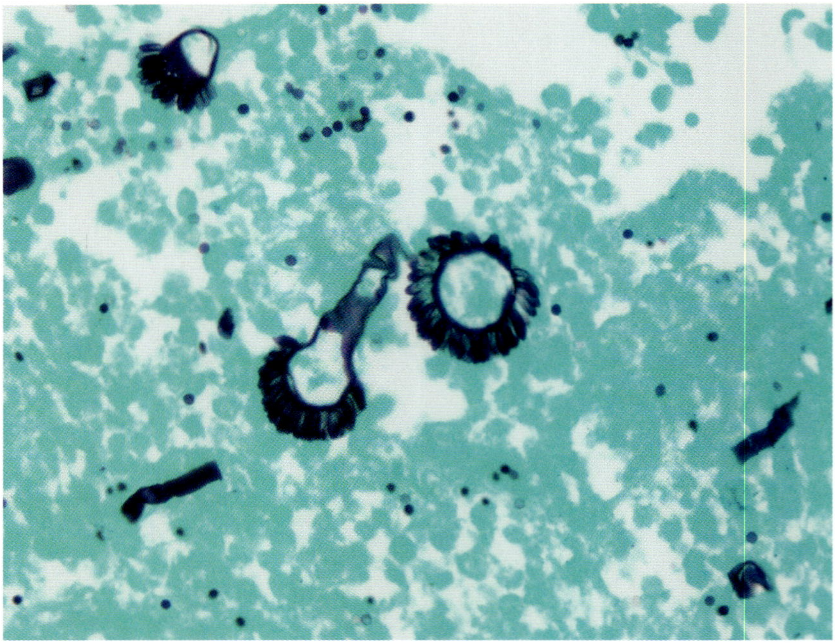

FIGURE 6.30 Gomori methenamine silver stain in pulmonary aspergilloma highlights fruiting bodies and conidial heads.

mass.[79] In acute invasive aspergillosis, there is extensive infarction of lung parenchyma with invasion of vessel walls and vascular occlusion by the organisms.

The diagnosis of pulmonary aspergillosis is usually straightforward in most cases; however, degenerative changes can make definitive diagnosis difficult in some cases (Table 6.2). In particular, it can be difficult to separate *Aspergillus* from *Zygomycetes*, *Fusarium*, and *Pseudallescheria boydii*, requiring confirmation of the diagnosis by culture, immunologic or molecular methods.[82]

Zygomycosis

Zygomycosis is caused by fungi belonging to the class of *Zygomycetes* that share with *Aspergillus* the capacity for angioinvasion leading to hemorrhagic infarcts. There are two orders of *Zygomycetes*: the Mucorales and the Entomophthorales; however, the majority of human disease is caused by the Mucorales, which includes the genera *Absidia*, *Rhizopus*, *Rhizomucor*, and *Mucor*, among others. Despite the fact that historically, the taxonomically incorrect term "mucormycosis" has been used for these infections, the majority of cases are caused by *Absidia* and *Rhizopus*.[83] Pulmonary infection occurs by inhalation of the spores or by percutaneous routes and is most often seen in the setting of immunosuppression,

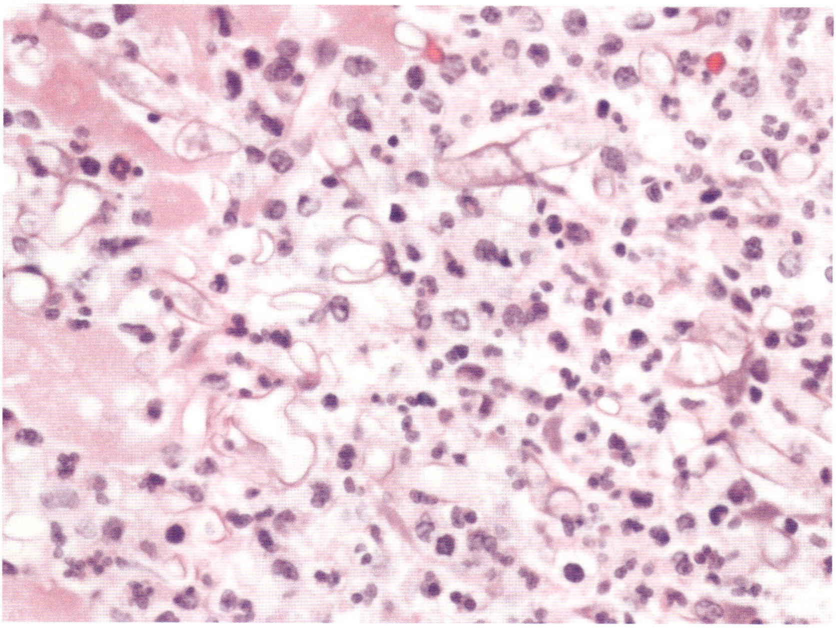

FIGURE 6.31 Necrotizing pneumonitis in zygomycosis owing to *Mucor* species shows broad, thin-walled hyphae that show irregular twisting and folding and show irregular branching.

hematopoietic malignancies, and diabetes mellitus with acidosis.[84] There is a broad spectrum of pulmonary disease that includes solitary or multiple nodular lesions, segmental or lobar consolidation, cavitary lesions, infarcts, and formation of fungus balls.[85] The lesions can undergo direct extension into the chest cavity and organs. Pulmonary zygomycosis is characterized by invasive growth, with angioinvasion, vascular thrombosis, and infarcts (Fig. 6.31).

Morphologically, the organisms are characterized by broad, thin-walled hyphae that range from 5 to 25 µm in width. The hyphae are usually twisted or folded and show irregular branching at wide angles and few or inconspicuous septae (eFig. 6.10).[6] On cross sections, the hyphae can appear as large, round, or oval structures with clear centers that may be confused for other organisms. The hyphae usually stain very weakly with H&E and can be highlighted with a GMS stain (Fig. 6.32). In cavitary lesions exposed to air, the hyphae may develop large, spherical, or ovoid, thick-walled chlamydospores at their ends. These are densely basophilic and positive for PAS. Culture or immunohistochemical methods are most commonly used to support the histopathologic diagnosis, though molecular testing may provide the most accurate way of speciating different mucormycosis species.[86]

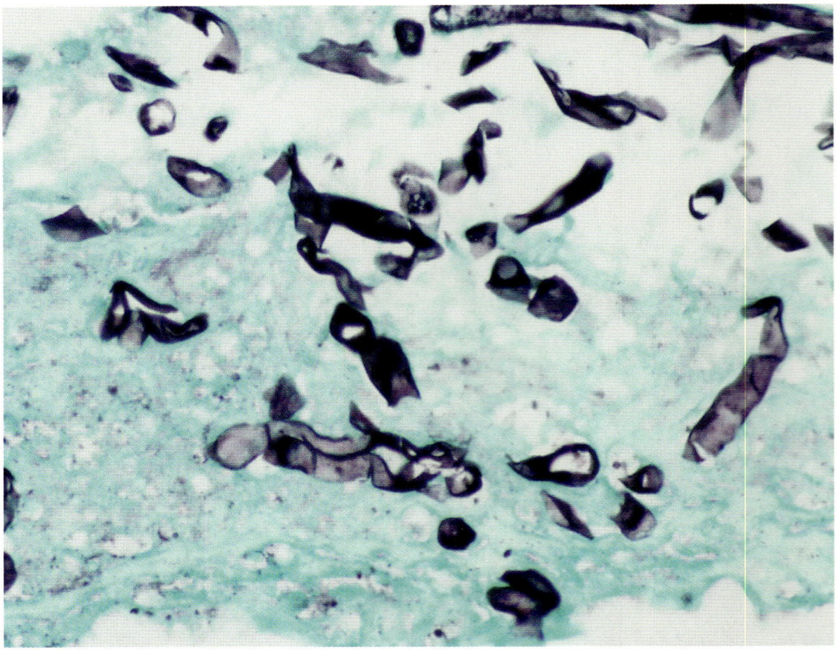

FIGURE 6.32 Gomori methenamine silver stain highlights the organisms in pulmonary infection by *Zygomycetes*.

OTHER RARE FUNGAL DISORDERS

A number of other less common fungal infections can be seen in the lungs, including sporotrichosis, phaeohyphomycosis, fusariosis, pseudallescheriasis, adiaspiromycosis, and malasseziosis. These are quite rare and definitive diagnosis requires culture, immunologic, or molecular testing methods.[87]

REFERENCES

1. El-Zammar OA, Katzenstein AL. Pathological diagnosis of granulomatous lung disease: a review. *Histopathology*. 2007;50:289-310.
2. Saubolle M. Fungal pneumonias. *Semin Respir Infect*. 2000;15:162-177.
3. Watts JC, Chandler FW. Morphologic identification of mycelia pathogens in tissue sections: a caveat. *Am J Clin Pathol*. 1998;109:1-2.
4. Cartun RW. Use of immunohistochemistry in the surgical pathology laboratory for the diagnosis of infectious disease. *Pathol Case Rev*. 1999;4:260-265.
5. Wolk D, Mitchell S, Patel R. Principles of molecular microbiology testing methods. *Infect Dis Clin N Am*. 2001;15:1157-1204.
6. Guarner J, Brandt ME. Histopathologic diagnosis of fungal infections in the 21st century. *Clin Microbiol Rev*. 2011;24(2):247-280.
7. Sangoi AR, Rogers WM, Longacre TA, Montoya JG, Baron EJ, Banaei N. Challenges and pitfalls of morphologic identification of fungal infections in histologic and cytologic specimens: a ten-year retrospective review at a single institution. *Am J Clin Pathol*. 2009;131(3):364-375.

8. Wheat J. Endemic mycoses in AIDS: a clinical review. *Clin Microbiol Rev*. 1995;8:146-159.
9. Kauffman CA. Diagnosis of histoplasmosis in immunosuppressed patients. *Curr Opin Infect Dis*. 2008;21(4):421-425.
10. Loulergue P, Bastides F, Baudouin V, et al. Literature review and case histories of *Histoplasma capsulatum* var. *duboisii* infections in HIV-infected patients. *Emerg Infect Dis*. 2007;13(11):1647-1652.
11. Rutjanawech S, Zuniga-Moya JC, George I, et al. Presentation and outcomes of histoplasmosis in transplant recipients: a retrospective single-centre cohort study. *Transpl Infect Dis*. 2024;27:e14421.
12. Abad CLR, Razonable RR. Clinical characteristics and outcomes of endemic mycoses after solid organ transplantation: a comprehensive review. *Open Forum Infect Dis*. 2024;11(3):ofae036.
13. Mukhopadhyay S, Katzenstein AL. Biopsy findings in acute pulmonary histoplasmosis: unusual histologic features in 4 cases mimicking lymphomatoid granulomatosis. *Am J Surg Pathol*. 2010;34(4):541-546.
14. Weydert JA, Van Natta TL, DeYoung BR. Comparison of fungal culture versus surgical pathology examination in the detection of *Histoplasma* in surgically excised pulmonary granulomas. *Arch Pathol Lab Med*. 2007;131(5):780-783.
15. Albandak M, Azar J, Ayyad M, et al. Chronic cavitary pulmonary histoplasmosis in an immunocompetent patient. *Cureus*. 2023;15(4):e37095.
16. Goodwin RA Jr, Shapiro JL, Thurman GH, Thurman SS, Prez RMD. Disseminated histoplasmosis: clinical and pathologic correlations. *Medicine (Baltimore)*. 1980;59:1-33.
17. Bialek R, Feucht A, Aepinus C, et al. Evaluation of two nested PCR assays for detection of *Histoplasma capsulatum* DNA in human tissue. *J Clin Microbiol*. 2002;40(5):1644-1647.
18. Chandler FW, Watts JC. *Pathologic Diagnosis of Fungal Infections*. American Society of Clinical Pathologists; 1987.
19. Trecourt A, Rabodonirina M, Donzel M, et al. *Cryptococcus neoformans/gattii* and *Histoplasma capsulatum* var. capsulatum infections on tissue sections: diagnostic pitfalls and relevance of an integrated histomolecular diagnosis. *Med Mycol*. 2024;63(1):myae126.
20. Chen J, Li Y, Li Z, Chen G, Liu X, Ding L. Metagenomic next-generation sequencing identified Histoplasma capsulatum in the lung and epiglottis of a Chinese patient: a case report. *Int J Infect Dis*. 2020;101:33-37.
21. Hennessee I, Palmer S, Reik R, et al. Epidemiological and clinical features of a large blastomycosis outbreak at a paper mill in Michigan. *Clin Infect Dis*. 2025;80(2):356-363.
22. Bagal UR, Ireland M, Gross A, et al. Molecular epidemiology of *Blastomyces gilchristii* clusters, Minnesota, USA. *Emerg Infect Dis*. 2022;28(9):1924-1926.
23. Lemos LB, Baliga M, Guo M. Blastomycosis: the great pretender can also be an opportunist. Initial clinical diagnosis and underlying disease in 123 patients. *Ann Diagn Pathol*. 2002;6:194-203.
24. Martynowicz MA, Prakash UB. Pulmonary blastomycosis: an appraisal of diagnostic techniques. *Chest*. 2002;121(3):768-773.
25. Gazzoni FF, Severo LC, Marchiori E, et al. Fungal diseases mimicking primary lung cancer: radiologic-pathologic correlation. *Mycoses*. 2014;57(4):197-208.
26. Glassroth J. Fungal infections complicating HIV infection. In: Sarosi GA, Davies SF, eds. *Fungal Diseases of the Lung*. 3rd ed. Lippincott Williams & Wilkins; 2002:213-218.
27. Lemos LB, Baliga M, Guo M. Acute respiratory distress syndrome and blastomycosis: presentation of nine cases and review of the literature. *Ann Diagn Pathol*. 2001;5:1-9.
28. Gullapalli D, Raza A, Khan A, Ganti SS, Pervaiz A. Battling the breath-stealers: *Blastomyces* and *Pseudomonas* triggering acute respiratory distress syndrome (ARDS). *Med Mycol Case Rep*. 2024;45:100655.

29. Hussain Z, Martin A, Youngberg GA. *Blastomyces dermatitidis* with large yeast forms. *Arch Pathol Lab Med.* 2001;125:663-664.
30. Bialek R, González GM, Begerow D, Zelck UE. Coccidioidomycosis and blastomycosis: advances in molecular diagnosis. *FEMS Immunol Med Microbiol.* 2005;45(3):355-360.
31. Setianingrum F, Rautemaa-Richardson R, Denning DW. Pulmonary cryptococcosis: a review of pathobiology and clinical aspects. *Med Mycol.* 2019;57:133-150.
32. Galanis E, Macdougall L, Kidd S, Morshed M; British Columbia *Cryptococcus gattii* Working Group. Epidemiology of *Cryptococcus gattii*, British Columbia, Canada, 1999-2007. *Emerg Infect Dis.* 2010;16(2):251-257.
33. Galanis E, MacDougall L, Rose C, et al. Predictors of *Cryptococcus gattii* clinical presentation and outcome: an international study. *Clin Infect Dis.* 2025;ciae640.
34. McDonnell JM, Hutchins GM. Pulmonary cryptococcosis. *Hum Pathol.* 1985;16:121-128.
35. Chang WC, Tzao C, Hsu HH, et al. Pulmonary cryptococcosis: comparison of clinical and radiographic characteristics in immunocompetent and immunocompromised patients. *Chest.* 2006;129(2):333-340.
36. Gazzoni AF, Severo CB, Salles EF, Severo LC. Histopathology, serology and cultures in the diagnosis of cryptococcosis. *Rev Inst Med Trop Sao Paulo.* 2009;51(5):255-259.
37. Huang J, Weng H, Ye L, et al. Bronchoalveolar lavage fluid and lung biopsy tissue metagenomic next-generation sequencing in the diagnosis of pulmonary cryptococcosis. *Front Cell Infect Microbiol.* 2024;14:1446814.
38. Pasley T, Baladad C, DeSear K, et al. Bridging echinocandin with azole antifungal therapy on prevention of invasive candidiasis post-lung transplantation. *Open Forum Infect Dis.* 2024;11(9):ofae525.
39. Luna MA. Candidiasis. In: Connor D, Chandler FW, Schwartz DA, Lack EE, eds. *Pathology of Infectious Diseases.* Appleton and Lange; 1997:953-964.
40. Feldman C. Pneumonia associated with HIV infection. *Curr Opin Infect Dis.* 2005;18:165-170.
41. Edman JC, Kovacs JA, Masur H, Santi DV, Elwood HJ, Sogin ML. Ribosomal RNA sequence shows *Pneumocystis carinii* to be a member of the fungi. *Nature.* 1988;334:519-522.
42. Stringer JR, Beard CB, Miller RF, Wakefield AE. A new name (*Pneumocystis jirovecii*) for pneumocystis from humans. *Emerg Infect Dis.* 2002;8:891-896.
43. Krajicek BJ, Thomas CF, Limper AH. Pneumocystis pneumonia: current concepts in pathogenesis, diagnosis, and treatment. *Clin Chest Med.* 2009;30(2):265-278.
44. Doyle L, Vogel S, Procop GW. Pneumocystis PCR: it is time to make PCR the test of choice. Open Forum. *Infect Dis.* 2017;4(4):ofx193. doi:10.1093/ofid/ofx193
45. Garg M, Prabhakar N, Gulati A, Agarwal R, Dhooria S. Spectrum of imaging findings in pulmonary infections. Part 2: fungal, mycobacterial, and parasitic. *Pol J Radiol.* 2019;84:e214-e223.
46. Schliep TC, Yarrish RL. *Pneumocystis carinii* pneumonia. *Semin Respir Infect.* 1999;14:333-343.
47. Blumenfeld W, Kovacs JA. Use of a monoclonal antibody to detect *Pneumocystis carinii* in induced sputum and bronchoalveolar lavage fluid by immunoperoxidase staining. *Arch Pathol Lab Med.* 1988;112:1233-1236.
48. Kobayashi M, Urata T, Ikezoe T, et al. Simple detection of the 5S ribosomal RNA of *Pneumocystis carinii* using in situ hybridisation. *J Clin Pathol.* 1996;49(9):712-716.
49. Brown L, Alanio A, Cruciani M, et al. Strengths and limitations of molecular diagnostics for *Pneumocystis jirovecii* pneumonia. *Expert Rev Mol Diagn.* 2024;24(10):899-911.
50. White PL. Progress on nonculture based diagnostic tests for invasive mould infection. *Curr Opin Infect Dis.* 2024;37(6):451-463.

51. Node J, Scherer E, Millon L, Bellanger AP. Commercial loop-mediated isothermal amplification (LAMP) assay for rapid diagnosis of pneumocystis pneumonia: an alternative to immunofluorescence assays. *J Mycol Med.* 2024;34(4):101508.

52. Xing F, Deng C, Luo Z, et al. Rapid diagnosis of *Pneumocystis jirovecii* pneumonia and respiratory tract colonization by next-generation sequencing. *Mycopathologia.* 2024;189(3):38.

53. Travis WD, Pittaluga S, Lipschick GY, et al. Atypical pathologic manifestations of *Pneumocystis carinii* pneumonia in the acquired immune deficiency syndrome. Review of 123 lung biopsies from 76 patients with emphasis on cysts, vascular invasion, vasculitis and granulomas. *Am J Surg Pathol.* 1990;14:615-625.

54. Weber WR, Askin FB, Dehner LP. Lung biopsy in *Pneumocystis carinii* pneumonia: a histopathologic study of typical and atypical features. *Am J Clin Pathol.* 1977;67:11-19.

55. Cupples JB, Blackie SP, Road JD. Granulomatous *Pneumocystis carinii* pneumonia mimicking tuberculosis. *Arch Pathol Lab Med.* 1985;113:1281-1284.

56. Hartel PH, Shilo K, Klassen-Fischer M, et al. Granulomatous reaction to *Pneumocystis jirovecii*: clinicopathologic review of 20 cases. *Am J Surg Pathol.* 2010;34(5):730-734.

57. Dutz W. *Pneumocystis carinii* pneumonia. *Pathol Annu.* 1970;5:309-341.

58. Feuerstain IM, Francis P, Raffeld M, Pluda J. Widespread visceral calcifications in disseminated *Pneumocystis carinii* infection: CT characteristics. *J Comput Assist Tomogr.* 1990;14:149-151.

59. Ng VL, Yajko DM, Hadley WK. Extrapulmonary pneumocystosis. *Clin Microbiol Rev.* 1997;10(3):401-418.

60. Deng ZL, Connor DH. Progressive disseminated penicilliosis caused by *Penicillium marneffei*: report of eight cases and differentiation of the causative organism from *Histoplasma capsulatum*. *Am J Clin Pathol.* 1985;84:323-327.

61. Chen J, Zhang R, Shen Y, et al. Clinical characteristics and prognosis of penicilliosis among human immunodeficiency virus-infected patients in eastern China. *Am J Trop Med Hyg.* 2017;96(6):1350-1354.

62. Cheng Y, Li WM, Wang SX, Shao D. PET/CT manifestations of a case of penicilliosis marneffei misdiagnosed as lung cancer. *Clin Nucl Med.* 2023;48(4):e167-e169. doi:10.1097/RLU.0000000000004531

63. Nishikubo M, Doi A, Takegawa H, Yamashita D, Ohira J, Nishioka H. Asymptomatic pulmonary penicilliosis with a lung mass in an HIV-infected patient. *J Gen Fam Med.* 2020;21(4):152-154. doi:10.1002/jgf2.325

64. Donovan FM, Ampel NM, Thompson GR III. Updates in coccidioidomycosis. *Infect Dis Clin N Am.* 2025;39(1):183-197. doi:10.1016/j.idc.2024.11.012

65. Davis SF, Sarosi GA. Fungal infections. In: Murray JF, Nadel JA, Mason RJ, Boushey H, eds. *Textbook of Respiratory Medicine.* 3rd ed. WB Saunders; 2000:1107-1141.

66. Ampel NM. Coccidioidomycosis: a review of recent advances. *Clin Chest Med.* 2009;30(2):241-251.

67. Adam RD, Elliott SP, Taljanovic MS. The spectrum and presentation of disseminated coccidioidomycosis. *Am J Med.* 2009;122(8):770-777.

68. Ampel NM. Coccidioidomycosis. In: Sarosi GA, Davis SF, eds. *Fungal Diseases of the Lung.* 3rd ed. Lippincott Williams & Wilkins; 2000:59-78.

69. Li L, Dial SM, Schmelz M, Rennels MA, Ampel NM. Cellular immune suppressor activity resides in lymphocyte cell clusters adjacent to granulomata in human coccidioidomycosis. *Infect Immun.* 2005;73(7):3923-3928.

70. Winn RE, Johnson R, Galgiani JN, Butler C, Pluss J. Cavitary coccidioidomycosis with fungus ball formation. Diagnosis by fiberoptic bronchoscopy with coexistence of hyphae and spherules. *Chest.* 1994;105:412-416.

71. van den Biggelaar R, Couwenbergh T, Leenders ACAP, van der Sloot CA, van der Lee H, Buil JB. Pulmonary coccidioidomycosis presenting as a fungal ball mimicking aspergilloma. *Med Mycol Case Rep*. 2024;47:100690.
72. Kaplan W, Kraft DE. Demonstration of pathogenic fungi in formalin-fixed tissues by immunofluorescence. *Am J Clin Pathol*. 1969;52:420-432.
73. Bialek R, Kern J, Herrmann T, et al. PCR assays for identification of *Coccidioides posadasii* based on the nucleotide sequence of the antigen 2/proline-rich antigen. *J Clin Microbiol*. 2004;42(2):778-783.
74. Taborda AB, Arechavala AI. Paracoccidioidomycosis. In: Sarosi GA, Davies SF, eds. *Fungal Diseases of the Lung*. 3rd ed. Lippincott William & Wilkins; 2000:79-90.
75. Peçanha-Pietrobom PM, Tirado-Sánchez A, Gonçalves SS, Bonifaz A, Colombo AL. Diagnosis and treatment of pulmonary coccidioidomycosis and paracoccidioidomycosis. *J Fungi (Basel)*. 2023;9(2):218.
76. Buitrago MJ, Merino P, Puente S, et al. Utility of real-time PCR for the detection of *Paracoccidioides brasiliensis* DNA in the diagnosis of imported paracoccidioidomycosis. *Med Mycol*. 2009;47(8):879-882.
77. Benedict K, Gold JAW, Toda M, Hsu J. Prevalence and features of allergic bronchopulmonary aspergillosis, United States, 2016-2022. *PLoS One*. 2025;20(1):e0317054.
78. Regnard JF, Icard P, Nicolosi M, Magdeleinat P, Jauffret B, Levasseur P. Aspergilloma: a series of 89 surgical cases. *Ann Thorac Surg*. 2000;69:898-903.
79. Yousem SA. The histological spectrum of chronic necrotizing forms of pulmonary aspergillosis. *Hum Pathol*. 1997;28:650-656.
80. Tron V, Churg A. Chronic necrotizing pulmonary aspergillosis mimicking bronchocentric granulomatosis. *Pathol Res Pract*. 1986;181:621-626.
81. Challa S, Uppin SG, Uppin MS, Pamidimukkala U, Vemu L. Diagnosis of filamentous fungi on tissue sections by immunohistochemistry using anti-aspergillus antibody. *Med Mycol*. 2015;53(5):470-476.
82. Gali V, Al-Ghanamah R, Finnigan K, et al. Evaluating the clinical utility of *Aspergillus, Mucorales,* and *Nocardia* bronchoalveolar PCRs for the diagnosis of invasive pulmonary infections in patients with hematological malignancies. *J Clin Microbiol*. 2025;63(2):e0135524.
83. Ribes JA, Vanover-Sams CL, Baker DJ. Zygomycetes in human disease. *Clin Microbiol Rev*. 2000;13:236-301.
84. Kontoyiannis DP, Wessel VC, Bodey GP, Rolston KV. Zygomycosis in the 1990s in a tertiary-care cancer center. *Clin Infect Dis*. 2000;30:851-856.
85. McAdams HP, Rosado-de-Christenson ML, Lesar M, Templeton PA, Moran CA. Thoracic mycoses from opportunistic fungi: radiologic–pathologic correlation. *Radiographics*. 1995;15:271-286.
86. Zacharias M, Thüringer A, Krause R, Kashofer K, Gorkiewicz G. The mutual value of histopathology and ITS sequencing in the diagnosis of mucormycosis. *Histopathology*. 2024;84(4):702-706.
87. Travis WD, Colby TV, Koss MN, Rosado-de-Christenson ML, Müller NL, King TE Jr. Non-neoplastic disorders of the lower respiratory tract. *Atlas of Nontumor Pathology*. Vol. 2. Armed Forces Institute of Pathology; 2002:592-638.

7

PARASITIC LUNG INFECTIONS

Pulmonary parasitic infections are rare and are hardly ever encountered in lung biopsy samples. However, tourism and increased travel to endemic areas can expose patients to a variety of parasites, thus posing a challenge for diagnostic surgical pathologist unfamiliar with these conditions. Several species of parasites migrate through the lungs as part of their life cycle, but few actually infect the lung. Most parasitic infections in the lung result from systemic dissemination in immunocompromised patients. Some of the more common parasitic lung pathogens are listed in Table 7.1. When parasites migrate to lung tissue, they usually elicit an intense inflammatory reaction with neutrophils, eosinophils, lymphocytes, histiocytes, and plasma cells that may produce various patterns of lung injury, including eosinophilic pneumonia, small or large nodular lesions, bronchitis and bronchiolitis, and abscess cavities and cysts.

PROTOZOAL INFECTIONS

Amebiasis

Amebiasis is one of the most common parasitic infections in underdeveloped tropical countries that is caused by *Entamoeba histolytica*. The

TABLE 7.1 Common Lung Parasitic Infections

Protozoa	Amebiasis
	Toxoplasmosis
	Cryptosporidiosis
	Microsporidiosis
Nematodes	Dirofilariasis
	Filariasis
	Strongyloidiasis
Trematodes	Paragonimiasis
	Schistosomiasis
Cestodes	Echinococcosis

disease is primarily acquired through ingestion of contaminated water and food and can also be transmitted sexually among homosexual men. The disease causes gastrointestinal infections with mucosal ulceration that may spread to the liver causing amebic liver abscess.[1] Pleuropulmonary complications of amebiasis occur in up to 20% of patients with hepatic infection. The organisms can reach the lung through direct invasion owing to rupture of a hepatic abscess into the lung or by hematogenous spread from the liver.[2,3] Rupture of an amebic liver abscess into the thoracic cavity may also cause a bronchopulmonary fistula. Pulmonary amebiasis may also be associated with empyema or masslike lesions that are rarely confused for malignancy.[4,5] Pulmonary amebiasis is characterized by the formation of multiple abscesses that contain yellow-brown fluid.[6,7] The center of the abscess shows inflammatory cells admixed with necrotic debris and contains scattered trophozoites (Fig. 7.1; eFig. 7.1). In histologic sections, the trophozoites measure approximately 15 to 25 μm in diameter and display a sharply defined cell membrane with clear to lightly eosinophilic cytoplasm that may contain red blood cells or other cellular debris and a small nucleus showing accentuation of the nuclear membrane. The cytoplasm also contains abundant glycogen that stains strongly with periodic acid-Schiff (PAS) stain (Fig. 7.2). The trophozoites may be difficult to visualize on routine examination and can be confused with histiocytes, but they have smaller nuclei and are slightly larger than histiocytes.

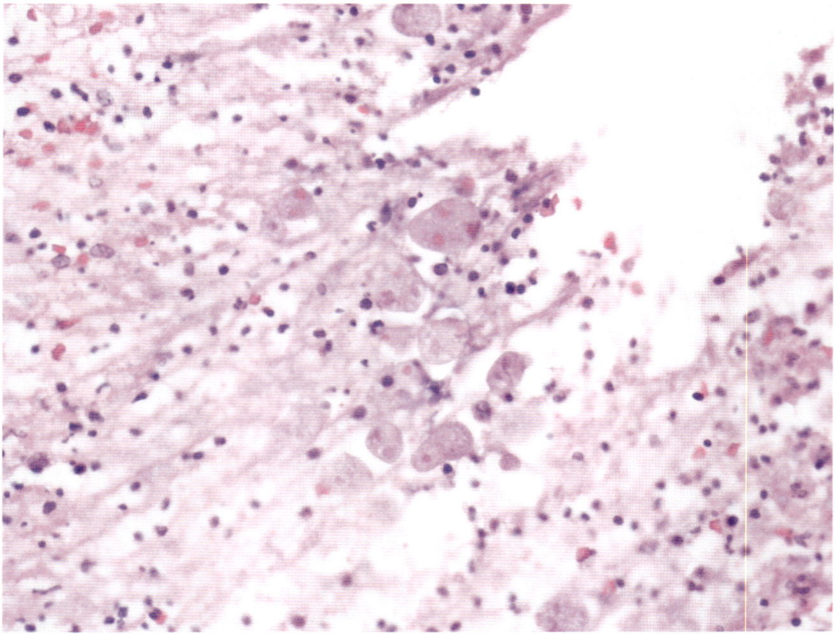

FIGURE 7.1 **Pulmonary abscess caused by amebiasis.** Notice scattered necrotic debris and large trophozoites with sharply defined cell membranes, abundant lightly eosinophilic cytoplasm, and occasional ingested red blood cells.

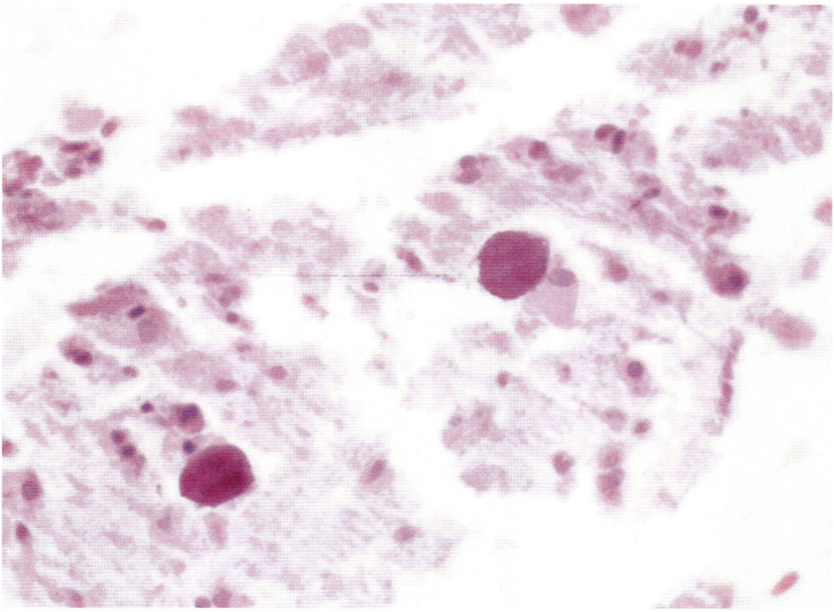

FIGURE 7.2 Periodic acid-Schiff stain highlights the organisms in amebic abscess of the lung.

Toxoplasmosis

Toxoplasmosis is caused by an obligate intracellular protozoan with worldwide distribution, *Toxoplasma gondii*. The infection is transmitted by cats through their feces but can also be acquired by eating raw meat or by perinatal exposure from an infected mother.[8] Acute toxoplasmosis most often causes a painless, self-limited lymphadenopathy. Systemic dissemination occurs in immunocompromised patients or in patients with defective cell-mediated immunity.[9] The organisms are transported to the lungs through the bloodstream and lymphatics. In the lung, the organisms cause diffuse acute bronchopneumonia with occasional cavitation. Toxoplasmosis is a common opportunistic infection in acquired immunodeficiency syndrome (AIDS) patients.[10] In AIDS patients, the diffuse pulmonary opacities caused by toxoplasmosis must be distinguished from pneumocystosis. Histologically, the organisms (tachyzoites) invade the host cells and grow within the cytoplasm, forming cysts and pseudocysts. The cysts are slightly larger than histiocytes and contain numerous bradyzoites that appear as dark, uniform dots within the cytoplasm. The organisms can be readily visualized on hematoxylin and eosin (H&E) and can be highlighted with the PAS stain. Serologic tests are very helpful for diagnosis (Sabin-Feldman dye test; differential agglutination test).[11] Immunohistochemistry using a monoclonal antibody or polymerase chain reaction can also help identify the organism in tissue sections.[12,13]

Cryptosporidiosis

Cryptosporidiosis is caused by an intestinal protozoan, *Cryptosporidium parvum*, which rarely affects the lungs. The main clinical manifestation is acute diarrhea owing to colonization of the gastrointestinal tract epithelium. It is a common opportunistic infection in AIDS patients; approximately 10% to 15% of AIDS patients will develop pulmonary cryptosporidiosis.[14,15] Pulmonary involvement is rare and most likely secondary to aspiration associated with fecal-oral spread in debilitated patients. Rare cases associated with lung cancer have been documented.[16] Respiratory infection is characterized by tracheitis, bronchitis, and bronchiolitis. Patients will present with nonspecific symptoms, including cough, fever, and dyspnea that may or may not be present.[17] There is usually a very mild chronic inflammatory reaction, but the organisms are most commonly seen in the luminal aspect of the respiratory mucosa.[18] The organisms comprise small (4-6 µm), round to oval, basophilic structures that can be very easily missed on cursory examination. They appear to be lying in a single row on the surface of the respiratory mucosa and can be highlighted with the PAS, Giemsa, or Gomori methenamine silver stain. The biggest challenge for diagnosis is overlooking the organisms in tissue sections.

Microsporidiosis

Microsporidiosis is an infection caused by various protozoans, including, *Encephalitozoon intestinalis*, *Encephalitozoon cuniculi*, and *Enterocytozoon bieneusi*. Microsporidium is a well-recognized opportunistic pathogen in AIDS and transplant patients that can affect the kidney, gastrointestinal and biliary tracts, cornea, and brain. In the lungs, the disease is most often the result of dissemination from the gastrointestinal or biliary tract.[19] The diagnosis is most often established by cytologic examination of bronchioalveolar lavage fluid.[20] Molecular techniques are useful for identifying the species as well.[21,22] In tissue sections from lung biopsies, the organisms are found within bronchial and bronchiolar epithelial cells, where they grow within vacuoles in the apical aspect of the cells. A mild acute and chronic inflammatory reaction is seen in the mucosa. The intracytoplasmic spores are very small (1-1.5 µm) and appear as slightly basophilic small dots on H&E stains. They are gram-positive and weakly acid-fast. Some organisms can also stain with Gomori methenamine silver, but the Brown and Brenn stain is the most reliable for visualization in routine histologic sections. The parasites are also birefringent under polarized light.[21] Because of their small size and subtle appearance, it is very easy to miss them on cursory examination.

NEMATODES

Dirofilariasis

Dirofilariasis is a disease caused by a parasite of dogs and other mammals, *Dirofilaria immitis* (aka dog heartworm). The disease is transmitted by

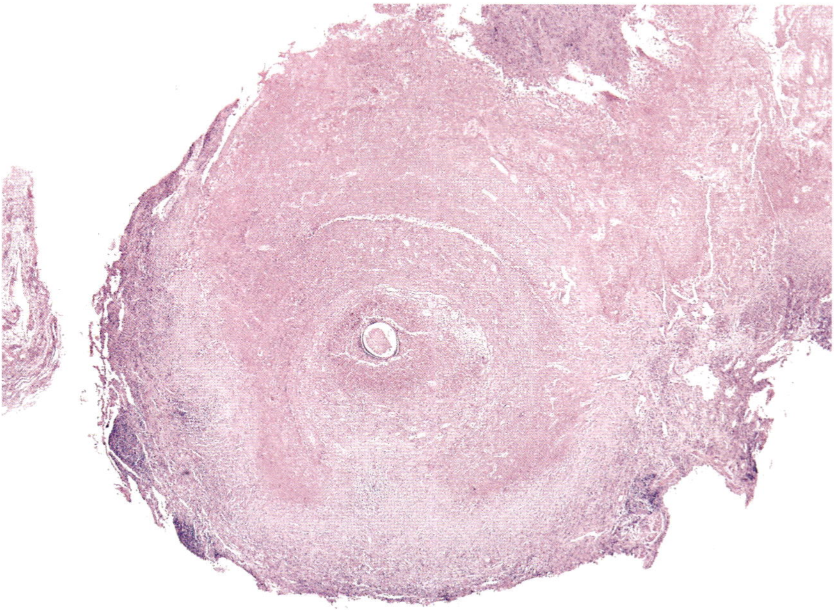

FIGURE 7.3 **Pulmonary *Dirofilaria* granuloma.** Notice centrally necrotic granuloma surrounded by a rim of epithelioid histiocytes and a single dead worm in the center.

mosquitoes that inject the larvae into the skin and from there the larvae migrate to the heart. The parasites enter the pulmonary arterial circulation and become implanted in the periphery of the lungs where they form a small nodule containing a central zone of infarction surrounded by a rim of fibrosis (eFigs. 7.2-7.4). These solitary nodules may clinically resemble malignancy.[23-25] A dead worm can be usually identified within the lumen of a vessel. The worm elicits an intense granulomatous reaction (Fig. 7.3). The organism measures approximately 120 to 300 μm in diameter, is densely eosinophilic, and is surrounded by a smooth cuticle with prominent external striations (Figs. 7.4 and 7.5). The lesions are usually stable and do not progress over time. Because of their peripheral location, dirofilariasis is not diagnosed on endoscopic biopsies but may rarely be seen in core biopsies or video-assisted thoracoscopic surgery biopsies done to rule out malignancy.[26]

Filariasis

Filariasis is an infection of the lung caused by *Wuchereria bancrofti*, *Brugia malayi*, and *Onchocerca volvulus*. The parasites are transmitted by infected mosquitoes. Lymphadenopathy and the formation of subcutaneous nodules are the primary manifestation of the disease.[27] However, microfilaria can migrate to the lung and other internal tissues. Pulmonary

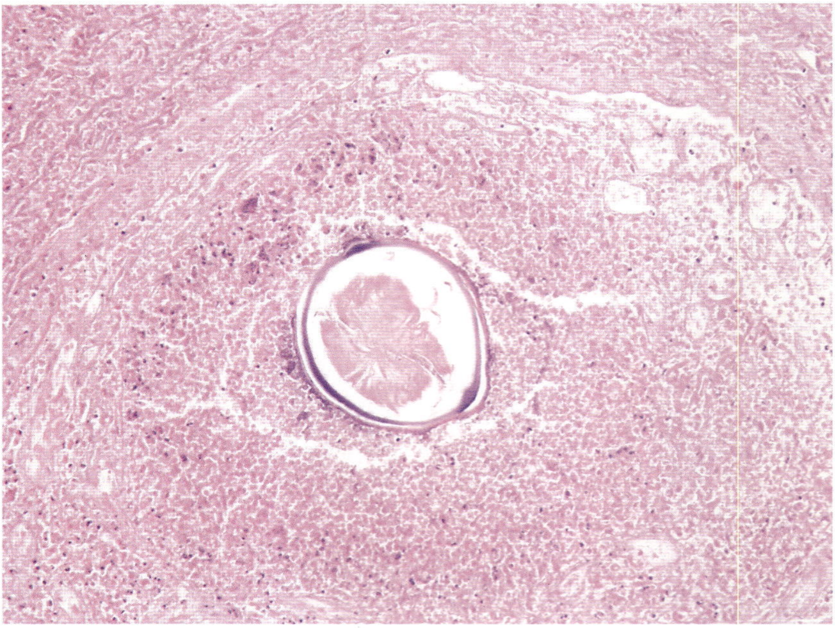

FIGURE 7.4 Higher magnification of *Dirofilaria* granuloma showing cross section of dead worm in the center.

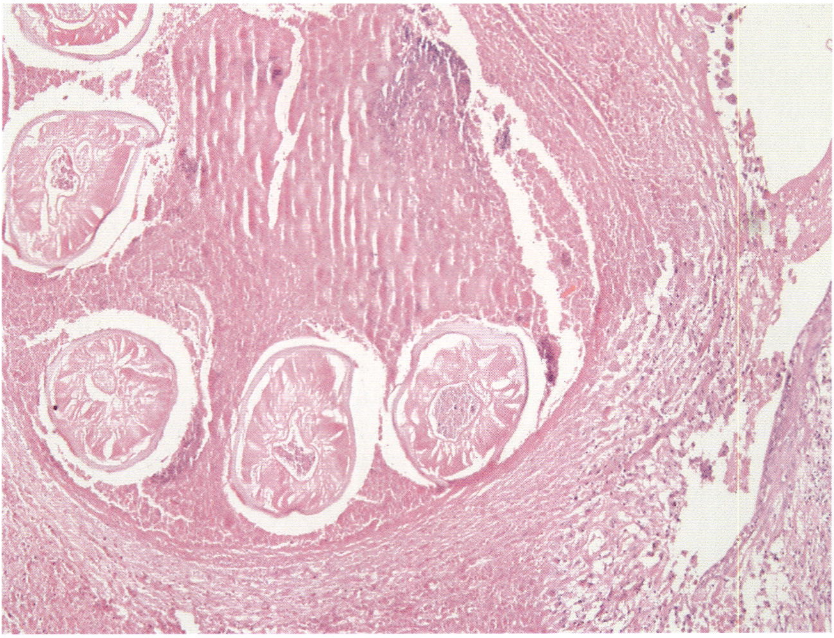

FIGURE 7.5 Another example of pulmonary *Dirofilaria* containing the worm surrounded by a smooth cuticle with extensive tissue necrosis of the surrounding parenchyma.

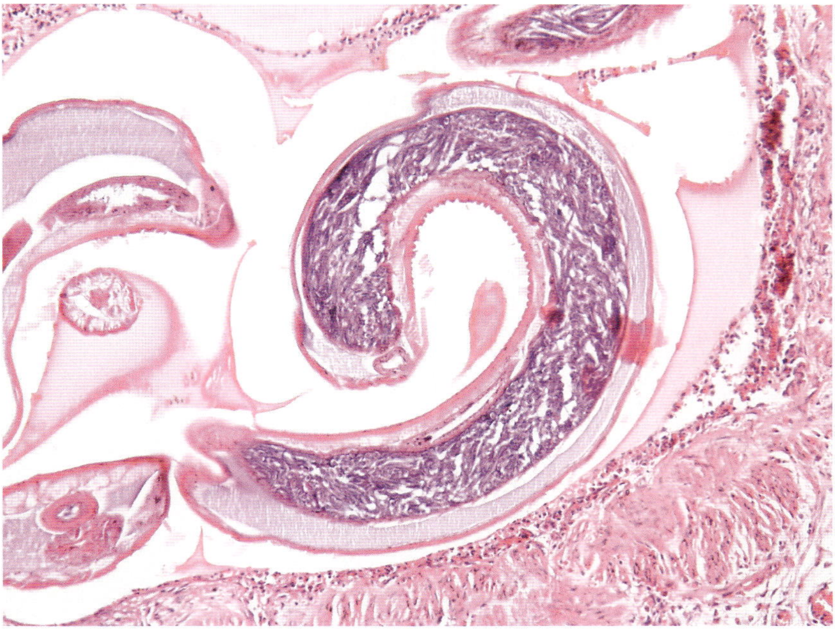

FIGURE 7.6 **Pulmonary involvement by *Wuchereria bancrofti* shows a coiled adult worm.** Notice thin eosinophilic cuticle surrounding the organism.

involvement may take the form of eosinophilic pneumonia, or a pulmonary nodule resembling a mass can develop owing to the nodular infarcts caused by the adult worm (eFigs. 7.5 and 7.6).[28,29] The worms range from 100 to 250 µm in length and show tight coils with multiple cross sections that are surrounded by a thin, finely striated cuticle (Figs. 7.6-7.8). In the diffuse form, the histologic appearance is that of an eosinophilic pneumonia; microfilariae showing a fine, pointed tail can sometimes be identified within lymphatics.

Strongyloidiasis

Strongyloidiasis is an infection caused by the threadworm *Strongyloides stercoralis*. The organism penetrates the skin from the soil, and the larvae migrate through the bloodstream into the lungs and then to the gastrointestinal tract where they mature and produce rhabditiform (noninfective) and filariform (infective) larvae. Hyperinfection owing to endogenous reinfection can lead to massive larval infection of the lungs, leading to consolidation and acute respiratory distress.[30,31] Patients may present with acute respiratory distress syndrome, superimposed bacterial pneumonia, alveolar hemorrhage, and hemoptysis.[32,33] Histologically, diffuse alveolar damage and pulmonary hemorrhage are seen. The filariform larvae are 300 to 600 µm long and 10 to 20 µm wide, basophilic, S-shaped,

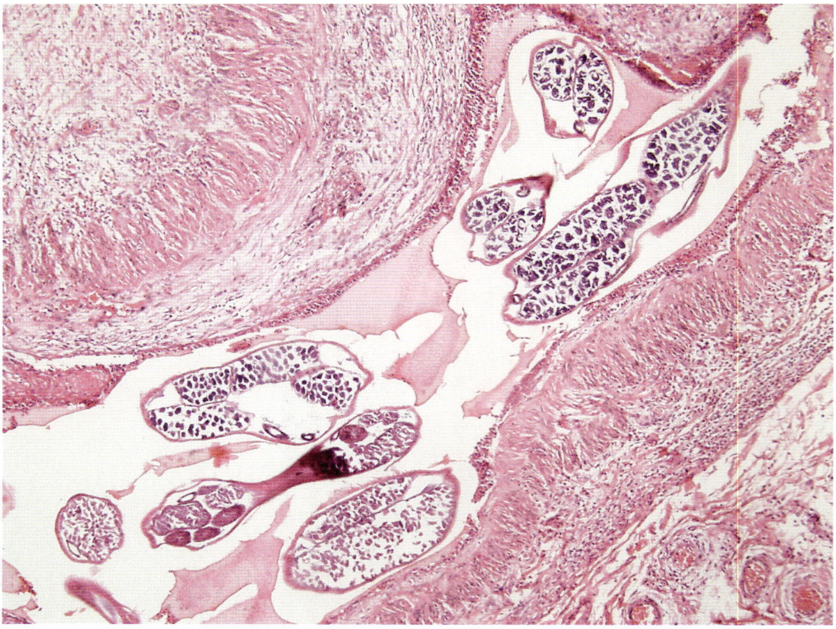

FIGURE 7.7 Another example of pulmonary filariasis showing multiple worms in cross section surrounded by thin eosinophilic cuticles.

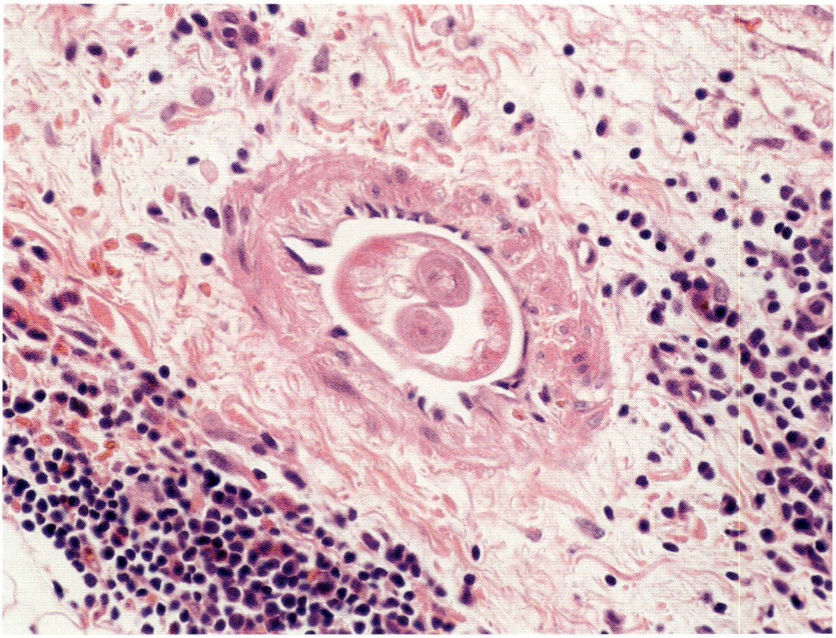

FIGURE 7.8 Cross section of a worm in filariasis caused by *Wuchereria bancrofti* lying within the lumen of small pulmonary vessel.

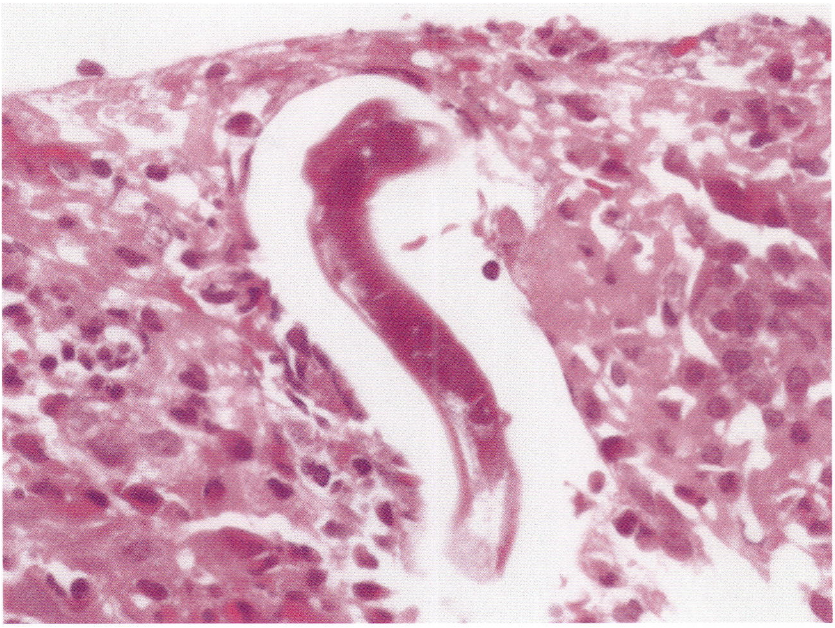

FIGURE 7.9 Larval infection of the lung by *Strongyloides stercoralis* showing S-shaped, basophilic filiform larva lying within alveolar space.

and usually found within the alveolar spaces or bronchioles (Fig. 7.9). Pulmonary strongyloidiasis can be effectively diagnosed on open lung biopsy.[34]

TREMATODES

Paragonimiasis

Paragonimiasis is an infection caused by the Asian lung fluke *Paragonimus westermani*. Infection is acquired by eating raw or undercooked crabs or crayfish and is most common in Asia. The life cycle starts with a snail that infects a crustacean, where the cercaria develop into cysts (metacercaria), which are later ingested by the definitive host leading to human infection. The larvae pass from the intestines into the peritoneum, through the diaphragm into the chest cavity, and from there to the lungs.[35] In the lungs, the worms are found adjacent to large bronchioles and are surrounded by fibrinopurulent exudate admixed with eosinophils and fibrosis forming a cyst.[36] The cysts are 1.5 cm in diameter and can rupture into the airways, spilling eggs that will elicit a granulomatous and fibrosing reaction (Fig. 7.10). The disease can clinically simulate other infectious disorders such as tuberculsosis.[37-39] The eggs measure 75 to 100 μm, are yellow to brown and oval, have a flattened operculum at one end and a thick birefringent shell, a feature that permits distinction

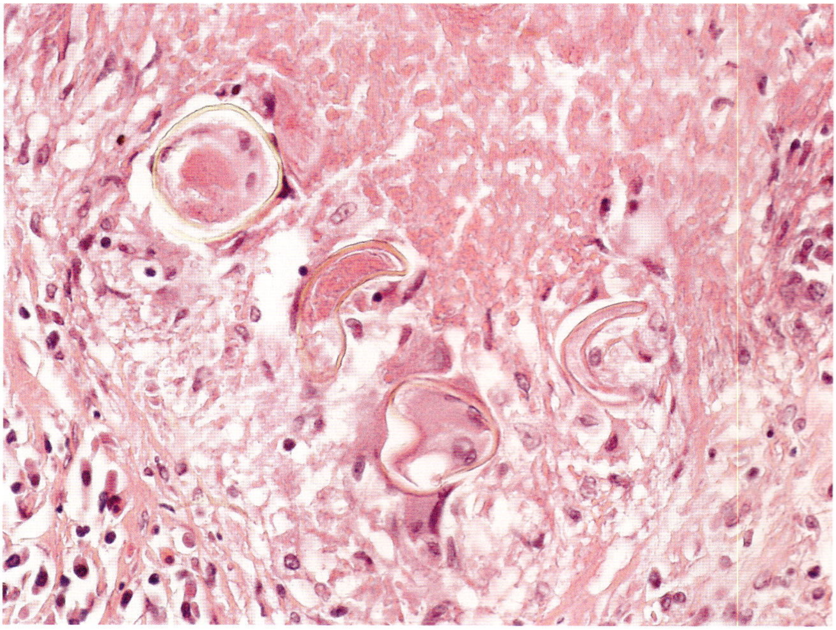

FIGURE 7.10 Cyst of *Paragonimus westermani* in the lungs shows oval eggs with thick birefringent shell surrounded by granulomatous and fibrosing reaction.

from nonbirefringent *Schistosoma* eggs. In addition, antibody serology and molecular assays are available to aid in diagnosis.[40]

Schistosomiasis

Schistosomiasis is an infection caused by tropical flukes, namely *Schistosoma mansoni*, *Schistosoma japonicum*, and *Schistosoma haematobium*. Human infection occurs through exposure to contaminated water infected with cercariae. The cercariae enter the circulation through the skin where they mature into adult worms. The female worm produces eggs that migrate into tissue, causing disease. The eggs of *S mansoni* and *S japonicum* infect the gut, liver, and lung, whereas the eggs of *S haematobium* reside mostly in the bladder, ureter, and pelvis. Larval pneumonitis can occur following heavy cercarial exposure and presents with peripheral eosinophilia and basilar patchy consolidation.[41] Chronic disease can present in the form of miliary nodular infiltrates.[42] A now well-recognized complication of pulmonary schistosomiasis is pulmonary artery hypertension.[43-45] Histologically, in chronic infection, the *Schistosoma* eggs are seen in association with a granulomatous reaction and fibrosis (Fig. 7.11).[46] The eggs are usually deposited in perivascular location and can be recognized by their morphology (Fig. 7.12; eFig. 7.7). The eggs in *S haematobium* are characterized by a terminal spine, those of *S mansoni* have a large lateral spine, and those of *S japonicum* have a small lateral spine. The eggs may

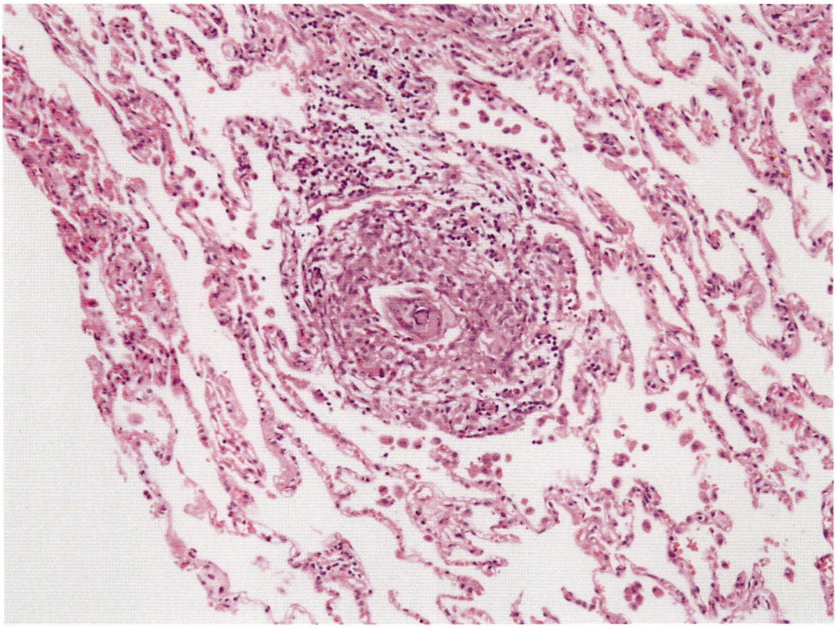

FIGURE 7.11 Pulmonary involvement in schistosomiasis shows pulmonary parenchyma containing a small egg surrounded by prominent granulomatous reaction.

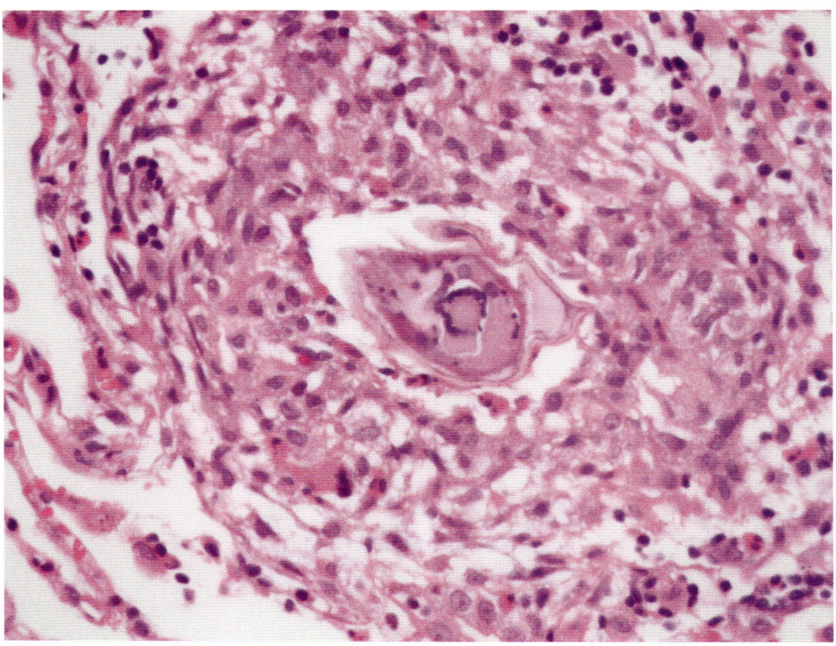

FIGURE 7.12 Higher magnification of *Schistosoma* granuloma showing the organism with a nonrefringent capsule and a short lateral spine.

range in size from 100 to 170 µm in diameter. They can be distinguished from those of *Paragonimus* by the smaller size, nonbirefringence of the capsule, and absence of a spine in the latter.

CESTODES

Echinococcosis

Echinococcosis, also known as hydatid disease or hydatidosis, is an infection of the lung caused by the larval tapeworms *Echinococcus granulosus*, *Echinococcus multilocularis*, and *Echinococcus vogeli*. The dog/sheep strain of *E granulosus* is the most common. The most frequent site of infection following ingestion of the parasites is the liver, followed by the lung.[47,48] In the lung, the echinococcal cyst presents as a unilocular or multilocular cyst that can vary in size from a few millimeters to 20 cm.[49-51] The cyst wall in *E granulosus* is thick with a hyaline appearance and is lined by a laminated germinal layer that is approximately 1 mm thick (Figs. 7.13 and 7.14; eFig. 7.8). Attached to the germinal layer are multiple brood capsules that contain protoscolices (Figs. 7.15 and 7.16; eFigs. 7.9 and 7.10). The protoscolices may lose their teethlike hooklets that can be found floating in the vicinity of the cyst wall (Fig. 7.17). The hooklets are best identified

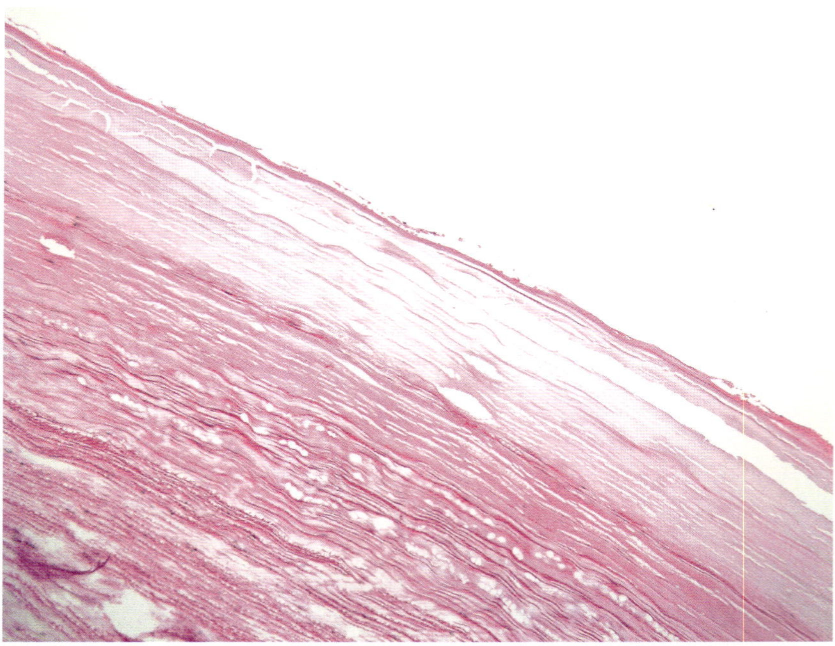

FIGURE 7.13 **Hydatid disease of the lung owing to *Echinococcus granulosus* showing characteristic thick hyaline wall of the cyst.** Occasionally, this may be the only structure identified in the biopsy.

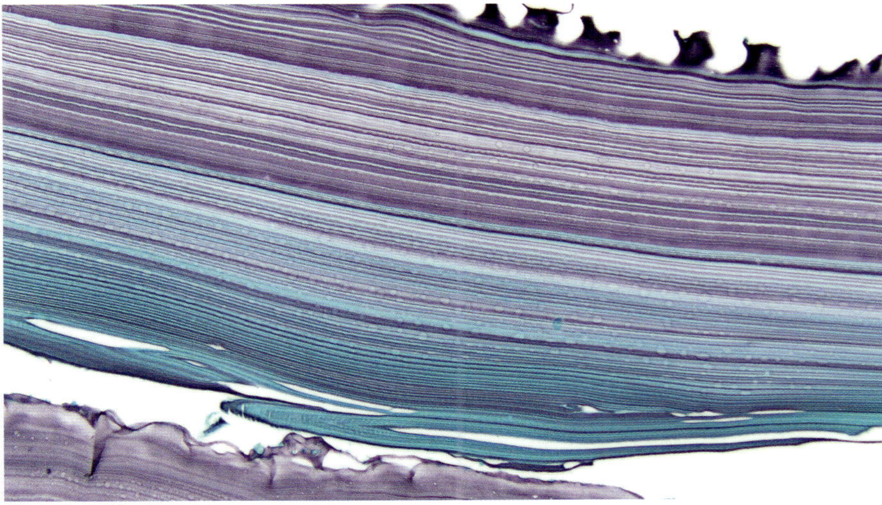

FIGURE 7.14 **Gomori methenamine silver (GMS) special stain highlights the laminated layers within the wall of an echinococcal cyst.** Though GMS does not stain the parasites, it can be useful in highlighting the concentric layers within the cyst walls.

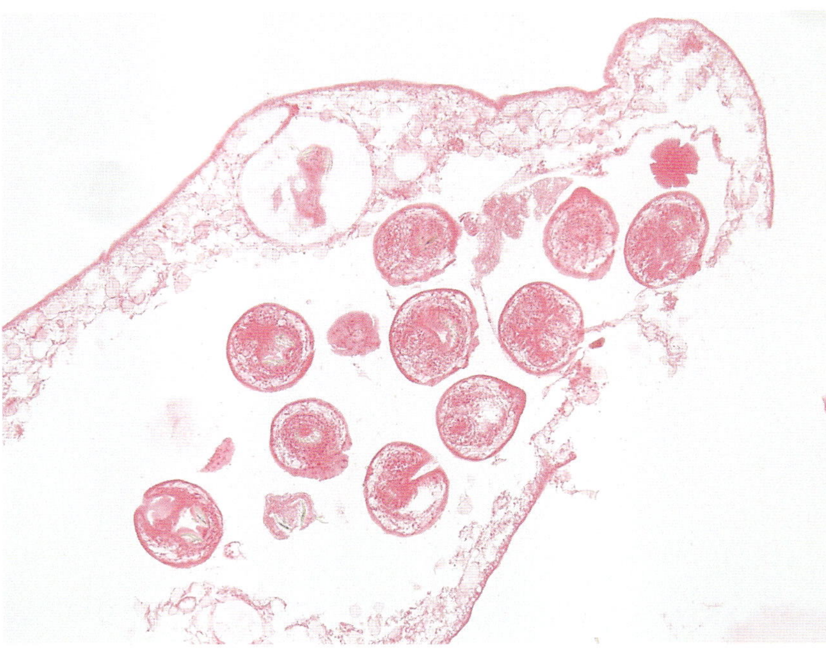

FIGURE 7.15 **Fragment of the wall in hydatid cyst lined by hyaline germinal layer and multiple brood capsules.**

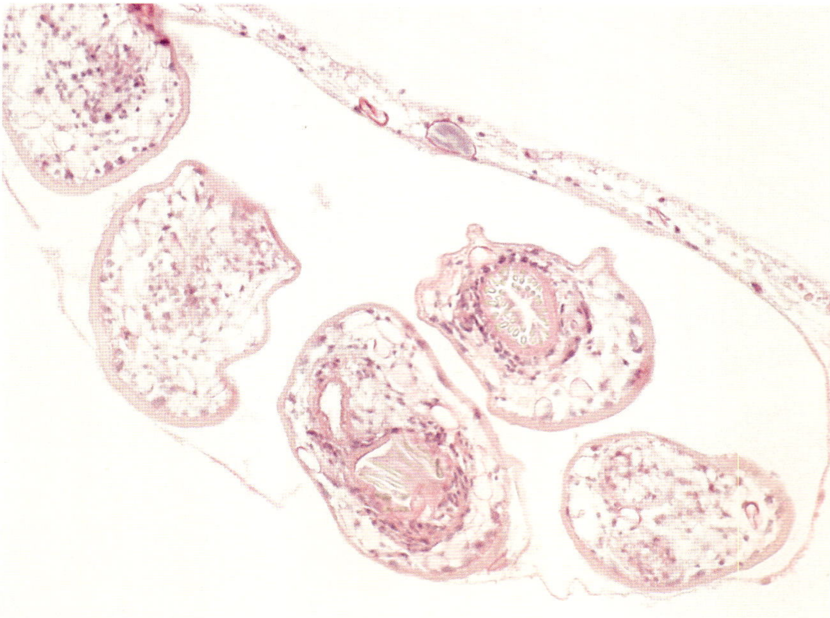

FIGURE 7.16 **Higher magnification of brood cysts in hydatidosis showing protoscolices with multiple hooklets.**

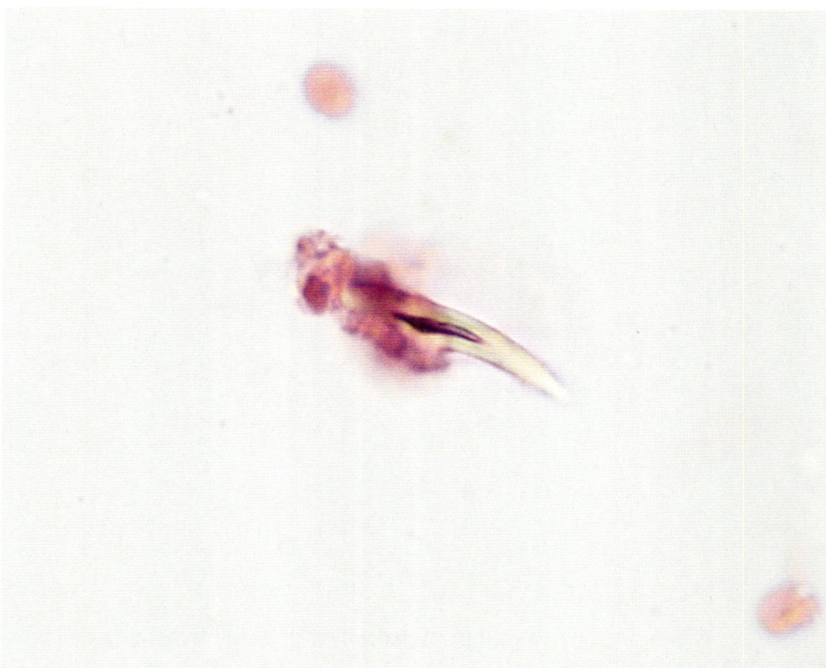

FIGURE 7.17 **Toothlike hooklet in pulmonary hydatidosis.** In the absence of brood cysts, the hooklets may be the only clue to the nature of the process.

by lowering the condenser on the microscope, which highlights their refringent appearance. The cyst wall may elicit a necrotizing granulomatous response in the surrounding lung parenchyma.

REFERENCES

1. Stanley SL. Amoebiasis. *Lancet*. 2003;361(9362):1025-1034.
2. Gopinath R, Nutman TB. Parasitic diseases. In: Murray JF, Nadel JA, Mason RJ, Boushey HA, eds. *Textbook of Respiratory Medicine*. 3rd ed. WB Saunders; 2000:1143-1171.
3. Ismail M, Elaskandrany MA, Singh S, Chmielewska N, Wang W. A novel case of a massive amebic liver abscess in the setting of uncontrolled diabetes mellitus and concurrent pulmonary embolism. *Cureus*. 2024;16(1):e52533.
4. Zakaria A, Al-Share B, Al-Asad K. Primary pulmonary amebiasis complicated with multicystic empyema. *Case Rep Pulmonol*. 2016;2016:8709347.
5. Putra AC, Chyntia B, Winardi E, et al. Primary pulmonary amoebiasis mimicking lung tumour in immunocompromised patient: a case report. *Respirol Case Rep*. 2023;11(8):e01199.
6. Lyche KD, Jensen WA. Pleuropulmonary amebiasis. *Semin Respir Infect*. 1997;12:106-112.
7. Gottschling M, Lerzer C, Geismann F, et al. Seltene Ursache einer einschmelzenden Pneumonie: Ein Fallbericht [rare cause of necrotizing pneumonia: a case report]. *Inn Med (Heidelb)*. 2023;64(11):1119-1122.
8. Saadatnia G, Golkar M. A review on human toxoplasmosis. *Scand J Infect Dis*. 2012;44(11):805-814.
9. Pomeroy C, Filice GA. Pulmonary toxoplasmosis: a review. *Clin Infect Dis*. 1992;14:863-870.
10. Nash G, Kerschmann RL, Herndier B, Dubey JP. The pathological manifestations of pulmonary toxoplasmosis in the acquired immunodeficiency syndrome. *Hum Pathol*. 1994;25:652-658.
11. Zhang K, Lin G, Han Y, Li J. Serological diagnosis of toxoplasmosis and standardization. *Clin Chim Acta*. 2016;461:83-89.
12. Desoubeaux G, Cabanne É, Franck-Martel C, et al. Pulmonary toxoplasmosis in immunocompromised patients with interstitial pneumonia: a single-centre prospective study assessing PCR-based diagnosis. *J Clin Pathol*. 2016;69(8):726-730.
13. Robert-Gangneux F, Belaz S. Molecular diagnosis of toxoplasmosis in immunocompromised patients. *Curr Opin Infect Dis*. 2016;29(4):330-339.
14. Soave R, Johnson WD Jr. *Cryptosporidium* and *Isospora belli* infections. *J Infect Dis*. 1988;157:225-229.
15. Topan A, Ionică AM, Binder A, Briciu V, Lupse M. A rare case of pulmonary cryptosporidiosis associated with pulmonary tuberculosis in a patient with advanced HIV infection. *Parasitol Int*. 2025;104:102983.
16. Ulusan Bagci O, Guldaval F, Muftuoglu C, Magalhães V. A pilot study on the evaluation of *Cryptosporidium* infection in patients with lung cancer: respiratory cryptosporidiosis. *Jpn J Infect Dis*. 2022;75(6):569-574.
17. Albuquerque YM, Silva MC, Lima AL, Magalhães V. Pulmonary cryptosporidiosis in AIDS patients: an underdiagnosed disease [in Portuguese]. *J Bras Pneumol*. 2012;38(4):530-532.
18. Ma P, Villanueva TG, Kaufman D, Gillooley JF. Respiratory cryptosporidiosis in the acquired immune deficiency syndrome. Use of modified cold Kinyoun and Hemacolor stains for rapid diagnoses. *JAMA*. 1984;252:1298-1301.
19. Weber R, Bryan RT, Schwartz DA, Owen RL. Human microsporidial infections. *Clin Microbiol Rev*. 1994;7:426-461.

20. Remadi S, Dumais J, Wafa K, MacGee W. Pulmonary microsporidiosis in a patient with the acquired immunodeficiency syndrome. A case report. *Acta Cytol*. 1995;39:1112-1116.
21. Ramanan P, Pritt BS. Extraintestinal microsporidiosis. *J Clin Microbiol*. 2014;52(11):3839-3844.
22. Bagci OU, Muftuoglu C, Guldaval F, et al. Molecular prevalence of microsporidia infection in patients with lung cancer. *Am J Trop Med Hyg*. 2023;108(5):895-900.
23. Silva MJ, Costa AR, Calvinho P. Human pulmonary dirofilariasis: a pitfall in solitary pulmonary nodule. *Pulmonology*. 2022;28(5):413-414.
24. Theodore SG, Sawkins HJ, Mathew M, Yadav S, Norton R. Human pulmonary dirofilariasis: an unexpected differential diagnosis for a solitary lung lesion. *Med J Aust*. 2023;219(10):455-456.
25. Tsai CC, Chang YC, Chang IW. Human pulmonary dirofilariasis mimicking a metastatic disease in a cancer patient. *Asian J Surg*. 2024;47(1):538-539.
26. Flieder DB, Moran CA. Pulmonary dirofilariasis: a clinicopathologic study of 41 lesions in 39 patients. *Hum Pathol*. 1999;30:251-256.
27. Meyers WM, Neafie RC, Connor DH. Bancroftian and Malayan filariasis. In: Binford CH, Connor DH, eds. *Pathology of Tropical and Extraordinary Diseases*. 2nd ed. Armed Forces Institute of Pathology; 1976:340-355.
28. Atsumi E, Matsumoto H, Taira N, et al. Thirteen cases of pulmonary dirofilariasis in a single institution in Okinawa Island. *Virchows Arch*. 2019;475(3):335-340.
29. Jacob S, Parameswaran A, Santosham R, Santosham R. Human pulmonary dirofilariasis masquerading as a mass. *Asian Cardiovasc Thorac Ann*. 2016;24(7):722-725.
30. Upadhyay D, Corbridge T, Jain M, Shah R. Pulmonary hyperinfection syndrome with *Strongyloides stercoralis*. *Am J Med*. 2001;111:167-179.
31. Fan W, Fu Q, Yu Y. Pulmonary strongyloidiasis and hyperinfection in a patient with idiopathic inflammatory myopathy: a case report. *Heliyon*. 2023;10(1):e23484.
32. Nabeya D, Haranaga S, Parrott GL, et al. Pulmonary strongyloidiasis: assessment between manifestation and radiological findings in 16 severe strongyloidiasis cases. *BMC Infect Dis*. 2017;17(1):320.
33. Barkati S, Greenaway C, Libman M. Strongyloidiasis-related lung involvement: too much of a bad thing. *Curr Opin Infect Dis*. 2023;36(3):203-208.
34. Byard RW, Bourne AJ, Matthews N, et al. Pulmonary strongyloidiasis in a child diagnosed on open lung biopsy. *Surg Pathol*. 1993;5:55-61.
35. Blair D. Paragonimiasis. *Adv Exp Med Biol*. 2019;1154:105-138.
36. Kagawa FT. Pulmonary paragonimiasis. *Semin Respir Infect*. 1997;12:149-158.
37. Sun B, Deng J, Kuang R, Zhou J. The great masquerader: pulmonary paragonimiasis. *Surg Infect*. 2025;26:49-50.
38. Villanueva-Villegas R, Diaz-Mendoza J, Salas-Lopez J, Espiche C. Paragonimiasis misdiagnosed as pulmonary tuberculosis: a case report. *Cureus*. 2023;15(3):e36169.
39. Poudyal BS, Paudel B, Bista B, Shrestha GS, Pudasaini P. Clinical, laboratory and radiological features of paragonimiasis misdiagnosed as pulmonary tuberculosis. *Iran J Parasitol*. 2022;17(3):410-414.
40. Fischer PU, Weil GJ. North American paragonimiasis: epidemiology and diagnostic strategies. *Expert Rev Anti-Infect Ther*. 2015;13(6):779-786.
41. Cooke GS, Lalvani A, Gleeson FV, Conlon CP. Acute pulmonary schistosomiasis in travelers returning from Lake Malawi, sub-Saharan Africa. *Clin Infect Dis*. 1999;29:836-839.
42. Gerber V, Biry M, Sohler S, et al. Multiple lung nodules revealing chronic pulmonary schistosomiasis. *J Travel Med*. 2025;32(1):taae144.
43. Gavilanes F, Fernandes CJ, Souza R. Pulmonary arterial hypertension in schistosomiasis. *Curr Opin Pulm Med*. 2016;22(5):408-414.

44. Botoni FA, Marinho CC, Carvalho VT, Mickael CS, Graham BB. A retrospective study of schistosomiasis-associated pulmonary hypertension from an endemic area in Brazil. *Int J Cardiol Heart Vasc*. 2019;24:100387.
45. Bobrovski VG, Pinheiro AL, de-Castro JAL, et al. Schistosomiasis: a neglected cause of pulmonary arterial hypertension in Brazil. *Curr Probl Cardiol*. 2024;49(3):102340.
46. Bethlem EP, Schettino Gde P, Carvalho CR. Pulmonary schistosomiasis. *Curr Opin Pulm Med*. 1997;3:361-365.
47. Mao T, Chungda D, Phuntsok L, et al. Pulmonary echinococcosis in China. *J Thorac Dis*. 2019;11(7):3146-3155.
48. Aydin Y, Ogul H, Topdagi O, et al. Pulmonary alveolar echinococcosis: a report of thirty-four cases from a reference center. *Arch Bronconeumol*. 2019;56(12): doi:10.1016/j.arbres.2019.07.014
49. Bhatia G. Echinococcus. *Semin Respir Infect*. 1997;12:171-186.
50. Greenberg DJ, Canoy J, Tomac Pavosevic H, Epelbaum O. Pulmonary cystic echinococcosis. *Mayo Clin Proc*. 2022;97(4):752-753.
51. Weber TF, Junghanss T, Stojković M. Pulmonary cystic echinococcosis. *Curr Opin Infect Dis*. 2023;36(5):318-325.

8

VIRAL LUNG INFECTIONS

Viruses are a common cause of infection in the upper and lower respiratory tracts. Most respiratory viral infections are self-limited, however, serious life-threatening disease can also be caused by these agents in both previously healthy and immunocompromised individuals. Outbreaks of respiratory illness are caused every year by certain viruses, including influenza, parainfluenza, respiratory syncytial virus (RSV), coronavirus, and adenovirus.[1] These can be responsible for serious, life-threatening disease in the elderly and in immunocompromised patients. Certain viruses, however, are more commonly associated with respiratory infections in immunocompromised patients, such as cytomegalovirus (CMV) and herpes simplex virus (HSV).

Viral infection of the pulmonary tract may manifest in a variety of ways, with several possible patterns of lung injury, including diffuse alveolar damage (DAD), acute bronchitis, organizing pneumonia, diffuse interstitial pneumonia, and acute fibrinous and organizing pneumonia.[2] The histologic diagnosis of specific viral infections, however, can be made only by recognizing their characteristic cytopathic effects, including nuclear and cytoplasmic alterations as seen on hematoxylin- and eosin-stained histologic slides on routine light microscopy.[3] Several specific antibodies have been developed for use by immunohistochemistry to identify several common pulmonary viral pathogens. Laboratory testing for viral infections includes antigen detection methods and viral cell culture. In addition, next-generation sequencing and polymerase chain reaction (PCR) assays have become available over the last decade, which can also aid in the diagnosis of viral infections.[4,5]

The most common pattern of lung injury owing to viruses is DAD. However, this is a very nonspecific injury pattern in the lung that can be caused by many other insults, including infections by bacteria, mycobacterial and fungal pneumonias, various forms of lung toxicity, drugs, and inhalation of toxic fumes. A careful search for viral cytopathic effect as well as correlation with the clinical history is indispensable for correct interpretation. The commonest cytopathic effect caused by viruses in the lung is the presence of cytoplasmic or intranuclear inclusions within the infected cells. A summary of the various types of inclusions in the lung is presented in Table 8.1. It is of note that some viral infections affecting the lung, such as hantavirus, influenza virus, and severe acute respiratory

TABLE 8.1 Cytopathic Effect in Pulmonary Viral Infections

Virus	Location	Cytopathic Effect
Cytomegalovirus	Intranuclear and cytoplasmic	Large cells containing large, round, or oval eosinophilic to basophilic intranuclear or cytoplasmic inclusions
Herpes simplex virus/varicella-zoster virus	Intranuclear	Ground-glass amphophilic intranuclear inclusion (early stage); single eosinophilic intranuclear inclusion surrounded by a halo (later stage)
Adenovirus	Intranuclear	Smudgy eosinophilic intranuclear inclusion (early stage); basophilic smudged nucleus (later stage)
Respiratory syncytial virus	Cytoplasmic	Syncytial giant cells with small eosinophilic inclusions, halo may be present
Measles	Intranuclear and cytoplasmic	Giant cells with intranuclear and cytoplasmic eosinophilic inclusions; halo may be present

syndrome (SARS) due to coronavirus, do not produce any inclusions that are discernible on routine histologic examination.

CYTOMEGALOVIRUS INFECTION

CMV infection represents an acquired infection that is generally asymptomatic in healthy children and adults but can lead to severe and sometimes fatal illness in immune-deficient individuals. The organism is a double-stranded DNA herpesvirus that replicates in the host cell nucleus. CMV is one of the most common opportunistic viral infections in patients with acquired immunodeficiency syndrome and in organ transplant patients.[6-8] Lung infection by CMV can be minimal, with only a few scattered alveolar lining cells showing the cytopathic viral changes, or it may progress to a hemorrhagic and necrotizing pneumonia. There are four main patterns of lung infection: minimal infection with isolated viral inclusions, a miliary pattern of lung involvement, a diffuse interstitial pneumonia pattern, and hemorrhagic pneumonia. The diffuse interstitial pattern may range from mild to severe DAD (Fig. 8.1). In the mild form, there is interstitial chronic inflammation with pneumocyte hyperplasia and intra-alveolar macrophages (Fig. 8.2). In the severe form, the main findings are those of DAD with abundant intra-alveolar fibrin deposition, hyaline membranes, fibroblastic proliferation, and necrosis (Fig. 8.3). In some immunocompromised patients, the

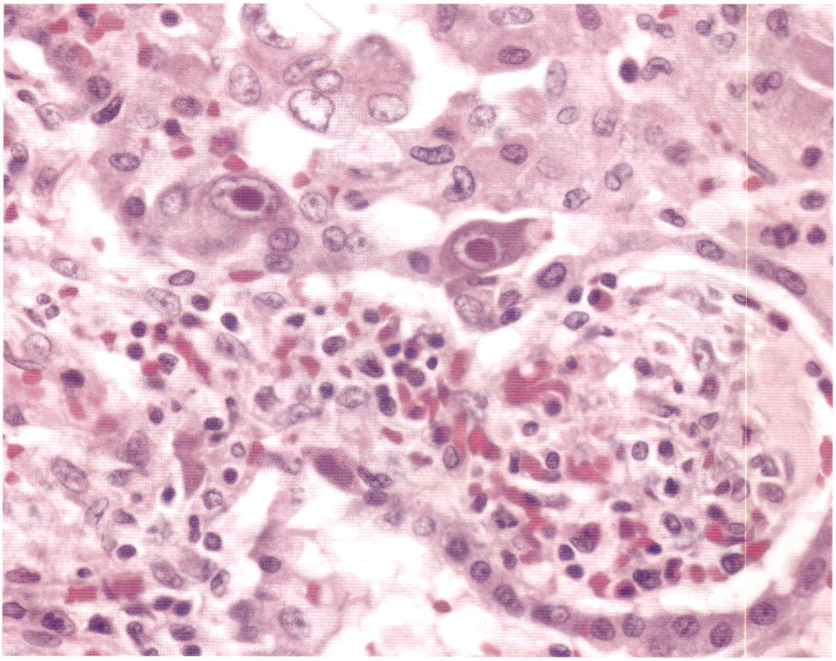

FIGURE 8.1 **Diffuse interstitial pattern of lung involvement in cytomegalovirus infection.** There is diffuse alveolar damage with organizing pneumonia and scattered pneumocytes containing eosinophilic viral inclusions.

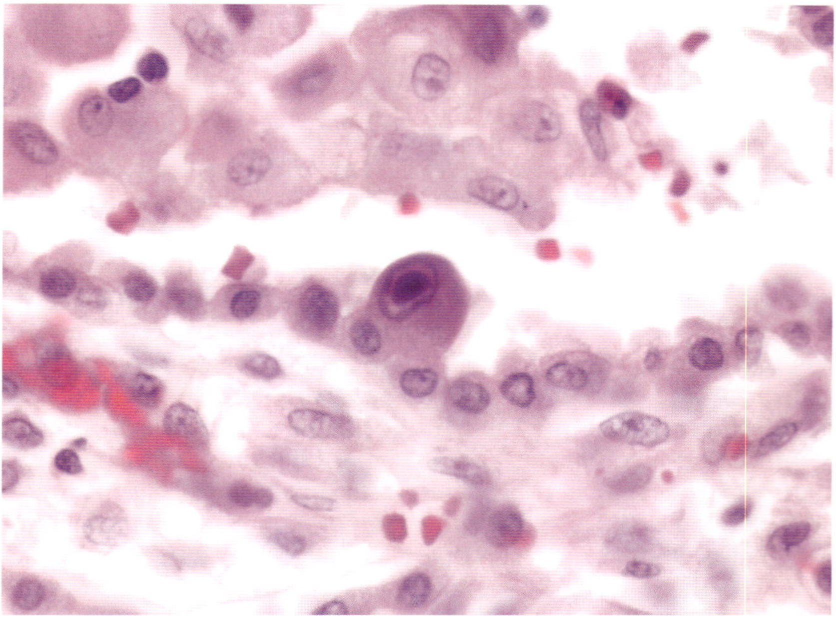

FIGURE 8.2 **Mild form of cytomegalovirus infection of the lung showing isolated infected cells in a minimally damaged lung.**

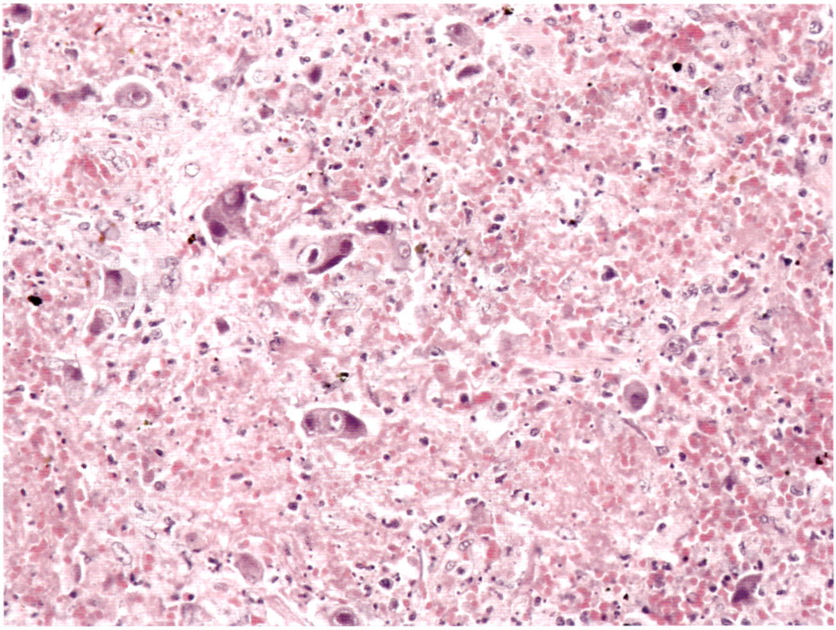

FIGURE 8.3 Severe form of cytomegalovirus pneumonitis with extensive hemorrhagic and necrotizing pneumonia with scattered cells containing viral inclusions.

infection can be quite massive, with sheets of infected cells against a background of necrotizing bronchopneumonia (Fig. 8.4). Diagnosis requires the identification of the characteristic viral inclusions known as Cowdry type A inclusions (also referred to as "owl's eye" inclusions). CMV can infect a wide variety of cell types, including alveolar pneumocytes, fibroblasts, macrophages, and endothelial cells. The cytopathic effects of CMV can be present in both the nucleus and the cytoplasm of infected cells (eFigs. 8.1-8.3). Infected cells usually show marked enlargement. The characteristic nuclear inclusions are large, single, and measure approximately 20 μm in diameter (Fig. 8.5). The cytoplasmic inclusions are usually much smaller and more difficult to identify; they can be stained with periodic acid-Schiff and Gomori methenamine silver (Fig. 8.6). The intranuclear inclusions are usually round to oval and may be basophilic or eosinophilic; they usually show a peripheral clear halo with accentuation of the nuclear membrane. The inclusions are easy to visualize using antibodies to CMV by immunohistochemistry (Fig. 8.7). In patients treated with antiviral agents, the inclusions may be very scant and difficult to identify on routine microscopy; use of anti-CMV antibodies by immunohistochemistry is recommended in such cases for adequate identification.

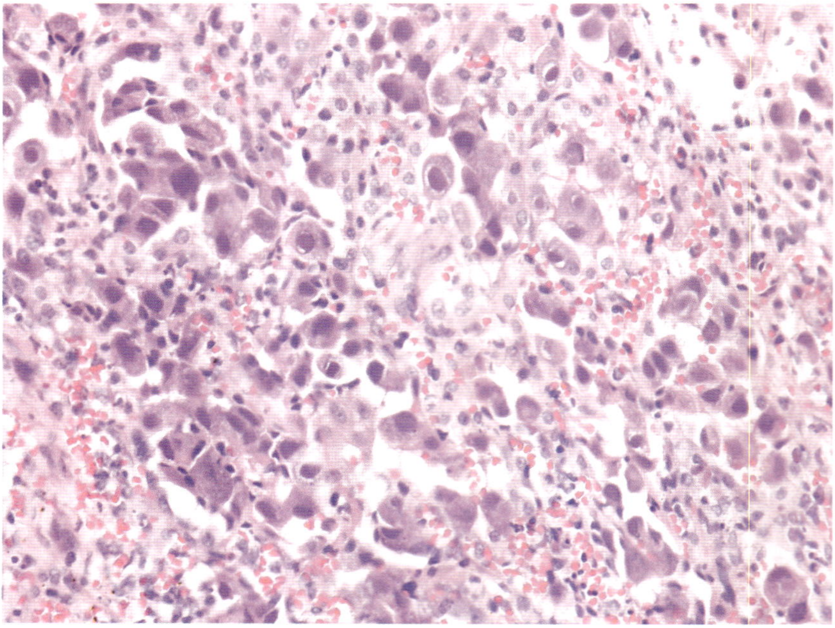

FIGURE 8.4 **Massive infection by cytomegalovirus in immunocompromised patient showing dense sheets of virally infected cells with large eosinophilic inclusions.**

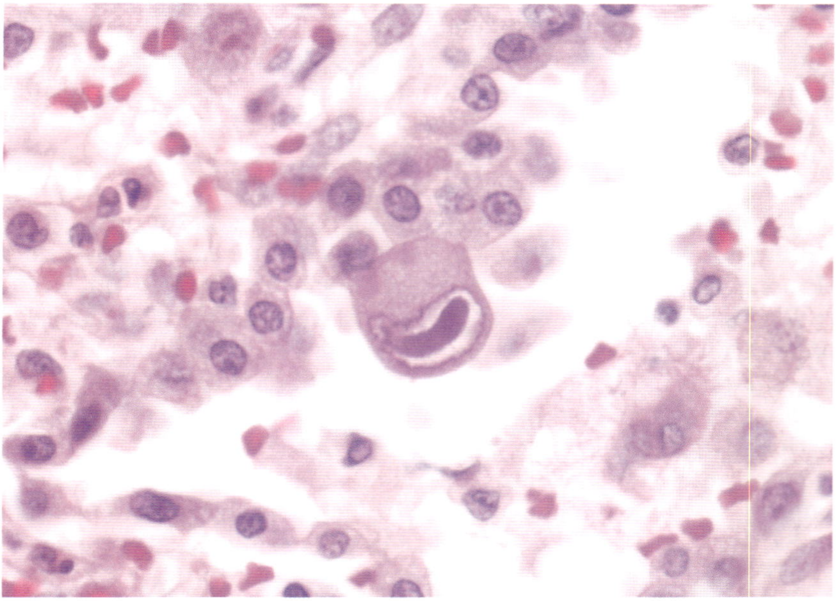

FIGURE 8.5 **Characteristic intranuclear eosinophilic inclusion in cytomegalovirus pneumonia.** Notice the peripheral clear halo surrounding the inclusion.

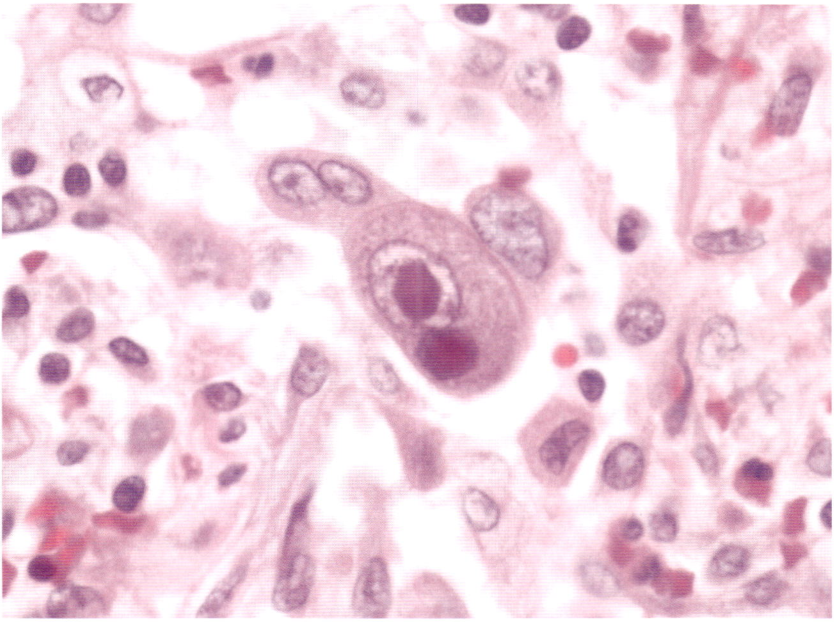

FIGURE 8.6 Cytomegalovirus-infected cell showing both nuclear and cytoplasmic inclusions.

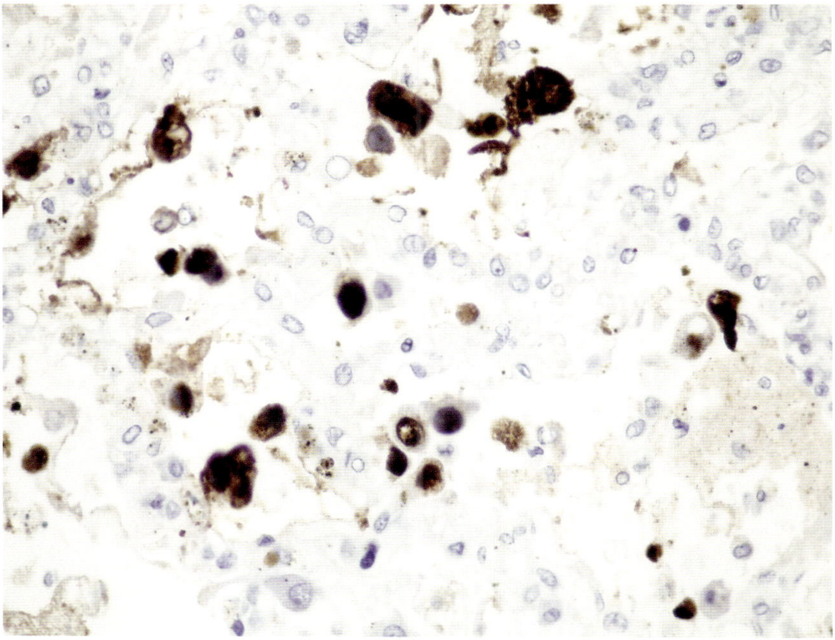

FIGURE 8.7 Immunohistochemical stain with anti-cytomegalovirus (anti-CMV) antibodies highlights infected cells in CMV pneumonitis.

HERPES SIMPLEX PNEUMONIA

Herpes simplex pneumonia is caused by HSV-1 and HSV-2, a double-stranded DNA virus that measures 100 nm in diameter. HSV pneumonia is seen in neonates as well as in adults who are immunosuppressed.[9,10] The organisms usually reach the lungs through contiguous spread from mucocutaneous lesions in the oral cavity and upper airways. There are three principal patterns of involvement in the lungs: necrotizing tracheobronchitis, necrotizing pneumonia, and interstitial pneumonitis.[11] Necrotizing tracheobronchitis owing to HSV is usually manifested by extensive ulceration and necrosis of the surface mucosa with production of abundant fibrinopurulent exudate (Fig. 8.8; eFigs. 8.4 and 8.5). Necrotizing HSV pneumonia is usually distributed around the bronchi and is characterized by extensive suppurative necrosis of the surrounding lung parenchyma (Fig. 8.9). The diffuse interstitial pneumonitis pattern of HSV infection shows the histologic features of DAD, with interstitial edema, interstitial inflammation, and hyaline membrane formation or can sometimes show features of acute fibrinous and organizing pneumonia (Figs. 8.10 and 8.11).

The viral inclusions of HSV can be either large, eosinophilic, and surrounded by a halo or homogeneous and glassy (amphophilic) (Fig. 8.12). The infected epithelial cells may be multinucleated and contain multiple viral nuclear inclusions (eFig. 8.6); these nuclear inclusions will push the

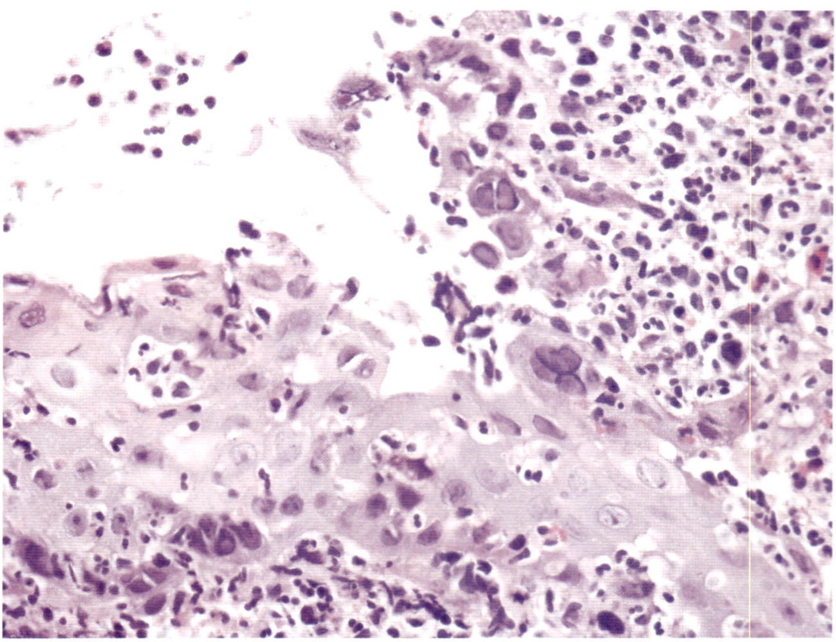

FIGURE 8.8 **Necrotizing herpes simplex virus tracheobronchitis.** Notice the infected cells showing hyaline nuclear inclusions with multinucleation, margination, and molding ("The 3 M's").

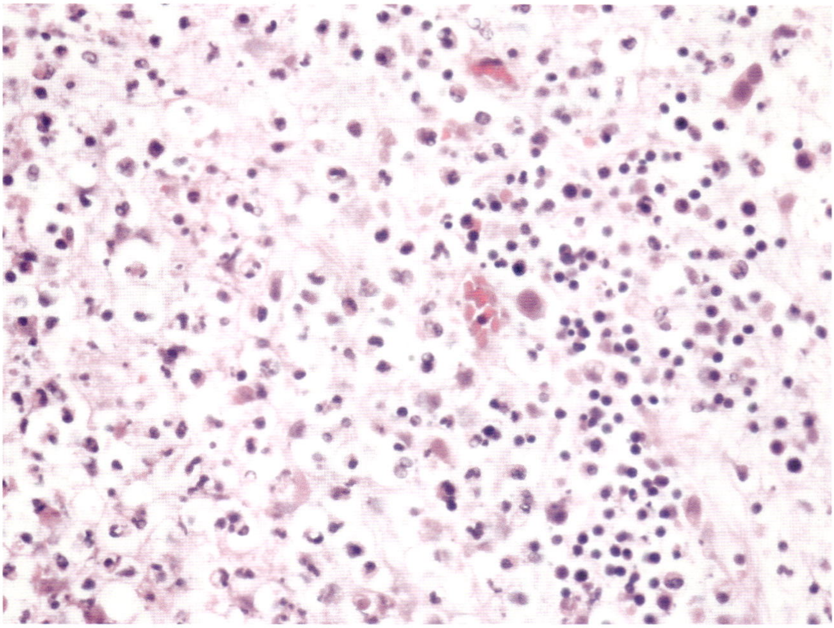

FIGURE 8.9 Necrotizing herpes simplex virus pneumonia showing diffuse alveolar damage with inflammation and scattered infected cells containing eosinophilic viral inclusions.

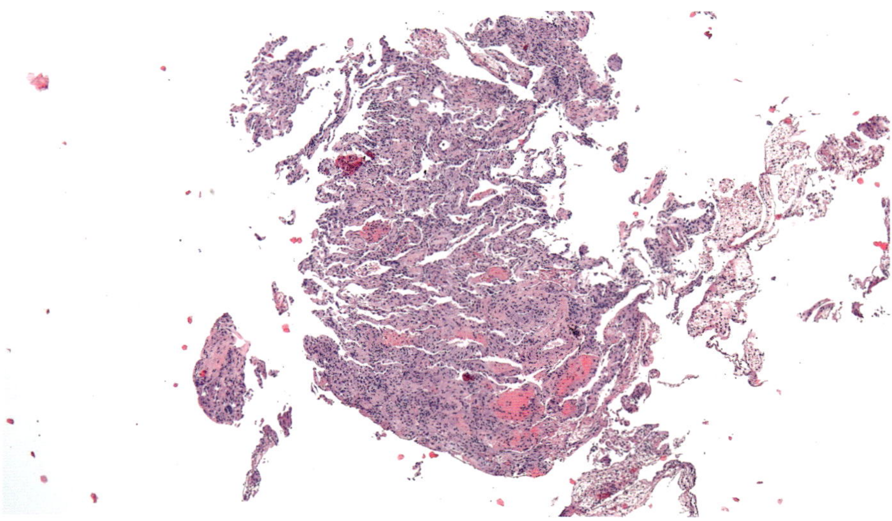

FIGURE 8.10 Transbronchial biopsy in a patient with herpes simplex virus pneumonia shows inflamed lung parenchyma with areas of acute fibrinous and organizing pneumonia.

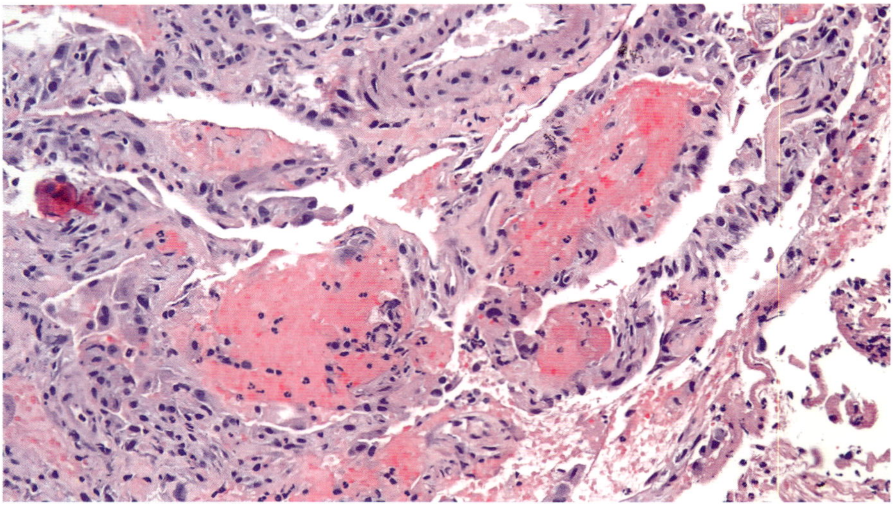

FIGURE 8.11 **Higher magnification of the area shows admixed acute inflammatory cells and focal evidence hyaline membrane formation (*top left*).** Definitive viral cytopathic effect is difficult to visualize even at higher power in some cases, and the diagnosis was confirmed by polymerase chain reaction analysis.

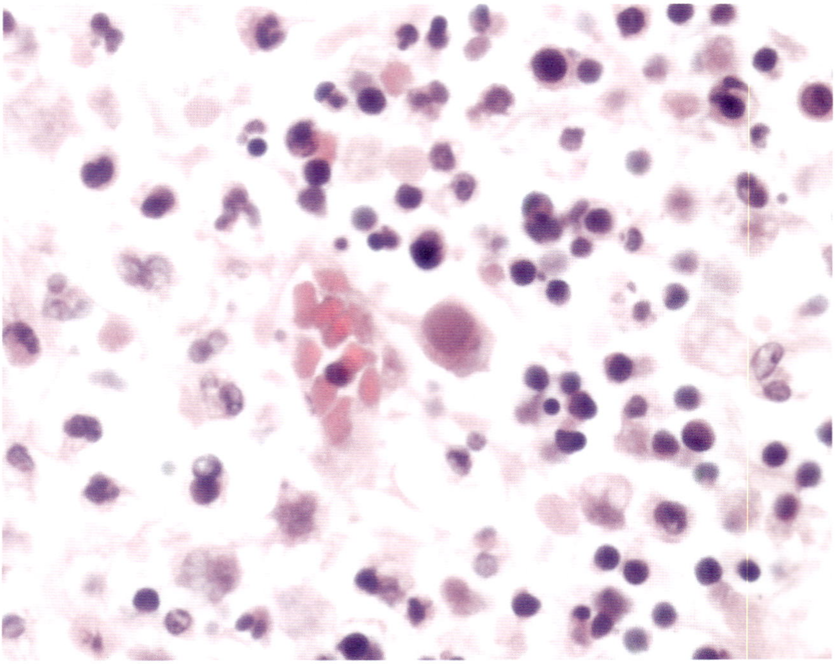

FIGURE 8.12 **Higher magnification of herpes simplex virus pneumonitis showing a large eosinophilic inclusion surrounded by a halo.**

chromatin to the periphery of the nuclei (a process known as margination). The cells may also display molding of the nuclei. The intranuclear inclusions are best appreciated in cells located at the periphery of the necrotic foci. The inclusions can closely resemble those of adenovirus. Immunohistochemical staining can be extremely useful for properly identifying the viral inclusions of HSV, particularly in cases with extensive necrosis. In recent years, application of multiplex PCR for HSV-1, Epstein-Barr virus, CMV, human herpesvirus 6, and human herpesvirus 7 has been used with success in bronchoalveolar lavage fluid to make a specific diagnosis in patients with acute lung injury or respiratory distress syndrome.[12] Metagenomic next-generation sequencing can also successfully identify HSV infections within the lung.[13,14]

VARICELLA-ZOSTER PNEUMONIA

Varicella-zoster pneumonia is a lung infection caused by a virus that is structurally very similar to HSV. Infection with the varicella-zoster virus (VZV) causes two clinical syndromes: varicella (chickenpox) and herpes zoster (shingles). In children and adults with impaired cell-mediated immunity, particularly bone marrow transplant recipients and acute leukemia patients, disseminated infection including pneumonia can occur.[15] VZV pneumonia may also affect individuals with chronic autoimmune disorders.[16,17] VZV pneumonia in immunocompromised patients is a common complication and has a particularly poor prognosis, with mortality rates between 30% and 50%.[18] The pathologic findings are very similar to those of HSV lung infection. The viral inclusions are identical to those of HSV but may be harder to identify. A more specific diagnosis can be attained by the use of specific antibodies by immunohistochemistry against VZV or by molecular analysis for viral nucleic acid. Isolation of the virus in cell culture, however, remains the gold standard for identification.

ADENOVIRUS

Adenovirus is a cause of respiratory infection owing to a double-stranded DNA virus found normally in the upper respiratory tract of humans. There are more than 50 known serotypes. In adults, the most common serotypes involved in causing pneumonia are 3, 4, 7, and 14.[19,20] The virus may cause latent infection that becomes reactivated during immunosuppression. The infection can spread quickly and be the cause of epidemics, particularly in military personnel, day care, and school and college students.[21] Lung involvement with adenovirus can display acute necrotizing pneumonia with severe bronchitis and bronchiolitis or an interstitial pattern characterized by DAD with hemorrhage and necrosis (Figs. 8.13 and 8.14).[22] Admixtures of the two are common. Involvement of secondary or medium-sized bronchi is characteristic and usually leads to striking necrosis with karyorrhexis and abundant cellular debris (Fig. 8.15). The intranuclear inclusions in adenoviral pneumonia closely resemble those of HSV and are characterized by small, dense eosinophilic round or oval inclusions surrounded by a clear halo (Figs. 8.16 and 8.17; eFigs. 8.7-8.9). As the

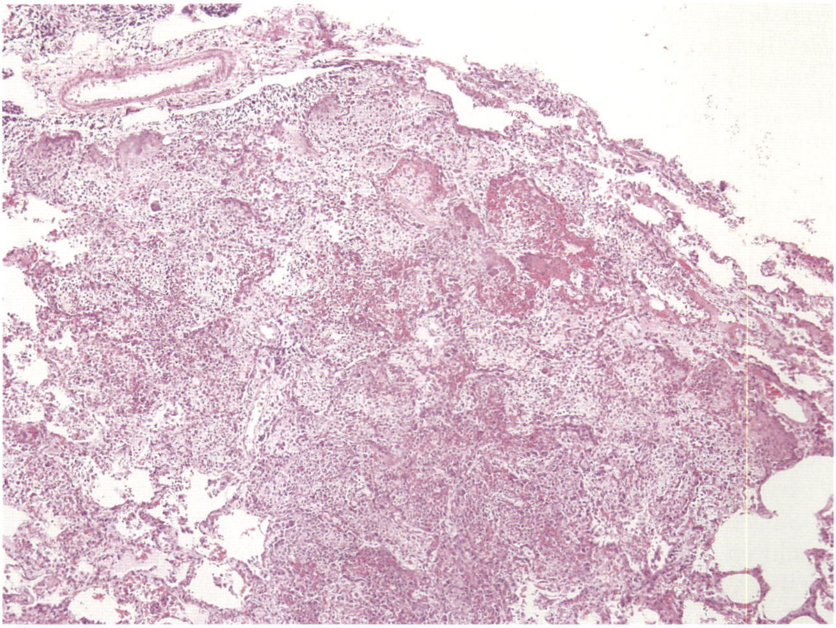

FIGURE 8.13 Acute necrotizing pneumonia in adenovirus infection characterized by extensive hemorrhage and diffuse alveolar damage.

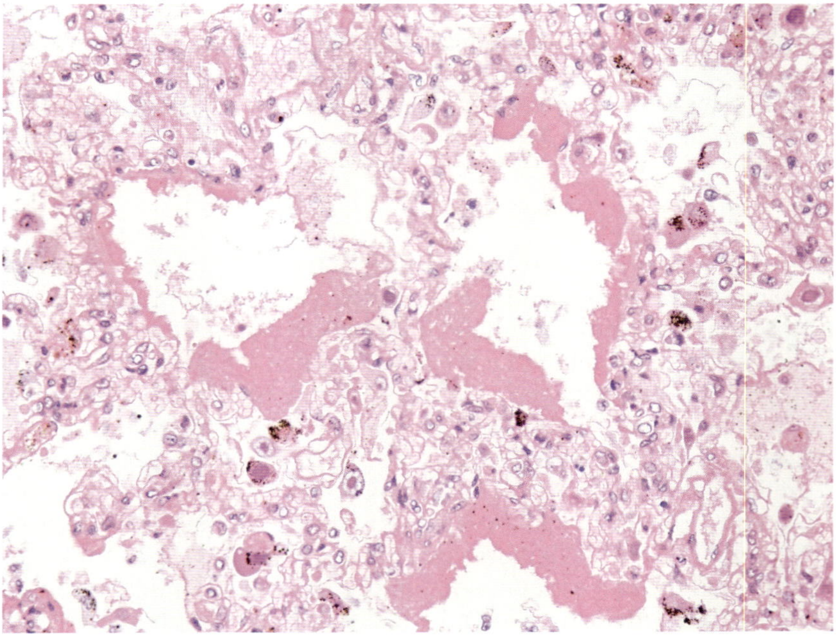

FIGURE 8.14 Interstitial pattern of involvement in adenoviral pneumonia showing fibrin deposition in alveolar lumens with hyaline membrane formation and scattered infected cells containing viral inclusions.

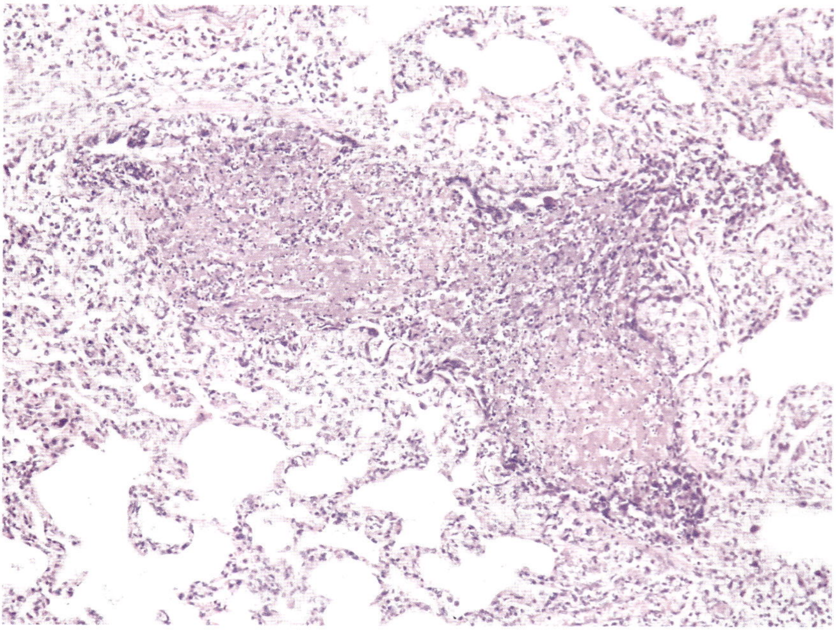

FIGURE 8.15 Adenoviral pneumonia showing acute necrotizing bronchiolitis.

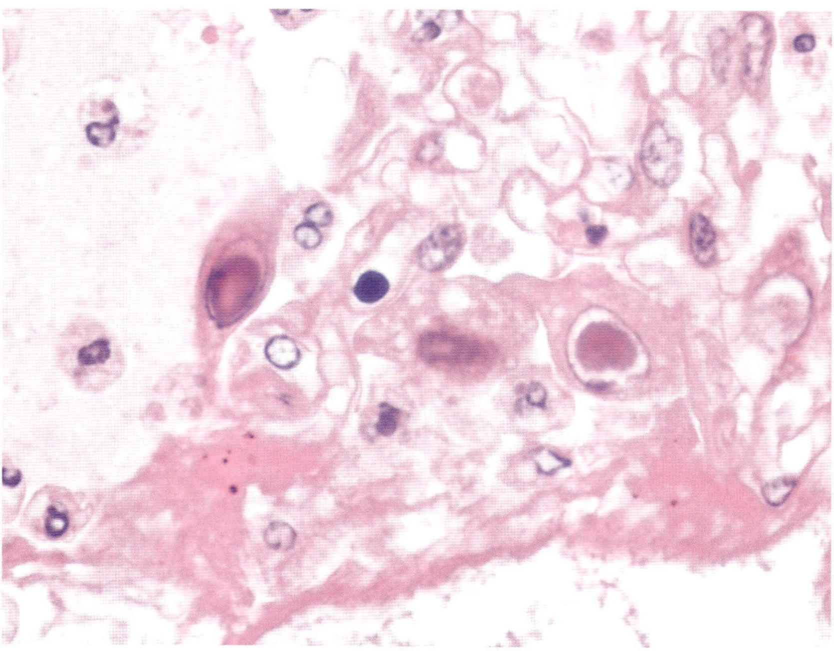

FIGURE 8.16 Small, dense, and eosinophilic round or oval inclusions surrounded by a halo are seen in the early lesions of adenovirus pneumonia.

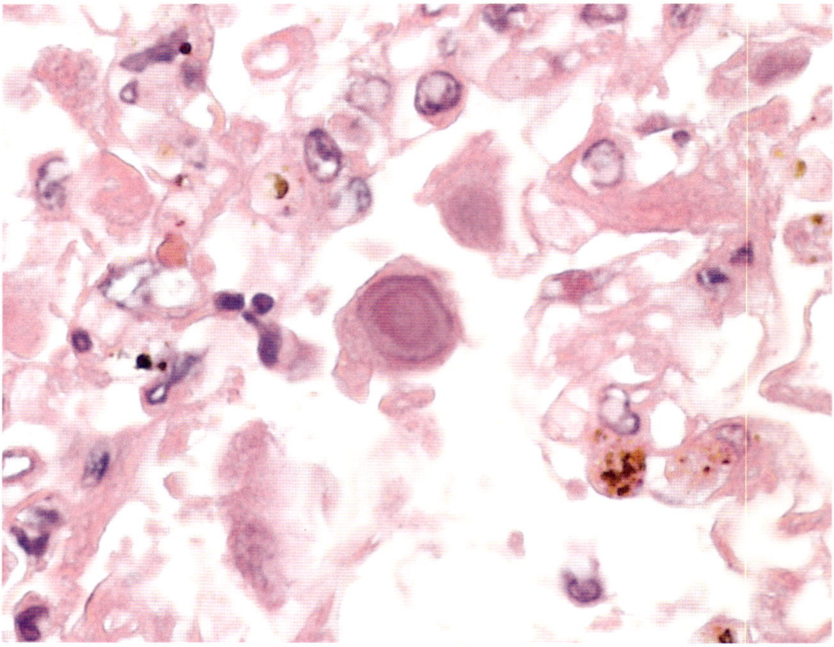

FIGURE 8.17 Characteristic adenovirus inclusion showing round eosinophilic structure surrounded by a distinct clear halo.

infection progresses, the inclusions become larger and more basophilic, and the halo disappears, leading to a blurring of the margins between the inclusion and the nuclear membrane resulting in a smudged appearance (so-called smudge cell) (Fig. 8.18). The inclusions may be hard to find and are best identified at the leading edge of the necrotic zones. Infected cells can be easily identified by the use of specific antibodies by immunohistochemistry on routine formalin-fixed paraffin-embedded tissues or by molecular techniques (Fig. 8.19; eFig. 8.10).

RESPIRATORY SYNCYTIAL VIRUS

RSV is a single-stranded RNA paramyxovirus that is a common cause of bronchiolitis and pneumonia in infants and children under 1 year of age. It has also been found to cause a small percentage (<5%) of community-acquired pneumonia in adults and more rarely is found in young adults, immunocompromised patients, and patients with underlying heart and lung conditions such as chronic obstructive pulmonary disease and asthma.[23] It is one of the leading global causes of respiratory infections responsible for 100,000 or more deaths annually in children younger than 5 years old.[24] The symptoms may be difficult to distinguish from other pulmonary viral infections and include coughing, wheezing, fevers,

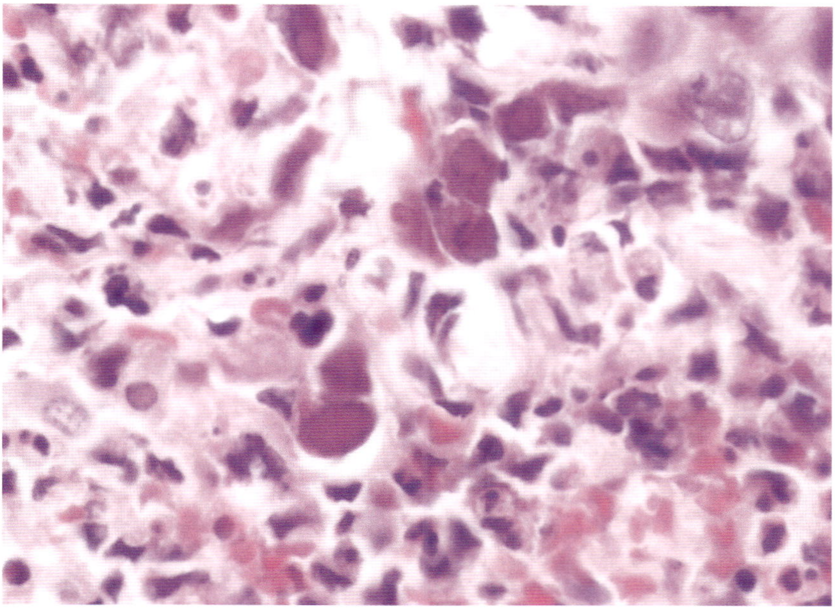

FIGURE 8.18 Late adenovirus inclusions are larger, more basophilic, and without a halo (smudge cells).

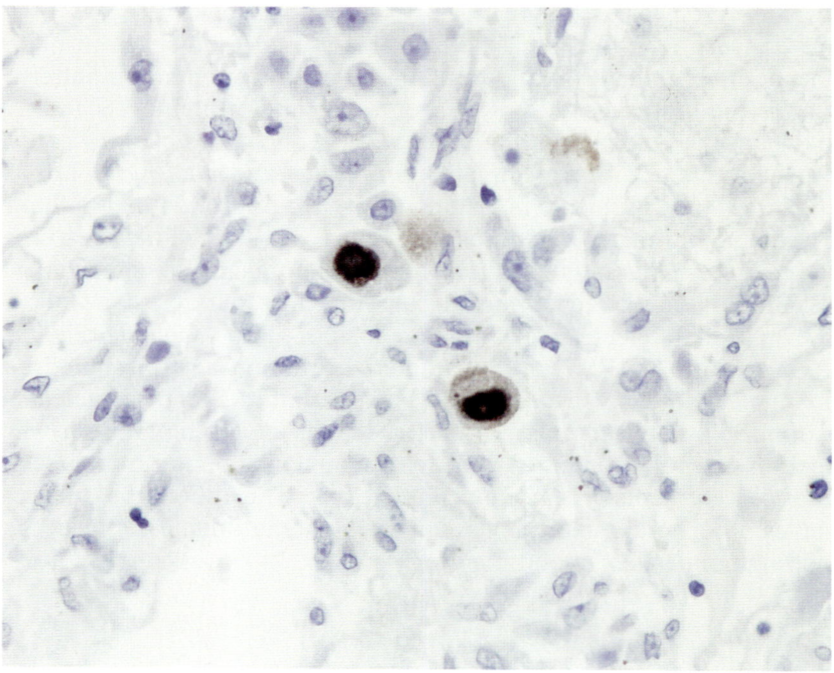

FIGURE 8.19 Immunohistochemical staining in adenoviral pneumonia highlights the viral cytopathic inclusions.

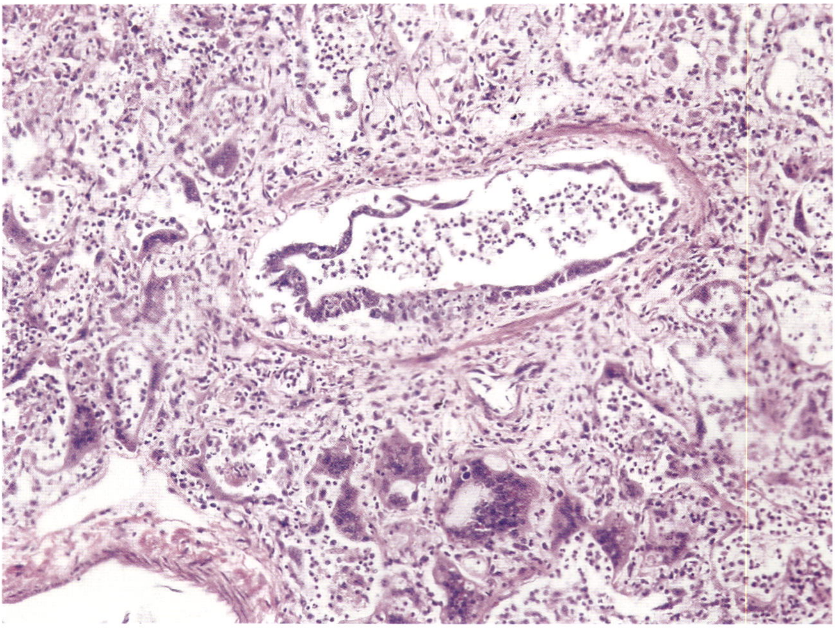

FIGURE 8.20 Necrotizing bronchiolitis surrounded by syncytial giant cells is seen in respiratory syncytial virus pneumonia.

sinus congestion, rhinorrhea, and severe respiratory distress in patients with underlying medical conditions.[23] The two most common patterns of injury to the lung caused by RSV are necrotizing bronchiolitis and interstitial giant cell pneumonia.[25] The involved bronchial lumens and airways are usually filled with inflammatory infiltrates and necrotic debris (Fig. 8.20). The terminal bronchioles show severe peribronchiolar inflammation comprising mainly lymphocytes. Some cases may show features of giant cell interstitial pneumonia with prominent DAD. The syncytial giant cells comprise enlarged epithelial cells that line the alveolar walls and show multiple nuclei and may contain eosinophilic inclusions (Fig. 8.21). The inclusions in RSV are characteristically intracytoplasmic rather than nuclear and are usually small, eosinophilic, and paranuclear and surrounded by a clear halo. A specific diagnosis can be made by direct detection of viral antigens in clinical specimens by immunofluorescence, immunohistochemistry, or molecular assays. The differential diagnosis involves other viral pneumonias that produce multinucleated giant cells, including parainfluenza and measles.

HUMAN METAPNEUMOVIRUS INFECTION

Human metapneumovirus (HMPV) infection is caused by a paramyxovirus that creates a very similar pattern of lung injury in children and

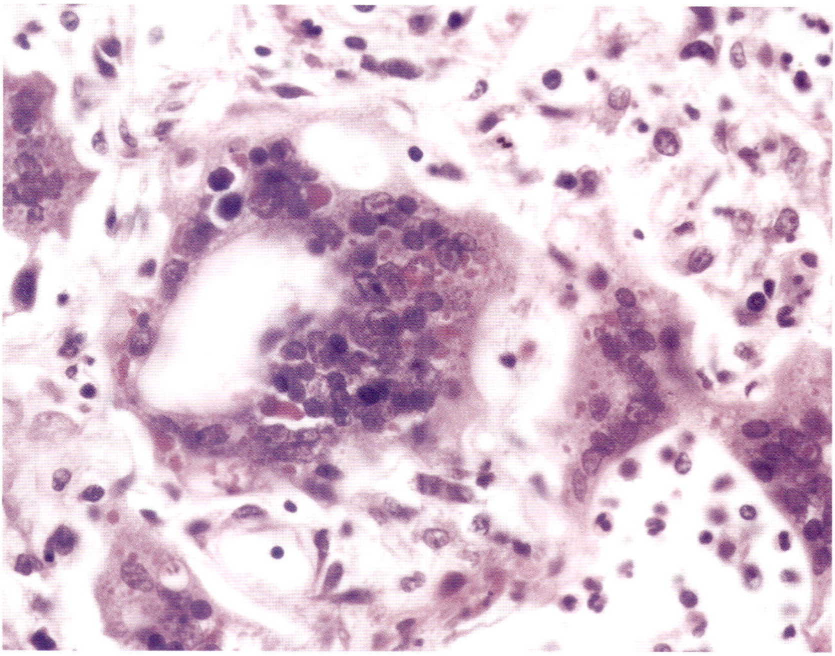

FIGURE 8.21 Syncytial giant cell in respiratory syncytial virus pneumonia containing multiple small eosinophilic intracytoplasmic inclusions.

adults as that of RSV, particularly in immunosuppressed patients and in patients with hematologic malignancies.[26-28] Few studies have examined the histopathologic characteristics of HMPV pulmonary infections. Vargas et al[29] described the pathologic findings in six patients, three of which had biopsy specimens available for review; they noted epithelial cells with degenerative changes, eosinophilic cytoplasmic inclusions, and multinucleated giant cells in the bronchoalveolar lavage specimens, and noted chronic airway inflammation and intra-alveolar foamy macrophages in the biopsy specimens. A single case reported describing the cytologic changes of HMPV was also recently published describing multinucleation, nuclear enlargement, homogenized nuclei, basophilic nuclear inclusions with perinuclear halos, and small eosinophilic cytoplasmic inclusions.[30] Antibodies to HMPV are not yet widely available; most cases have been identified using reverse transcription PCR assays or by demonstration of a rise in HMPV-specific antibodies by serology.

MEASLES

Measles is caused by a single-stranded RNA paramyxovirus. The disease (rubeola) is an acute febrile viral illness characterized by fever, upper

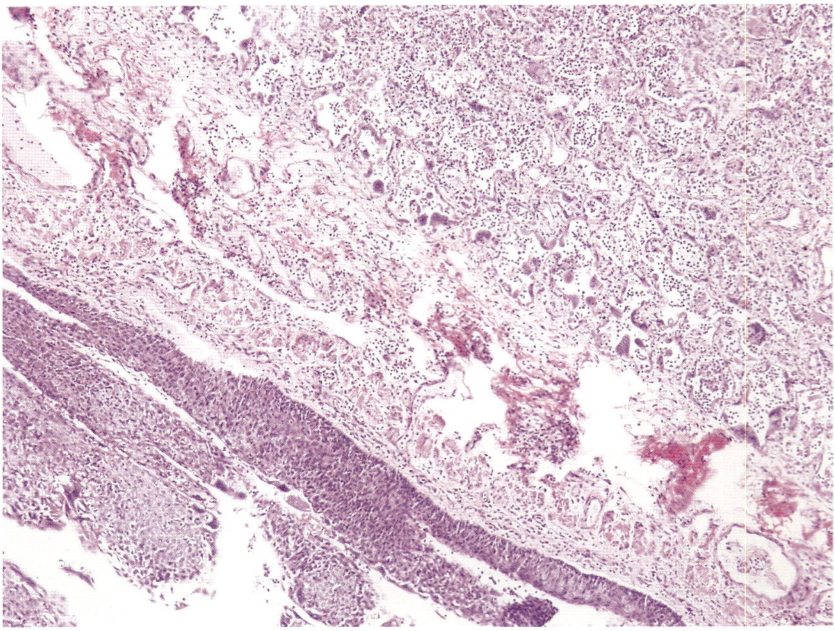

FIGURE 8.22 **Measles pneumonia showing necrotizing bronchiolitis with prominent squamous metaplasia.**

respiratory tract symptoms, and a maculopapular rash. The disease is highly contagious, spreads through respiratory secretions, and usually affects young children. There has been a global resurgence in cases of measles over the past decade.[31-33] Measles infection of the lungs can cause acute necrotizing bronchiolitis or a diffuse interstitial pneumonia with features of giant cell pneumonia.[34] The necrotizing bronchiolitis may be associated with regenerative changes of the epithelium including squamous metaplasia (Fig. 8.22). The interstitial giant cell pneumonitis will be characterized by DAD with prominent formation of syncytial giant cells (Fig. 8.23). The characteristic cytopathic change in measles pneumonia is the presence of large (100 μm) multinucleated epithelial cells in the bronchial mucosa and alveolar epithelium that have nuclear and cytoplasmic eosinophilic inclusions (Fig. 8.24). The nuclear inclusions are homogeneous and are usually surrounded by a clear halo. The presence of the measles virus can be confirmed in tissues by immunohistochemistry or in situ hybridization.[35] The differential diagnosis of giant cell viral pneumonias involves RSV, VZV, and parainfluenza virus; the various features of these infections are compared in Table 8.2.

VIRUSES THAT DO NOT PRODUCE CYTOPATHIC EFFECTS

Several viruses that can affect the lungs will not produce any cytopathic effects. Identification of such viruses is more difficult to establish on biopsy

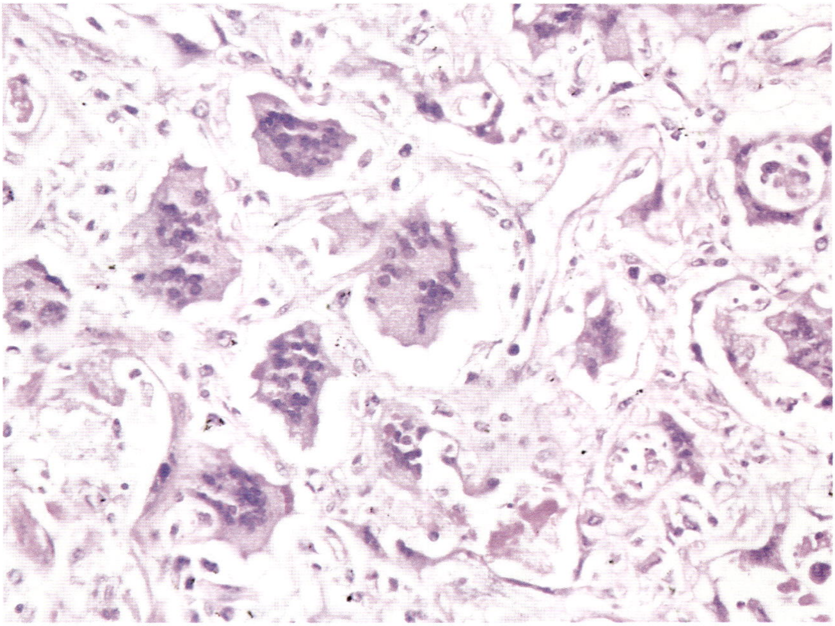

FIGURE 8.23 Measles giant cell interstitial pneumonia with multiple scattered multinucleated giant cells.

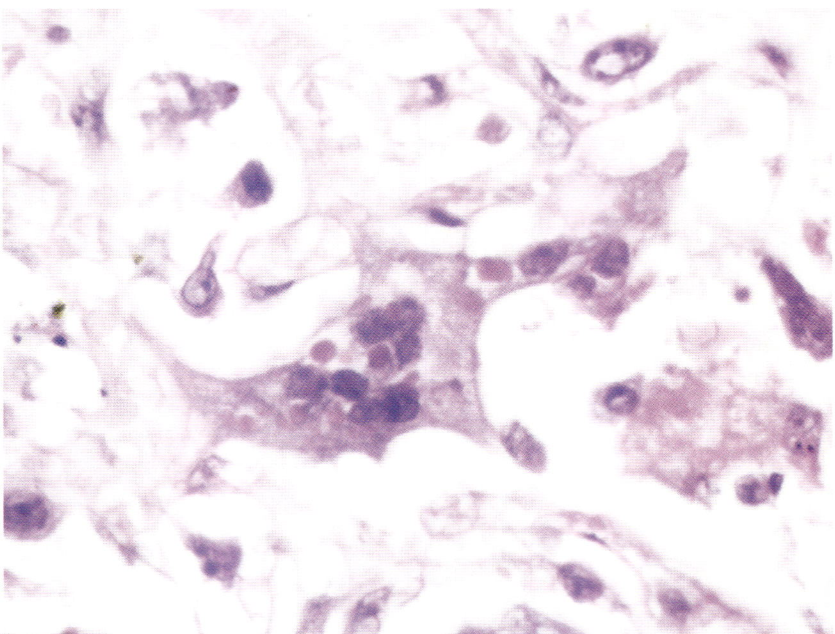

FIGURE 8.24 Higher magnification of multinucleated giant cell in interstitial pneumonia secondary to measles showing small, round eosinophilic inclusions similar to those seen in respiratory syncytial virus pneumonia.

TABLE 8.2 Differential Diagnosis of Giant Cell Viral Pneumonias

Virus	Location	Features
Measles	Nuclear and cytoplasmic inclusions (numerous)	Large multinucleated epithelial cells with nuclear and cytoplasmic inclusions. Diagnosis can be confirmed by immunohistochemistry and in situ hybridization
Respiratory syncytial virus	Cytoplasmic inclusions (few)	Small, eosinophilic, paranuclear inclusions surrounded by a clear halo. Diagnosis can be confirmed by culture or immunofluorescent techniques
Herpes simplex virus/varicella-zoster virus	Nuclear inclusions (few). Giant cells are rare	Small, eosinophilic, or amphophilic, homogeneous, and glassy. Diagnosis can be established by immunohistochemistry or molecular methods
Parainfluenza virus	Small cytoplasmic inclusions (numerous)	The cytoplasmic inclusions are very small and consist of aggregates of viral nucleocapsids. Diagnosis is established by cultures or immunofluorescent techniques

material and will generally require epidemiologic, serologic, and other types of studies for confirmation including viral cultures, direct fluorescent antibody detection, molecular testing, or immunohistochemistry. These include coronavirus, hantavirus, and influenza virus.

Severe Acute Respiratory Syndrome

Severe acute respiratory syndrome (SARS) is a severe influenzalike illness characterized by acute onset of fever, malaise, myalgia, dry cough, chills, and sore throat that can quickly progress to acute respiratory distress syndrome (ARDS). The causative agent is a positive-strand RNA virus belonging to the genus *Coronavirus*. SARS was first recognized during a global outbreak originating in China in 2002, from where it spread to Asia, Europe, and the Americas.[36,37] The typical computed tomography findings include peripheral subpleural ground-glass opacities or consolidation. The main histopathologic finding is DAD with scattered mononuclear cell infiltrates in the interstitium.[38] The affected parenchyma may also show intra-alveolar hemorrhage, suppurative inflammation, and organizing pneumonia.

Multinucleated syncytial cells may be present in alveolar spaces, but no viral inclusions are identified. The histopathologic findings are entirely nonspecific, and diagnosis will require laboratory tests such as serology, viral cultures, molecular techniques, or direct fluorescent antibody detection.

COVID-19

In December 2019, an outbreak of a second *Coronavirus*, SARS-CoV-2/"COVID-19," was detected in Wuhan, Hubei Province, China. This outbreak quickly became a global pandemic lasting approximately 4 years and causing untold social and economic disruption around the world with nearly 700 million cases reported.[39] During this time, the virus spread to nearly all parts of the world including Europe, Africa, Asia, the Middle East, and the Americas. Though official death counts are lower, it is estimated that the true number of deaths from COVID-19 during the pandemic ranged from approximately 15 to 20 million people.[40,41] COVID-19 is primarily a respiratory disease with patients most commonly presenting with upper and/or lower respiratory tract symptoms including cough, dyspnea, chest pain, wheezing and hemoptysis, congestion, sore throat, and rhinorrhea.[42] However, the disease presents with a wide variety of extra-pulmonary manifestations including fever, fatigue, myalgias, rash, gastrointestinal symptoms, and others.[42] A wide spectrum of postacute sequelae of COVID-19 have also been documented and termed "long COVID-19."[43,44] Unlike the original SARS virus, patients generally follow a milder clinical course and present asymptomatically or with fevers and mild respiratory symptoms. However, 15% to 20% of patients, usually the ill or elderly, present with severe illness requiring respiratory support.[45]

The histologic features of COVID-19 infection in the lungs are variable. Infected lungs show overlap with some types of other respiratory viral infections, and the early phase of the disease is characterized by pulmonary edema and congestion (Fig. 8.25).[46] Organizing pneumonia may be seen in some cases (Fig. 8.26). The latter stages of the disease can progress to acute fibrinous and organizing pneumonia and DAD with widespread destruction of lung tissue and deposition of hyaline membranes (Fig. 8.27).[47] Fibrin microthrombi may be identified within small pulmonary arteries, and approximately 50% of fatal cases demonstrate vascular congestion and features of capillary angiomatosis or capillaritis with microvessel destruction and neutrophilic infiltrates (Fig. 8.28).[48-50] Scattered multinucleated giant cells may be seen, and cases presenting with extensive histiocytic infiltrates have been described (Fig. 8.29).[51,52] Viral cytopathic effects are exceptionally rare, though have been reported in some cases as small eosinophilic intracytoplasmic inclusions. The infection is most commonly encountered in autopsy material though small biopsies may be taken in certain scenarios, such as in the posttransplant setting. The histologic findings overall are not entirely specific and diagnosis requires ancillary diagnostic tests, such as in situ hybridization or molecular based assays, to confirm the presence of virus.[53-55]

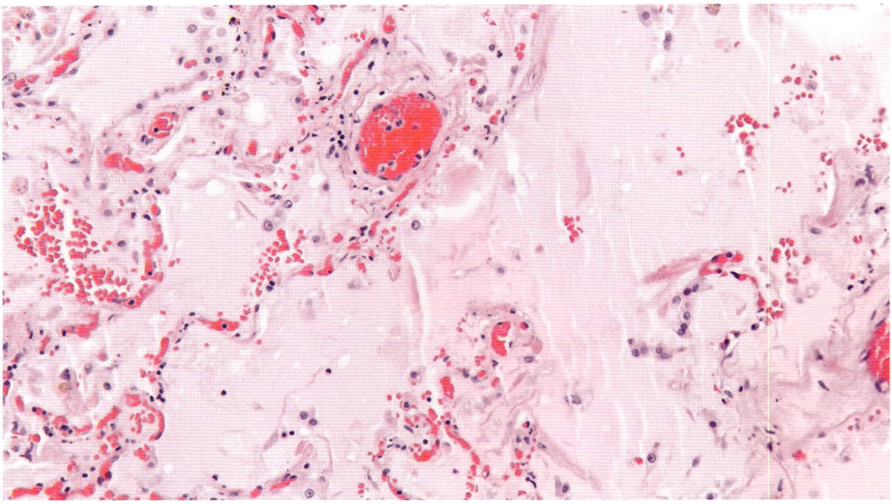

FIGURE 8.25 **Early stage of COVID-19 pneumonia shows alveoli filled with homogeneous, acellular lightly eosinophilic edema.** Small fibrin fragments are present without definitive evidence of hyaline membrane disease.

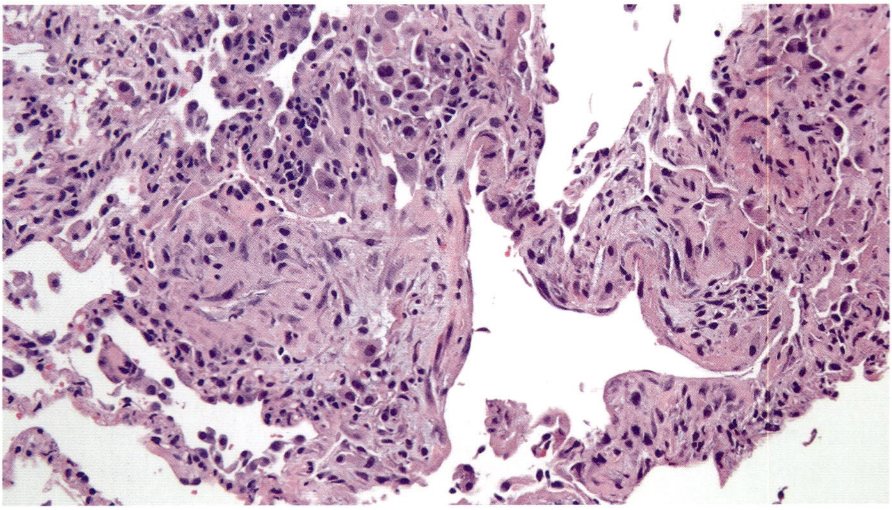

FIGURE 8.26 **Posttransplant lung biopsy from a patient with COVID-19 pneumonia showing only focal organizing pneumonia with subtle myxoid stromal changes.** There is background pneumocyte hyperplasia.

Influenza Virus

Influenza viruses are RNA orthomyxoviruses with segmented genomes. Influenza viruses A and B are most commonly associated with human disease.[56] Influenza virus is a major cause of respiratory illness in adults and children. Uncomplicated influenza is characterized by the onset of

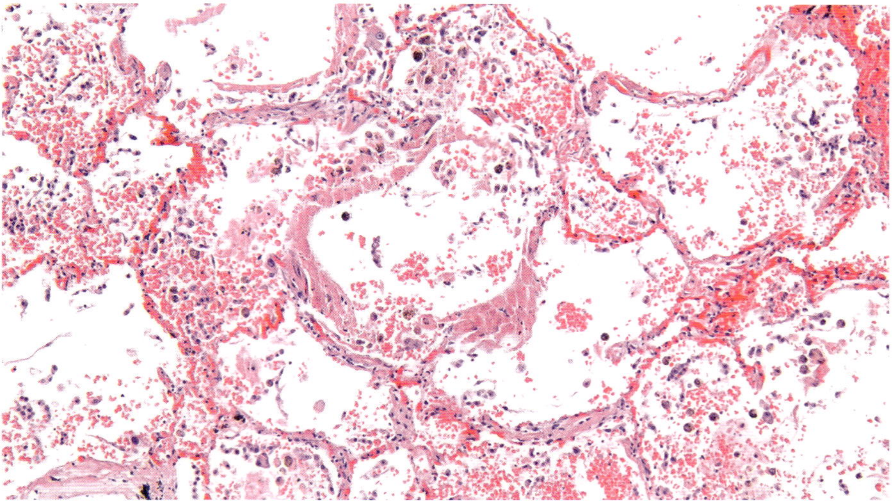

FIGURE 8.27 Advanced stage of COVID-19 pneumonia shows damaged lung parenchyma with vascular congestion and prominent hyaline membrane formation.

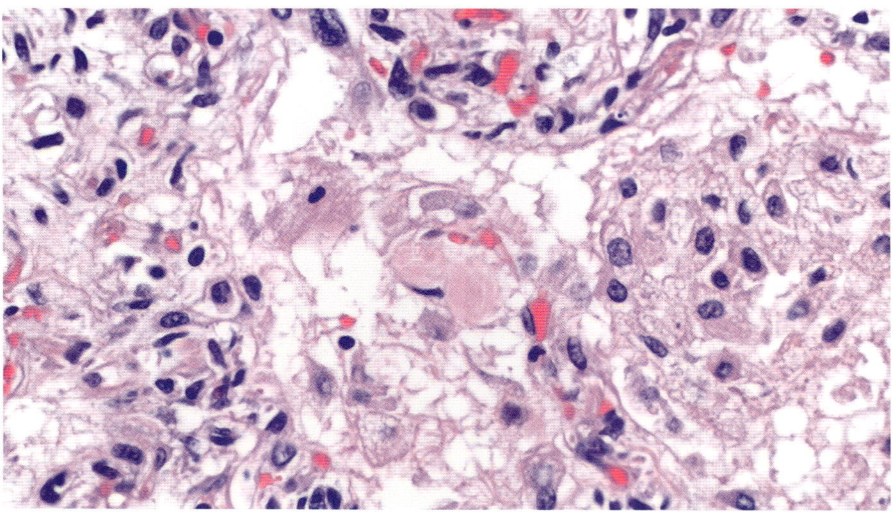

FIGURE 8.28 High-power examination of the lungs from a patient with COVID-19 demonstrates microthrombus formation with a small fibrin thrombus occluding an interstitial arteriole.

constitutional symptoms, including chills, myalgia, fever, sore throat, headache, and malaise. The symptoms usually resolve after 3 to 7 days. When complications supervene, patients will develop secondary bacterial pneumonias and, less commonly, seizures, Reye syndrome, encephalopathy, myositis, myocarditis, and pericarditis. Risk of death because of influenza

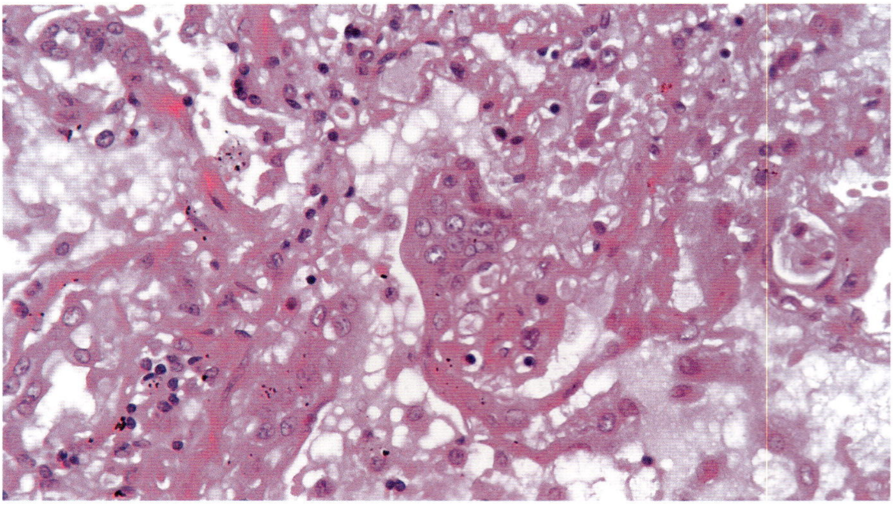

FIGURE 8.29 High-power magnification demonstrates a large multinucleated giant cell.

is highest among children and the elderly. Radiologically, the disease presents with patchy consolidation of lung parenchyma.[57,58] The histologic features in the lung of patients with severe influenza infections include DAD, intra-alveolar hemorrhage, and necrotizing bronchitis.[59,60] No viral inclusions are present. The pathologic changes associated with the primary viral infection are often obscured by secondary bacterial pneumonia. Because the pathologic findings are so nonspecific, diagnosis requires laboratory tests such as direct fluorescent antibody, in situ hybridization, serology, viral cultures, and molecular techniques.

Of historical interest, a novel influenza A virus (H1N1) of swine origin was identified in 2009. After global spread, it was declared by the World Health Organization the first influenza pandemic in 41 years. Patients with the disease developed respiratory illness that could progress to acute respiratory distress syndrome.[61] Fatal cases were characterized by tracheitis, bronchiolitis, and DAD, not unlike other severe influenza infections. In those cases, PCR was also able to detect the virus in the epithelium of the tracheobronchial tree and alveolar epithelial cells.[62]

Hantavirus

Hantavirus is responsible for the hantavirus pulmonary syndrome (HPS), a disease characterized by malaise, fever, myalgia, headache, vomiting, weakness, and cough.[63,64] The initial phase is followed by acute pulmonary edema, respiratory distress, and shock. Large, bilateral pleural effusions are characteristic of HPS. The disease is caused by a negative-sense RNA virus of the genus *Hantavirus*. The pathologic findings include mild to moderate interstitial pneumonitis with prominent interstitial mononuclear cell infiltrates.[65] There may be focal hyaline membranes, but damage to the alveolar lining is not a prominent feature. No inclusions are seen. Specific diagnosis is made by serology, molecular testing, or immunohistochemistry with antibodies to hantaviral antigens. HPS should be suspected in cases of acute respiratory distress without a known precipitating cause among previously healthy individuals. Exposure to rodents in endemic areas also should raise the level of suspicion.

Viral Hemorrhagic Fever

Viral hemorrhagic fever (VHF) represents infection caused by a group of viruses transmitted to humans by rodents and arthropods. The syndrome of VHF is caused by RNA viruses that may belong to four different families, including *Arenaviridae*, *Bunyaviridae*, *Flaviviridae*, and *Filoviridae*. Hemorrhagic fever can occur worldwide, and the diseases are usually named after the place where they were first described, such as Thailand hemorrhagic fever and Crimean-Congo hemorrhagic fever. The oldest and best-known cause of VHF is yellow fever; others include Ebola, Lassa, and Dengue viruses.[66,67] The clinical manifestations of hemorrhagic fever are dominated by hemorrhage, which most commonly affects the mucosal surfaces. The most common findings in the lung include intra-alveolar hemorrhage, edema, interstitial pneumonia, and DAD.[68] No viral inclusions are seen. The diagnosis is suspected in patients who have a history of travel to endemic areas. Definitive diagnosis can be made only by laboratory tests such as serology, cell culture, molecular techniques, and immunohistochemistry.

REFERENCES

1. De Roux A, Marcos MA, Garcia E, et al. Viral community-acquired pneumonia in non-immunocompromised adults. *Chest*. 2004;125:1343-1351.
2. Otto C, Huzly D, Kemna L, et al. Acute fibrinous and organizing pneumonia associated with influenza A/H1N1 pneumonia after lung transplantation. *BMC Pulm Med*. 2013;13:30.
3. Fields BN, Knipe DM, Howley PM, eds. *Fields Virology*. 4th ed. Lippincott Williams & Wilkins; 2001.
4. Marcos MA, Esperatti M, Torres A. Viral pneumonia. *Curr Opin Infect Dis*. 2009;22(2):143-147.
5. Scagnolari C, Turriziani O, Monteleone K, Pierangeli A, Antonelli G. Consolidation of molecular testing in clinical virology. *Expert Rev Anti Infect Ther*. 2017;15(4):387-400.
6. Ison MG, Fishman JA. Cytomegalovirus pneumonia in transplant recipients. *Clin Chest Med*. 2005;26:691-705.
7. Ljungman P, Griffiths P, Paya C. Definitions of cytomegalic infection and disease in transplant recipients. *Clin Infect Dis*. 2002;34:1094-1097.
8. Stewart AG, Kotton CN. What's new: updates on cytomegalovirus in solid organ transplantation. *Transplantation*. 2024;108(4):884-897.
9. Singer DB. Pathology of neonatal herpes simplex virus infection. *Perspect Pediatr Pathol*. 1981;6:243-278.

10. Patrucco F, Curtoni A, Sidoti F, et al. Herpes virus infection in lung transplantation: diagnosis, treatment and prevention strategies. *Viruses*. 2023;15(12):2326.
11. Ramsey PG, Fife KH, Hackman RC, Meyers JD, Corey L. Herpes simplex virus pneumonia: clinical, virologic, and pathologic features in 20 patients. *Ann Intern Med*. 1982;97:813-820.
12. Tachikawa R, Tomil K, Seo R, et al. Detection of herpes viruses by multiplex and real-time polymerase chain reaction in bronchoalveolar lavage fluid of patients with acute lung injury or acute respiratory distress syndrome. *Respiration*. 2014;87:279-286.
13. Gao Q, Li L, Su T, et al. A single-center, retrospective study of hospitalized patients with lower respiratory tract infections: clinical assessment of metagenomic next-generation sequencing and identification of risk factors in patients. *Respir Res*. 2024;25(1):250.
14. Shi W, Zhu S. The application of metagenomic next-generation sequencing in detection of pathogen in bronchoalveolar lavage fluid and sputum samples of patients with pulmonary infection. *Comput Math Methods Med*. 2021;2021:7238495.
15. Karre T. Herpes virus infections. In: Procop GW, Pritt BS, eds. *Pathology of Infectious Diseases*. Elsevier; 2015:17-36.
16. Eshak N, Abdelnabi M, Nugent K, Pixely J. Varicella-zoster virus pneumonia presenting as diffuse alveolar haemorrhage in a patient with a history of systemic lupus erythematosus. *BMJ Case Rep*. 2022;15(5):e250148.
17. Urrutia Royo B, Robles-Perez A. Fatal pneumonia due to disseminated infection by reactivated varicella zoster virus in a patient with interstitial lung disease associated with rheumatoid arthritis. *Arch Bronconeumol*. 2022;58(11):772.
18. Inokuchi R, Nakamura K, Sato H, et al. Bronchial ulceration as a prognostic indicator for varicella pneumonia: case report and systematic literature review. *J Clin Virol*. 2013;56(4):360-364.
19. Ison MG, Hayden RT. Adenovirus. *Microbiol Spectr*. 2016;4:4.
20. Radke JR, Cook JL. Human adenovirus lung disease: outbreaks, models of immune-response-driven acute lung injury and pandemic potential. *Curr Opin Infect Dis*. 2023;36(3):164-170.
21. Lion T. Adenovirus infections in immunocompetent and immunocompromised patients. *Clin Microbiol Rev*. 2014;27(3):441-462.
22. Becroft DM. Histopathology of fatal adenovirus infection of the respiratory tract in young children. *J Clin Pathol*. 1967;20:561-569.
23. Falsey AR, Walsh EE. Respiratory syncytial virus infection in adults. *Clin Microbiol Rev*. 2000;13(3):371-384.
24. Zhang XL, Zhang X, Hua W, et al. Expert consensus on the diagnosis, treatment, and prevention of respiratory syncytial virus infections in children. *World J Pediatr*. 2024;20(1):11-25.
25. Delage G, Brochu P, Robillard L, Jasmin G, Joncas JH, Lapointe N. Giant cell pneumonia due to respiratory syncytial virus. Occurrence in severe combined immunodeficiency syndrome. *Arch Pathol Lab Med*. 1984;108:623-625.
26. Van den Hoogen BG, de Jong JC, Groen J, et al. A newly discovered human pneumovirus isolated from young children with respiratory tract disease. *Nat Med*. 2001;7:719-724.
27. Godet C, Le Goff J, Beby-Defaux A, et al. Human metapneumovirus pneumonia in patients with hematological malignancies. *J Clin Virol*. 2014;61:593-596.
28. Wang X, Li Y, Deloria-Knoll M, et al. Global burden of acute lower respiratory infection associated with human metapneumovirus in children under 5 years in 2018: a systematic review and modelling study. *Lancet Glob Health*. 2021;9(1):e33-e43.
29. Vargas SO, Kozakewich HP, Perez-Atayde AR, McAdam AJ. Pathology of human metapneumovirus infection: insights into the pathogenesis of a newly identified respiratory virus. *Pediatr Dev Pathol*. 2004;7(5):478-486.

30. Tang E, Gador-Whyte AP, Newman MR. Viral cytopathic changes in sputum cytology in a patient with known human metapneumovirus. *Acta Cytol.* 2024;68(4):374-378.
31. Turaiche M, Grigoras ML, Bratosin F, et al. Disease progression, clinical features, and risk factors for pneumonia in unvaccinated children and adolescents with measles: a re-emerging disease in Romania. *Int J Environ Res Public Health.* 2022;19(20):13165.
32. Cherry JD. Ongoing measles in the developed and developing world. *J Pediatric Infect Dis Soc.* 2024;13(4):233-236.
33. Parums DV. A Review of the resurgence of measles, a vaccine-preventable disease, as current concerns contrast with past hopes for measles elimination. *Med Sci Monit.* 2024;30:e944436.
34. Radoycich GE, Zuppan CW, Weeks DA, Krous HF, Langston C. Patterns of measles pneumonia. *Pediatr Pathol.* 1992;12:773-786.
35. Sata T, Kurata T, Aoyama Y, Sakaguchi M, Yamanouchi K, Takeda K. Analysis of viral antigens in giant cells of measles pneumonia by immunoperoxidase method. *Virchows Arch A Pathol Anat Histopathol.* 1986;410:133-138.
36. Ding Y, Wang H, Shen H, et al. The clinical pathology of severe acute respiratory syndrome (SARS): a report from China. *J Pathol.* 2003;200:282-289.
37. Chong PY, Chui P, Ling AE, et al. Analysis of deaths during the severe acute respiratory syndrome (SARS) epidemic in Singapore: challenges in determining a SARS diagnosis. *Arch Pathol Lab Med.* 2004;128:195-204.
38. Franks TJ, Chong PY, Chui P, et al. Lung pathology of severe acute respiratory syndrome (SARS): a study of 8 autopsy cases from Singapore. *Hum Pathol.* 2003;34:743-748.
39. John Hopkins Coronavirus Resource Center. Accessed January 20, 2025. https://coronavirus.jhu.edu/us-map
40. COVID-19 Excess Mortality Collaborators. Estimating excess mortality due to the COVID-19 pandemic: a systematic analysis of COVID-19-related mortality, 2020-21. *Lancet.* 2022;399(10334):1513-1536.
41. Msemburi W, Karlinsky A, Knutson V, Aleshin-Guendel S, Chatterji S, Wakefield J. The WHO estimates of excess mortality associated with the COVID-19 pandemic. *Nature.* 2023;613(7942):130-137.
42. Grant MC, Geoghegan L, Arbyn M, et al. The prevalence of symptoms in 24,410 adults infected by the novel coronavirus (SARS-CoV-2; COVID-19): a systematic review and meta-analysis of 148 studies from 9 countries. *PLoS ONE.* 2020;15(6):e0234765.
43. Toepfner N, Brinkmann F, Augustin S, Stojanov S, Behrends U. Long COVID in pediatrics-epidemiology, diagnosis, and management. *Eur J Pediatr.* 2024;183(4):1543-1553. doi: 10.1007/s00431-023-05360-y. PMID: 38279014; PMCID: PMC11001657.
44. Herman E, Shih E, Cheng A. Long COVID: rapid evidence review. *Am Fam Physician.* 2022;106(5):523-532.
45. Wang D, Hu B, Hu C, et al. Clinical characteristics of 138 hospitalized patients with 2019 novel coronavirus-infected pneumonia in Wuhan, China. *JAMA.* 2020;323(11):1061-1069.
46. Tian S, Hu W, Niu L, Liu H, Xu H, Xiao S-Y. Pulmonary pathology of early phase 2019 novel coronavirus (COVID-19) pneumonia in two patients with lung cancer. *J Thorac Oncol.* 2020;15(5):700-704. doi:10.1016/j.jtho.2020.02.010
47. Bryce C, Grimes Z, Pujadas E, et al. Pathophysiology of SARS-CoV-2: the Mount Sinai COVID-19 autopsy experience. *Mod Pathol.* 2021;34(8):1456-1467.
48. Burkhard-Koren NM, Haberecker M, Maccio U, et al. Higher prevalence of pulmonary macrothrombi in SARS-CoV-2 than in influenza A: autopsy results from 'Spanish flu' 1918/1919 in Switzerland to Coronavirus disease 2019. *J Pathol Clin Res.* 2021;7(2):135-143.
49. Nuovo GJ, Magro C, Shaffer T, et al. Endothelial cell damage is the central part of COVID-19 and a mouse model induced by injection of the S1 subunit of the spike protein. *Ann Diagn Pathol.* 2021;51:151682.

50. Magro CM, Mulvey J, Kubiak J, et al. Severe COVID-19: a multifaceted viral vasculopathy syndrome. *Ann Diagn Pathol.* 2021;50:151645.
51. Suster D, Tili E, Nuovo GJ. The differential immune response in mild versus fatal SARS-CoV2 infection. *Ann Diagn Pathol.* 2022;61:152032.
52. Felix JC, Sheinin YM, Suster D, et al. Diffuse interstitial pneumonia-like/macrophage activation syndrome-like changes in patients with COVID-19 correlate with length of illness. *Ann Diagn Pathol.* 2021;53:151744.
53. Kevadiya BD, Machhi J, Herskovitz J, et al. Diagnostics for SARS-CoV-2 infections. *Nat Mater.* 2021;20(5):593-605.
54. Nuovo GJ, Suster D, Tili E, Awad H, Magro C. A standardization protocol for the in situ detection of SARS-CoV2 RNA and proteins. *Appl Immunohistochem Mol Morphol.* 2022;30(2):83-90.
55. Nuovo G, Tili E, Suster D, Matys E, Hupp L, Magro C. Strong homology between SARS-CoV-2 envelope protein and a *Mycobacterium* sp. antigen allows rapid diagnosis of mycobacterial infections and may provide specific anti-SARS-CoV-2 immunity via the BCG vaccine. *Ann Diagn Pathol.* 2020;48:151600.
56. Pritt BS, Aubry MC. Histopathology of viral infections of the lung. *Semin Diagn Pathol.* 2017;34(6):510-517.
57. Jané M, Vidal MJ, Soldevila N, et al. Epidemiological and clinical characteristics of children hospitalized due to influenza A and B in the south of Europe, 2010-2016. *Sci Rep.* 2019;9(1):12853.
58. Jia L, Xie J, Zhao J, et al. Mechanisms of severe mortality-associated bacterial co-infections following influenza virus infection. *Front Cell Infect Microbiol.* 2017;7:338.
59. Guarner J, Paddock CD, Shieh WJ, et al. Histopathologic and immunohistochemical features of fatal influenza virus infections in children during the 2003–2004 season. *Clin Infect Dis.* 2006;43:132-140.
60. Yeldandi AV, Colby TV. Pathologic features of lung biopsy specimens from influenza pneumonia cases. *Hum Pathol.* 1994;25:47-53.
61. Lai AR, Keet K, Yong CM, Diaz JV. Severe H1N1-associated acute respiratory distress syndrome: a case series. *Am J Med.* 2010;123:282-285.
62. Gill JR, Sheng ZM, Ely SF, et al. Pulmonary pathologic findings of fatal 2009 pandemic influenza A/H1N1 viral infections. *Arch Pathol Lab Med.* 2010;134:235-243.
63. Duchin JS, Koster FT, Peters CJ, et al. Hantavirus pulmonary syndrome: a clinical description of 17 patients with a newly recognized disease. The Hantavirus Study Group. *N Engl J Med.* 1994;330:949-955.
64. Thorp L, Fullerton L, Whitesell A, Dehority W. Hantavirus pulmonary syndrome: 1993-2018. *Pediatrics.* 2023;151(4):e2022059352.
65. Nolte KB, Federsen RM, Foucar K, et al. Hantavirus pulmonary syndrome in the United States: a pathological description of a disease caused by a new agent. *Hum Pathol.* 1995;26:110-120.
66. Burke T. Dengue hemorrhagic fever: a pathological study. *Trans R Soc Trop Med Hyg.* 1968;62:682-692.
67. Walker DH, McCormick JB, Johnson KM, et al. Pathologic and virologic study of fatal Lassa fever in man. *Am J Pathol.* 1982;107:349-356.
68. de Almeida RR, Paim B, de Oliveira SA, et al. Dengue hemorrhagic fever: a state-of-the-art review focused in pulmonary involvement. *Lung.* 2017;195(4):389-395.

9

INTERSTITIAL LUNG DISEASE

Involvement of the interstitial compartment of the lung, with or without compromise of the airspaces, can be seen in a wide variety of circumstances and represents a major cause of lung morbidity and mortality. Interstitial pneumonias can be categorized, in broad terms, into idiopathic interstitial pneumonias (IIPs) and into those for which a known precipitating cause or agent can be demonstrated (Table 9.1).

IDIOPATHIC INTERSTITIAL PNEUMONIAS

The IIPs are a group of relatively rare conditions of unknown etiology that are generally characterized by insidious onset and progressive interstitial fibrosis with inflammation. Secondary involvement of the airspaces can also occur, but the principal pathology is centered in the interstitium of the alveolar walls. Our understanding of idiopathic interstitial lung diseases has progressed slowly, from the initial description by Liebow,[1] to the classification

TABLE 9.1 Types of Interstitial Lung Disease

Idiopathic Interstitial Pneumonias	Specific Interstitial Pneumonias
Idiopathic pulmonary fibrosis/usual interstitial pneumonia	Collagen vascular disease–related interstitial pneumonia
Idiopathic nonspecific interstitial pneumonia	Drug-mediated diffuse lung disease
Desquamative interstitial pneumonia	Hypersensitivity pneumonitis (extrinsic allergic alveolitis)
Cryptogenic organizing pneumonia (bronchiolitis obliterans organizing pneumonia)	Respiratory bronchiolitis–associated interstitial lung disease
Acute interstitial pneumonia	Langerhans cell histiocytosis
Lymphoid interstitial pneumonia	Giant cell interstitial pneumonia (hard metal disease)
Idiopathic pleuroparenchymal fibroelastosis	Smoking-related interstitial fibrosis

proposed by Katzenstein[2] and to the more recent international workshop on the classification of these conditions.[3,4] There has even been some advances on understanding the genetic underpinnings of some of these conditions including familial forms of the diseases.[5,6] IIP is generally a diffuse and bilateral process, and the various specific categories that comprise this spectrum of disorders represent various reaction patterns of lung parenchyma to the underlying injury. In general, such reaction patterns are nonspecific and often blend into each other or may show significant overlap. The diagnosis is established strictly on the basis of clinicopathologic and radiologic correlation and not on the basis of the histopathologic findings alone. Because the lesions are usually not localized but diffuse/patchy and also because there can be considerable variation in the stage of evolution of the lesions, proper evaluation of these disorders, particularly in the case of fibrosing interstitial lung disorders, generally cannot be reliably accomplished by performing a single transbronchial biopsy.[7] In recent years, cryobiopsy has been increasingly used in the diagnosis and management of interstitial lung disease.[8-10] Cryobiopsy has been demonstrated to have an enhanced tissue yield and is a good option for certain types of interstitial lung disease, such as sarcoidosis. Though cryobiopsy taken from the correct location may provide some information regarding a fibrotic process, in general the evaluation of conditions that require overall larger pattern recognition may still not be diagnosed with the use of cryobiopsy.[11,12] For now it seems that the best way to evaluate patients suspected of having an idiopathic fibrosing interstitial lung disease remains through multiple video-assisted thoracoscopic lung biopsies; though it is possible that through advanced molecular testing biopsy may one day not even be required.[13] It is important to obtain at least three samples involving all lobes, taking care to avoid areas of scarring particularly in the apices or the lingula. The damage in these conditions often affects the periphery of the lungs, and these areas cannot be adequately sampled through transbronchial biopsies. The changes described in this chapter will thus focus on features that can be observed in open or thoracoscopic wedge biopsies rather than in bronchoscopic or transbronchial biopsies.

Idiopathic Pulmonary Fibrosis/Usual Interstitial Pneumonia

Idiopathic pulmonary fibrosis (IPF) represents a clinical pulmonary disease in which there is progressive fibrosing lung damage with no known etiology. Usual interstitial pneumonia (UIP) refers to the histologic correlate to IPF, which comprises a reaction pattern of inflammation and lung fibrosis that can be observed in a variety of conditions. The histopathologic changes observed are nonspecific and must be correlated with the clinical and radiologic changes before a diagnosis of UIP can be established. UIP-like changes can be observed in a variety of specific conditions, such as collagen vascular disease (CVD), asbestosis, and drug reactions. The term *idiopathic pulmonary fibrosis–UIP pattern* should be applied only when no underlying causes for the changes are observed clinically.[14] Patients are usually middle aged to older adults with a slight male predominance who present with slowly progressive dyspnea and nonproductive cough.

High-resolution computed tomography (HRCT) shows distinctive findings in more than 50% of cases. There is a predominantly reticular pattern of ground-glass opacities with honeycombing showing basal and peripheral predominance.[15] The findings are patchy and heterogeneous in distribution. Traction bronchiectasis is another distinctive finding. Chest X-ray in patients with UIP typically shows a bilateral reticular pattern predominantly involving the lung bases. A normal chest X-ray can be seen in some cases.

If the characteristic HRCT findings are present, a diagnosis of idiopathic interstitial fibrosis can be made without a need for lung biopsy (Table 9.2).[16-18] A lung biopsy should generally be undertaken only in patients suspected of UIP who do not have the characteristic HRCT findings or an "indeterminate" pattern on HRCT. IPF is a progressive disorder that leads to death as a result of respiratory failure in the majority of instances, with a median survival of less than 4 years from the time of initial diagnosis and a 30% to 50% 5-year survival.[16] The standard of therapy is with immunosuppressants or corticosteroids, including agents such as colchicine, azathioprine, and cyclophosphamide. More recently, some new antifibrinolytic agents have become available, although there are questions as to their efficacy and other approaches, including antibiotic therapy in combination with antioxidant therapy have been explored.[19,20] Despite some improvement or delay to the disease process with these treatments, the disease continues to have a progressive course with poor overall outcomes.[21]

The histopathologic hallmark of UIP is the presence of areas of lung parenchyma showing the fibrosing and inflammatory changes adjacent to areas displaying early involvement or perfectly normal parenchyma (Fig. 9.1; eFigs. 9.1 and 9.2). This has been referred to as "spatial heterogeneity" and refers essentially to the variegated appearance of the lung caused by areas showing lung parenchyma with fibrosis alternating with areas of uninvolved, normal lung parenchyma.[22] The fibrosis is usually subpleural and paraseptal. In the early stages of fibrosis, foci containing spindled fibroblasts or myofibroblasts admixed with loose connective tissue are usually present (so-called fibroblastic foci; Fig. 9.2). Marked thickening secondary to fibrosis with widening of the alveolar septa is seen in well-established lesions (Fig. 9.3; eFig. 9.3); the difference in the character of the fibrosis between the early lesions and later lesions is referred to as "temporal heterogeneity." Mild interstitial chronic inflammation and scattered lymphoid aggregates can also be found. Accumulation of alveolar macrophages can be seen focally resulting in a "desquamative interstitial pneumonia (DIP)-like" appearance (Fig. 9.4). Bronchiolization ("lambertosis") and squamous metaplasia of alveolar spaces can be observed in the areas of scarring and fibrosis (Fig. 9.5; eFigs. 9.4 and 9.5). Smooth muscle proliferation may accompany the scarring, a process referred to in the old literature as "muscular cirrhosis" (Fig. 9.6). The fibrosis may progress, resulting in scarring and the formation of cystic spaces containing mucus or inflammatory cells, a process that has been termed *honeycombing* (Fig. 9.7; eFig. 9.6). Histologic criteria to go with the newly established radiologic criteria have also now been created, which require certain specific features to be present to make the diagnosis of UIP (Table 9.3).[16,17]

TABLE 9.2 Radiologic Criteria for Diagnosis of UIP on HRCT Scan

CT Feature	Typical UIP Pattern	Probably UIP Pattern	Indeterminate UIP Pattern	Not-UIP Pattern
Pattern	Predominantly reticular pattern of ground-glass opacities with honeycombing with traction bronchiectasis	• Predominantly reticular pattern of ground-glass opacities with traction bronchiectasis • No honeycombing	Evidence of fibrosis without cardinal features of UIP-like pattern	Findings suggestive of alternative diagnoses: • Consolidations • Masses • Diffuse nodules • Cysts • Mosaic attenuation with extensive sharply defined lobular air trapping on expiration
Distribution	Basal (lower lung) and peripheral predominance	Basal (lower lung) and peripheral predominance	Variable or diffuse distribution of findings	• Upper or middle lung predominant, lower lung generally clear • Subpleural sparing

UIP, usual interstitial pneumonia.

Reprinted from Lynch DA, Sverzellati N, Travis WD, et al. Diagnostic criteria for idiopathic pulmonary fibrosis: a Fleischner Society white paper. *Lancet Respir Med*. 2018;6(2):138-153, with permission from Elsevier.

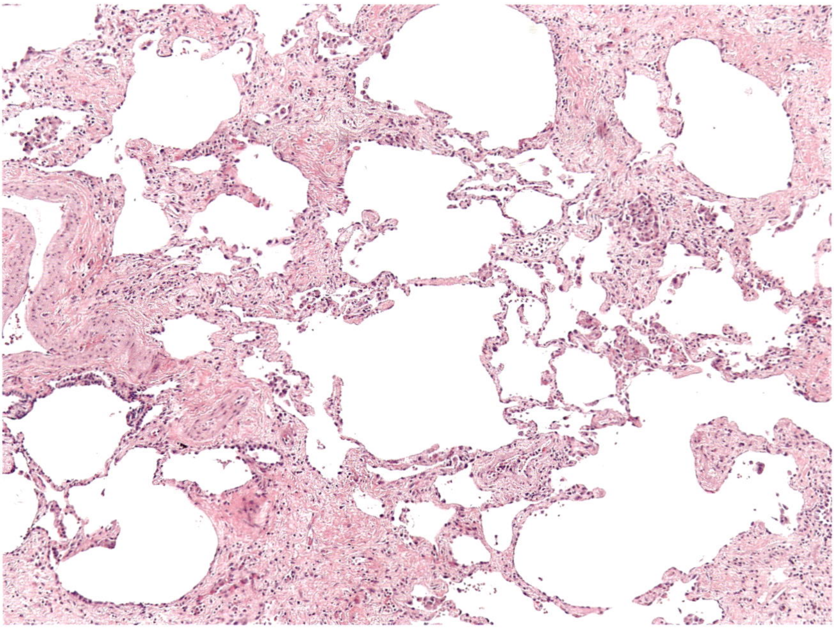

FIGURE 9.1 **Scanning magnification of lung biopsy in usual interstitial pneumonia.** Notice areas containing thickened and fibrotic alveolar septa alternating with areas of normal lung parenchyma.

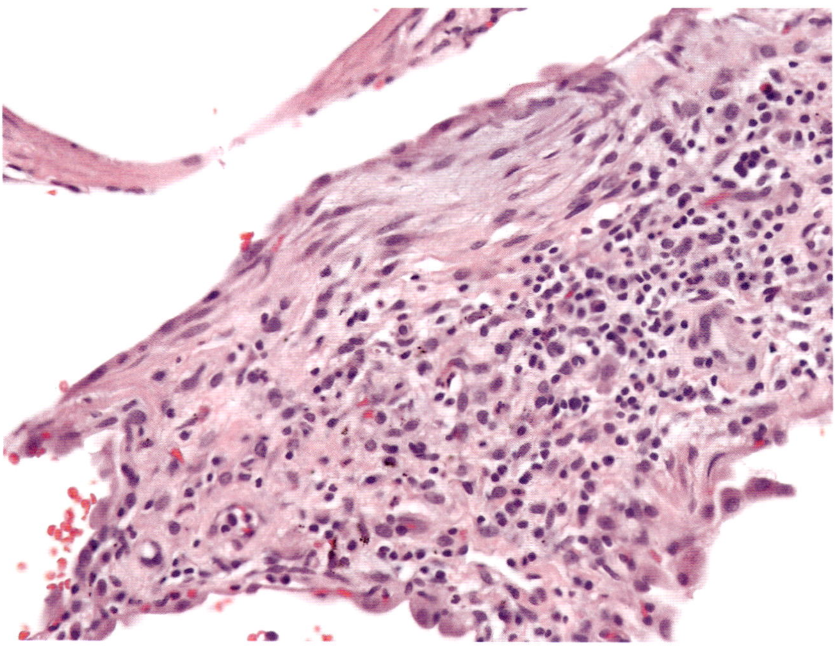

FIGURE 9.2 **Usual interstitial pneumonia showing thickening of the alveolar wall because of fibrosis and chronic inflammation with early fibroblastic focus comprising young fibroblasts admixed with a myxoid matrix.**

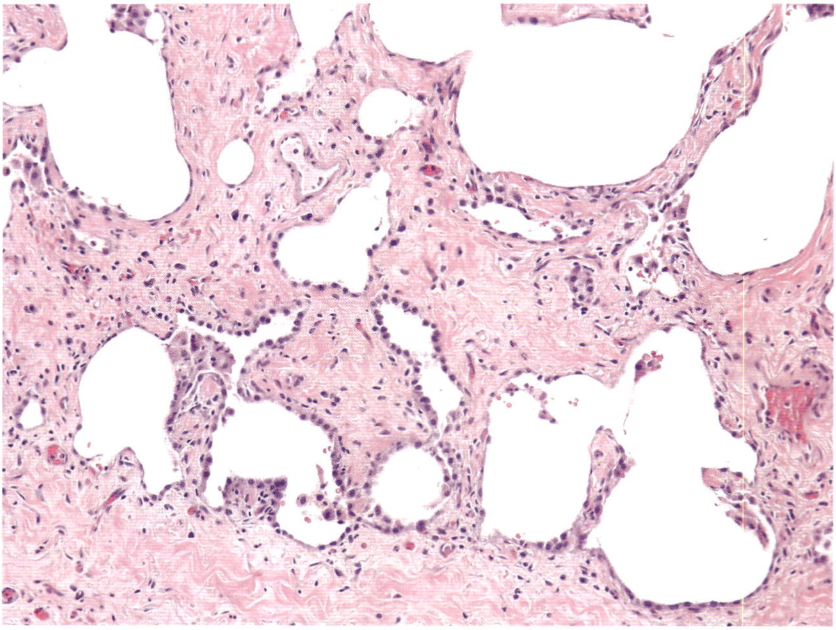

FIGURE 9.3 **Marked thickening of alveolar septa because of fibroblastic proliferation and collagen deposition is seen in usual interstitial pneumonia.** Notice focal hyperplasia of type II pneumocytes lining the alveolar spaces.

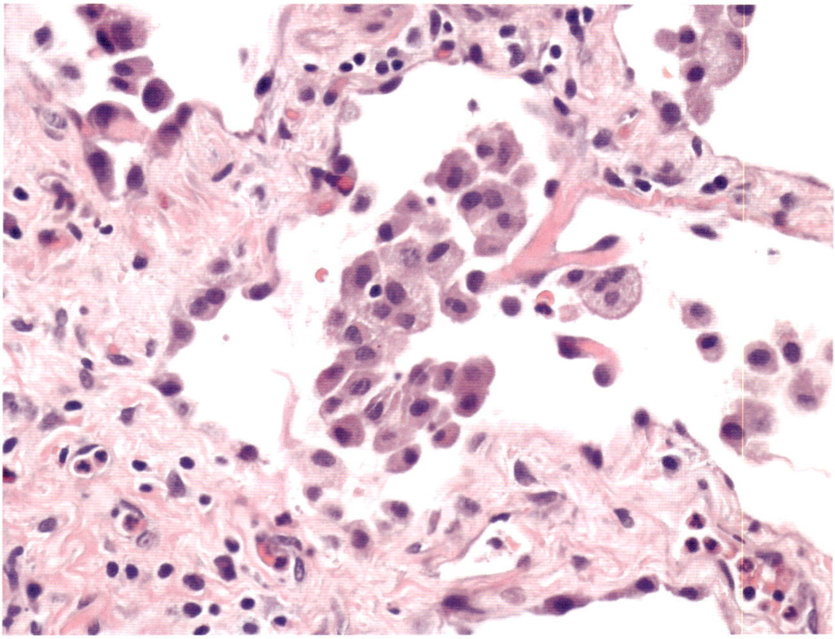

FIGURE 9.4 **Desquamative interstitial pneumonia–like changes can be seen in usual interstitial pneumonia, with accumulation of macrophages in alveolar lumina.**

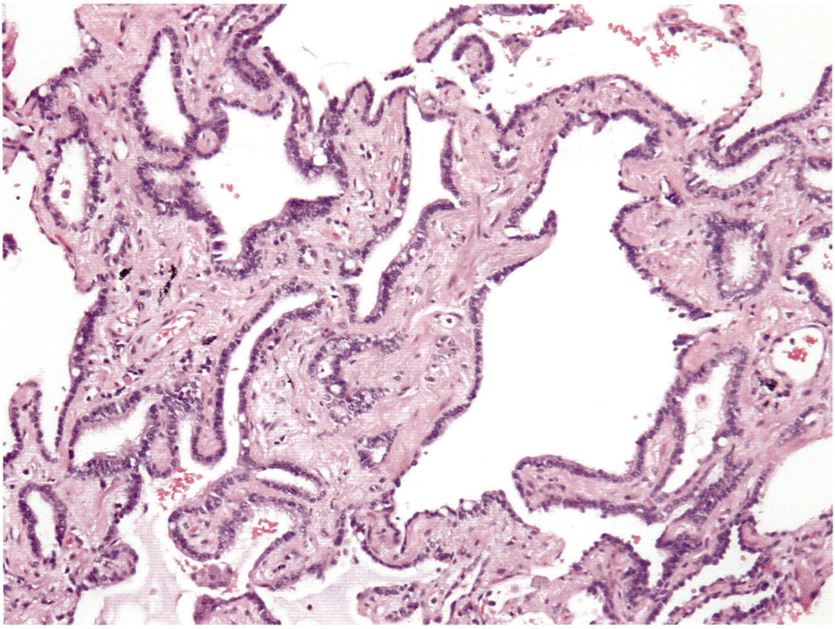

FIGURE 9.5 Extensive bronchiolization is seen in this example of usual interstitial pneumonia characterized by replacement of the alveolar lining by columnar ciliated epithelium.

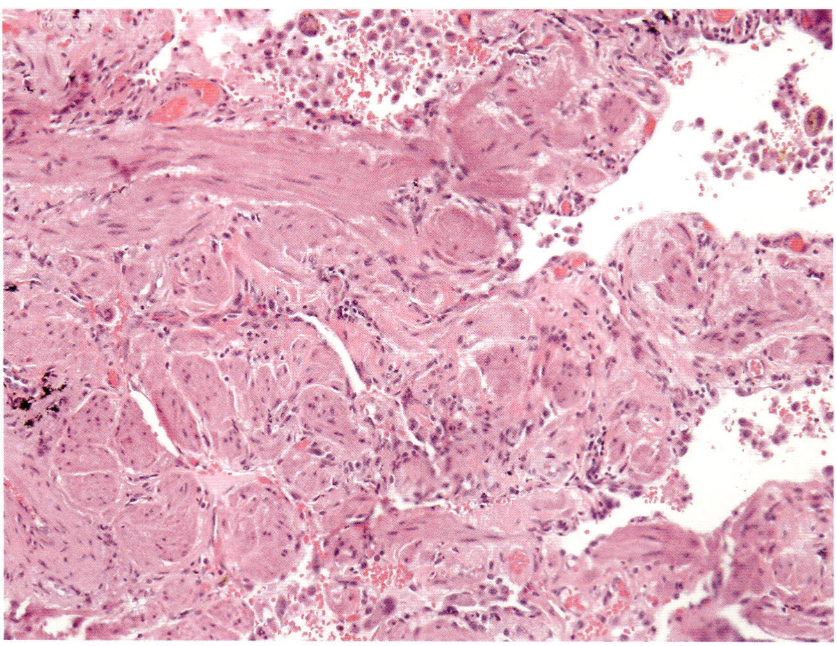

FIGURE 9.6 Prominent smooth muscle proliferation is seen in the walls of the alveolar septa in advanced stages of usual interstitial pneumonia.

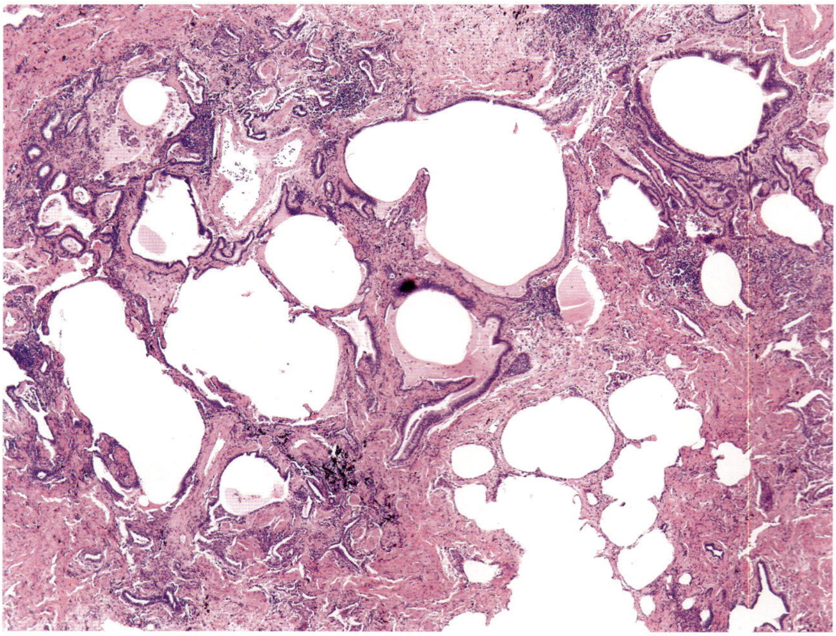

FIGURE 9.7 Extensive "honeycombing" of the lung is seen in advanced stages of usual interstitial pneumonia characterized by cystic dilatation of alveolar spaces that sometimes become filled with mucin.

TABLE 9.3 Histologic Criteria for Diagnosis of UIP

UIP Pattern Confirmed (All Four Criteria Present)	Probably UIP Pattern (Less Than Four Criteria Present)	Indeterminate for UIP (Only One or Two Criteria Present)	Not UIP
1. Dense fibrosis with honeycombing 2. Temporal heterogeneity 3. Spatial heterogeneity 4. Subpleural/ paraseptal distribution	1. Dense fibrosis with honeycombing 2. Temporal heterogeneity 3. Spatial heterogeneity Or 1. Only honeycombing fibrosis	Fibrosis is present with some potential features of UIP; however, other features may suggest alternative diagnosis	1. No criteria for UIP pattern identified Or 2. UIP-like pattern present in the context of other features highly suggestive of alternative diagnosis

UIP, usual interstitial pneumonia.

Reprinted from Lynch DA, Sverzellati N, Travis WD, et al. Diagnostic criteria for idiopathic pulmonary fibrosis: a Fleischner Society white paper. *Lancet Respir Med.* 2018;6(2):138-153, with permission from Elsevier.

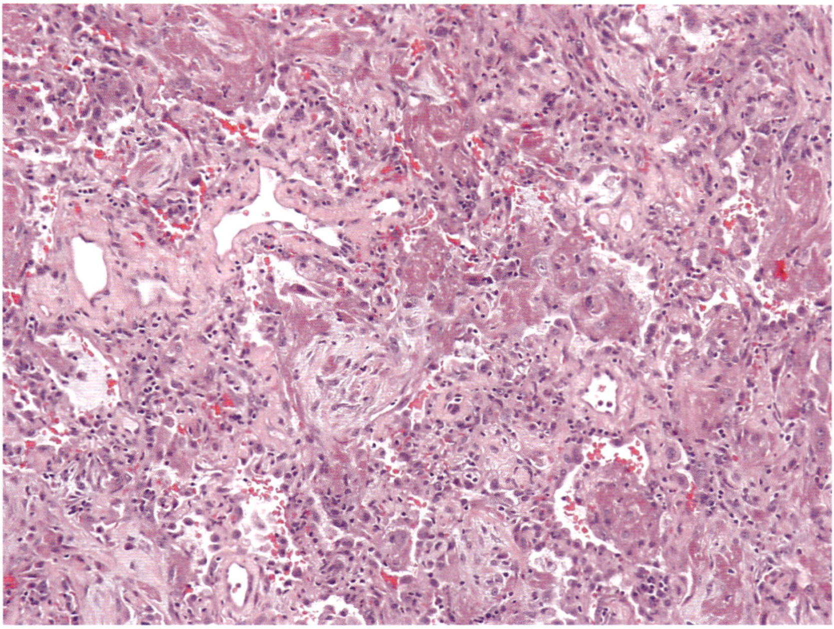

FIGURE 9.8 Acute exacerbation in usual interstitial pneumonia shows changes of diffuse alveolar damage superimposed in a background of alveolar wall fibrosis.

Another complication is episodes of acute exacerbation, which can be seen in patients with UIP, leading to foci of diffuse alveolar damage and organizing pneumonia superimposed on the chronic changes of UIP (Fig. 9.8).[23] Additionally, cases of malignancy arising in association with the fibrotic lung disease have been reported; in these situations, patients tend to have higher rates of respiratory complications.[24] As mentioned in the introduction, cryobiopsy may pick up areas that are histologically consistent with IPF/UIP and show many of the features such as dense scarring of the lung and extensive bronchiolar metaplasia, but the lack of ability to assess the overall pattern of fibrosis precludes a definitive diagnosis in most scenarios (Figs. 9.9-9.12).

Nonspecific Interstitial Pneumonia

The term *nonspecific interstitial pneumonia* (NSIP) was proposed in 1994 by Katzenstein and Fiorelli[22,25] for patients presenting with slowly progressive cough and dyspnea, bilateral interstitial infiltrates, and a histopathologic picture on open lung biopsy that differed significantly from UIP. Advanced fibrosis is rare in this condition and portends a worse prognosis. The NSIP pattern of fibrosis may be secondary to various causes, particularly some types of autoimmune conditions, or it may be idiopathic NSIP without a known underlying cause.[26] The prognosis for NSIP tends

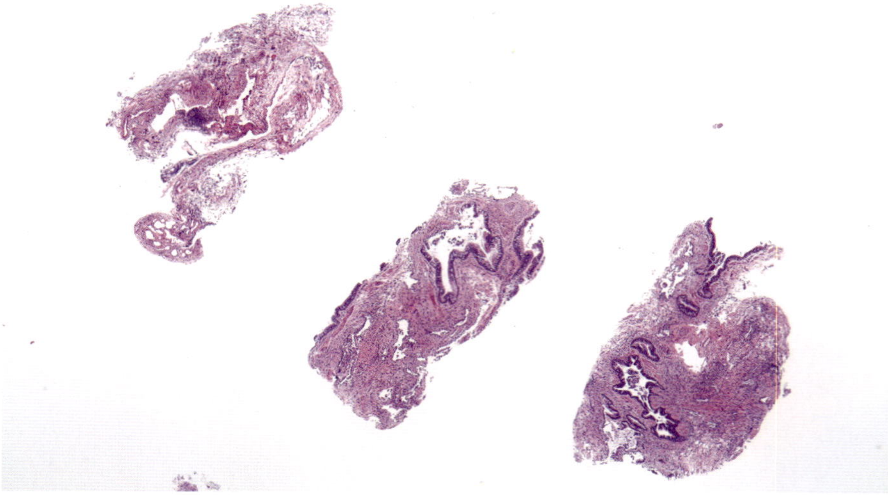

FIGURE 9.9 **Intermediate magnification of a cryobiopsy taken from a patient with suspected fibrosing lung disease.** There is three relatively large fragments of distorted lung parenchyma with evidence of fibrosis; however, note that it is difficult to tell the anatomic position of where this biopsy was taken from and thus the true distribution of fibrosis.

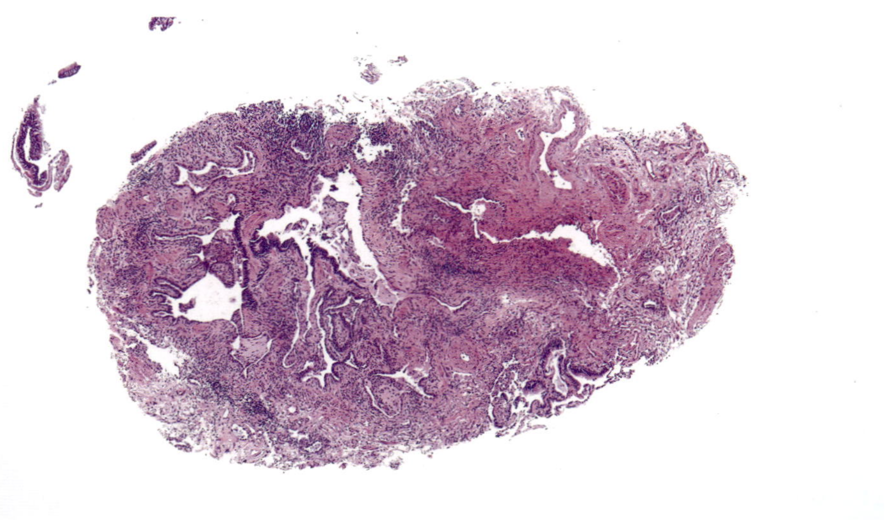

FIGURE 9.10 **Higher magnification of the cryobiopsy shows an area of sampling near a bronchovascular bundle with bronchiolar metaplasia, interstitial fibrosis, and chronic inflammation; all features that may be present in lungs with idiopathic pulmonary fibrosis/usual interstitial pneumonia.**

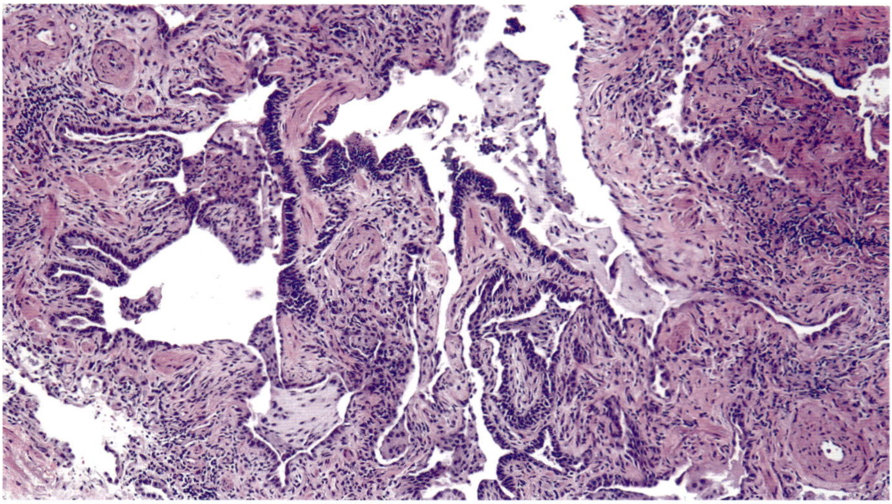

FIGURE 9.11 High-power magnification of the cryobiopsy shows the bronchiolar metaplasia with widening of the interstitial walls by fibrosis and possible fibroblastic foci (*bottom left*).

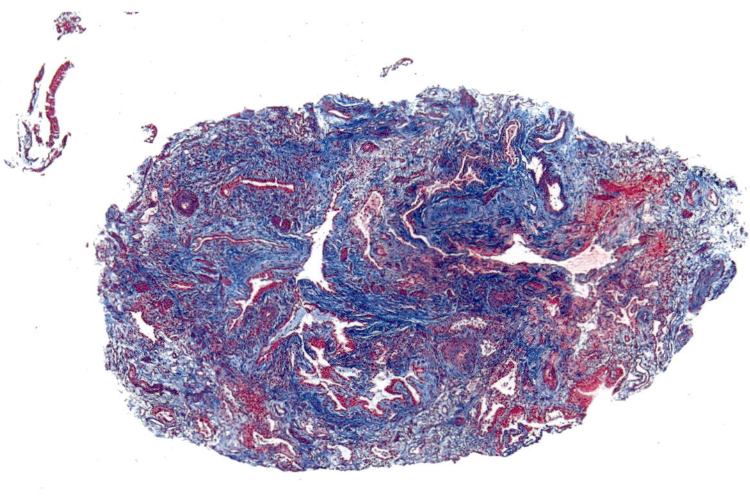

FIGURE 9.12 Trichrome special stain highlights the increase in fibrotic stroma within the alveolar walls.

to be better than that for UIP, and most patients will respond favorably to corticosteroid therapy. About 50% to 70% of patients will recover completely after treatment.[27] The prognosis for "cellular" NSIP (ie, NSIP with increased interstitial inflammation) is much better than that seen in fibrosing NSIP as cellular NSIP will respond better to steroids (Figs. 9.13 and 9.14).

The histologic picture is one of a uniform process throughout, with identical findings in all areas of the biopsy (eFigs. 9.7 and 9.8). In contrast with UIP, which is characterized by "temporal and spatial heterogeneity," NSIP is characterized by a temporally uniform pattern of changes (Figs. 9.15 and 9.16). The inflammatory process in cellular NSIP is diffuse and uniform and involves mainly the alveolar septa (Fig. 9.17). The temporal uniformity of the changes (ie, all lesions are in the same stage of evolution) is the most important histologic feature of NSIP. The interstitial inflammatory infiltrate is mainly composed of plasma cells and small lymphocytes and can be accompanied by mild interstitial fibrosis (Fig. 9.18). Fibroblastic foci and honeycombing are less commonly seen.[27-29] Small areas showing organizing pneumonia or obliterative bronchiolitis–like changes can be found in nearly half the cases. Focal, patchy accumulation of intra-alveolar macrophages can also be observed.

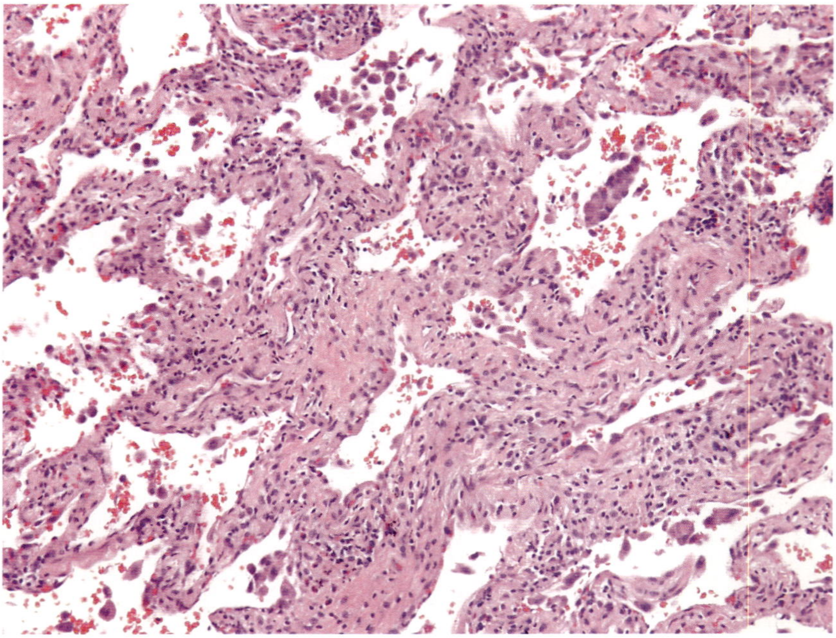

FIGURE 9.13 "Cellular" nonspecific interstitial pneumonia showing predominance of inflammatory cells in alveolar walls.

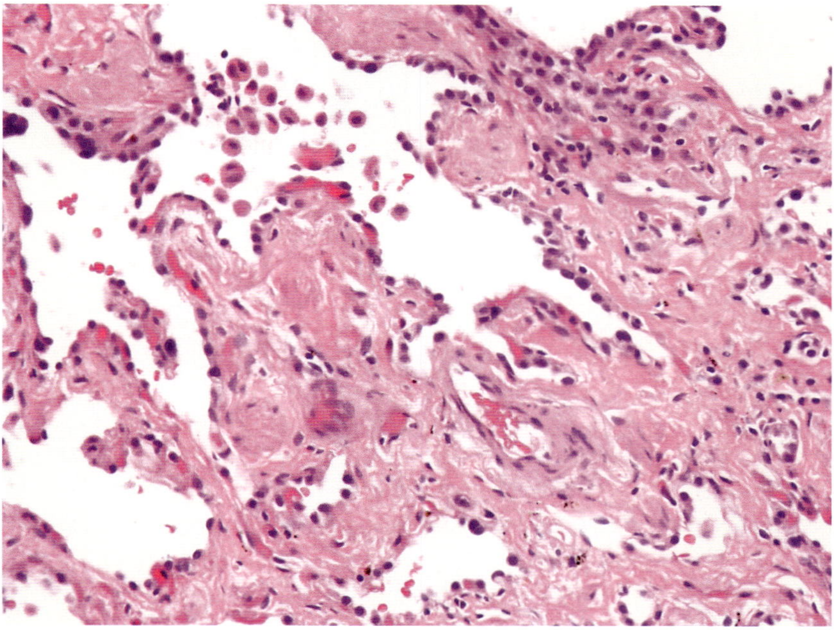

FIGURE 9.14 **Fibrotic nonspecific interstitial pneumonia showing widening of alveolar septa secondary to fibrosis with scant inflammatory elements.**

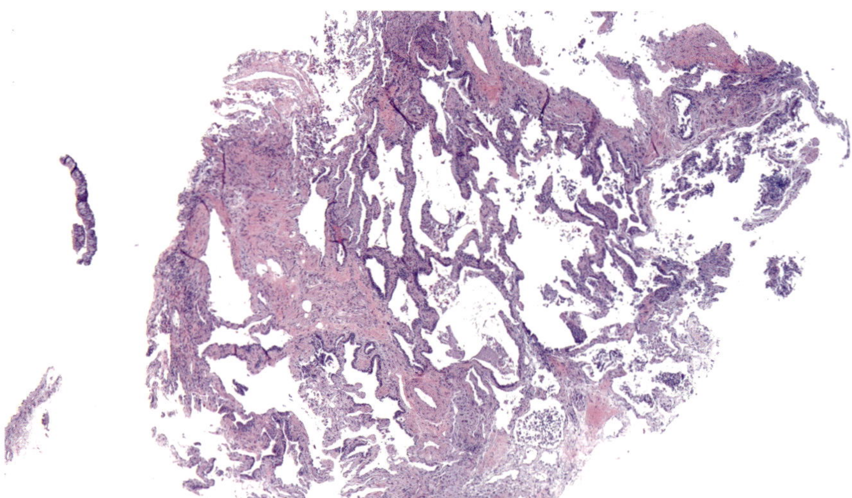

FIGURE 9.15 **Scanning power magnification from a cryobiopsy taken from a patient with suspect pulmonary fibrosis.** Note the relatively uniform expansion of the alveolar septal walls.

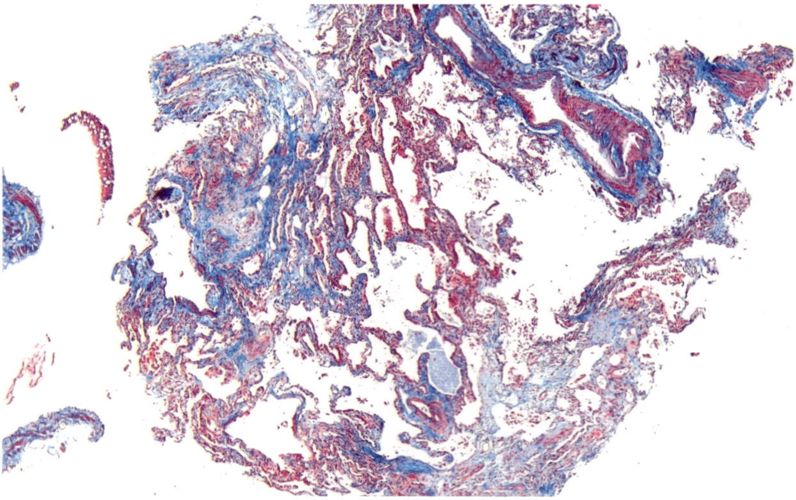

FIGURE 9.16 Trichrome special stain in the same biopsy highlights the interstitial fibrosis.

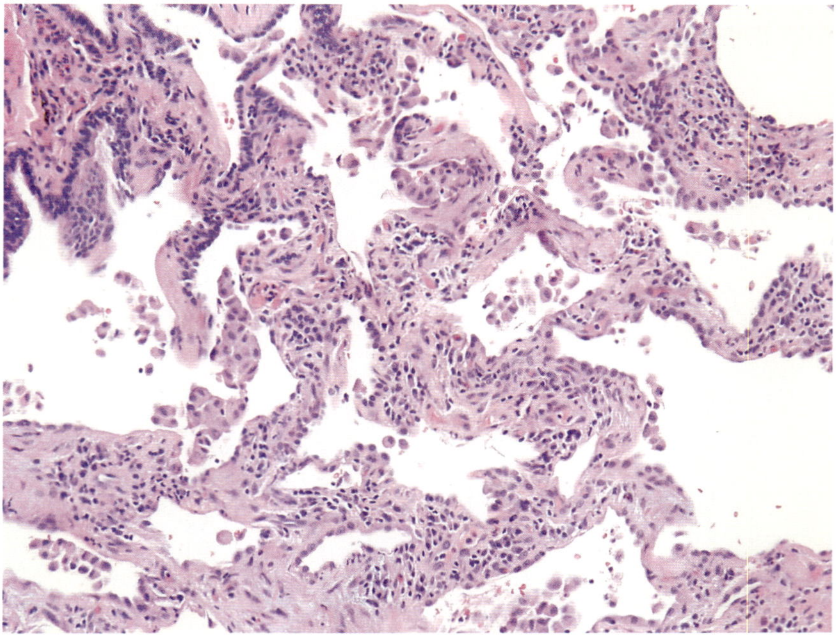

FIGURE 9.17 Cellular nonspecific interstitial pneumonia pattern showing uniform thickening and fibrosis of alveolar septa without intervening normal areas.

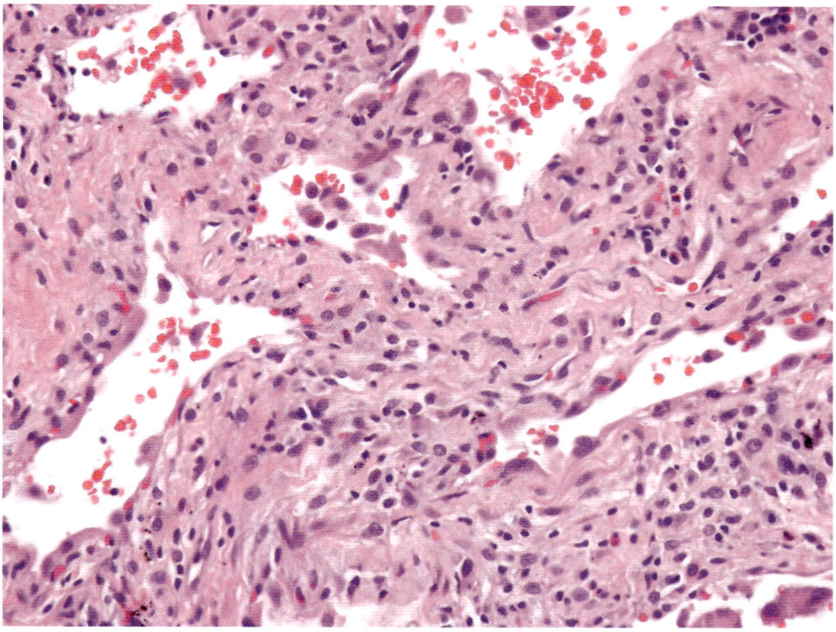

FIGURE 9.18 Higher magnification of nonspecific interstitial pneumonia showing inflammatory infiltrate and fibrosis producing widening of alveolar walls.

Desquamative Interstitial Pneumonia

Initially reported by Liebow[1] as a disease characterized by "desquamated" epithelial cells filling the alveolar lumens, DIP represents a very rare lung process characterized by accumulation of macrophages within the air-spaces. DIP usually occurs in patients at least 10 years younger than those with UIP. The process has an insidious onset, is strongly associated with cigarette smoking, and is usually grouped under the category of smoking-related interstitial lung diseases.[30-32] Patients develop slowly progressive cough and dyspnea over several weeks or months, with mild restriction in lung function and moderate reduction in diffusing capacity. Digital clubbing can be seen in approximately half of the patients. Chest films and CT may be normal in some patients but more often show patchy areas of ground-glass opacification in the lung bases and at the periphery.[33-35] The most striking histologic finding is distention of the alveolar spaces by sheets of macrophages containing abundant eosinophilic cytoplasm with or without pigmentation (Figs. 9.19-9.22; eFig. 9.9). The alveolar walls show mild thickening owing to fibrosis and chronic inflammation (Figs. 9.23 and 9.24). The histiocytic nature of the intra-alveolar infiltrate can be demonstrated by immunohistochemistry with antibodies to CD68 or CD163 (Fig. 9.25). The process shows an even and diffuse distribution throughout the lung fields with temporal uniformity (ie, all lesions are in

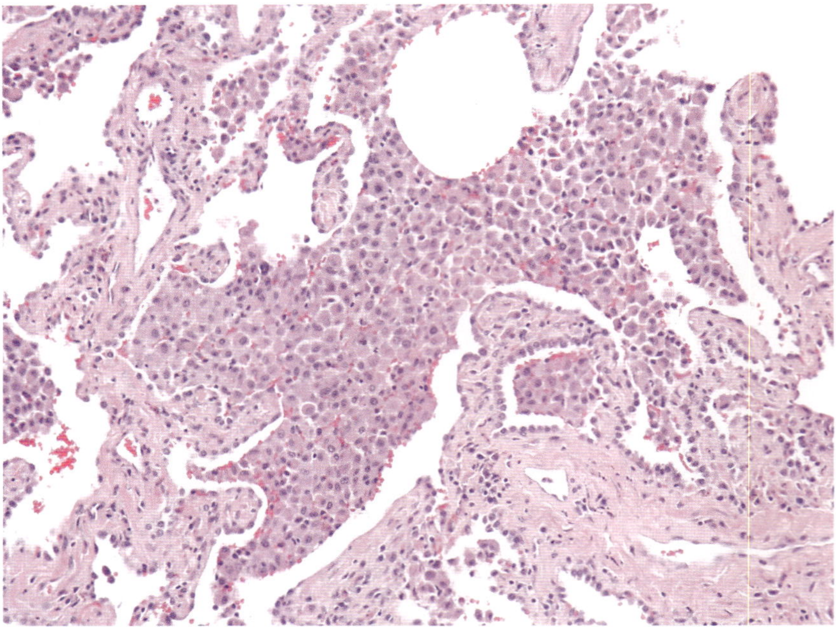

FIGURE 9.19 **Scanning magnification of lung biopsy in desquamative interstitial pneumonia showing distention of alveolar spaces by macrophages.**

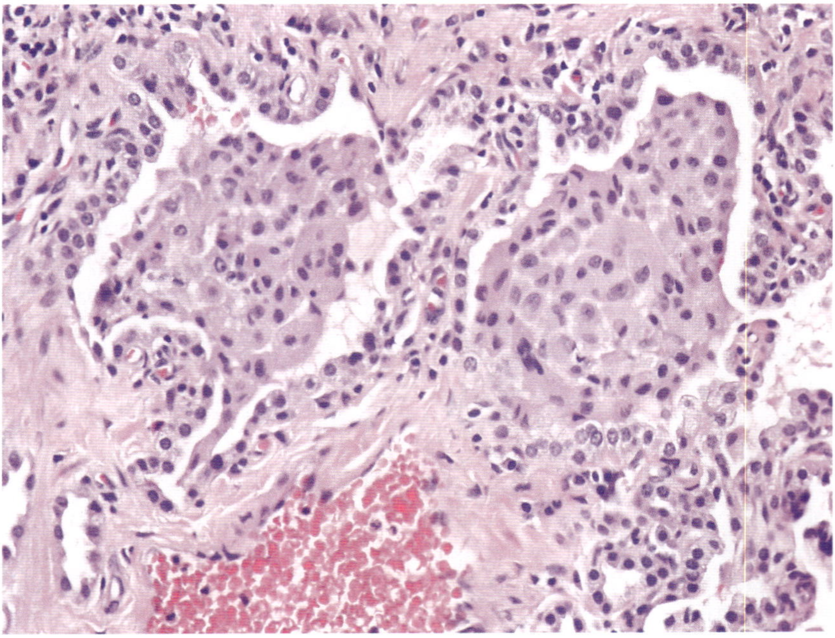

FIGURE 9.20 **High-power magnification of desquamative interstitial pneumonia showing almost complete filling of alveolar lumina by a monotonous population of macrophages.** Mild thickening and fibrosis/inflammation of alveolar walls is present.

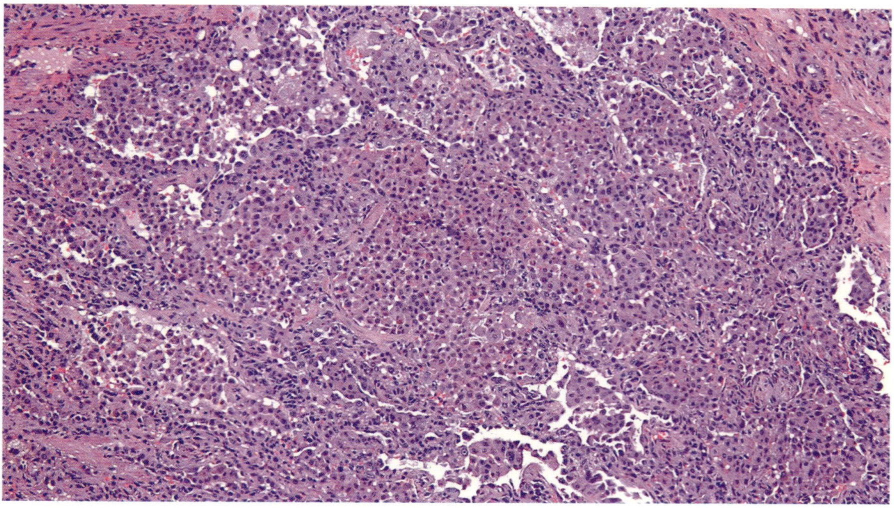

FIGURE 9.21 **Scanning magnification from a patient with desquamative interstitial pneumonia shows innumerable pigment-laden macrophages filling the alveolar spaces.** Most of the macrophages are characterized by eosinophilic cytoplasm although numerous scattered macrophages show cytoplasmic brown pigment.

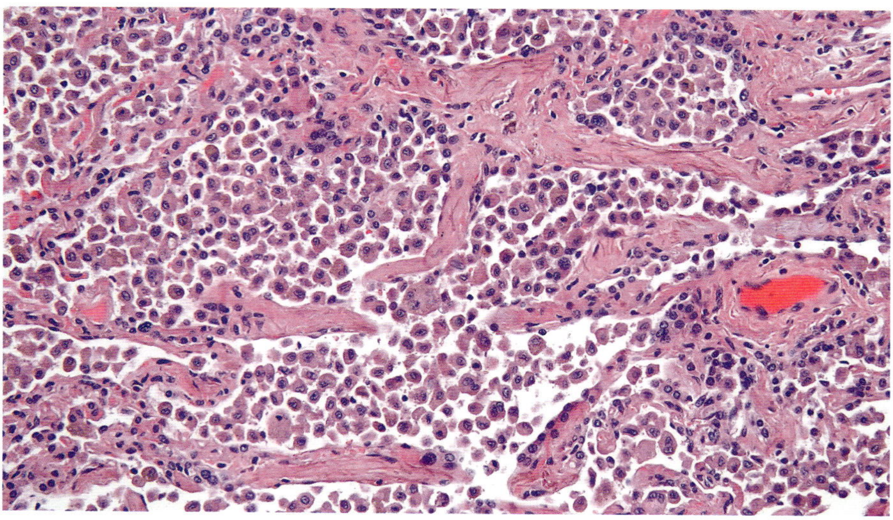

FIGURE 9.22 **High-power magnification of a case of desquamative interstitial pneumonia shows numerous brown-tinged pigment-laden macrophages filling alveolar spaces.** Notice the mild interstitial fibrosis expanding the alveolar septa.

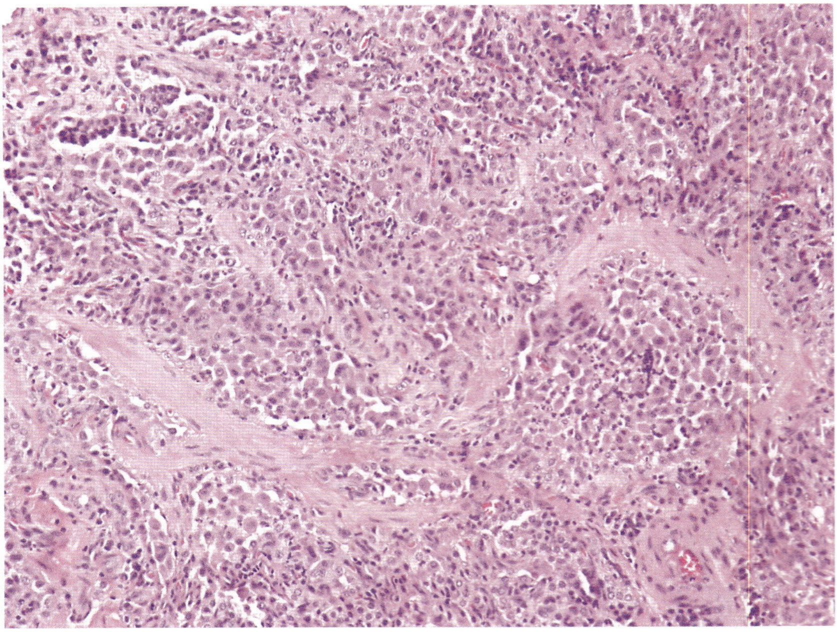

FIGURE 9.23 Another example of desquamative interstitial pneumonia showing mild thickening of alveolar septa by fibrosis.

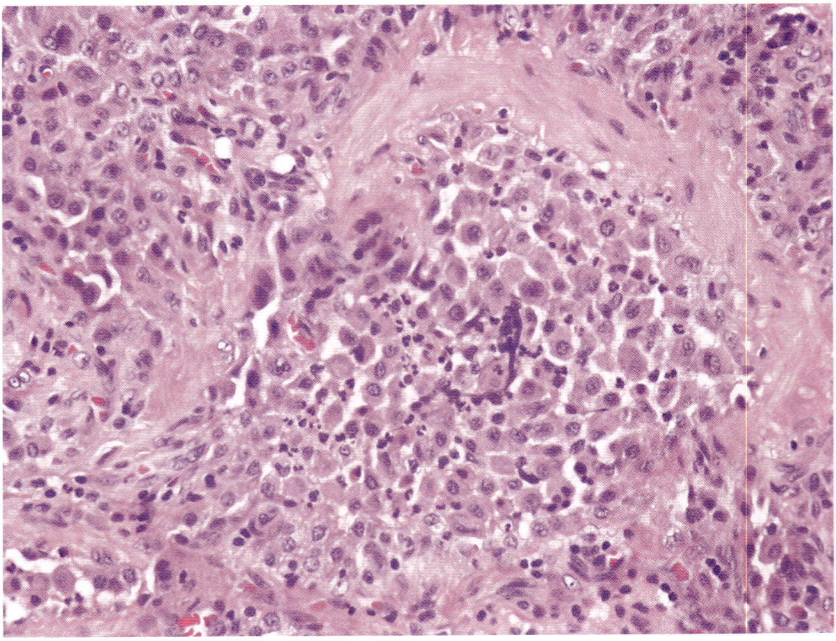

FIGURE 9.24 Higher magnification from the same field showing complete filling of the alveolar lumen by monotonous sheets of macrophages.

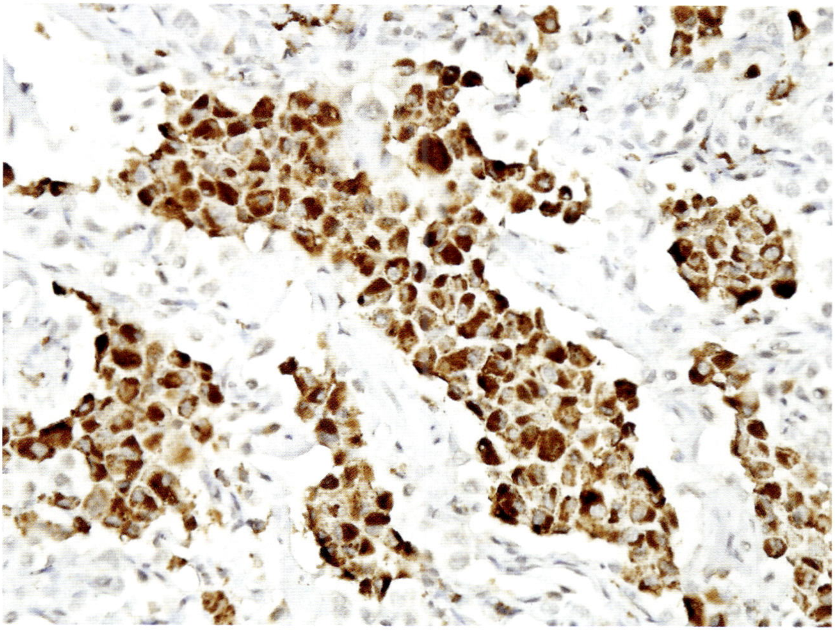

FIGURE 9.25 Immunohistochemical staining shows CD68+ (KP-1 macrophage marker) alveolar macrophages in desquamative interstitial pneumonia.

the same stage of evolution).[35,36] The prognosis for DIP is much better than that of UIP. A favorable response to steroids and smoking cessation with complete recovery is observed in most patients. DIP-like reactions can be observed focally in other conditions, including UIP, Langerhans cell histiocytosis (LCH), and respiratory bronchiolitis–associated interstitial lung disease (RB-ILD). Proper distinction from these conditions is important because of the differences in prognosis and treatment.[37]

Cryptogenic Organizing Pneumonia

The term *bronchiolitis obliterans organizing pneumonia* (BOOP) was first proposed for patients who presented with organizing pneumonia of unexplained etiology.[38] This pattern of airspace organization is an extremely common and nonspecific manifestation of lung injury that can be seen in a variety of conditions, from infections to neoplasia. Because of the nonspecific nature of the changes, the term *BOOP* has been increasingly abandoned in recent years and replaced by the term *cryptogenic organizing pneumonia* (COP) when the changes are extensive and no etiology can be recognized.[3,39] COP is associated with a favorable clinical evolution and responds well to corticosteroid administration although some patients will relapse.[40-42] The term *COP* or *BOOP* should not be used in the setting of extensive interstitial fibrosis, as the finding in such instances is secondary to the underlying fibrosing process and will be associated with a poor prognosis. COP often occurs after an upper respiratory tract infection with slowly progressive symptoms of cough and shortness of breath. Some cases have been described following treatment with drugs for other conditions.[43,44] Patients are usually middle-aged and nonsmokers. Three different patterns have been described on imaging: patchy airspace consolidation with ground-glass attenuation (the most common radiologic finding), a solitary nodule or mass, or diffuse infiltrative opacities.[39] COP is histologically characterized by filling of the airspaces by plugs comprising loose fibroblasts admixed with a myxoid ground substance (Fig. 9.26).[40] The surrounding alveolar walls may contain a mild interstitial inflammatory infiltrate made up of small lymphocytes, plasma cells, and histiocytes (Fig. 9.27). Fibrin may also be seen focally in association with the fibroblastic plugs, and more advanced lesions may display more prominent fibrosis (Fig. 9.28). Interstitial fibrosis and honeycombing should not be present in the idiopathic form of organizing pneumonia.

Lymphoid Interstitial Pneumonia

Lymphoid interstitial pneumonia is generally included in the rare IIP category, but it is accepted today that this often represents a precursor lesion to

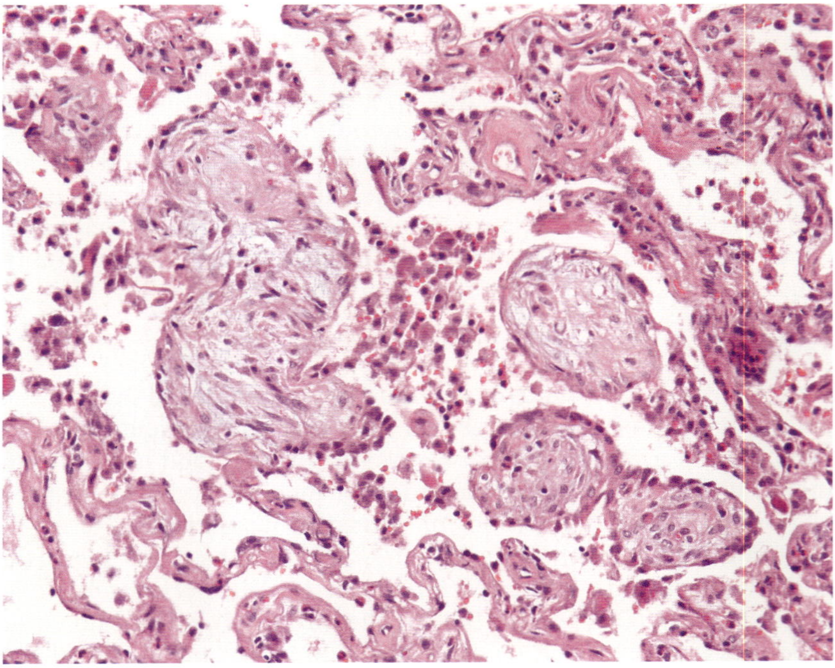

FIGURE 9.26 **Cryptogenic organizing pneumonia shows multiple fibroblastic plugs filling the alveolar lumens.** Notice the absence of fibrosis in surrounding alveolar walls.

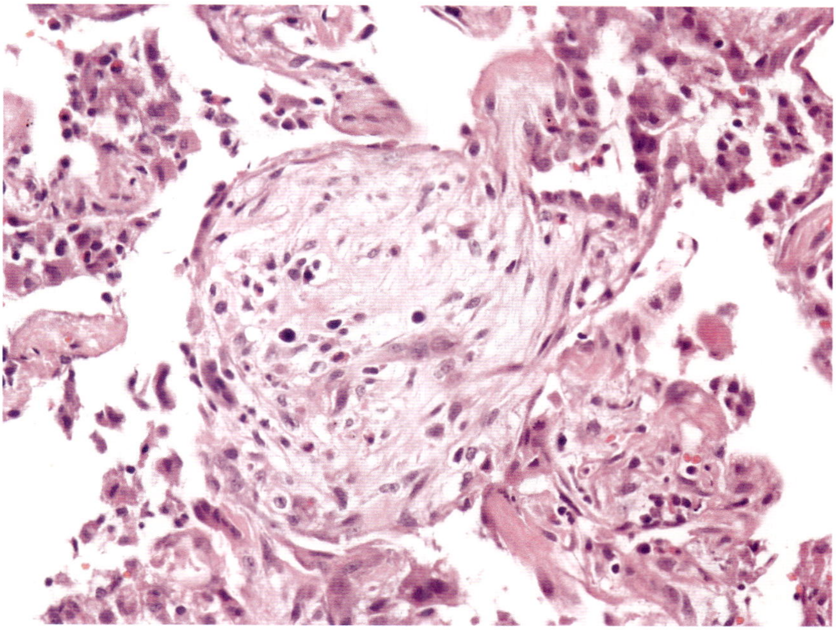

FIGURE 9.27 Early stage of organization in cryptogenic organizing pneumonia shows abundant myxoid matrix with granulation tissue plugging the alveolar space.

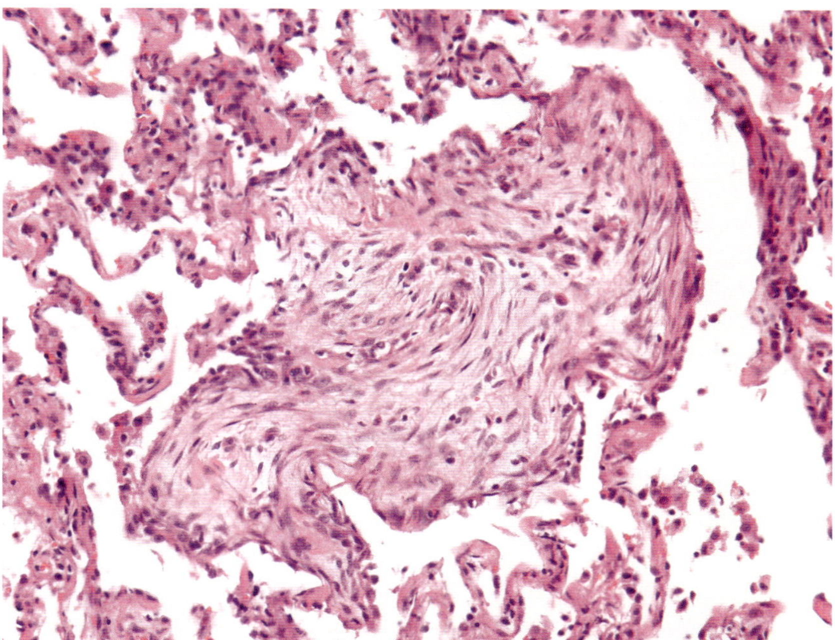

FIGURE 9.28 More advanced stage of cryptogenic organizing pneumonia shows plugging of alveolar lumens by a predominantly fibroblastic proliferation with minimal inflammation.

a lymphoproliferative disorder that may progress to a low-grade extranodal marginal zone lymphoma (so-called bronchus-associated lymphoid tissue lymphoma).[45] As such, it will be discussed in more detail under the heading "lymphoproliferative disorders." Some cases categorized as examples of lymphoid interstitial pneumonia may also overlap morphologically with cases of "cellular" NSIP.

Pleuroparenchymal Fibroelastosis

Pleuroparenchymal fibroelastosis (PPFE) is a fibrosing lung disease currently characterized as a rare IIP.[17] This term was first coined in 2004 in a study by Frankel et al.,[46,47] although the entity was likely described prior to this as "idiopathic pulmonary upper lobe fibrosis" in Japan. It is often idiopathic, although some cases may have an identifiable underlying cause. The condition involves fibrosis of the pleura and subpleural lung parenchyma within the upper lobes with sparing of the lower lobes. HRCT usually shows the subpleural fibrosis along with upper lobe volume loss, distortion, and traction bronchiectasis.[48] It presents in middle-aged adults, usually with a nonproductive cough and exertional dyspnea, with pneumothorax and bacterial infections as common complications. It is a progressive disease in approximately 60% of patients with as high as 40% of patients dying from the disease.[49] While some radiologic and histologic diagnostic criteria have been proposed, the disease is often difficult to diagnose with a variable clinical course and heterogenous clinical scenarios in which it occurs.[50] This is compounded by the fact that surgical lung biopsies in PPFE patients tend to have worse complications as compared to other interstitial lung diseases.[51] Histologically, it presents with some characteristic findings that include fibrosis of the visceral pleura, subpleural fibroelastosis, sparing of the parenchyma distant from the pleura, mild patchy chronic inflammation, and fibroblastic foci at the leading edge of the fibrosis (Figs. 9.29 and 9.30).[46] Although the diagnosis is primarily made based on larger resection specimens, with proper clinical-pathologic correlation, it can be made on wedge biopsies especially if the distribution of the fibrosis is within the upper lobes. The process is unresponsive to steroids or immunosuppressive agents, although one study did find that the antifibrotic drug nintedanib may reduce the rate of pulmonary function decline in patients with PPFE.[52,53] In some cases, lung transplant has been attempted, though patients tended to have high postoperative morbidity and mortality.[54]

Acute Interstitial Pneumonia

Acute interstitial pneumonia (AIP) is a rapidly progressive form of interstitial pneumonia that affects young adults and is usually preceded by flu-like symptoms. The histopathologic findings are similar to those seen in organizing diffuse alveolar damage and have been detailed in Chapter 2. The condition has also been termed *idiopathic adult respiratory distress*

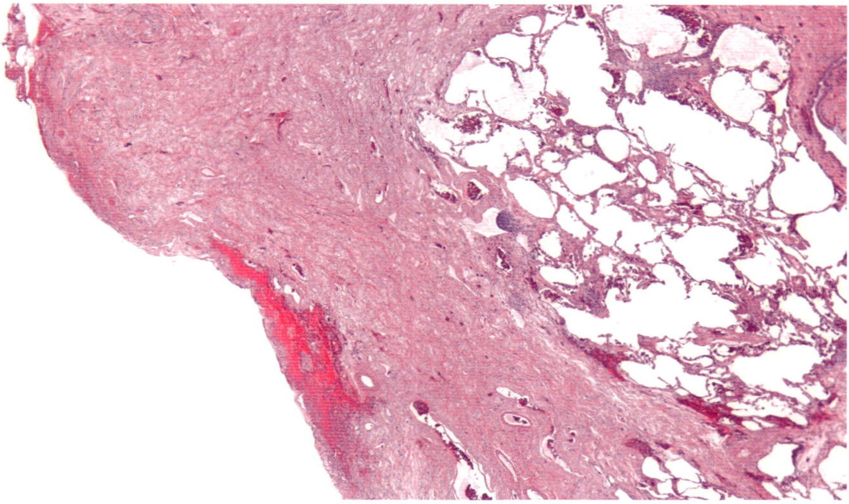

FIGURE 9.29 **Low-power magnification in a patient with pleuroparenchymal fibroelastosis shows a portion of a wedge biopsy demonstrating a dense band of subpleural fibroelastosis that shows a sharp transition with the remaining alveolated lung parenchyma.**

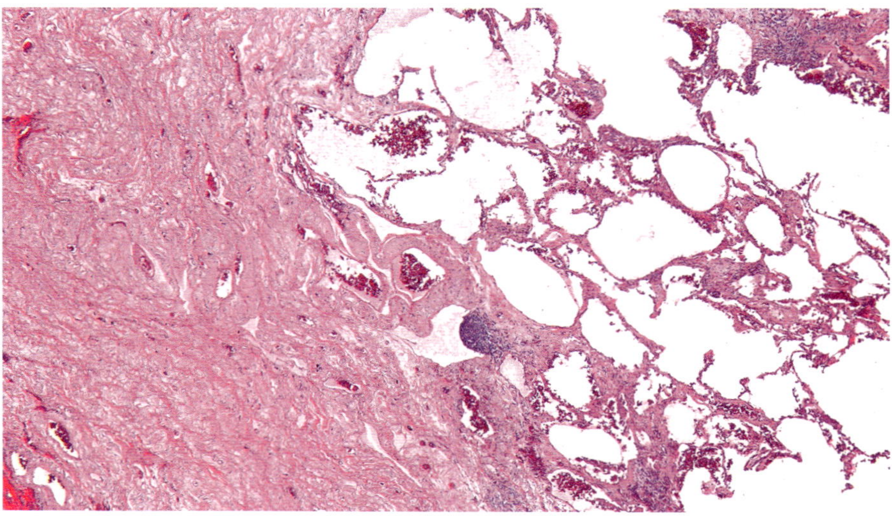

FIGURE 9.30 **Higher-power magnification shows the fibroelastotic scarring process as it pushes into the alveolated lung parenchyma.** Small patches of chronic inflammatory infiltrates can be identified at the leading edge of the fibrosis.

syndrome. The term *AIP* should not be used in cases where an inciting event such as shock, sepsis, or drugs has been documented. Patients present with acute symptoms of short duration (1 or 2 days), including dyspnea, fever, and bilateral opacities on chest X-rays. The clinical course is rapidly progressive with more than 70% mortality. Briefly, the histologic findings are characterized by thickening of alveolar septa because of the fibroblastic proliferation admixed with chronic inflammation.[55] There is usually hyperplasia of alveolar pneumocytes with squamous metaplasia. There may be residual hyaline membranes lining alveolar spaces. The process closely resembles the organizing stage of diffuse alveolar damage. The diagnosis of AIP requires strict clinical-pathologic correlation and demonstration of absence of an underlying cause for the acute respiratory distress.

SPECIFIC INTERSTITIAL PNEUMONIAS

Diffuse interstitial lung disease may often be the result of various specific underlying conditions that are amenable to specific therapeutic strategies (Table 9.1). One of the most common causes of diffuse lung disease is connective tissue disorders (CTD), also known as CVD, which accounts for approximately 15% to 25% of all cases of interstitial lung diseases and 2% of deaths from respiratory causes (Table 9.4).[56,57] The histopathologic findings in the acute and chronic phases of the various CVDs have been detailed in Chapters 2 and 3, including rheumatoid arthritis, progressive systemic sclerosis, systemic lupus erythematosus, polymyositis/dermatomyositis, and Sjögren syndrome. The findings in these conditions can often be confused

TABLE 9.4 Diffuse Lung Manifestations of Systemic Collagen Vascular Disease

Disease	Pulmonary Manifestation
Rheumatoid arthritis	Follicular bronchiolitis, diffuse alveolar damage, organizing pneumonia, diffuse fibrosing interstitial pneumonia (UIP pattern), granulomatous interstitial pneumonia, vasculitis
Systemic lupus erythematosus	Follicular bronchiolitis, diffuse alveolar damage, organizing pneumonia, diffuse fibrosing interstitial pneumonia (UIP pattern), granulomatous interstitial pneumonia, vasculitis
Progressive systemic sclerosis	Diffuse alveolar damage, organizing pneumonia, diffuse fibrosing interstitial pneumonia (UIP and NSIP patterns), vasculitis
Dermatomyositis/polymyositis	Bronchiolitis, diffuse alveolar damage, organizing pneumonia, diffuse fibrosing interstitial pneumonia (UIP and NSIP patterns), vasculitis
Sjögren syndrome	Follicular bronchiolitis, diffuse alveolar damage, organizing pneumonia, diffuse fibrosing interstitial pneumonia (UIP pattern), vasculitis

UIP, usual interstitial pneumonia.

for UIP, NSIP, or other types of IIPs. In fact, the histology of interstitial pneumonia because of CTD/CVD can be nearly indistinguishable from that of idiopathic interstitial fibrosis, although some authors have suggested that prominence of plasma cells in the infiltrate and presence of lymphoid follicles with germinal centers statistically favors CTD/CVD.[58] Clinical history and laboratory tests are indispensable for arriving at the correct diagnosis.

A similar situation applies to diffuse lung disease associated with drugs.[59,60] The various pathologic manifestations of drug-induced lung changes are detailed in Chapters 2, 3, and 4 and include acute lung injury associated with drug administration, interstitial fibrosis, alveolar hemorrhage, and vascular disease produced by medications. The most common offending agents include methotrexate, amiodarone, carmustine, busulfan, and bleomycin.

Four other types of diffuse lung disease that can have a treatable and identifiable underlying cause will be dealt with here in more detail: hypersensitivity pneumonitis (extrinsic allergic alveolitis), respiratory bronchiolitis–interstitial lung disease, LCH, and giant cell interstitial pneumonia due to heavy metal exposure.

Chronic Hypersensitivity Pneumonitis

Chronic hypersensitivity pneumonitis (CHP) is a distinctive type of diffuse interstitial lung process caused by airway inhalation exposure to environmental antigens. Typical examples include "farmer's lung," caused by inhalation of *actinomyces* in hay, and "pigeon breeder's lung," caused by inhalation of avian antigens.[61,62] The pathologic and immunologic features of acute hypersensitivity pneumonitis were discussed in more detail in Chapter 3.

A chronic form of this disease may result from lower levels of long-term exposure to antigens and may be progressive and lead to death because of diffuse lung fibrosis. HRCT scans show upper- and middle-lobe predominant fibrosis, peribronchovascular fibrosis, mosaic attenuation, air trapping, centrilobular nodule formation, and sparing of the bases of the lung.[63,64] In very late stages, honeycombing resembling that of UIP can be seen. Treatment of the condition involves removal of exposure to the offending antigen. Patients may not respond well to corticoids if the offending antigen is not removed. Even with the removal of the offending agent, some cases of CHP may progress to lung fibrosis with a potentially fatal outcome.[65] Standardized diagnostic criteria are beginning to emerge, but the diagnosis of CHP continues to have a high degree of subjective variability among clinical centers.[66,67] With the advent of antifibrotic agents for fibrosing interstitial lung diseases, recent consensus guidelines have recommended separating CHP into fibrotic and nonfibrotic forms.[68-70]

The classical histologic picture of CHP shows changes of chronic interstitial inflammation associated with the production of small, nonnecrotizing interstitial granulomas and multinucleated giant cells located in association with the airways. The chronic interstitial inflammation may resemble NSIP and other forms of cellular inflammatory interstitial pneumonias. The lung biopsy typically shows widening of the alveolar walls by a dense interstitial inflammatory infiltrate comprising small lymphocytes and plasma cells. Foci of organizing pneumonia with airspace fibroblastic plugs can be seen in more than half of cases. Focal bronchiolization of airspaces (lambertosis) can also result from chronic injury to airway spaces, as well as bronchiolitis with aggregates of plasma cells and small lymphocytes surrounding terminal airways.[71] The chronic inflammatory changes will eventually give rise to interstitial fibrosis; the histologic spectrum of fibrosis in CHP is quite varied and can include patterns that resemble UIP (including honeycombing of the lung), NSIP, and patterns seen in CTD/CVDs.[72] An indispensable component for the histologic diagnosis of the process is the presence of ill-formed epithelioid granulomas in the interstitium, especially near the airways (Fig. 9.31). The granulomas may be extremely subtle and easy to overlook on cursory examination.[73] Sometimes, only scattered multinucleated giant cells will be seen in the interstitium, which should prompt a search for the microgranulomas. Refractile oxalate crystals may be found within giant cells; these should not be interpreted as evidence of aspiration pneumonia. Prominent, well-formed epithelioid granulomas should point in the direction of an alternate diagnosis.

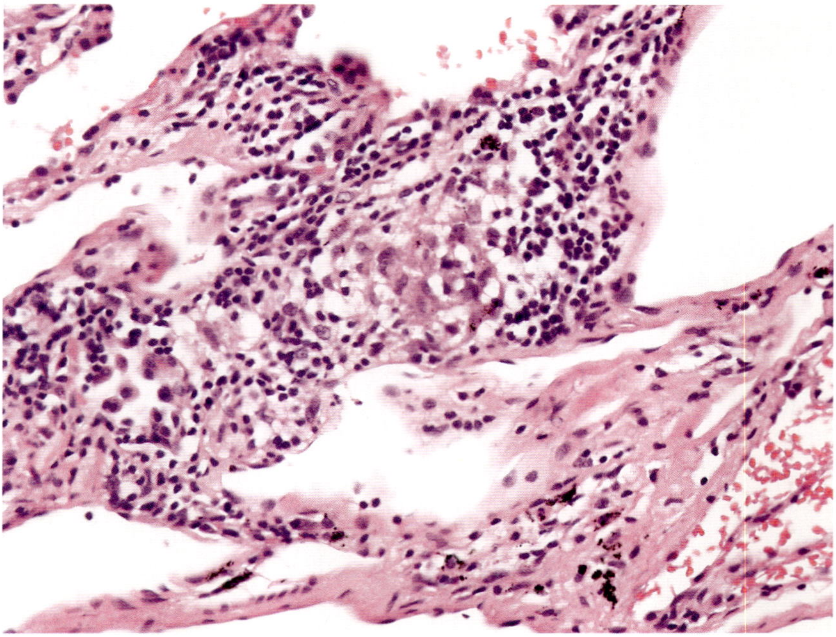

FIGURE 9.31 **Thickening of alveolar septa by dense lymphoid infiltrate and incipient fibrosis in chronic hypersensitivity pneumonitis.** Notice the small, ill-defined epithelioid granuloma admixed with the lymphocytes within the alveolar wall.

The differential diagnosis for hypersensitivity pneumonitis includes cellular interstitial pneumonias caused by drug reactions, infection, idiopathic fibrosing lung diseases, and CVD. Perhaps the most important differential diagnosis though is between CHP with a UIP-like pattern and UIP. Studies have shown that there are poor kappa values when pulmonary pathologists are presented with this scenario. Some features such as bronchiolitis, organizing pneumonia, granulomas or multinucleated giant cells, and peribronchiolar fibrosis may help support CHP with UIP-like changes.[66,72,73] However, strict clinical correlation, including a detailed clinical history and exposure history, is critical for eliciting the proper diagnosis in this context, especially in cases where the histologic picture resembles that of another fibrosing lung disease.

Respiratory Bronchiolitis–Associated Interstitial Lung Disease

RB-ILD is a disorder strictly related to cigarette smoking that generally leads to a mild form of interstitial lung disease.[37] This process is currently believed to be closely related to smoking, akin to DIP and LCH, and is generally limited to the upper lung lobes. Respiratory bronchiolitis (RB) is a microscopic incidental finding in the small airways of cigarette smokers characterized by mild peribronchiolar inflammation with deposition of pigment-laden macrophages within the lumen of the bronchioles.[74] It should be noted that some authors have begun to move away from the term "respiratory bronchiolitis" in favor of more descriptive terms that better describe the intra-alveolar accumulation of pigmented macrophages such as "pigmented airspace macrophages".[32,75] In some patients, an exuberant form of this process will develop leading to clinical and radiographic manifestations of disease. RB, RB-ILD, and DIP have been regarded by some as a continuous spectrum of disease, with RB representing the asymptomatic end of the spectrum and DIP corresponding to the other end.[76] Patients with RB-ILD are usually 10 years younger than those with DIP (30-40 years old) and present with symptoms of shortness of breath and cough. Chest X-rays and CT will show ground-glass opacities. Histologic changes reminiscent of RB-ILD can be seen in smokers in the vicinity of other processes and may represent an incidental finding. A diagnosis of RB-ILD should be established only in the appropriate clinical and radiographic contexts. The main histologic findings comprise mild chronic inflammation around bronchioles with variable numbers of hemosiderin-laden macrophages in the lumen and metaplastic bronchiolar epithelium extending into the alveolar ducts (Fig. 9.32).[77] Scant peribronchiolar fibrosis may also be present (Fig. 9.33). RB-ILD has an excellent prognosis, and the symptoms may subside with cessation of smoking or use of immunosuppressive therapy.[78,79] Of note, a separate smoking-related interstitial lung disease, labeled smoking-related interstitial fibrosis, has been more recently described.[75] Histologically, this process is characterized by the presence of RB and bright pink, dense, ropelike interstitial wall fibrosis

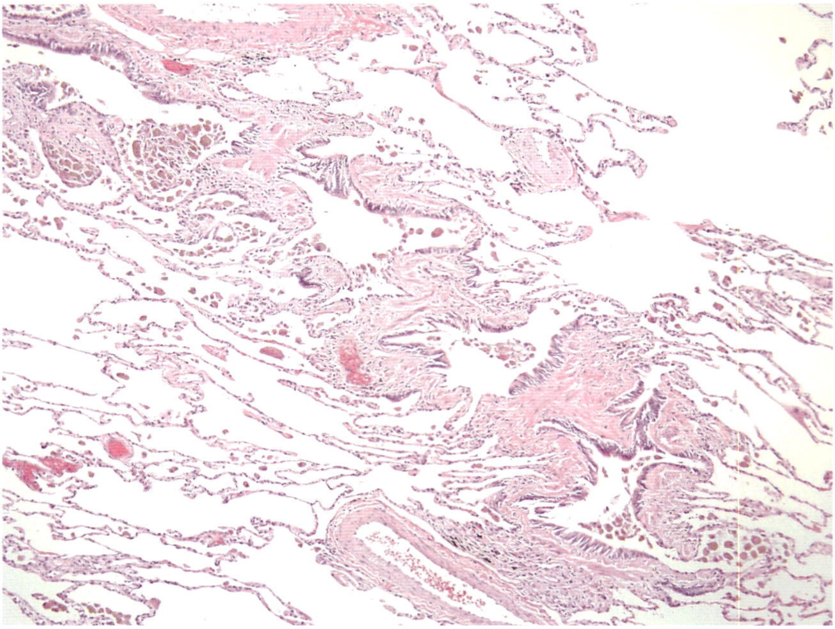

FIGURE 9.32 Lung changes in respiratory bronchiolitis–associated interstitial lung disease characterized by mild chronic peribronchiolar inflammation with metaplastic bronchiolar epithelium extending into alveolar ducts and collections of hemosiderin-laden macrophages.

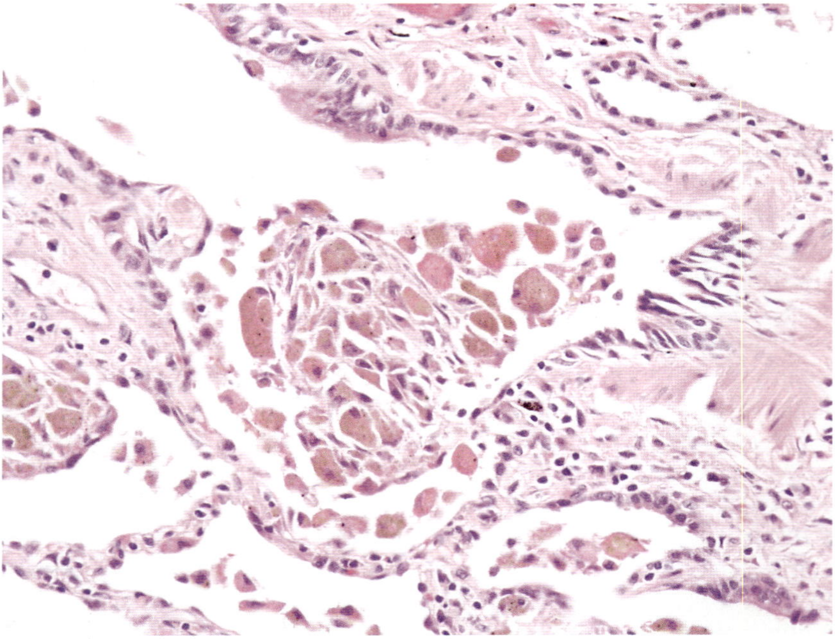

FIGURE 9.33 Higher magnification in lung biopsy from patient with respiratory bronchiolitis–associated interstitial lung disease showing respiratory bronchiolitis characterized by mild peribronchiolar inflammation with variable numbers of hemosiderin-laden macrophages in the lumen.

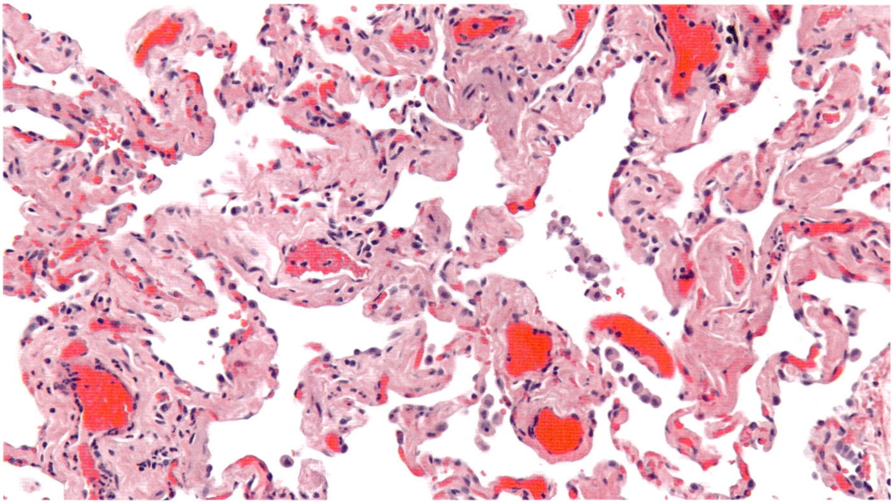

FIGURE 9.34 Wedge biopsy of the lung in a patient with subclinical smoking-related interstitial fibrosis demonstrating widening of the interalveolar septa by eosinophilic collagen deposition.

that is not bronchiolocentric (Fig. 9.34). The condition may be subclinical although in some cases presents as diffuse parenchymal lung disease with clinical and radiologic abnormalities that trigger a lung biopsy.

Langerhans Cell Histiocytosis

Formerly known as pulmonary eosinophilic granuloma or "histiocytosis-X," LCH is another smoking-related condition that can lead to chronic lung disease.[80,81] It is a rare disorder of unknown etiology caused by a neoplastic proliferation of Langerhans cells. The disease occurs almost exclusively in smokers. Affected individuals are usually young adults, between 20 and 40 years of age, and present with slowly progressive cough and dyspnea. In the early stages of the disease, imaging studies show small, bilateral nodules that form "tree-in-bud" lesions distributed in the upper lobes. In the late stages, the nodules are replaced by cysts, eventually ending in fibrosis and honeycombing.[82] Molecular studies have proven the neoplastic nature of the disease and have demonstrated *BRAF* V600E mutations in approximately 50% to 70% of cases as well as mutations in the *TP53*, *NRAS*, *KRAS*, and *MAP2K1* genes in approximately 25% of cases.[83-86] There has been some evidence in the literature that the different mutational profiles may also help stratify LCH into clinically distinct risk groups.[86,87] Molecular testing has been shown to be effective in both lung biopsies as well as fluid from bronchoalveolar lavages in the diagnosis of LCH.[88] Smoking cessation is the most effective treatment and usually results in disappearance of the symptoms. Some have utilized immunosuppressive agents with or without the addition of a cytotoxic agent. Most patients recover spontaneously; however, in some cases, it may progress to fibrosis with development of honeycomb lung.[82]

The histology mirrors the radiologic findings, with the early lesions showing a cellular process and the late lesions showing mainly fibrosis. In the late stages, the disease can be very difficult to recognize because the characteristic Langerhans cells may not be present in the fibrotic areas. The cellular form of the disease is characterized on scanning magnification by small, irregular, stellate nodules centered on the small airways (Fig. 9.35; eFig. 9.10). Small cysts may be formed adjacent to the nodules because of traction on the surrounding alveolar walls. The nodules comprise eosinophils in variable numbers admixed with a population of Langerhans cells and small lymphocytes (Fig. 9.36). Langerhans cells are characterized by pale, irregular oval to spindle nuclei displaying striking nuclear convolutions and infoldings imparting them a "cerebriform" appearance (Fig. 9.37). The cytoplasm of the Langerhans cells is mildly eosinophilic with indistinct cell borders. The surrounding small airways may display features of RB. The late, fibrotic lesions are characterized by residual, stellate, parenchymal scars that may be completely depleted of Langerhans cells. The Langerhans cells, when present, can be highlighted by the use of immunohistochemical stains. Antibodies to CD1a, S-100 protein, and CD207 (Langerin) will stain these cells very strongly, facilitating the diagnosis (Fig. 9.38A and B). In addition, antibodies specifically targeting the *BRAF* V600E mutation are now available and may be of help as well.[89]

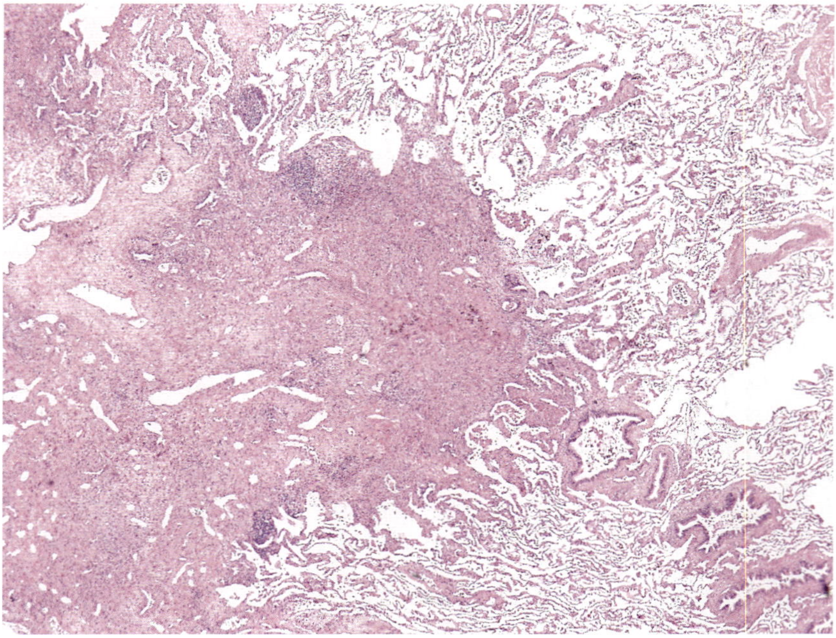

FIGURE 9.35 **Scanning magnification in lung biopsy of patient with Langerhans cell histiocytosis showing a stellate scar adjacent to the small airways.**

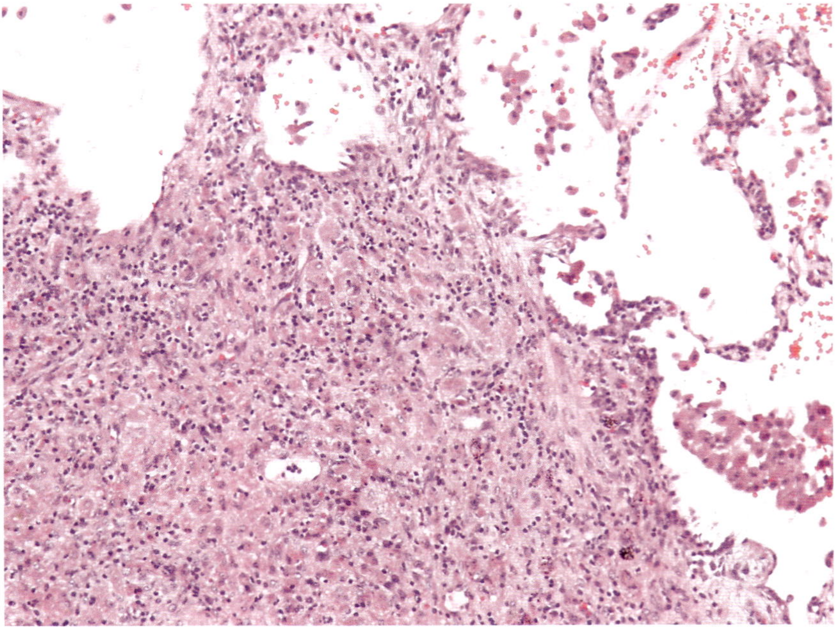

FIGURE 9.36 **Higher magnification from fully developed lesion in Langerhans cell histiocytosis of the lung shows a dense population of inflammatory and mononuclear cells admixed with histiocytes.**

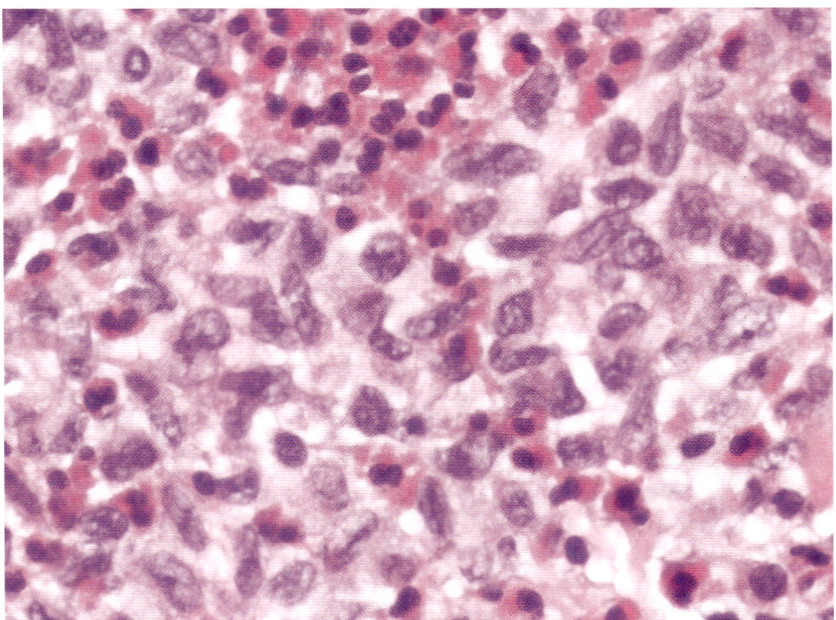

FIGURE 9.37 **High-power magnification of Langerhans cell histiocytosis showing eosinophils admixed with Langerhans cells.** The latter are characterized by their striking nuclear convolutions, longitudinal nuclear grooves, and small inconspicuous nucleoli.

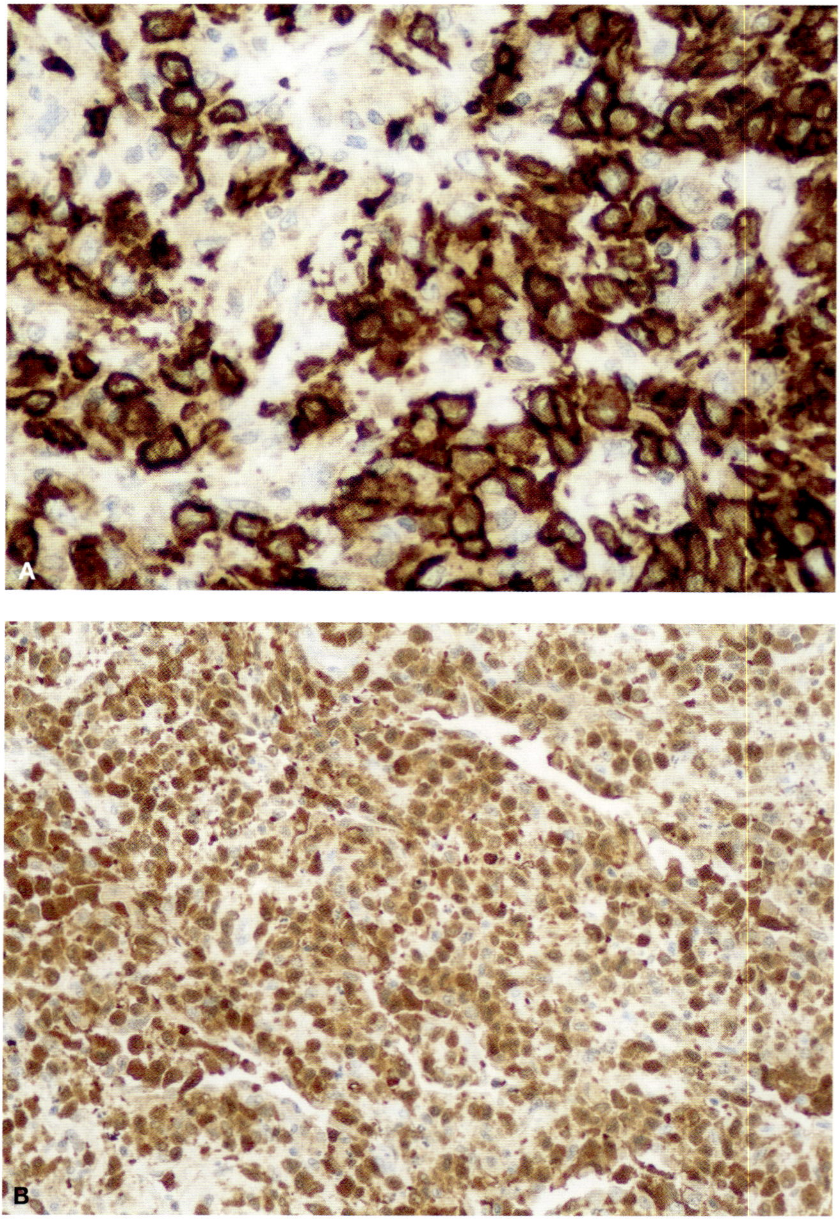

FIGURE 9.38 **A.** Immunohistochemical stain for CD1a shows strong diffuse membranous positivity of the Langerhans cells. **B.** Immunohistochemical stain for S-100 protein highlights the Langerhans cells in Langerhans cell histiocytosis of the lung.

Giant Cell Interstitial Pneumonitis Due to Hard Metal Pneumoconiosis

Originally described as "giant cell interstitial pneumonia" by Liebow,[90] this disorder is now known to be related primarily to inhalation of dust containing hard metal particles, such as tungsten carbide, titanium, and cobalt. Exposure to hard metals can occur during the manufacturing process of products containing hard metals or in certain industries such as the diamond-polishing industry. Patients usually present with progressive dyspnea. Cessation of the exposure is usually effective in controlling the symptoms and leads to full recovery in most patients. In a few cases, the disease may follow a progressive course to death. It is believed that the pathogenetic mechanism of disease is because of hypersensitivity; less than 1% of those exposed to hard metals develop the disease. Rare cases with unknown exposures have been documented and may indicate that other contributory factors play a role in the disease course.[91] The histologic findings were described in detail in Chapter 3. Briefly, they include thickening of alveolar septa secondary to fibrosis, chronic inflammation, and hyperplasia of type II alveolar pneumocytes. The most distinctive feature, however, is the presence of abundant multinucleated giant cells within the alveolar lumens and lining the alveolar septa (Fig. 9.39). The giant cells are found

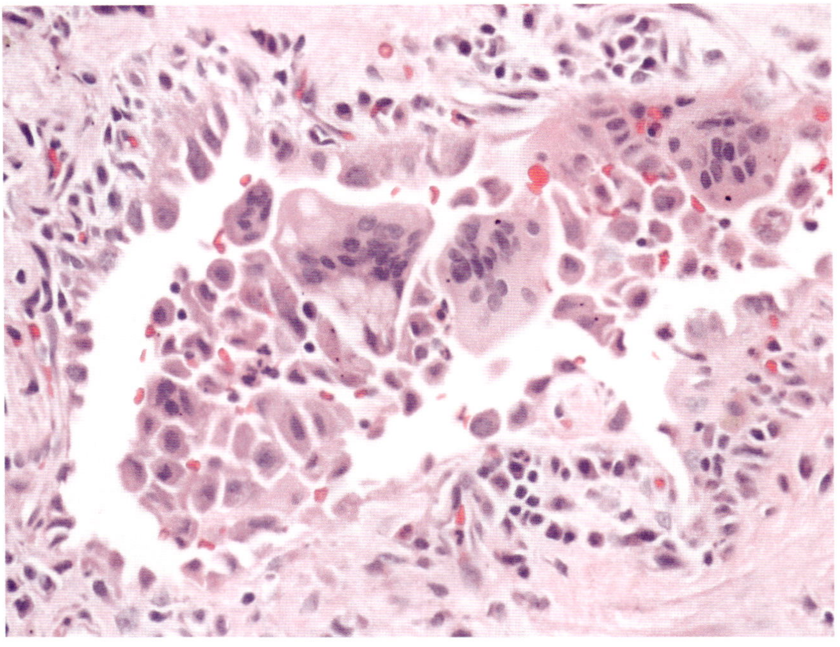

FIGURE 9.39 Lung biopsy in patient with giant cell interstitial pneumonia due to exposure to dust with hard metal particles (hard metal pneumoconiosis) showing abundant macrophages within the alveolar lumen admixed with large, multinucleated giant cells.

admixed with numerous macrophages, resulting in a histologic appearance that is reminiscent of DIP. In advanced stages, there is severe interstitial fibrosis with bronchiolar metaplasia and honeycombing resembling UIP. The metal particles can be observed by using analytical electron microscopy.[92,93] Transbronchial biopsy and bronchioloalveolar lavage may be useful in the diagnosis of this condition.[94,95]

REFERENCES

1. Liebow A, Carrington C. The interstitial pneumonias. In: Simon M, Potchen E, LeMay M, eds. *Frontiers of Pulmonary Radiology: Pathophysiologic, Roentgenographic and Radioisotopic Considerations*. Grune & Stratton; 1969:109-141.
2. Katzenstein AL. Idiopathic interstitial pneumonia: classification and diagnosis. *Monogr Pathol.* 1993;36:1-31.
3. Travis W, King TJ, Bateman E, et al. American Thoracic Society/European Respiratory Society international multidisciplinary consensus classification of the idiopathic interstitial pneumonias. *Am Rev Respir Crit Care Med.* 2002;165:227-304.
4. Raghu G, Rochwerg B, Zhang Y, et al. An official ATS/ERS/JRS/ALAT clinical practice guideline: treatment of idiopathic pulmonary fibrosis. An update of the 2011 clinical practice guideline. *Am J Respir Crit Care Med.* 2015;192(2):e3-e19.
5. Cerri S, Manzini E, Nori O, et al. Genetic risk factors in idiopathic and non-idiopathic interstitial lung disease: similarities and differences. *Medicina (Kaunas).* 2024;60(12):1967.
6. Adegunsoye A, Kropski JA, Behr J, et al. Genetics and genomics of pulmonary fibrosis: charting the molecular landscape and shaping precision medicine. *Am J Respir Crit Care Med.* 2024;210(4):401-423.
7. Wall CP, Gaensler EA, Carrington CB. Comparison of transbronchial and open biopsies in diffuse infiltrative lung disease. *Am Rev Respir Dis.* 1981;123:280-285.
8. Kida R, Yoshida R, Nitanai K, et al. Viability and diagnostic potential of tissues obtained through cryobiopsy. *Respir Investig.* 2024;62(6):1220-1226.
9. Kaburaki S, Tanaka T, Kamio K, Tanaka Y, Kasahara K, Seike M. Transbronchial lung cryobiopsy for interstitial lung disease: early experience, learning curve, and the impact of sedation on complication rates at a single centre in Japan. *BMC Pulm Med.* 2024;24(1):540.
10. Ueoka M, Ronaghi R, Khauli S, Channick CL. Cryoprobe biopsy versus mechanical biopsies in pulmonary diagnostics. *Curr Opin Pulm Med.* 2025;31(1):19-27.
11. Churg A, Poletti V, Ravaglia C, et al. Pathological features of connective tissue disease-associated interstitial lung disease in transbronchial cryobiopsies. *Histopathology.* 2025;86(2):260-267.
12. Avasarala SK, Wells AU, Colby TV, Maldonado F. Transbronchial cryobiopsy in interstitial lung diseases: state-of-the-art review for the interventional pulmonologist. *J Bronchology Interv Pulmonol.* 2021;28(1):81-92.
13. Kim SY, Diggans J, Pankratz D, et al. Classification of usual interstitial pneumonia in patients with interstitial lung disease: assessment of a machine learning approach using high-dimensional transcriptional data. *Lancet Respir Med.* 2015;3(6):473-482.
14. Crystal R, Fulmer J, Roberts W, Moss ML, Line BR, Reynolds HY. Idiopathic pulmonary fibrosis. Clinical, histologic, radiographic, physiologic, scintigraphic, cytologic and biochemical aspects. *Ann Intern Med.* 1976;85:769-788.
15. Muller N, Staples C, Miller R, Vedal S, Thurlbeck WM, Ostrow DN. Disease activity in idiopathic pulmonary fibrosis. CT and pathologic correlation. *Radiology.* 1987;165:731-743.

16. Gal AA, Staton GW. Current concepts in the classification of interstitial lung disease. *Am J Clin Pathol.* 2005;123(suppl):S67-S81.
17. Lynch DA, Sverzellati N, Travis WD, et al. Diagnostic criteria for idiopathic pulmonary fibrosis: a Fleischner Society white paper. *Lancet Respir Med.* 2018;6(2):138-153.
18. Funke-Chambour M, Guler SA, Geiser T, et al. New radiological diagnostic criteria—impact on idiopathic pulmonary fibrosis diagnosis. *Eur Respir J.* 2019;54:1900905. doi:10.1183/13993003.00905-2019
19. Teirstein AS. The elusive goal of therapy for usual interstitial pneumonia. *N Engl J Med.* 2004;350(2):181-183.
20. Varone F, Gibiino G, Gasbarrini A, et al. Evaluation of the lung microbiome as a therapeutic target in the management of idiopathic pulmonary fibrosis: role of antioxidant/antibiotic combination therapy. *Eur Rev Med Pharmacol Sci.* 2019;23(14):6379-6386.
21. Inoue Y, Ogura T, Azuma A, et al. Real-world safety, tolerability and effectiveness of nintedanib in patients with idiopathic pulmonary fibrosis: final report of post-marketing surveillance in Japan. *Adv Ther.* 2025;42(2):1075-1093.
22. Katzenstein ALA. Idiopathic interstitial pneumonia. In: Katzenstein ALA, ed. *Katzenstein and Askin's Surgical Pathology of Non-Neoplastic Lung Disease*. 3rd ed. WB Saunders; 1990:48-80.
23. Ryerson CJ, Cottin V, Brown KK, Collard HR. Acute exacerbation of idiopathic pulmonary fibrosis: shifting the paradigm. *Eur Respir J.* 2015;46(2):512-520.
24. Masai K, Tsuta K, Motoi N, et al. Clinicopathological, immunohistochemical, and genetic features of primary lung adenocarcinoma occurring in the setting of usual interstitial pneumonia pattern. *J Thorac Oncol.* 2016;11(12):2141-2149.
25. Katzenstein AL, Fiorelli RF. Nonspecific interstitial pneumonia/fibrosis: histologic features and clinical significance. *Am J Surg Pathol.* 1994;18:136-147.
26. Jo YS, Lee HK, Park SH, Joh JS, Jang HJ, Park JS. Korean guidelines for diagnosis and management of idiopathic nonspecific interstitial pneumonia. *Tuberc Respir Dis (Seoul).* 2025;88(2):237-246.
27. Danil ZD, Gilchrist FC, Nicholson AG, et al. A histologic pattern of nonspecific interstitial pneumonia is associated with a better prognosis than usual interstitial pneumonia in patients with cryptogenic fibrosing alveolitis. *Am J Respir Crit Care Med.* 1999;160:899-905.
28. Belloli EA, Beckford R, Hadley R, Flaherty KR. Idiopathic non-specific interstitial pneumonia. *Respirology.* 2016;21(2):259-268.
29. Churg A, Bilawich A. Confluent fibrosis and fibroblast foci in fibrotic non-specific interstitial pneumonia. *Histopathology.* 2016;69(1):128-135.
30. Carrington CB, Gaensler EA, Coutu RE, FitzGerald MX, Gupta RG. Natural history and treated course of usual and desquamative interstitial pneumonia. *N Engl J Med.* 1978;298:801-803.
31. Tazelaar HD, Wright JL, Churg A. Desquamative interstitial pneumonia. *Histopathology.* 2011;58(4):509-516.
32. Mukhopadhyay S, Sansano I. Smoking-related interstitial lung disease: historical perspective and advances in the twenty-first century. *Surg Pathol Clin.* 2024;17(2):159-171.
33. Hartman TE, Primack SL, Swensen SJ, Hansell D, McGuinness G, Müller NL. Desquamative interstitial pneumonia: thin-section CT findings in 22 patients. *Radiology.* 1993;187:787-790.
34. Medenica M, Medenica M. Desquamative interstitial pneumonia with clinical, radiological and histologic correlation. *Radiol Case Rep.* 2019;14(4):505-509.
35. Diken ÖE, Şengül A, Beyan AC, Ayten Ö, Mutlu LC, Okutan O. Desquamative interstitial pneumonia: risk factors, laboratory and bronchoalveolar lavage findings, radiological and histopathological examination, clinical features, treatment and prognosis. *Exp Ther Med.* 2019;17(1):587-595.

36. Carrington CB, Gaensler EA, Coutu RE, Fitzgerald MX, Gupta RG. Usual and desquamative interstitial pneumonia. *Chest.* 1976;69(suppl):261-263.
37. Konopka KE, Myers JL. A review of smoking-related interstitial fibrosis, respiratory bronchiolitis, and desquamative interstitial pneumonia: overlapping histology and confusing terminology. *Arch Pathol Lab Med.* 2018;142(10):1177-1181.
38. Epler GR, Colby TV, McLoud TC, Carrington CB, Gaensler EA. Bronchiolitis obliterans organizing pneumonia. *N Engl J Med.* 1985;312:152-158.
39. Cottin V, Cordier JF. Cryptogenic organizing pneumonia. *Semin Respir Crit Care Med.* 2012;33(5):462-475.
40. Zhou Y, Wang L, Huang M, et al. A long-term retrospective study of patients with biopsy-proven cryptogenic organizing pneumonia. *Chron Respir Dis.* 2019;16: 1479973119853829.
41. Paknejad O, Loni S, Mirshafiee S, Varpaei HA, Gharabaghi MA. Disease course, treatment response and relapse in a group of patients with a primary diagnosis of cryptogenic organizing pneumonia: a cohort study. *Tanaffos.* 2024;23(1):3-10.
42. Taniguchi Y, Arai T, Tsuji T, et al. Cryptogenic organizing pneumonia: clinical outcomes of 60 consecutive cases. *J Thorac Dis.* 2024;16(5):3129-3141.
43. Gans A, Verrengia EP, Ricchiuti E, et al. Ocrelizumab-associated cryptogenic organizing pneumonia in multiple sclerosis: two case reports and comprehensive literature review. *Mult Scler.* 2025;31(6):740-743.
44. Wang L, Zhang L, Ying C, et al. Cryptogenic organizing pneumonia caused by solanine: a case report. *Medicine (Baltimore).* 2024;103(39):e39807.
45. Herbert A, Walters MT, Crawley MI, Godfrey RC. Lymphocytic interstitial pneumonia identified as lymphoma of mucosa associated lymphoid tissue. *J Pathol.* 1985;146:129-138.
46. Frankel SK, Cool CD, Lynch DA, Brown KK. Idiopathic pleuroparenchymal fibroelastosis. Description of a novel clinicopathologic entity. *Chest.* 2004;126:2007-2013.
47. Amitani R, Niimi A, Kuse F. Idiopathic pulmonary upper lobe fibrosis. *Kokyu.* 1992;11:693-699.
48. Reddy TL, Tominaga M, Hansell DM, et al. Pleuroparenchymal fibroelastosis: a spectrum of histopathological and imaging phenotypes. *Eur Respir J.* 2012;40:377-385.
49. Travis WD, Costabel U, Hansell DM, et al. An official American Thoracic Society/European Respiratory Society statement: update of the international multidisciplinary classification of the idiopathic interstitial pneumonias. *Am J Respir Crit Care Med.* 2013;188(6):733-748.
50. Watanabe K, Ishii H, Kiyomi F, et al. Criteria for the diagnosis of idiopathic pleuroparenchymal fibroelastosis: a proposal. *Respir Investig.* 2019;57:312-320.
51. Shiiya H, Nakamura T, Ujiie H, et al. Outcomes of surgical lung biopsy in pleuroparenchymal fibroelastosis: a single-center retrospective study. *Arch Bronconeumol.* 2025;61(3):176-179.
52. Watanabe K. Pleuroparenchymal fibroelastosis: its clinical characteristics. *Curr Respir Med Rev.* 2013;9(4):229-237.
53. Nasser M, Chebib N, Philit F, et al. Treatment with nintedanib in patients with pleuroparenchymal fibroelastosis. *Eur Respir J.* 2017;50(suppl 61):PA4876.
54. Clermidy H, Mercier O, Brioude G, et al. Outcomes of lung transplantation for pleuroparenchymal fibroelastosis: a French multicentric retrospective study. *J Heart Lung Transplant.* 2024;43:1727-1736.
55. Olson J, Colby TV, Elliott C. Hamman-Rich syndrome revisited. *Mayo Clin Proc.* 1998;65:1538-1548.
56. Black I, Katz S. *Respiratory Disease: Task Force Report on Problems, Research Approaches, Needs.* National Heart and Lung Institute; 1977.

57. Strange C, Highland KB. Interstitial lung disease in the patient who has connective tissue disease. *Clin Chest Med.* 2004;25(3):549-559.
58. Ozasa M, Ichikawa H, Sato S, et al. Proposed method of histological separation between connective tissue disease-associated interstitial pneumonia and idiopathic interstitial pneumonias. *PLoS One.* 2018;13:1-11.
59. Cooper JA Jr. Drug-induced lung disease. *Adv Intern Med.* 1997;42:231-268.
60. Camus PH, Foucher P, Bounniaud PH, Ask K. Drug-induced infiltrative lung disease. *Eur Respir J Suppl.* 2001;32:93s-100s.
61. Braun SR, Pico GA, Tsiatis S, et al. Framer's lung disease: long-term clinical and physiologic outcome. *Am Rev Respir Dis.* 1979;119:185-191.
62. Suda T, Sato A, Ida M, Gemma H, Hayakawa H, Chida K. Hypersensitivity pneumonitis associated with home ultrasonic humidifiers. *Chest.* 1995;107:711-719.
63. Hansell DM, Wells AU, Padley SP, Müller NL. Hypersensitivity pneumonitis: correlation of individual CT patterns with functional abnormalities. *Radiology.* 1996;199:123-128.
64. Vasakova M, Morell F, Walsh S, Leslie K, Raghu G. Hypersensitivity pneumonitis: perspectives in diagnosis and management. *Am J Respir Crit Care Med.* 2017;196(6):680-689.
65. Wang P, Jones KD, Urisman A, et al. Pathological findings and prognosis in a large prospective cohort of chronic hypersensitivity pneumonitis. *Chest.* 2017;152(3):502-509.
66. Churg A, Bilawich A, Wright JL. Pathology of chronic hypersensitivity pneumonitis what is it? What are the diagnostic criteria? Why do we care? *Arch Pathol Lab Med.* 2018;142(1):109-119.
67. Morisset J, Johannson KA, Jones KD, et al. Identification of diagnostic criteria for chronic hypersensitivity pneumonitis: an international modified Delphi survey. *Am J Respir Crit Care Med.* 2018;197(8):1036-1044.
68. Fernández Pérez ER, Travis WD, Lynch D, et al. Diagnosis and evaluation of hypersensitivity pneumonitis: CHEST Guideline and Expert Panel Report. *Chest.* 2021;160(2):e97-e156.
69. Raghu G, Remy-Jardin M, Ryerson CJ, et al. Diagnosis of hypersensitivity pneumonitis in adults. An official ATS/JRS/ALAT clinical practice guideline. *Am J Respir Crit Care Med.* 2020;202(3):e36-e69.
70. Churg A. Hypersensitivity pneumonitis: new concepts and classifications. *Mod Pathol.* 2022;35(Suppl 1):15-27.
71. Botelho AB, Ferreira RG, Coletta ENAM, et al. Transbronchial biopsy in chronic hypersensitivity pneumonitis. *Sarcoidosis Vasc Diffuse Lung Dis.* 2021;38(2):e2021018.
72. Takemura T, Akashi T, Kamiya H, et al. Pathological differentiation of chronic hypersensitivity pneumonitis from idiopathic pulmonary fibrosis/usual interstitial pneumonia. *Histopathology.* 2012;61(6):1026-1035.
73. Coleman A, Colby TV. Histologic diagnosis of extrinsic allergic alveolitis. *Am J Surg Pathol.* 1988;12:514-518.
74. Niewoehner D, Kleinerman J, Rice D. Pathologic changes in the peripheral airways in young cigarette smokers. *N Engl J Med.* 1974;291:755-758.
75. Vehar SJ, Yadav R, Mukhopadhyay S, Nathani A, Tolle LB. Smoking-related interstitial fibrosis (SRIF) in patients presenting with diffuse parenchymal lung disease. *Am J Clin Pathol.* 2023;159(2):146-157.
76. Heyneman LE, Ward S, Lynch DA, Remy-Jardin M, Johkoh T, Müller NL. Respiratory bronchiolitis, respiratory bronchiolitis-associated interstitial lung disease, and desquamative interstitial pneumonia: different entities or part of the spectrum of the same disease process? *Am J Roentgenol.* 1999;173:1617-1622.
77. Ryu JH, Myers JL, Capizzi SA, Douglas WW, Vassallo R, Decker PA. Desquamative interstitial pneumonia and respiratory bronchiolitis-associated interstitial lung disease. *Chest.* 2005;127:178-184.

78. Myers J, Veal C, Shin M, Katzenstein AL. Respiratory bronchiolitis causing interstitial lung disease. A clinicopathologic study of six cases. *Am Rev Respir Dis.* 1987;135:880-884.
79. Portnoy J, Veraldi KL, Schwarz MI, et al. Respiratory bronchiolitis-interstitial lung disease: long-term outcome. *Chest.* 2007;131(3):664-671.
80. Vasallo R, Ryu JH, Colby TV, Hartman T, Limper AH. Pulmonary Langerhans'-cell histiocytosis. *N Engl J Med.* 2000;342:1969-1978.
81. Travis WD, Borok Z, Roum JH, et al. Pulmonary Langerhans cell granulomatosis (histiocytosis X). A clinicopathologic study of 48 cases. *Am J Surg Pathol.* 1993;17:971-986.
82. Radzikowska E. Pulmonary Langerhans' cell histiocytosis in adults. *Adv Respir Med.* 2017;85(5):277-289.
83. Thierry AR, Mouliere F, El Messaoudi S, et al. Clinical validation of the detection of KRAS and BRAF mutations from circulating tumor DNA. *Nat Med.* 2014;20(4):430-435.
84. Badalian-Very G, Vergilio JA, Degar BA, et al. Recurrent BRAF mutations in Langerhans cell histiocytosis. *Blood.* 2010;116(11):1919-1923.
85. McGinnis LM, Nybakken G, Ma L, Arber DA. Frequency of MAP2K1, TP53, and U2AF1 mutations in BRAF-mutated Langerhans cell histiocytosis: further characterizing the genomic landscape of LCH. *Am J Surg Pathol.* 2018;42(7):885-890.
86. Méhes G, Irsai G, Bedekovics J, et al. Activating BRAF V600E mutation in aggressive pediatric Langerhans cell histiocytosis: demonstration by allele-specific PCR/direct sequencing and immunohistochemistry. *Am J Surg Pathol.* 2014;38(12):1644-1648.
87. Berres ML, Lim KP, Peters T, et al. BRAF-V600E expression in precursor versus differentiated dendritic cells defines clinically distinct LCH risk groups. *J Exp Med.* 2014;211(4):669-683.
88. Pierry C, Caumont C, Blanchard E, et al. Assessment of BRAFV600E mutation in pulmonary Langerhans cell histiocytosis in tissue biopsies and bronchoalveolar lavages by droplet digital polymerase chain reaction. *Virchows Arch.* 2018;472(2):247-258.
89. Ballester LY, Cantu MD, Lim KP, et al. The use of BRAF V600E mutation-specific immunohistochemistry in pediatric Langerhans cell histiocytosis. *Hematol Oncol.* 2018;36(1):307-315.
90. Liebow AA. Definition and classification of interstitial pneumonias in human pathology. *Prog Resp Res.* 1975;8:1-33.
91. Fortarezza F, Perilli M, Della Barbera M, et al. Giant cell interstitial pneumonia: case series with comprehensive ultrastructural analyses of "not only" hard metal pneumoconiosis. *Histopathology.* 2025;86(3):450-459.
92. Stettler LE, Groth DH, Platek SF. Automated characterization of particles extracted from human lungs: three cases of tungsten carbide exposure. *Scan Electron Microsc.* 1983;(pt 1): 439-448.
93. Tabatowski K, Roggli VL, Fulkerson WJ, Langley RL, Benning T, Johnston WW. Giant cell interstitial pneumonia in a hard-metal worker: cytologic, histologic and analytical electron microscopic investigation. *Acta Cytol.* 1988;32:240-246.
94. Seaman DM, Meyer CA, Kanne JP. Occupational and environmental lung disease. *Clin Chest Med.* 2015;36(2):249-269.
95. Mizutani RF, Terra-Filho M, Lima E, et al. Hard metal lung disease: a case series. *J Bras Pneumol.* 2016;42(6):447-452.

10

LUNG TRANSPLANT PATHOLOGY

Lung transplantation has been utilized over the past years for the management of advanced-stage lung disease, including emphysema, cystic fibrosis, chronic obstructive pulmonary disease, primary pulmonary hypertension, and idiopathic pulmonary fibrosis. Unlike some other transplant organs, complications of lung transplants occur with high frequency, and about half of the patients suffer from chronic rejection. In a 2001 report, the figures for 5-year survival in lung transplant patients were below 50%,[1] which rose slightly in the 2015 report by the Registry of the International Society for Heart and Lung Transplantation. This report indicated that 45,542 adults underwent lung transplantation between January 1990 and June 2013 with survival rates of 89% at 3 months, 80% at 1 year, 65% at 3 years, 54% at 5 years, and 31% at 10 years.[2] Patients who survived to at least 1 year had a median survival of 7.9 years after lung transplantation.[2,3]

Several complications can ensue after lung transplant leading to primary graft dysfunction, including vascular complications, airway anastomosis complications, ischemia-reperfusion injury, and complications related to immunosuppressive therapy. The development of neoplastic processes has also been demonstrated to occur following lung transplantation. Vascular complications include acute postsurgical obstruction of the arterial or venous anastomosis by thrombus, which constitutes a medical emergency, or chronic obstruction because of organizing thrombosis with progressive stenosis. The site of anastomosis may develop a superimposed infection with necrosis or dehiscence of the anastomosis. Ischemia-reperfusion injury can occur in up to 20% of patients, resulting in endothelial injury and pulmonary edema with or without alveolar damage. Recovery occurs in a few days in most patients with supportive therapy alone. Complications of lung transplant can occur immediately in the early postoperative period, within the first month of transplant or later (Table 10.1).[4,5] The most common complication of lung transplant, however, is allograft rejection.

Transbronchial lung biopsy has traditionally been the method of choice for evaluating pulmonary complications in transplant patients.[6] Bronchioloalveolar lavage fluid should also be obtained at the time of the procedure for cultures and to be stained with silver stains and Gram stain for the identification of fungi and bacteria. Obtaining adequate

TABLE 10.1 Complications of Lung Transplantation

Period	Complication
Immediate (0-5 days)	Primary graft failure
	Vascular complications (bleeding, obstruction)
	Ischemia-reperfusion injury
	Hyperacute rejection
	Lobar torsion
	Pneumothorax
	Aspiration
Early (7-30 days)	Infection (*Aspergillus*, cytomegalovirus, *Pneumocystis jirovecii*)
	Dehiscence of anastomosis
	Acute rejection
	Aspiration
Late (>30 days)	Lung infection
	Airway stenosis
	Chronic rejection
	Posttransplant lymphoproliferative disease
	Aspiration

Modified and reproduced in part by permission from Yousem SA, Berry GJ, Cagle PT, et al. Revision of the 1990 working formulation for the classification of pulmonary allograft rejection: Lung Rejection Study Group. The International Society for Heart Transplantation. *J Heart Lung Transplant.* 1996;15:1-15.

tissue samples by the endoscopist is critical for proper evaluation of the process. Multiple tissue samples are preferable and should contain sufficient alveoli and at least one bronchiole in each fragment for proper evaluation. Current consensus recommendations state that there should be a minimum of five biopsies that display evaluable alveolated lung parenchyma for optimal assessment.[7,8] If fewer than five evaluable fragments are received, morphologic assessment for rejection can still be performed; if the features of rejection are present, they should be reported as such; however, if no features are identified, a note should be included indicating that fewer than five fragments were received and that the results may be a false-negative finding. In cases where there is high clinical concern for rejection (ie, extremely ill patient with acute decline in pulmonary function) with negative findings, discussion and correlation with the clinical transplant team is required. A minimum of three levels per tissue block are recommended for examination, although more levels may be needed in many instances.[7] Biopsies of the site of anastomosis may also be indicated if infection is suspected to evaluate whether microorganisms are present. In general, infectious etiology should be rigorously ruled out morphologically and clinically because the morphologic and clinical features of an infectious process can closely mimic rejection. In cases where significant inflammation is present, silver stains, tissue Gram stains, and virus specific immunohistochemistry should be applied.

Recent studies have demonstrated that an alternative technique for the procurement of lung transplant biopsy material is cryobiopsy.[9,10] Studies have demonstrated that cryobiopsy yields better diagnostic material (increased evaluable tissue area and better preservation of histology), and the technique has seen wider adoption in recent years.[11,12]

Multiple studies have now shown the safety and efficacy of cryobiopsy in the transplantation setting indicating that the biopsy-related complication rate is comparable to traditional transbronchial forceps biopsy.[13-16] This biopsy technique is a useful new tool for evaluation of both acute and chronic manifestations of posttransplant complications. In the future, molecular diagnostics and noninvasive measurement of circulating biomarkers may play a role in rejection diagnostics.[17]

REPERFUSION INJURY

Ischemia-reperfusion injury occurs early in the transplant process as a result of capillary injury leading to noncardiogenic pulmonary edema. The injury is produced by the ischemia induced during the procedure but becomes manifested only when the circulation to the lung is reestablished. This complication has been observed clinically in up to 80% of patients undergoing lung or lung-heart transplant.[18] This condition manifests clinically within the first 3 to 4 days posttransplant with worsening oxygenation and decreased lung compliance. Imaging studies show diffuse alveolar and perihilar interstitial infiltrates. Severe ischemia-reperfusion injury leads to primary graft dysfunction, which is a major source of morbidity in lung transplantation patients, particularly within the first 72 hours of transplant.[19-21] Transbronchial biopsy may be required to exclude acute rejection in this scenario. The main histologic finding is that of diffuse alveolar damage (DAD), with congestion, interstitial edema, hyperplasia of alveolar type-II pneumocytes, and hyaline membrane formation (Fig. 10.1).[22] A few neutrophils can be observed in the interstitium. In the healing phase of reperfusion injury, the hyaline membranes are replaced by intra-alveolar plugs of loose fibrous tissue with myxoid matrix (Masson bodies) with fibrous thickening of the alveolar septa (Fig. 10.2). The features of reperfusion injury can also occur in conjunction with acute rejection and can mask the rejection process. The presence of small lymphocytes in the interstitium, particularly when showing a dense perivascular location and in association with eosinophils, should raise the suspicion of acute rejection superimposed on reperfusion injury (Fig. 10.3). Severe acute rejection typically contains a component of DAD; however, acute rejection generally manifests after the first week posttransplant. Attention to the time of the biopsy is therefore critical to assess the presence of DAD in the biopsy sample. Biopsies taken early in the course of the first week

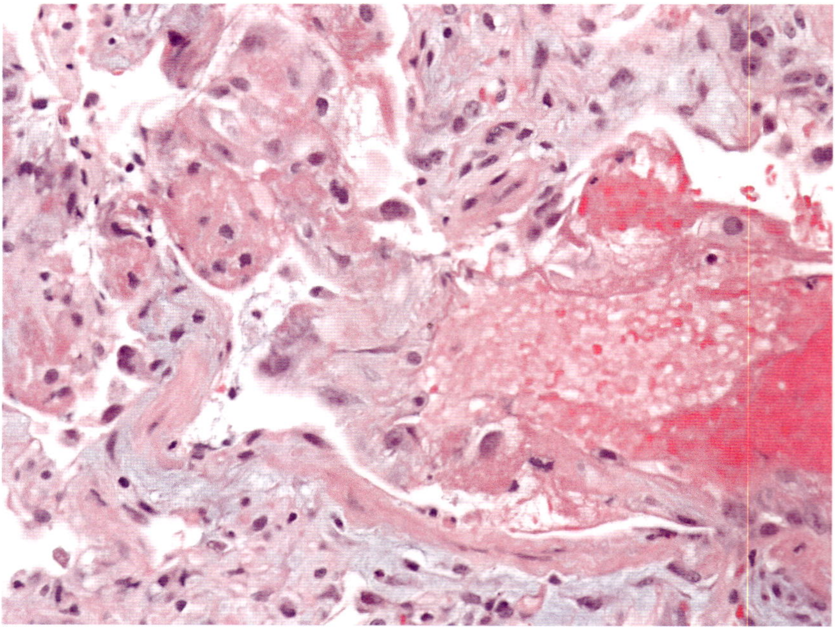

FIGURE 10.1 Reperfusion injury in heart-lung transplant showing diffuse alveolar damage with hyaline membranes and scattered inflammatory cells.

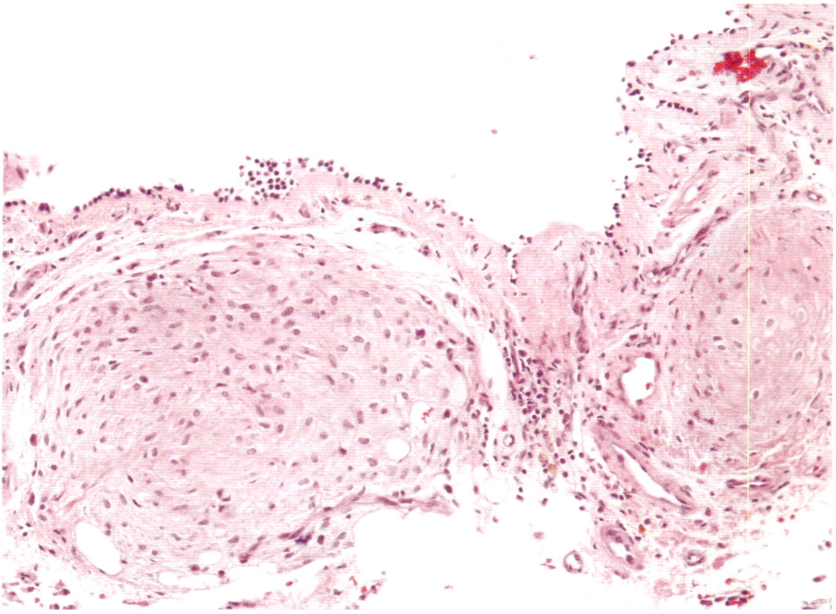

FIGURE 10.2 Healing phase of reperfusion injury showing intra-alveolar plugs of fibromyxoid tissue with fibrous thickening of alveolar septa.

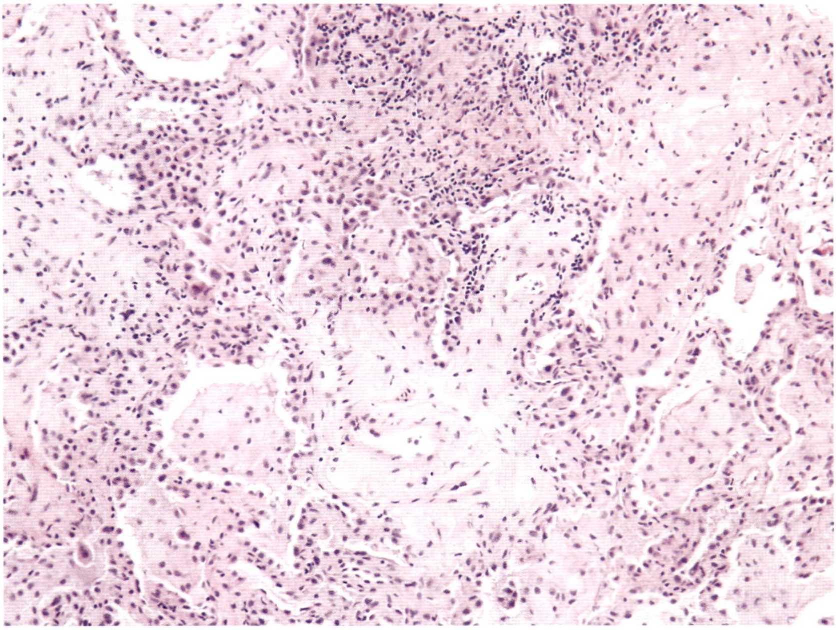

FIGURE 10.3 Acute rejection superimposed on reperfusion injury showing dense interstitial lymphoid infiltrate in alveolar septa.

posttransplant and that show DAD with lymphoid infiltrates restricted to perivascular areas with minimal interstitial component most likely correspond to combined reperfusion injury with mild rejection. When the lymphoid infiltrates are perivascular and also extend prominently into the interstitium, the process most likely corresponds to severe acute rejection. If the biopsy is done after 2 weeks posttransplant, reperfusion injury would be highly unlikely, and the process will most likely correspond to acute rejection. Fortunately, acute rejection is becoming less frequent in the immediate posttransplant period. Infection is another cause of DAD and should also be considered in such cases.

HYPERACUTE REJECTION

Hyperacute rejection represents a hyperacute response to the lung transplant and occurs within minutes to a few hours after transplantation. It is a rare, but potentially fatal complication of lung transplant caused by a humoral-mediated response by antibodies generated against the donor (donor-specific antibodies [DSAs]) that develop in the recipient. Recipients with high titers of these antiendothelial antibodies are at the highest risk for developing hyperacute rejection.[23] Hyperacute rejection has been reported to be caused by both antihuman leukocyte antigen (anti-HLA) and non–anti-HLA antibodies.[24,25] Clinical features include respiratory failure

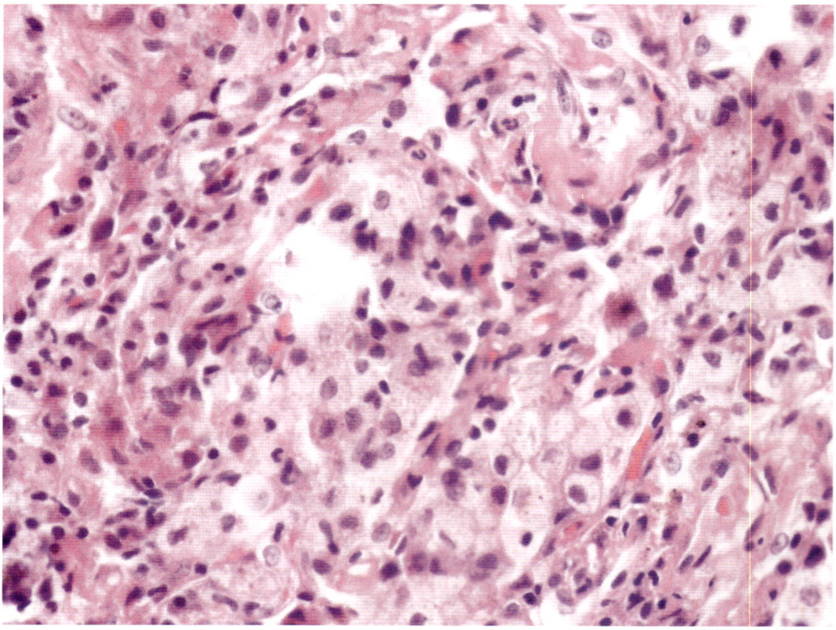

FIGURE 10.4 **Acute injury with diffuse alveolar damage and capillaritis in humoral response to hyperacute rejection.** The diagnosis is established by demonstrating IgG and complement deposition in the alveolar septa by immunofluorescence.

and pulmonary edema with complete opacification of the transplanted lung on imaging studies. The diagnosis is based on the clinical findings and a positive donor-specific IgG cross-match.[23] Histologic features of hyperacute rejection may be variable and include DAD, neutrophilic infiltration, vasculitis, and fibrin thrombi (Fig. 10.4).[23,26] Immunofluorescent studies will show deposition of IgG and complement in the alveolar septa.[23] DSAs may also be involved in chronic rejection (see "Humoral Rejection [Antibody-Mediated Rejection]" section).

ACUTE CELLULAR REJECTION

Acute cellular rejection (ACR) refers to a cell-mediated response that causes rejection of the allograft and is common in the first 3 to 6 months after lung transplantation. A revised working formulation for the classification of pulmonary allograft rejection was proposed in 1996.[26] This was revised again more recently in 2007; the suggested criteria are currently regarded as the accepted standard for the grading of pulmonary allograft rejection.[7] The immune cell activation in acute rejection causes the release of chemokines with progressive infiltration of the graft by host mononuclear cells. Various risk factors including HLA discrepancies, age, transplant type, and recipient telomere length have been identified.[27-29] Patients can experience multiple episodes of acute rejection. The symptoms include cough, fever, and shortness of breath, but some patients can be asymptomatic. The most important challenge lies in distinguishing acute rejection from infection. Endobronchial forceps biopsy is the method of choice for establishing this distinction, although other methods such as cryobiopsy are emerging as mentioned above.[30] Imaging studies show nonspecific changes that simulate those of interstitial pulmonary edema. There can be pleural effusion, and up to 50% of patients may show normal radiographic findings. Minimal rejection generally does not require treatment unless the patient is symptomatic (this also may vary by center and practice group), but mild-to-severe rejection is treated by increasing the immunosuppression.

Histologically, acute rejection is graded on the basis of the intensity and composition of the mononuclear cell infiltrates. It is generally divided into acute rejection (A grade) and small airway rejection (B grade)[7,8] (Table 10.2). Acute rejection usually affects multiple vessels, although because of sampling error, it may only be identified within a single vessel in a biopsy–sometimes only on a single level of the tissue block. Per the revised criteria–in cases where multiple foci of rejection are present–the highest-grade focus should be used for grading.[7]

Grade A0—No Acute Rejection

Grade A0 acute rejection indicates the presence of completely normal pulmonary parenchyma with none of the features of ACR, such as inflammation or hemorrhage.

Grade A1—Minimal Acute Rejection

The earliest manifestation of acute rejection is perivascular mononuclear cell infiltrates. The infiltrate comprises predominantly small lymphocytes; occasionally, immunoblasts or plasma cells may be present. In minimal acute rejection (A1), the perivascular mononuclear cell infiltrate is usually less than three cells thick (Figs. 10.5-10.7). The cuffing of vessels is generally circumferential, although it may have a loose appearance. Generally, only small vessels will be involved in grade A1 rejection.[7] Discriminating between grade A1 and grade A2 rejection on low-power magnification may be difficult; though A2 rejection can usually be identified from low-power magnification, in some cases, grade A1 rejection may also be identified on low power, particularly in well-preserved biopsy specimens. In any case, careful examination of vessels is indicated for evidence of focal areas of rejection as a single involved vessel is sufficient to establish the diagnosis (eFigs. 10.1 and 10.2).

Grade A2—Mild Acute Rejection

Mild acute rejection (A2) is characterized by increased density of the perivascular mononuclear cell infiltrate that can be up to seven or eight cells thick (Fig. 10.8; eFig. 10.3). The infiltrates are prominent enough

TABLE 10.2 Grading of Acute Cellular Rejection and Airway Inflammation

Grade	Histologic Features	Cell Composition
A0–none	Normal lung parenchyma	–
A1–minimal acute rejection	Perivascular mononuclear cell infiltrates, two to three cells thick (usually not apparent on scanning magnification)	Small lymphocytes (predominantly T cells), plasma cells, occasional larger, transformed lymphocytes
A2–mild acute rejection	Perivascular mononuclear cell infiltrates, more than three cells thick (already visible at scanning magnification)	Same as A1, with macrophages and eosinophils
A3–moderate acute rejection	Perivascular mononuclear cell infiltrates more than three cells thick with extension into alveolar septa and air spaces	Same as A2, with occasional neutrophils
A4–severe acute rejection	Diffuse mononuclear cell infiltrates similar to A3, with prominent pneumocyte damage (diffuse alveolar damage)	Same as A3
B0–no small airway inflammation	Normal airway architecture, no inflammation	–
B1R–low-grade small airway inflammation	Submucosal/subepithelial mononuclear cell infiltrate, no evidence of epithelial damage	Predominantly lymphocytes, eosinophils may be present
B2R–high-grade small airway inflammation	Submucosal/subepithelial mononuclear cell infiltrate, infiltration of epithelium by inflammatory infiltrates, possible necrosis, metaplasia, ulceration	Lymphocytes, activated lymphocytes, plasmacytoid cells, eosinophils
BX–ungradable	No small airways present for evaluation or overt evidence of infection	–

Reprinted from Stewart S, Fishbein MC, Snell GI, et al. Revision of the 1996 working formulation for the standardization of nomenclature in the diagnosis of lung rejection. *J Heart Lung Transplant.* 2007;26(12):1229-1242, with permission from Elsevier.

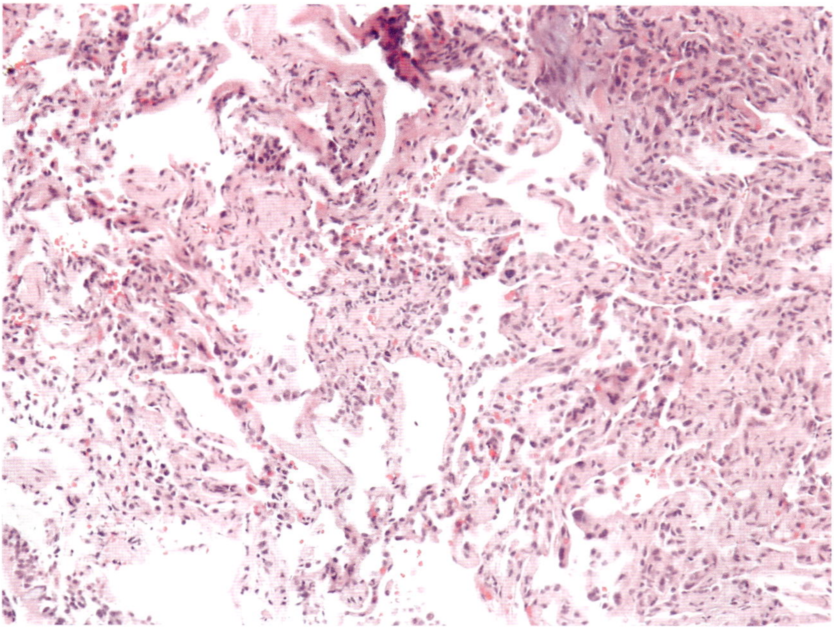

FIGURE 10.5 Scanning magnification in patient with minimal acute rejection (A1) does not reveal any significant abnormalities.

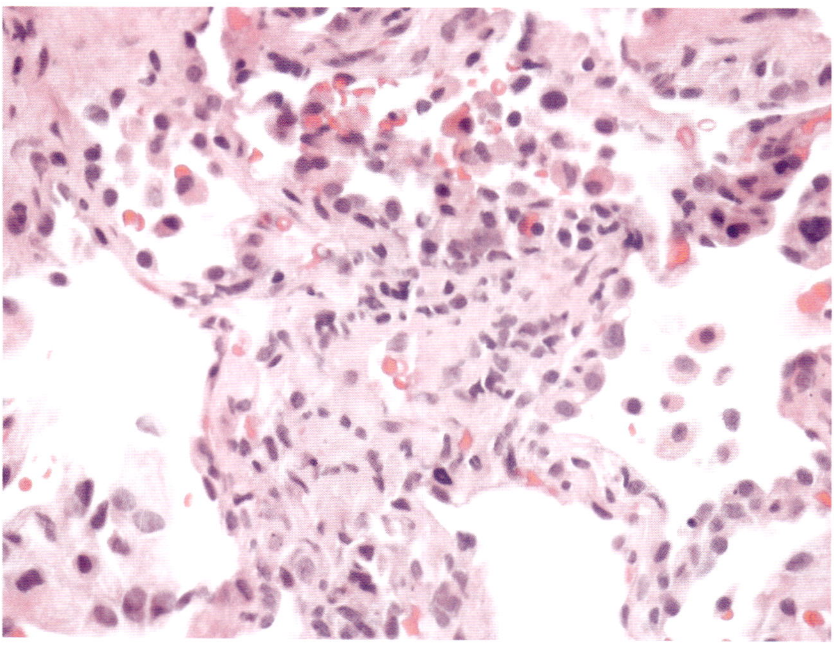

FIGURE 10.6 Higher magnification from preceding field shows a small vessel (*center*) displaying a mild perivascular lymphoid cell infiltrate less than three cells thick.

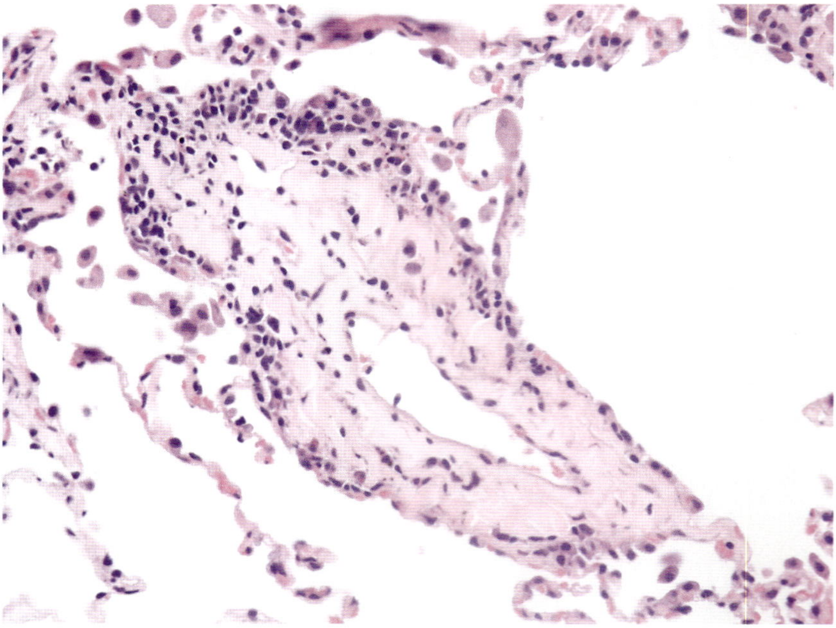

FIGURE 10.7 Another example of minimal acute rejection (A1) showing a small blood vessel surrounded by small lymphocytes that are less than three cells in thickness.

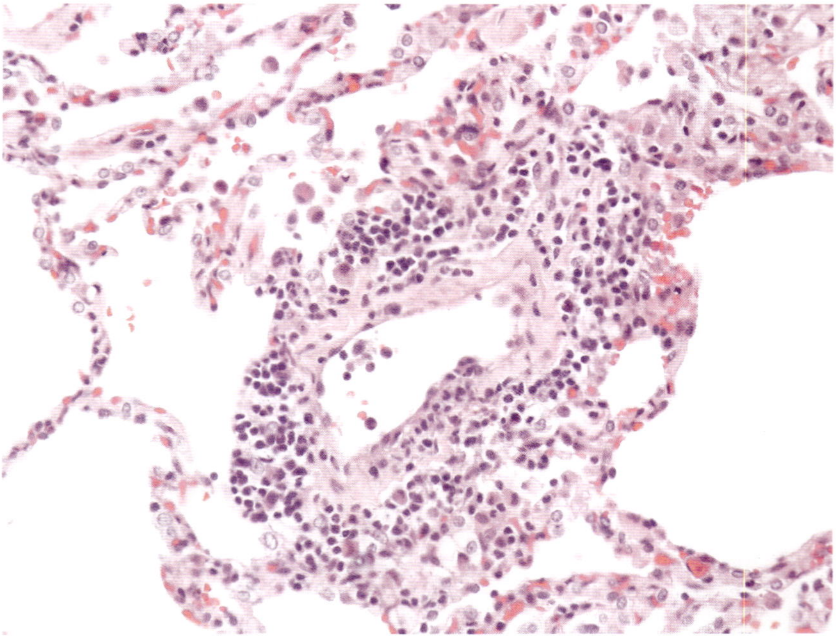

FIGURE 10.8 Mild acute rejection (A2) showing a small vessel surrounded by a lymphoid cell infiltrate that is more than three cells thick.

that they can usually be identified from low-power magnifications.[7] In addition to the predominantly lymphocytic infiltrates seen in grade A1, macrophages, eosinophils (which should generally not be seen in grade A1), endothelialitis, and lymphocytic bronchiolitis may be present. The presence of more prominent mononuclear infiltrates with the addition of the features listed above allow for the distinction between grade A1 and grade A2 rejection.

Grade A3—Moderate Acute Rejection

Moderate acute rejection (A3) shows extension of the mononuclear cell infiltrate into the alveolar septa and airspaces (Figs. 10.9 and 10.10; eFig. 10.4), in addition to the features of A2. Neutrophils may be present in limited numbers in grade A3 rejection as well. There can be variability in the extent of mononuclear cell infiltration into the alveolar septa, and there may be admixed intra-alveolar macrophages with pneumocyte hyperplasia.[7]

Grade A4—Severe Acute Rejection

In severe acute rejection (A4), the mononuclear cell infiltrate is diffuse and is associated with pneumocyte damage that essentially shows the features of DAD, with severe interstitial edema, fibrin deposition, and hyaline

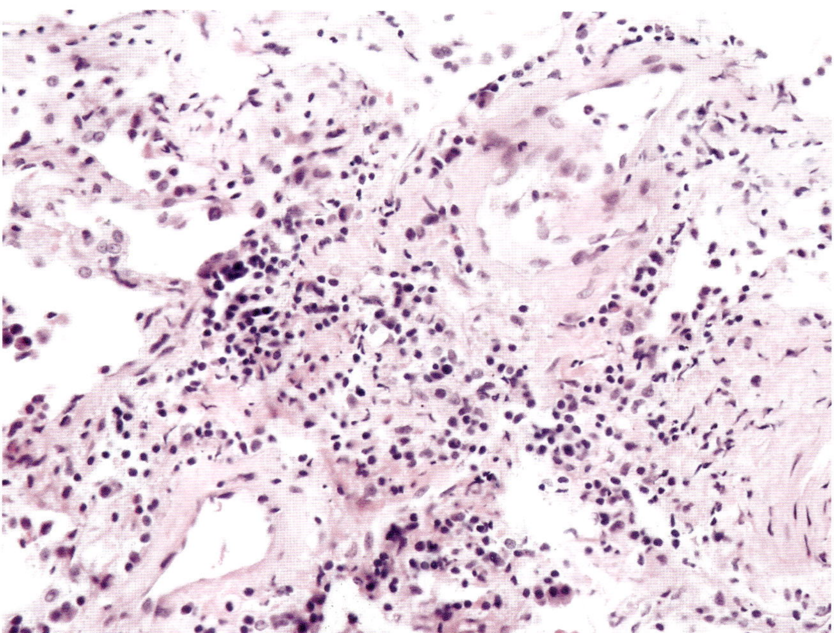

FIGURE 10.9 Moderate acute rejection (A3) shows a vessel wall surrounded by a mononuclear cell infiltrate thicker than three cells and with extension into the surrounding alveolar septa and airspaces.

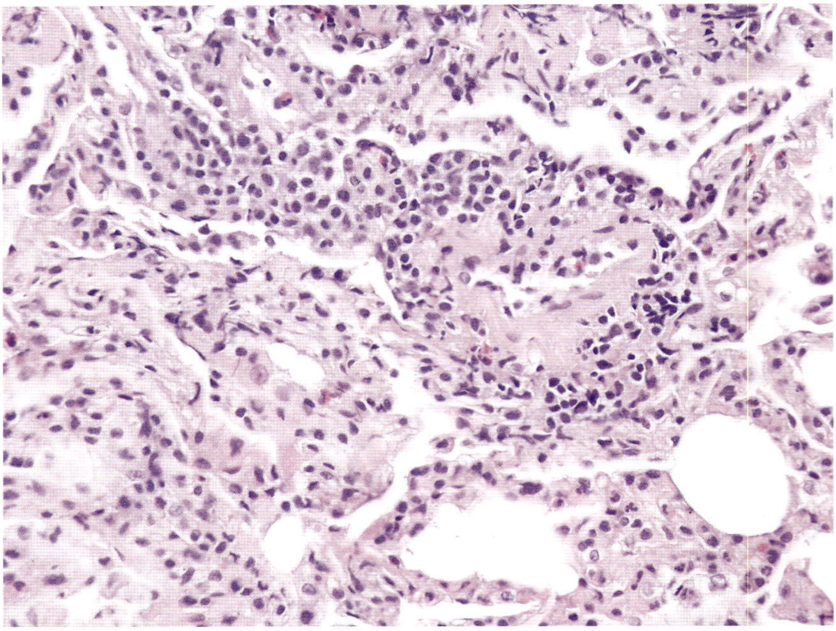

FIGURE 10.10 Another example of moderate acute rejection (A3) showing a thick cuff of lymphocytes surrounding the vessel wall and extending into adjacent alveolar septa.

membranes (Fig. 10.11). Necrosis and hemorrhage may be present as well. There is perivascular, interstitial, and airspace involvement. The cell composition of the infiltrate also varies in the different stages. In the early stages, the infiltrate primarily comprises small lymphocytes, plasma cells, and occasional larger, transformed lymphocytes (lymphoblasts) (Figs. 10.12 and 10.13; eFigs. 10.5 and 10.6). As the process advances, the infiltrate also displays macrophages, eosinophils, and neutrophils. A rare and unusual variant of acute rejection is characterized by dense eosinophilic infiltration, which can obscure the mononuclear cells in the perivascular infiltrates.[31] ACR in general may present with increased peripheral blood eosinophilia, though levels tend to be higher in moderate and severe rejection.[32]

Grade B—Small Airway Inflammation/Lymphocytic Bronchiolitis

Acute rejection can also be accompanied by lymphocytic bronchitis or bronchiolitis, with variable subepithelial lymphocytic infiltrates in the submucosa of the bronchial or bronchiolar walls, which may occasionally extend into the epithelium (Fig. 10.14).

This airway inflammation is graded based on the presence of inflammation within smaller bronchioles. The grading schema for airway inflammation is divided into grade B0 (no airway inflammation), grade B1R (lymphocytes located within the submucosa of the airway, without

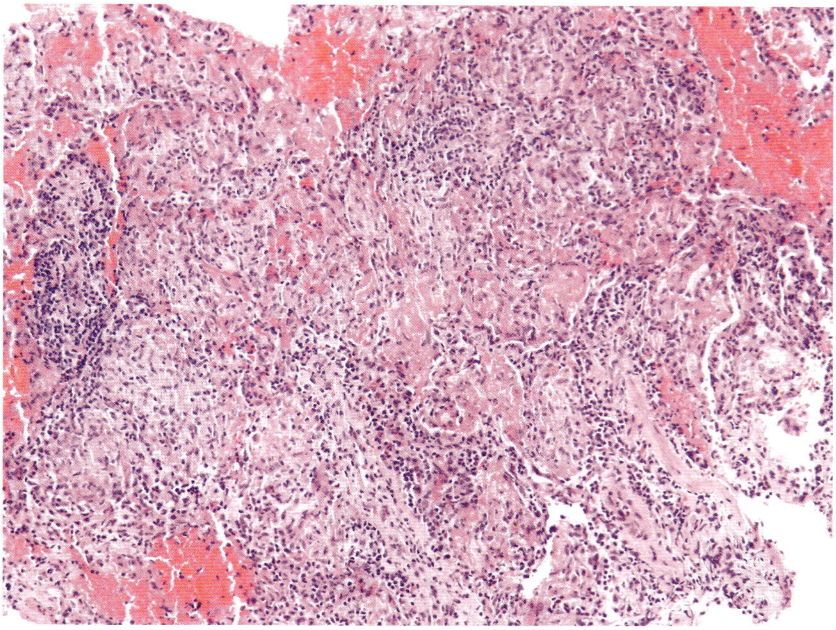

FIGURE 10.11 Severe acute rejection (A4) shows dense perivascular lymphoid infiltrates (*left*) associated with diffuse alveolar damage in surrounding parenchyma.

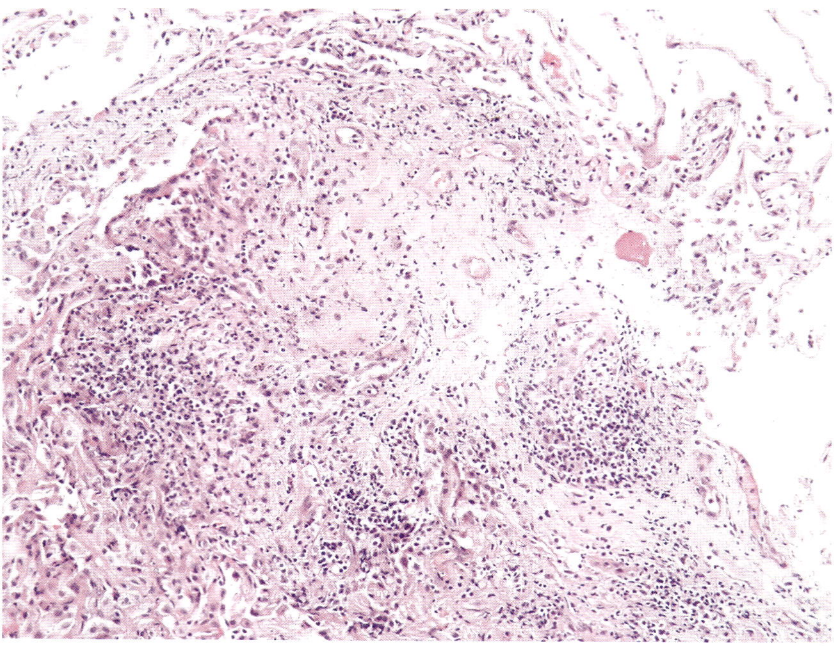

FIGURE 10.12 Another example of severe acute rejection (A4) showing dense perivascular mononuclear cell infiltrates with interstitial edema and fibrin deposition.

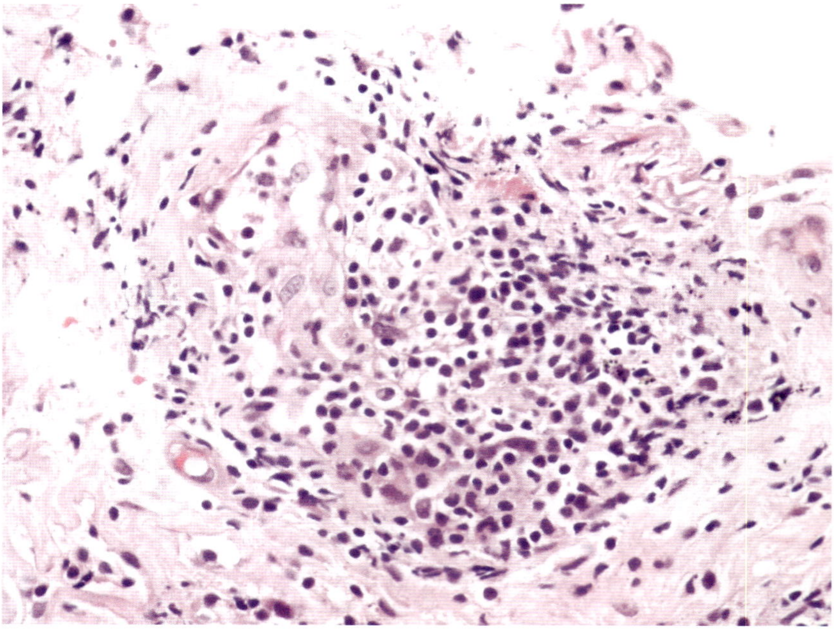

FIGURE 10.13 Higher magnification from preceding field shows a small vessel with a dense perivascular cuff of lymphocytes admixed with plasma cells and histiocytes.

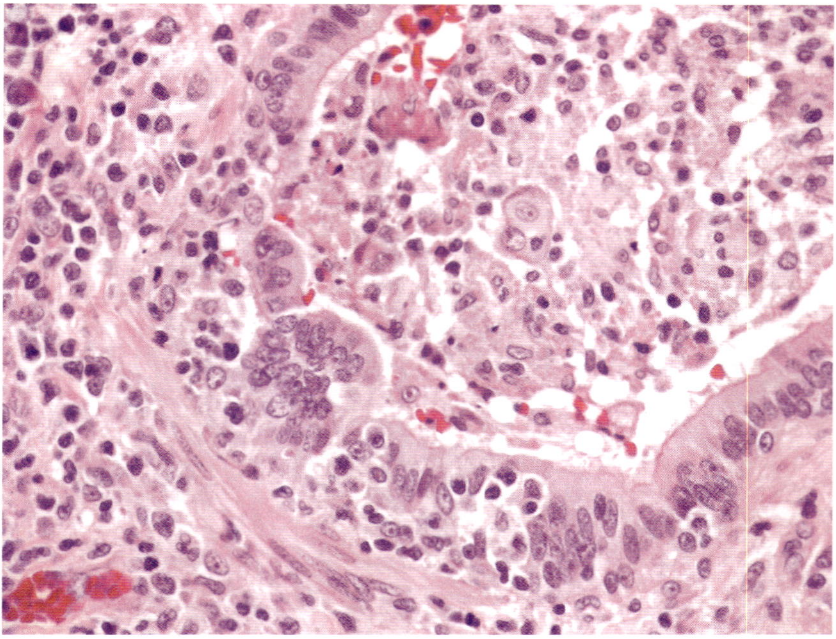

FIGURE 10.14 Small airway inflammation (grade B2R) showing lymphocytic bronchiolitis causing destruction of the bronchiolar wall with infiltration of the overlying mucosa by small mononuclear cells.

involvement of the epithelium), grade B2R (lymphocytes located within the submucosa, with involvement of the overlying epithelium), and grade BX (no small airways present or the presence of obvious evidence of infection as a source of the inflammation is identified).[7,8]

ADDITIONAL CONSIDERATIONS REGARDING THE DIAGNOSIS OF ACUTE CELLULAR REJECTION

Many other processes can produce histology that overlaps with ACR, including drug toxicity, infections, antibody-mediated rejection (AMR), post-transplant lymphoproliferative disorders (PTLDs), the presence of bronchus-associated lymphoid tissue, and ischemia–reperfusion injury.[8] Acute rejection is diagnosed only after infection is excluded.[7,8,33] Perivascular lymphoid infiltrates are not specific for rejection and can also be seen in infection with *Pneumocystis*, cytomegalovirus (CMV), *Candida*, and *Aspergillus* among others.[34] In some cases of *Pneumocystis* pneumonia, the characteristic intra-alveolar infiltrates may be diminished or only partially sampled and may resemble intra-alveolar fibrin seen in acute fibrinous and organizing pneumonia (AFOP). Infection and rejection may both generate areas that resemble AFOP on biopsy material (Figs. 10.15 and 10.16).[35] Stains for microorganisms, including viruses, need to be routinely performed on lung transplant biopsies in addition to correlation with culture results from lavage or peripheral blood specimens. Another commonly encountered confounder

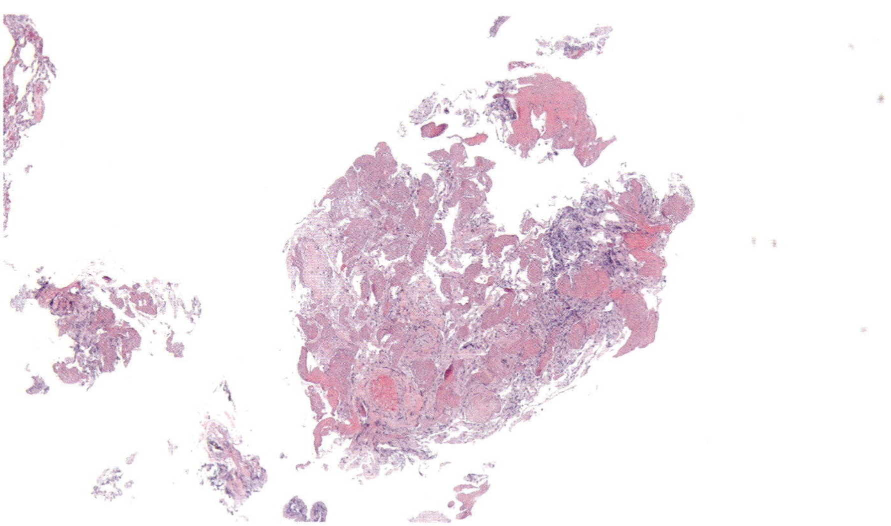

FIGURE 10.15 **Cryobiopsy, on low-power magnification, from an acutely ill transplant patient with suspected acute rejection shows numerous intra-alveolar aggregates of eosinophilic material consistent with acute fibrinous and organizing pneumonia.** The primary differential from low power would be with *Pneumocystis* pneumonia and require silver stains and culture to exclude infectious etiology.

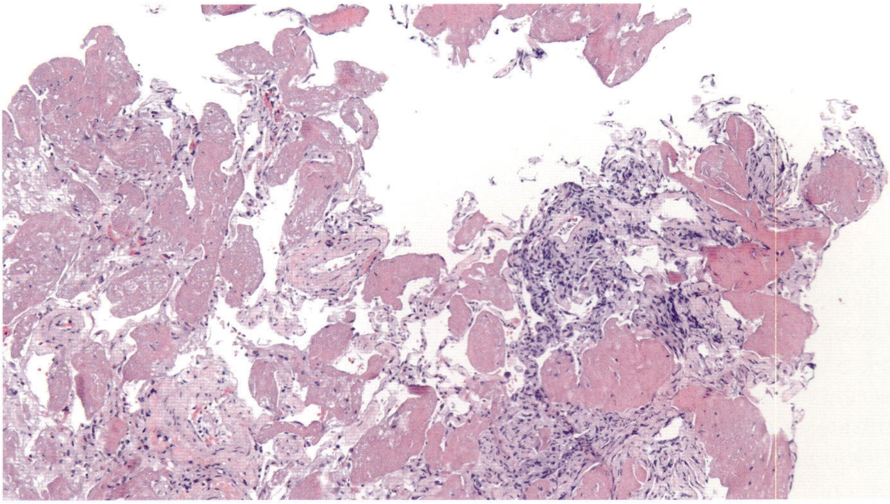

FIGURE 10.16 **Higher magnification demonstrates the intra-alveolar fibrin deposition.** Note that on the *right* side of the image, there was a small arteriole identified with a circumferential mononuclear cell infiltrate suggestive of at least A2 acute rejection.

is the presence of aspiration. Patients with severe lung disease as well as patients who have undergone lung transplantation often have compromised airway defense mechanisms, dysphagia, and gastroesophageal reflux leading to recurrent bouts of aspiration.[36-38] Approximately 50% of patients may show no evidence of aspiration during bedside examination (so-called "silent aspiration").[39] Pathologists examining transplant biopsy material should be aware of this and understand that aspiration can lead to inflammatory changes that mimic ACR. The presence of multinucleated giant cells, foamy histiocytes, or foreign material should be noted in the pathology report if they are identified and correlated with the patient's clinical status. Finally, it has been demonstrated that significant interobserver variability exists with regard to the grading of ACR.[40] Despite this, attempting to follow a standardized criterion for the diagnosis of ACR helps in defining the disease and allowing comparison for diagnosis and treatment across different medical centers. It is also important to remember that the evaluation of transplant lung pathology is a complex task and requires evaluation of many factors beyond simply the histology present on biopsies. Careful attention to the patient's medical history, clinical status, laboratory testing results, and correlation with the clinical transplant teams should be taken into consideration when evaluating transplant lung pathology.

CHRONIC LUNG ALLOGRAFT DYSFUNCTION

Chronic lung allograft dysfunction (CLAD) is a clinical term used to describe a group of pathologies that lead to decreased lung function and graft failure.[41,42] It is most commonly caused by chronic rejection, which generally develops between 3 and 12 months posttransplant. The frequency and severity of episodes of acute rejection have been regarded as the most important risk factors for the subsequent development of chronic rejection.[43,44] Chronic rejection occurs in 30% to 50% of lung transplant patients and has been associated with a 25% mortality rate. It is the leading cause of death in patients who survive beyond 1 year posttransplant.[45,46] Clinically, chronic rejection is characterized by an insidious onset with cough and general symptoms of malaise, followed by progressive shortness of breath.[46,47] Chest imaging studies will show changes once the process is well advanced, characterized by distal airway obstruction with proximal bronchiectasis and overinflation. The airway obstruction in chronic rejection is usually progressive and unresponsive to treatment; however, the course can be highly variable.[48] Increasing the immunosuppression has been shown to improve outcomes in some patients. Currently, most efforts are in increasing the tolerance between donor and recipient and in applying preventive measures to avoid infections and airway ischemic injuries.

CHRONIC REJECTION (OBLITERATIVE BRONCHIOLITIS)

The terms *obliterative bronchiolitis (OB)* or *bronchiolitis obliterans* have most commonly been used in the transplantation literature to refer to the histologic changes in chronic rejection. Similar pathology may exist in nontransplant patients as well.[49,50] The diagnosis is established by demonstrating the characteristic changes on transbronchial biopsy. Sampling can often be a significant issue in the evaluation of chronic rejection; in one study, the sensitivity of transbronchial biopsy for this process was only 28%.[49] Adequate sampling, including the presence of bronchioles, is therefore necessary for proper evaluation. Currently, the reporting of chronic airway rejection is divided into two categories–C0 (absent airway rejection/OB) and C1 (airway rejection/OB present) (Table 10.3).[7] The histologic features of OB in chronic rejection include progressive deposition of fibrous tissue around the bronchioles with narrowing of the bronchiolar lumen as a result of fibrosis (Fig. 10.17; eFig. 10.7). The term *active OB* has been proposed to refer

TABLE 10.3 Classification of Chronic Airway Rejection/Obliterative Bronchiolitis

Category	Histologic Features
C0–absent	Normal airways
C1–present	Concentric or asymmetric deposition of hyaline fibrosis around bronchioles with narrowing or partial narrowing of the bronchiolar lumen, admixed inflammatory cells may be present in active obliterative bronchiolitis

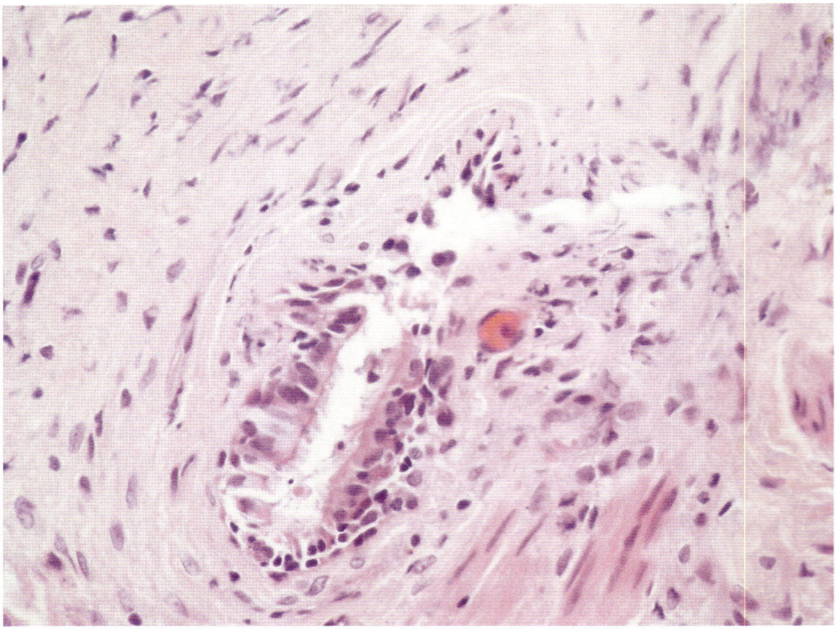

FIGURE 10.17 **Bronchiolitis obliterans in chronic rejection is characterized by progressive deposition of fibrous tissue around the bronchiole with narrowing of the lumen.**

to the presence of inflammatory cells admixed with the fibrosing process (Fig. 10.18) and the term *inactive OB* for those cases devoid of inflammation.[7,26] The submucosal fibrosis can be symmetrical and lead to concentric narrowing of the lumen, or can be asymmetric, causing bulging of the lumen with only partial obstruction. Elastic stains can be of aid in identifying late stages of peribronchiolar fibrosis by highlighting residual elastic fibers of bronchioles in areas showing extensive scarring.[51] Secondary changes can sometimes supervene, including mucostasis and endogenous lipid pneumonia. OB may be patchy in distribution and in severity. For this reason, the finding of a normal bronchiole does not entirely exclude the diagnosis.

A histologic mimic for OB is cryptogenic organizing pneumonia, which is characterized by concentric fibrous and fibrinous plugs within the airways comprising fibroblasts embedded in loose myxoid matrix. A trichrome stain can be helpful in distinguishing organizing pneumonia from OB, which is characterized by dense scar tissue surrounding the small airways rather than within the airspaces. Cryptogenic organizing pneumonia can occur in the setting of lung transplantation in patients with superimposed infection, following aspiration, or as a feature of acute rejection, but it is not generally associated with chronic rejection.[52,53] It is worthwhile noting that while the identification and reporting of any findings consistent with OB or fibrosis are important, that bronchial biopsy in general is a poor method for detecting chronic rejection. Studies

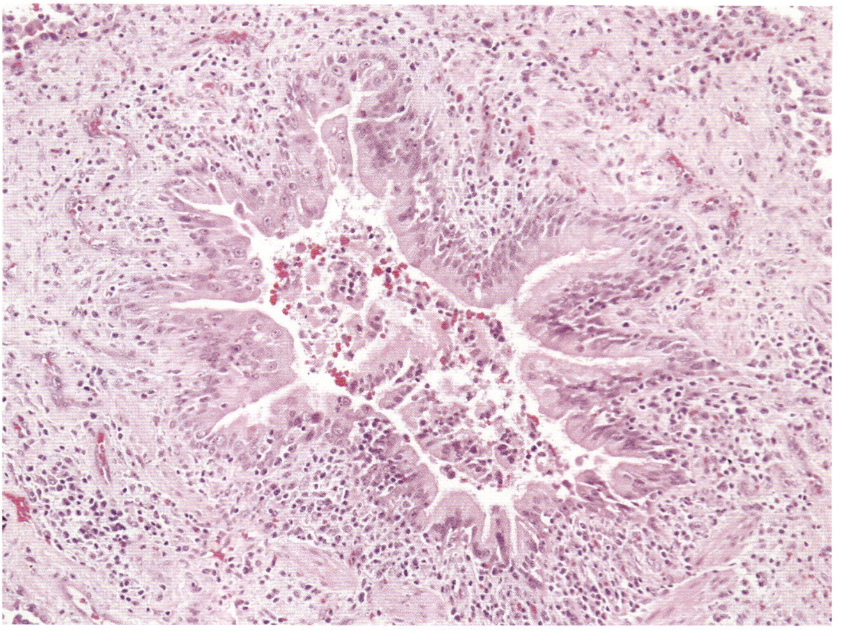

FIGURE 10.18 "Active" bronchiolitis obliterans in chronic rejection is characterized by a dense inflammatory infiltrate around the wall of the bronchiole.

have shown that long-standing chronic rejection can have a heterogeneous histologic picture, including OB, ACR-like changes, nonspecific interstitial pneumonia-like fibrosis, intra-alveolar fibroelastosis, and AFOP.[46,54-56] The use of the existing functional grading/classification systems for the diagnosis of the clinical correlates to chronic rejection (CLAD/bronchiolitis obliterans syndrome/restrictive allograft syndrome/neutrophilic reversible allograft dysfunction) is currently preferred for guiding the management of chronic airway rejection; however, biopsies may be helpful if positive findings are identified and should still be performed if there is a clinical suspicion to aid in the diagnosis.[7,41,42,46,55,56] Some authors have also advocated the use of mucosal or endobronchial biopsies in the evaluation of chronic allograft dysfunction, while others have noted that the identification of increased inflammatory infiltrates in large airways, particularly eosinophils, can help detect chronic allograft dysfunction earlier.[57,58]

Chronic vascular rejection with accelerated graft vascular sclerosis is another, but less frequent, manifestation of chronic rejection that can be reported accompanying chronic airway obstruction. The histologic features include fibrointimal and medial thickening of arteries and veins that may be accompanied by active lymphocytic inflammation (Fig. 10.19; eFig. 10.8).[59] The significance of this finding is uncertain, but it is believed that it does not contribute significantly to allograft dysfunction. Chronic vascular rejection is currently considered to not be applicable to transbronchial biopsies; however, it may be identified on open biopsy material.[7]

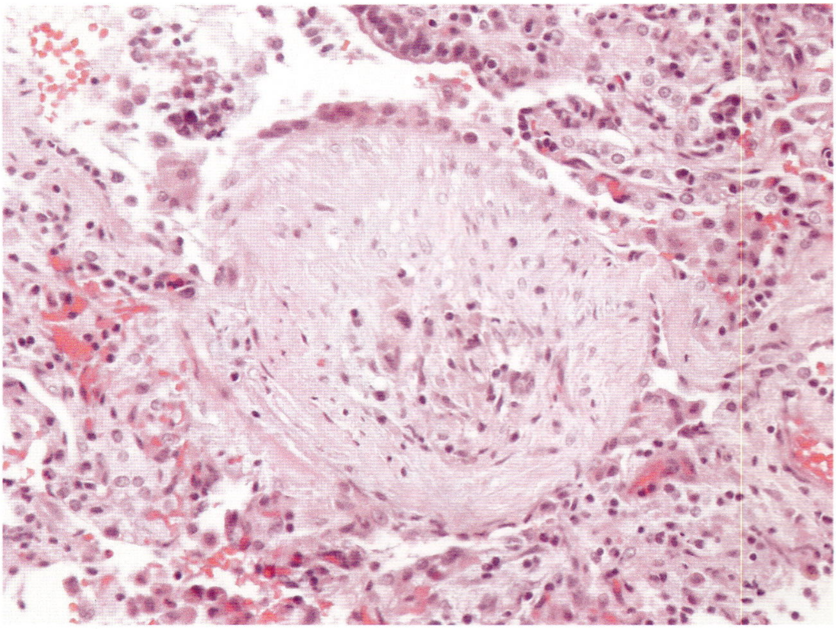

FIGURE 10.19 Sclerosing arteriopathy in chronic lung rejection shows thickening of the intima and the media of a small artery with mild chronic inflammation.

HUMORAL REJECTION (ANTIBODY-MEDIATED REJECTION)

In kidney and heart transplantation, the diagnostic criteria and features of AMR have been relatively well described; however, the exact role of AMR in lung transplantation is a topic that is still evolving. The pathophysiology is believed to be driven primarily by circulating preformed or newly formed anti-HLA antibodies by the recipient against the donor organ (referred to as donor specific antibodies [DSAs]), which are thought to interfere with the lung allograft through various mechanisms.[60-62] These DSAs can be involved in acute and chronic damage to lung allografts, and studies suggest that the presence of DSAs confer an increased risk for ACR, AMR, CLAD, and lymphocytic bronchiolitis.[63] The syndrome of AMR is associated with allograft dysfunction and generally poor outcomes with no standardized treatment regimens.[64-66] The clinical aspects have recently been better defined with a classification system meant to allow for standardization across medical centers; however, specific histopathologic findings have yet to be identified.[67-69] Identifying and monitoring for DSAs has allowed for better recognition of AMR over the past decade.[70-74] In addition, it has been recognized that in some cases, patients may develop non-HLA antibodies that can interfere with graft function.[75] As mentioned before, treatment regimens are not entirely standardized although they generally tend to revolve around detection of DSAs and immunosuppression including immunoglobulin therapy or complement inhibition.[76-82]

Histologic features that have been described in association with AMR include neutrophilic capillaritis/septal margination, high-grade acute rejection, acute lung injury, AFOP, lymphocytic bronchiolitis, arteritis, and OB.[8,83] Currently, the diagnosis of AMR is based on a combination of clinical features, serologic and pathologic features. C4d positivity by immunohistochemistry is one of the criteria that may be used for the diagnosis of AMR; however, there is debate as to whether it is reliable and reproducible. Although it has been well documented in renal and cardiac transplantation, its use is less clearly defined in lung transplantation.[84-86] It was originally suggested that C4d staining of small vessels in transplant biopsies may be used as a marker of chronic allograft dysfunction[87]; however, numerous subsequent studies have shown that (1) C4d positivity by immunohistochemistry is an extremely rare finding in conventional transplant populations (ie, when studies are not enriched for AMR patients), (2) AMR can occur without C4d positivity, and (3) interobserver variability in the assessment of C4d immunohistochemistry is high.[88-90] A general guideline has been established that greater than 50% C4d staining should be considered a positive result and, in the appropriate context, may be indicative of AMR. However, we believe that additional experience and stronger evidence with regard to the role of C4d is required to establish proper guidelines; for now, we recommend only ordering C4d staining if the clinical context is appropriate or if there is a histologic finding compatible with AMR (such as capillaritis) that cannot be explained by another process. A set of recent studies has also raised the possibility of using phosphorylated S6 ribosomal protein as evaluation in transplant biopsies as a surrogate for the detection of AMR.[91,92] Although the diagnosis of AMR is currently primarily a clinical and serologic diagnosis, biopsies may be helpful in the appropriate clinical context when they show the features discussed here. In the future, molecular genetic evaluation as part of the pretransplant workup may also help guide transplantation by identifying so called molecular rejection states in patients prior to transplantation.[93,94]

TRANSPLANT-RELATED INFECTION

Transplant-related infection represents a common complication of lung and heart-lung transplantations because of the immunosuppressed state of the individual.[95,96] Viral infections, in particular, are a common cause of morbidity and allograft dysfunction.[97] Patients may present with cough, fever, purulent sputum, dyspnea, and hypoxemia with peripheral leukocytosis. Bacterial infections have a tendency to be more common in the first month posttransplant, whereas viral and fungal infections tend to occur from 3 to 6 months following transplant. Distinguishing acute rejection from infection is of critical importance for patient management and can sometimes be problematic in transbronchial biopsies. Routine use of special stains for organisms and immunohistochemistry for viral etiology is therefore recommended in all transplant patients showing any findings suggestive of infection.

Bacterial infections commonly occur in the early posttransplant period. The most common types of bacteria involved in transplant-related infection are gram-negative organisms, particularly *Pseudomonas* species.[98] Bacterial infections in lung transplant patients are characterized by neutrophilic infiltrates within alveolar spaces and involvement of the bronchial mucosa, often with mucosal ulceration. Tissue Gram stains can be of aid in identifying bacteria. Cultures should be routinely done in such patients to identify microbiologic agents. The histologic findings are distinguished from acute rejection by the presence of neutrophils, instead of the perivascular mononuclear cells observed in acute rejection and by laboratory and clinical findings consistent with infection.

Viral infection by CMV is the most common type observed in lung and heart-lung transplant patients, followed by herpes simplex virus.[99-104] Other viruses implicated in posttransplant infections include influenza virus, respiratory syncytial virus, coronavirus, human metapneumovirus, and parainfluenza virus.[98] Most cases of CMV infection are characterized by a diffuse lymphoid interstitial pneumonia containing a mixed lymphocytic and polymorphonuclear infiltrate or they may show acute necrotizing pneumonia with DAD (Fig. 10.20; eFig. 10.9). The mononuclear cells will diffusely infiltrate the alveolar septa without perivascular accentuation. Careful search for the characteristic cytopathic effect with prominent nuclear and cytoplasmic

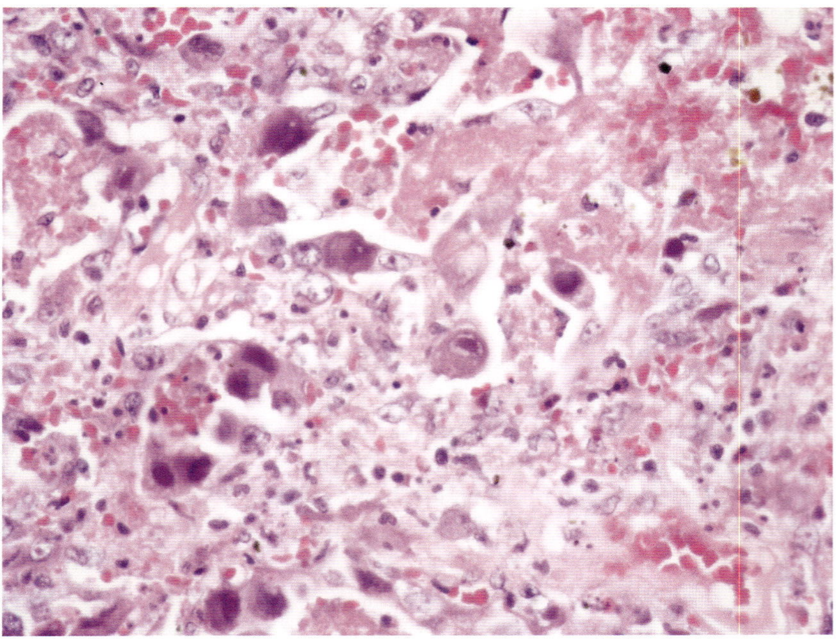

FIGURE 10.20 Cytomegalovirus infection in a lung transplant patient shows numerous infected cells with cytomegalic inclusions against a background of necrotizing pneumonia with diffuse alveolar damage.

eosinophilic inclusions is required for diagnosis. Use of immunohistochemical stains with anti-CMV antibodies can be helpful, particularly in treated cases in which the inclusions can become smudged and may be difficult to identify on routine microscopy. Areas of zonal necrosis may be observed with both CMV and herpes simplex virus. The differential diagnosis with acute rejection is based on the identification of the characteristic cytopathic effects or the use of immunohistochemical stains.[43] Immunohistochemistry, in situ hybridization, and molecular techniques can be used effectively for identifying many viruses and can be used for definitive diagnosis. A subtle histologic difference between viral infection and low to intermediate grade acute rejection is the fact that the mononuclear cell infiltrate in viral infection is predominantly interstitial, whereas in acute rejection, it is primarily perivascular.

Fungal infection in lung and heart-lung transplant patients is less frequent than viral and bacterial infection but is associated with a higher mortality when present. The most common organisms encountered in this setting are *Aspergillus* and *Candida*.[105-107] Other types of fungi have also been described, although less frequently. The organisms can be cultured from bronchoalveolar lavage samples, blood, or other body fluids. Transbronchial biopsy may be the fastest way to obtain a diagnosis. The organisms are easily identified by morphology on routine microscopy, although special stains such as periodic acid-Schiff and Gomori methenamine silver may be of help in highlighting them in small biopsy samples.

Pneumocystis pneumonia is another fungal infection of lung and heart-lung transplants. Without prophylaxis, *Pneumocystis* pneumonia occurs in nearly all transplant patients.[108] The histologic picture of *Pneumocystis* pneumonia is identical to that described in Chapter 6. As mentioned above, the frothy intra-alveolar infiltrates may be diminished or incompletely sampled in transplant biopsies requiring correlation with cultures. This condition should be separated primarily from AFOP, and silver stains should be routinely applied to any biopsies with eosinophilic intra-alveolar exudates/material. Routine prophylaxis has made this a relatively rare complication of lung transplantation.

POSTTRANSPLANT LYMPHOPROLIFERATIVE DISORDERS

PTLDs can occur in about 2% to 10% of all lung and heart-lung transplant patients, particularly among pulmonary allograft recipients.[109] Most PTLDs are associated with Epstein-Barr virus (EBV) infection and represent EBV-induced B-lymphocyte proliferations that develop secondary to solid organ or stem cell transplantation.[110,111] Approximately 20% of patients with PTLD can be EBV-negative. Very rare cases of T-cell PTLD have been reported.[112] There are many risk factors for PTLD, although the most important risk factor appears to be EBV seronegativity at the time of transplantation.[113] In addition, numerous underlying genetic abnormalities have been linked to PTLD, including gene rearrangements, copy number alterations, mutations, and polymorphisms.[114] The disease usually presents clinically between 3 and

7 months posttransplant. Patients usually develop shortness of breath, or the disease can be discovered incidentally on chest X-rays. Radiographic findings include single or multiple pulmonary nodules with or without mediastinal adenopathy. Histologically, the lesions of PTLD can show a variable spectrum, ranging from lymphoid hyperplasia to full-blown lymphoma.[115,116]

The most widely accepted classification for these disorders is that proposed by the World Health Organization (WHO), which traditionally divided them into early lesions, polymorphic PTLD, monomorphic PTLD, and Hodgkin lymphoma–like PTLD.[117] The latest 5th edition of the WHO blue book introduced slightly new terminology putting posttransplant PTLD into the larger overarching category of "lymphoid proliferations and lymphomas associated with immune deficiency and dysregulation (IDD)" that is subdivided into hyperplasias arising in IDD, polymorphic lymphoproliferative disorders arising in IDD, EBV+ mucocutaneous ulcer, lymphomas arising in IDD, and inborn error of immunity–associated lymphoid proliferations and lymphomas.[118] This novel terminology introduced by the WHO aims at alleviating inconsistencies in diagnostic criteria for similar lymphoid lesions in different immunodeficiency settings.

Recently, a second competing scheme was introduced in 2022–the International Consensus Classification (ICC)–originating from the WHO group's former clinical advisory committee, and this system uses similar terminology to the existing labels for PTLD and includes nondestructive PTLD (plasmacytic hyperplasia, infectious mononucleosis, and florid follicular hyperplasia subtypes), polymorphic PTLD, monomorphic PTLD (B-cell, T-cell/NK-cell subtypes), classic Hodgkin lymphoma PTLD, and other iatrogenic immunodeficiency-associated lymphoproliferative disorders.[119,120] Regardless of the ongoing division in hematopathology and the existence of multiple classification systems, this book will focus for simplicity on the criteria and terminology established in the prior edition of the WHO and continued forward in the ICC scheme.

Early lesions of PTLD involve mainly lymph nodes and lymphoid tissue outside of the lung and rarely involve the pulmonary parenchyma. They include plasmacytic hyperplasia, infectious mononucleosislike changes, and florid follicular hyperplasia. The infiltrates comprise small polyclonal B cells admixed with plasma cells and reactive T cells. Early lesions are generally EBV-positive. These lesions show rare or no genetic abnormalities.[121,122]

Polymorphic PTLD is a tissue destructive lesion comprising an admixture of mature lymphocytes, immunoblasts, plasma cells, and large transformed lymphocytes that show evidence of monoclonality by molecular testing (Fig. 10.21). The spectrum of lesions in this category is heterogeneous and may overlap with some monomorphic-type PTLDs that display polymorphic histology (eg, a T-cell/histiocyte-rich large B-cell lymphoma, which would technically fit the diagnostic criteria for a monomorphic PTLD). The lesions are nearly universally EBV-positive.[121,122]

Monomorphic PTLDs are lesions comprising a monomorphic population of atypical lymphoid cells indistinguishable from, and which fit the

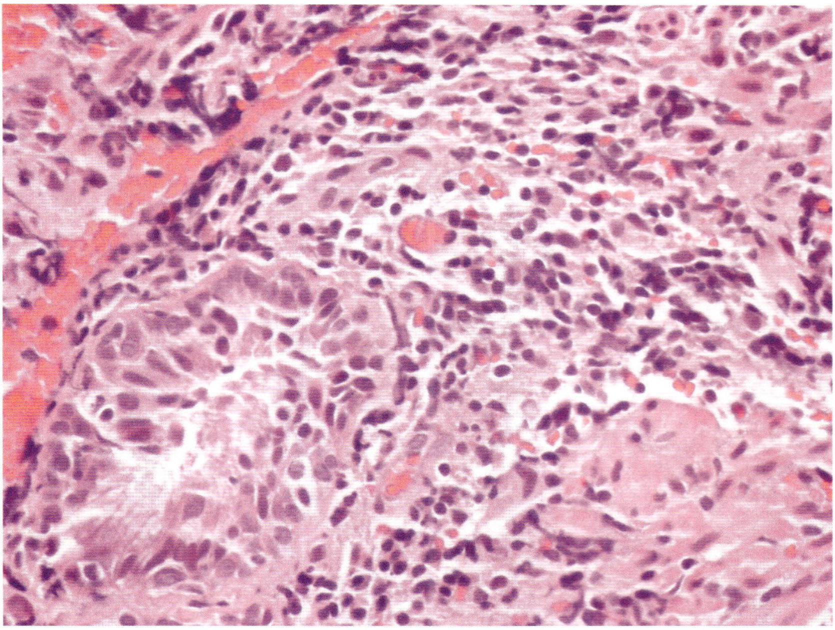

FIGURE 10.21 Polymorphic posttransplant lymphoproliferative disorder shows an admixture of small lymphocytes, immunoblasts, and plasma cells.

criteria for, conventional types of lymphoma which would be diagnosed in nontransplant patients (Figs. 10.22-10.26). They are classified using the same classification for malignant lymphoma into diffuse large B-cell lymphoma, Burkitt and Burkitt-like lymphoma, plasma cell myeloma, peripheral T-cell lymphoma, and other types of lymphoma. Most cases are monoclonal and demonstrate EBV positivity (Fig. 10.27). Monomorphic PTLD lesions commonly demonstrate cytogenetic abnormalities, including trisomy 9 and 11, and rearrangements involving *MYC*, 3q27, and 14q32. Some of these lesions may rarely demonstrate a polymorphic appearance despite fitting the diagnostic criteria for the monomorphic category.[121,123]

Hodgkin disease–type PTLD can show features of classical Hodgkin lymphoma or Hodgkin lymphoma–like PTLD with an atypical immunophenotype and B-cell antigen expression (Figs. 10.28-10.31). Virtually all cases are EBV-positive.[121,124]

EBV can be identified in the atypical lymphocytes in the majority of polymorphic and monomorphic PTLD cases. EBV can be detected using immunohistochemistry for latent membrane protein (LMP-1) or by in situ hybridization for EBV-encoded nuclear RNA-1. The latter test, however, is considered more reliable. EBV determination should be made in all lung transplant patients showing a suspicious dense polymorphic or monomorphic lymphoid infiltrate. In rare cases, early lesions may be confused with acute lung rejection; demonstration of EBV infection will help establish the diagnosis.[125] Early lesions of PTLD often regress spontaneously or with reduction of immunosuppressive

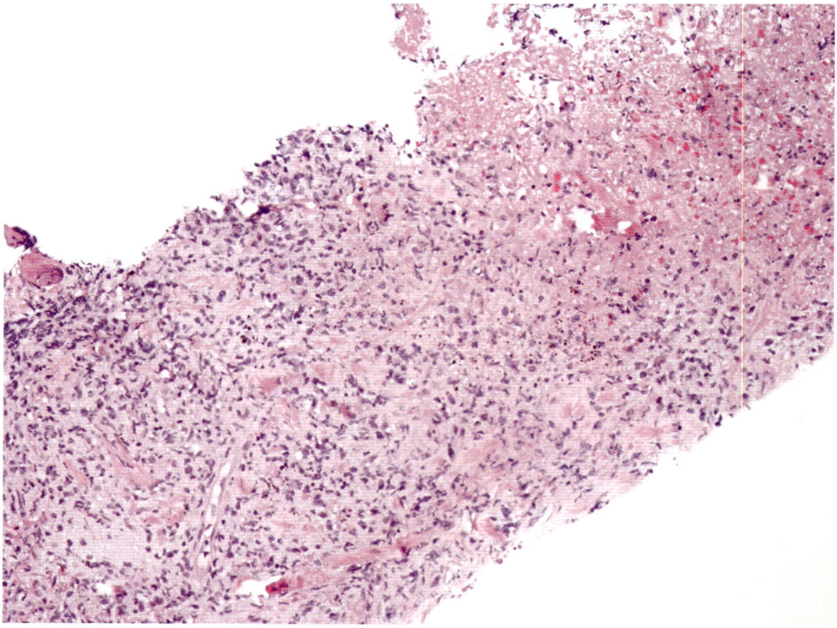

FIGURE 10.22 Biopsy in a posttransplant lymphoproliferative disorders patient demonstrates sheets of atypical cells with a prominent area of necrosis (*top right*).

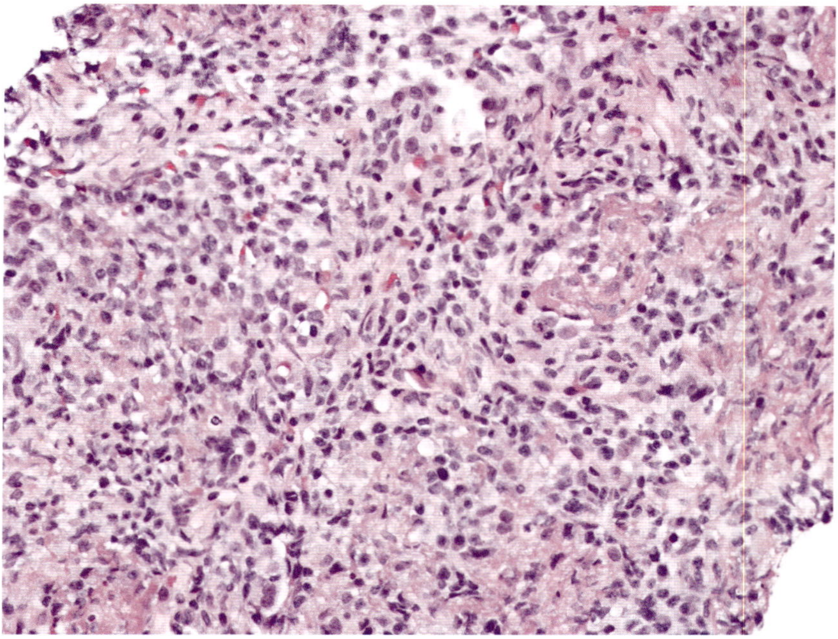

FIGURE 10.23 Higher-power magnification shows a sheetlike growth pattern with monomorphic population of numerous large atypical cells.

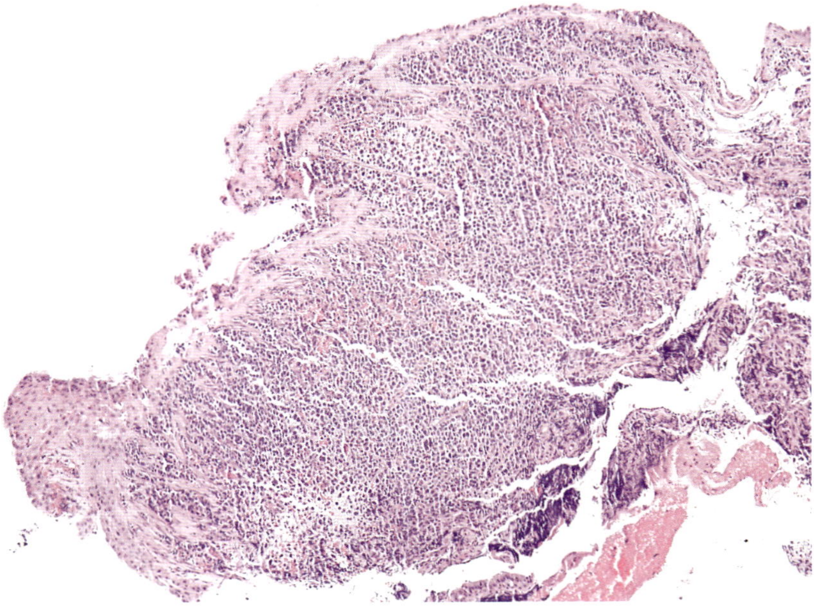

FIGURE 10.24 Transbronchial biopsy in patient with monomorphic posttransplant lymphoproliferative disorder shows a uniform, dense lymphoid cell population replacing the lung parenchyma.

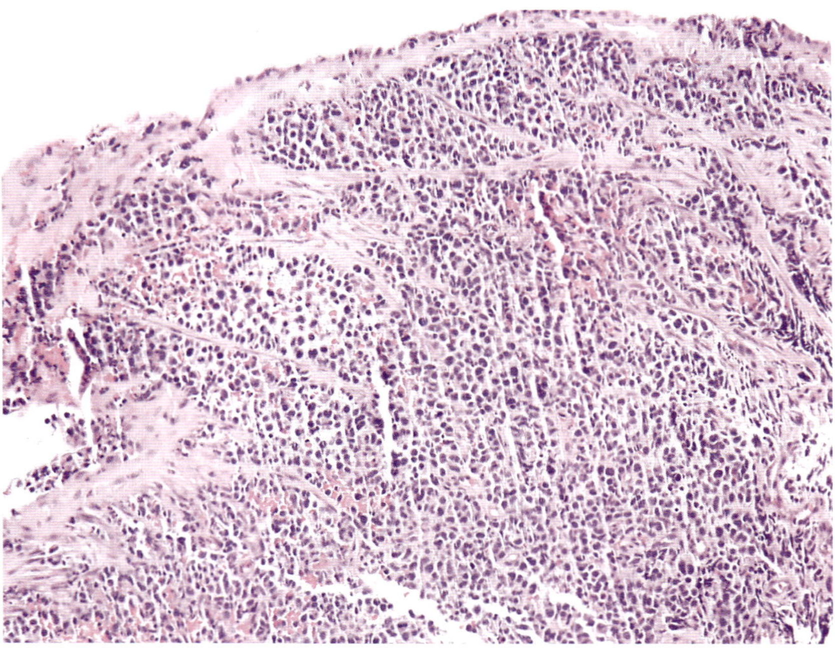

FIGURE 10.25 Higher magnification from preceding field shows large, atypical lymphocytes showing features of diffuse large cell lymphoma.

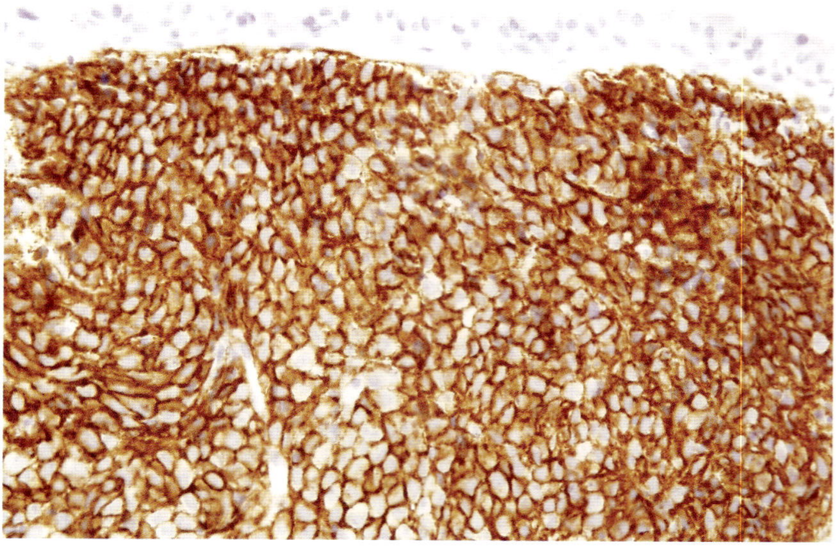

FIGURE 10.26 Immunohistochemical stain for CD20 shows strong positivity of the neoplastic lymphoid cells for this marker.

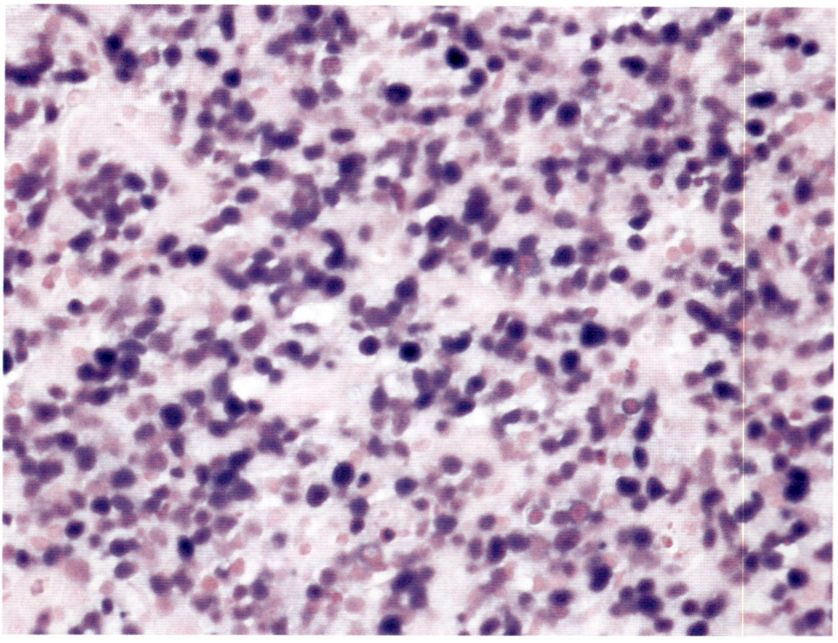

FIGURE 10.27 In situ hybridization for Epstein-Barr virus–encoded RNA-1 shows positive signal in the majority of the tumor cells.

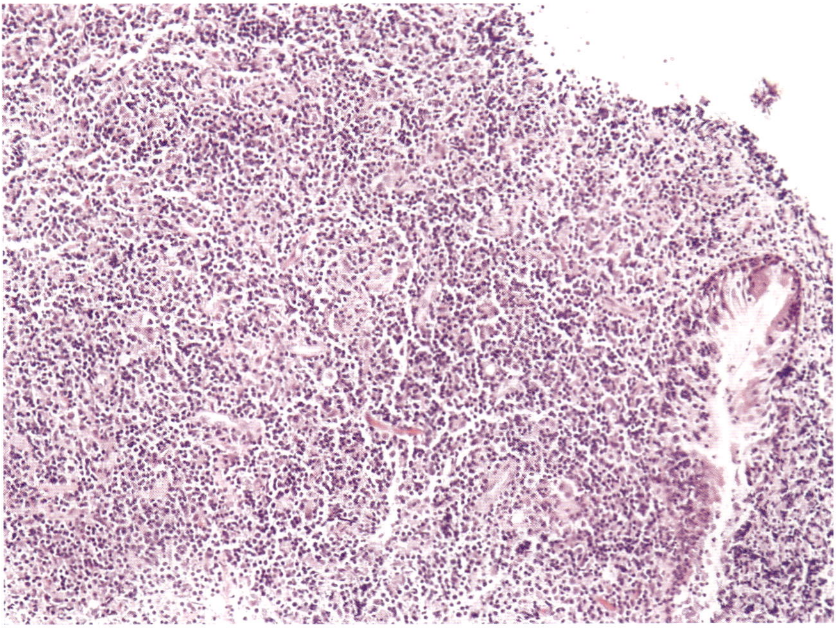

FIGURE 10.28 Transbronchial biopsy in patient with Hodgkin-type posttransplant lymphoproliferative disorder showing a mixed population of cells effacing underlying lung parenchyma.

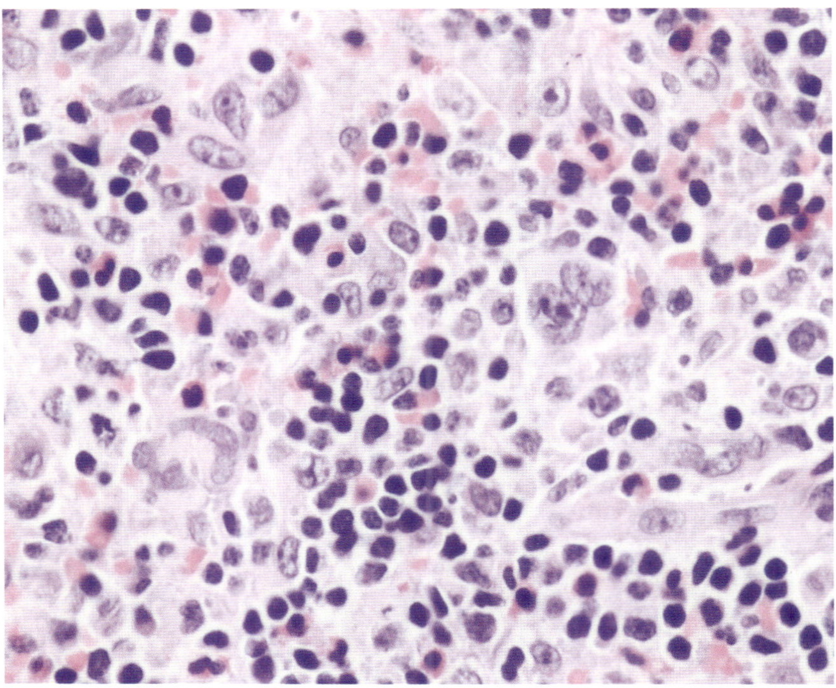

FIGURE 10.29 Higher magnification shows a mixed infiltrate comprising small lymphocytes, plasma cells, and scattered larger mono- and multinucleated cells with features of Reed-Sternberg cells.

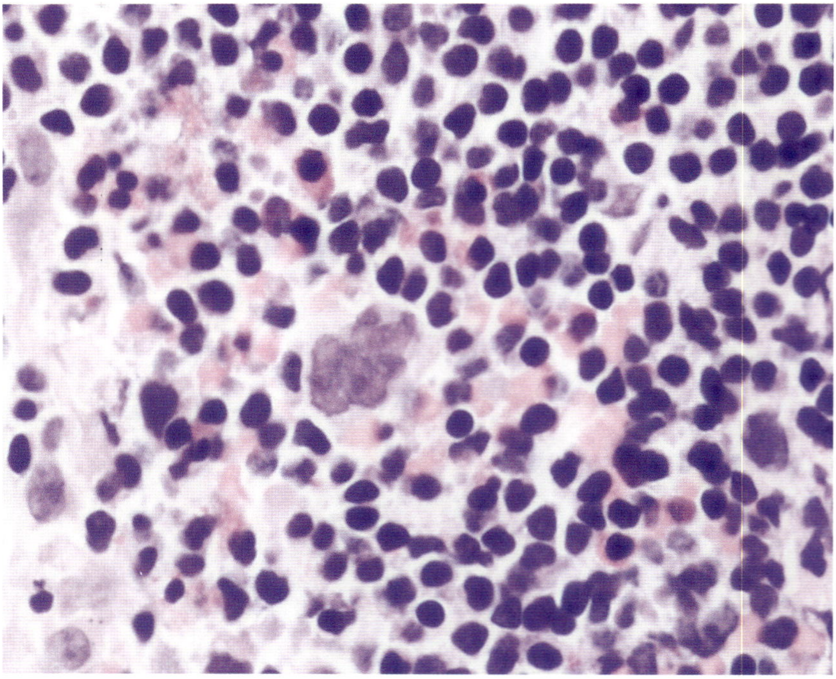

FIGURE 10.30 A multinucleated Reed-Sternberg cell is seen in the center of the field showing prominent eosinophilic nucleoli.

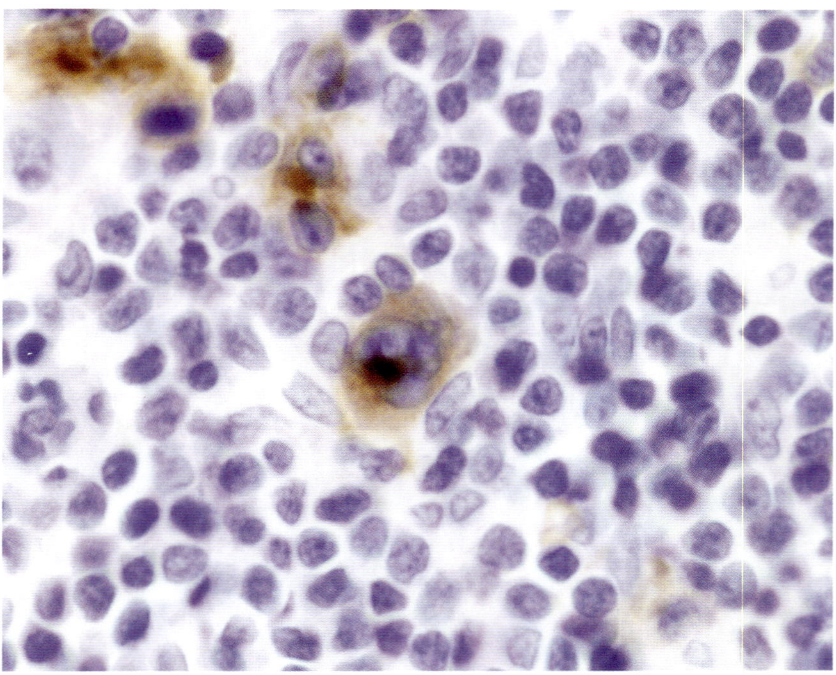

FIGURE 10.31 Immunohistochemical stain for CD30 shows characteristic cytoplasmic/membranous and dotlike paranuclear staining in a Reed-Sternberg cell.

therapy. Monomorphic lesions can progress and will require cytotoxic chemotherapy. The overall mortality of PTLD in solid organ allograft recipients has been reported to be approximately 60%.[121,126,127]

OTHER COMPLICATIONS

Other complications of lung transplant include graft versus host disease (GVHD) and recurrence of primary disease in the allograft.

Graft versus host disease is primarily a complication of hematopoietic stem cell transplants; however, it has been described secondary to solid organ transplantation as well.[128] Reported risk factors include donor HLA homozygosity, periorgan lymphoid tissue transfer, and immunosuppression.[128-130] The exact mechanisms of GVHD following solid organ transplantation are not known; however, it is thought that it is caused by the transfer of immune competent host cells contained within the graft that then attack foreign recipient antigens. The prognosis for patients who develop GVHD is generally poor with a large percentage of cases being fatal.[131] Pulmonary GVHD following lung transplantation is extremely rare with less than 20 cases reported in the literature, the diagnosis of which is complicated by the fact that many of the histologic and clinical features overlap with other forms of rejection as well as infection.[128,131] The histologic features of GVHD in lung biopsies are not well characterized; however, they can include similar features to ACR, infection, and OB depending on the stage of the process.[131-133] Common histologic findings across all patterns of GVHD in lung biopsies include intrabronchiolar lymphocytes, apoptotic cells, and perivenulitis, which have been suggested as features that can help distinguish GVHD from infection.[134] Given the rarity of the condition, morphologic overlap with other processes, and poorly defined criteria for diagnosis in lung transplant biopsies, the diagnosis of GVHD should only be entertained in the context of careful clinical correlation and after all other potential causes are excluded.

Recurrence of primary disease occurs in a small percentage of lung transplant patients. The most common disease that recurs in this setting is sarcoidosis.[135-137] Other conditions that have been reported to recur in lung transplant recipients include lymphangioleiomyomatosis, diffuse panbronchiolitis, desquamative interstitial pneumonia, giant cell pneumonitis, Langerhans cell histiocytosis, capillary hemangiomatosis, pulmonary alveolar proteinosis, hard metal lung disease, and neoplasia.[136,138,139] The diagnosis is made on transbronchial biopsy.

REFERENCES

1. Hopkins PM, Aboyoun CL, Chhajed PN, et al. Prospective analysis of 1,235 transbronchial lung biopsies in lung transplant recipients. *J Heart Lung Transplant.* 2002;21:1062-1067.
2. Yusen RD, Edwards LB, Kucheryavaya AY, et al. The Registry of the International Society for Heart and Lung Transplantation: thirty-second official adult lung and heart-lung transplantation report–2015; focus theme: early graft failure. *J Heart Lung Transplant.* 2015;34(10):1264-1277.

3. Hanks J, Girard C, Sehgal S. Acute rejection post lung transplant. *Curr Opin Pulm Med.* 2024;30(4):391-397.
4. Tejwani V, Panchabhai TS, Kotloff RM, Mehta AC. Complications of lung transplantation: a roentgenographic perspective. *Chest.* 2016;149(6):1535-1545.
5. Crespo MM, McCarthy DP, Hopkins PM, et al. ISHLT consensus statement on adult and pediatric airway complications after lung transplantation: definitions, grading system, and therapeutics. *J Heart Lung Transplant.* 2018;37(5):548-563.
6. Bierman MI, Satein KL, Stuart RS, Dauber JH. Critical care management of lung transplant recipients. *J Intensive Care Med.* 1991;6:135-142.
7. Stewart S, Fishbein MC, Snell GI, et al. Revision of the 1996 working formulation for the standardization of nomenclature in the diagnosis of lung rejection. *J Heart Lung Transplant.* 2007;26(12):1229-1242.
8. Roden AC, Aisner DL, Allen TC, et al. Diagnosis of acute cellular rejection and antibody-mediated rejection on lung transplant biopsies: a perspective from members of the Pulmonary Pathology Society. *Arch Pathol Lab Med.* 2017;141(3):437-444.
9. Yarmus L, Akulian J, Gilbert C, et al. Cryoprobe transbronchial lung biopsy in patients after lung transplantation: a pilot safety study. *Chest.* 2013;143(3):621-626.
10. Fruchter O, Fridel L, Rosengarten D, Raviv Y, Rosanov V, Kramer MR. Transbronchial cryo-biopsy in lung transplantation patients: first report. *Respirology.* 2013;18(4):669-673.
11. Luo Y, Li SP. Transbronchial cryobiopsy versus transbronchial forceps biopsy for acute cellular rejection detection in lung transplantation: a meta-analysis. *Arch Bronconeumol.* 2024;60(11):698-704.
12. Tosi D, Brivio M, Franzi S, et al. Transition from transbronchial forceps to cryobiopsy after lung transplantation: a single-centre experience. *Life (Basel).* 2024;14(11):1474.
13. Loor K, Culebras M, Sansano I, et al. Lung allograft transbronchial cryobiopsy for critical ventilated patients: a randomised trial. *Eur Respir J.* 2023;61(1):2102354.
14. Żegleń S, Karolak W, Mikołajczyk G, et al. Cryobiopsy as a new tool for complications diagnosis during follow-up after lung transplantation: single institution case series. *Transplant Proc.* 2021;53(6):2008-2012.
15. Steinack C, Gaspert A, Gautschi F, et al. Transbronchial cryobiopsy compared to forceps biopsy for diagnosis of acute cellular rejection in lung transplants: analysis of 63 consecutive procedures. *Life (Basel).* 2022;12(6):898.
16. Sadowska-Klasa A, Karolak W, Piekarska A, et al. The role of transbronchial cryobiopsy in the detection of pulmonary graft-versus-host disease. *Respiration.* 2025;104(4):264-271.
17. Goldberg JF, Truby LK, Agbor-Enoh S, et al. Selection and interpretation of molecular diagnostics in heart transplantation. *Circulation.* 2023;148(8):679-694.
18. Tazelaar HD, Yousem SA. The pathology of combined heart–lung transplantation: an autopsy study. *Hum Pathol.* 1988;19:1403-1416.
19. Laubach VE, Sharma AK. Mechanisms of lung ischemia-reperfusion injury. *Curr Opin Organ Transplant.* 2016;21(3):246-252.
20. den Hengst WA, Gielis JF, Lin JY, Schil PEV, De Windt LJ, Moens AL. Lung ischemia-reperfusion injury: a molecular and clinical view on a complex pathophysiological process. *Am J Physiol Heart Circ Physiol.* 2010;299(5):H1283-H1299.
21. Porteous MK, Diamond JM, Christie JD. Primary graft dysfunction: lessons learned about the first 72 h after lung transplantation. *Curr Opin Organ Transplant.* 2015;20(5):506-514.
22. Choi JK, Kearns J, Palevski HI, et al. Hyperacute rejection of a pulmonary allograft. Immediate clinical and pathologic findings. *Am J Respir Crit Care Med.* 1999;160:1015-1018.
23. Frost AE, Jammal CT, Cagle PT. Hyperacute rejection following lung transplantation. *Chest.* 1996;110:559-562.

24. Fernandez R, Chiu S, Raparia K, et al. Humoral human lung allograft rejection by tissue-restricted non-HLA antibodies. *Ann Thorac Surg*. 2016;102(4):e339-e341.
25. Masson E, Stern M, Chabod J, et al. Hyperacute rejection after lung transplantation caused by undetected low-titer anti-HLA antibodies. *J Heart Lung Transplant*. 2007;26(6):642-645.
26. Yousem SA, Berry GJ, Cagle PT, et al. Revision of the 1990 working formulation for the classification of pulmonary allograft rejection: Lung Rejection Study Group. The International Society for Heart Transplantation. *J Heart Lung Transplant*. 1996;15:1-15.
27. Snyder ME, Kitsios GD. Lung transplant outcomes keep bugging us: acute cellular rejection and the lung microbiome. *Am J Respir Crit Care Med*. 2024;209(12):1423-1425.
28. Renaud-Picard B, Koutsokera A, Cabanero M, Martinu T. Acute rejection in the modern lung transplant era. *Semin Respir Crit Care Med*. 2021;42:411-427.
29. Snyder ME, Anderson MR, Benvenuto LJ, et al. Impact of age and telomere length on circulating T cells and rejection risk after lung transplantation for idiopathic pulmonary fibrosis. *J Heart Lung Transplant*. 2023;42:1666-1677.
30. Roden AC, Kern RM, Aubry MC, et al. Transbronchial cryobiopsies in the evaluation of lung allografts: do the benefits outweigh the risks? *Arch Pathol Lab Med*. 2016;140(4):303-311.
31. Yousem SA. Graft eosinophilia in lung transplantation. *Hum Pathol*. 1992;23(10):1172-1177.
32. Ibáñez SA, Aguilar MP, Vicente AR, et al. Peripheral blood eosinophilia as a marker of acute cellular rejection in lung transplant recipients. *J Heart Lung Transplant*. 2022;41(4):501-507.
33. Hasegawa T, Iacono AT, Yousem SA. The anatomic distribution of acute cellular rejection in the allograft lung. *Ann Thorac Surg*. 2000;69:1529-1531.
34. Nakleh RE, Bolman RM III, Henke CA, Hertz MI. Lung transplant pathology. A comparative study of pulmonary acute rejection and cytomegaloviral infection. *Am J Surg Pathol*. 1991;15:1197-1201.
35. Abellan C, Ioakeim F, Casutt A, et al. Acute fibrinous and organizing pneumonia after lung transplantation: a case report of treatment with infliximab and tocilizumab and literature review. *Respir Med Case Rep*. 2024;53:102159.
36. Hu X, Lee JS, Pianosi PT, Ryu JH. Aspiration-related pulmonary syndromes. *Chest*. 2015;147(3):815-823.
37. Sweet MP, Patti MG, Hoopes C, Hays SR, Golden JA. Gastro-oesophageal reflux and aspiration in patients with advanced lung disease. *Thorax*. 2009;64(2):167-173.
38. Mendez BM, Davis CS, Weber C, Joehl RJ, Fisichella PM. Gastroesophageal reflux disease in lung transplant patients with cystic fibrosis. *Am J Surg*. 2012;204(5):e21-e26.
39. Baumann B, Byers S, Wasserman-Wincko T, et al. Postoperative swallowing assessment after lung transplantation. *Ann Thorac Surg*. 2017;104(1):308-312.
40. Bhorade SM, Husain AN, Liao C, et al. Interobserver variability in grading transbronchial lung biopsy specimens after lung transplantation. *Chest*. 2013;143(6):1717-1724.
41. Gauthier JM, Hachem RR, Kreisel D. Update on chronic lung allograft dysfunction. *Curr Transplant Rep*. 2016;3(3):185-191.
42. Todd JL, Weigt SS, Neely ML, et al. Prognosis and risks for probable chronic lung allograft dysfunction: a prospective multicenter study. *Am J Respir Crit Care Med*. 2024;211(2):239-247.
43. Martinu T, Howell DN, Palmer SM. Acute cellular rejection and humoral sensitization in lung transplant recipients. *Semin Respir Crit Care Med*. 2010;31:179-188.
44. Bando K, Paradis IL, Similo S, et al. Obliterative bronchiolitis after lung and heart–lung transplantation. An analysis of risk factors and management. *J Thorac Cardiovasc Surg*. 1995;110:4-14.

45. Colby TV. Bronchiolitis pathologic considerations. *Am J Clin Pathol.* 1998;109:101-109.
46. Meyer KC, Raghu G, Verleden GM, et al. An international ISHLT/ATS/ERS clinical practice guideline: diagnosis and management of bronchiolitis obliterans syndrome. *Eur Respir J.* 2014;44(6):1479-1503.
47. Pomerance A, Madden B, Burke MM, Yacoub MH. Transbronchial biopsy in heart and lung transplantation: clinicopathologic correlations. *J Heart Lung Transplant.* 1995;14:761-763.
48. Marchevsky A, Hartman G, Walts A, Ross D, Koerner S, Waters P. Lung transplantation: the pathologic diagnosis of pulmonary complications. *Mod Pathol.* 1991;4:133-138.
49. Myers JL, Colby TV. Pathologic manifestations of bronchiolitis, constrictive bronchiolitis, cryptogenic organizing pneumonia, and diffuse panbronchiolitis. *Clin Chest Med.* 1993;14:611-622.
50. Paradis I, Yousem S, Griffith B. Airway obstruction and bronchiolitis obliterans after lung transplantation. *Clin Chest Med.* 1993;14:751-763.
51. Schlesinger C, Meyer CA, Veeraraghavan S, Koss MN. Constrictive (obliterative) bronchiolitis: diagnosis, etiology, and a critical review of the literature. *Ann Diagn Pathol.* 1998;4:288-293.
52. Yousem SA, Duncan SR, Griffith BP. Interstitial and airspace granulation tissue reactions in lung transplant recipients. *Am J Surg Pathol.* 1992;16:877-884.
53. Abernathy ED, Hruban RH, Baumgartner WA, Reitz BA, Hutchins GM. The two forms of bronchiolitis obliterans in heart–lung transplant recipients. *Hum Pathol.* 1991;27:714-719.
54. Yousem SA, Paradis IL, Dauber JH, et al. Pulmonary arteriosclerosis in long-term human heart–lung transplant recipients. *Transplantation.* 1989;47:564-569.
55. Verleden GM, Glanville AR, Lease ED, et al. Chronic lung allograft dysfunction: definition, diagnostic criteria, and approaches to treatment–a consensus report from the Pulmonary Council of the ISHLT. *J Heart Lung Transplant.* 2019;38(5):493-503.
56. Glanville AR, Verleden GM, Todd JL, et al. Chronic lung allograft dysfunction: definition and update of restrictive allograft syndrome–a consensus report from the Pulmonary Council of the ISHLT. *J Heart Lung Transplant.* 2019;38(5):483-492.
57. Halloran K, Vos R, Snell G, Greenland JR. The lung transplant endobronchial biopsy: a forgotten specimen comes of age. *J Heart Lung Transplant.* 2025;44(2):293-297.
58. Patel T, Bemiss B, Panah E, et al. Airway associated inflammation in post-transplant cystic fibrosis patients as a predictor of chronic lung allograft dysfunction (CLAD). *J Clin Pathol.* 2025;78(4):251-258.
59. Weigt SS, Wallace WD, Derhovanessian A, et al. Chronic allograft rejection: epidemiology, diagnosis, pathogenesis, and treatment. *Semin Respir Crit Care Med.* 2010;31:189-207.
60. Appel JZ III, Hartwig MG, Davis RD, Reinsmoen NL. Utility of peritransplant and rescue intravenous immunoglobulin and extracorporeal immunoadsorption in lung transplant recipients sensitized to HLA antigens. *Hum Immunol.* 2005;66(4):378-386.
61. Colvin RB, Smith RN. Antibody-mediated organ-allograft rejection. *Nat Rev Immunol.* 2005;5(10):807-817.
62. Hadjiliadis D, Chaparro C, Reinsmoen NL, et al. Pre-transplant panel reactive antibody in lung transplant recipients is associated with significantly worse post-transplant survival in a multicenter study. *J Heart Lung Transplant.* 2005;24(7 Suppl):S249-S254.
63. Lobo LJ, Aris RM, Schmitz J, Neuringer IP. Donor-specific antibodies are associated with antibody-mediated rejection, acute cellular rejection, bronchiolitis obliterans syndrome, and cystic fibrosis after lung transplantation. *J Heart Lung Transplant.* 2013;32(1):70-77.
64. Hachem RR. Acute rejection and antibody-mediated rejection in lung transplantation. *Clin Chest Med.* 2017;38(4):667-675.

65. Muller YD, Aubert JD, Vionnet J, et al. Acute antibody-mediated rejection 1 week after lung transplantation successfully treated with eculizumab, intravenous immunoglobulins, and rituximab. *Transplantation.* 2018;102(6):e301-e303.
66. Roux A, Bendib Le Lan I, Holifanjaniaina S, et al. Antibody-mediated rejection in lung transplantation: clinical outcomes and donor-specific antibody characteristics. *Am J Transplant.* 2016;16(4):1216-1228.
67. Berry G, Burke M, Andersen C, et al. Pathology of pulmonary antibody mediated rejection: 2012 update from the Pathology Council of the ISHLT. *J Heart Lung Transplant.* 2013;32(1):14-21.
68. Roux A, Levine DJ, Zeevi A, et al. Banff lung report: current knowledge and future research perspectives for diagnosis and treatment of pulmonary antibody-mediated rejection (AMR). *Am J Transplant.* 2019;19(1):21-31.
69. Levine DJ, Glanville AR, Aboyoun C, et al. Antibody-mediated rejection of the lung: a consensus report of the International Society for Heart and Lung Transplantation. *J Heart Lung Transplant.* 2016;35(4):397-406.
70. Auner S, Hillebrand C, Boehm PM, et al. Impact of transient and persistent donor-specific antibodies in lung transplantation. *Transpl Int.* 2024;37:12774.
71. Benden C, Wikenheiser-Brokamp KA. Antibody-mediated rejection (AMR) in pediatric lung transplantation-current state and future directions. *Pediatr Transplant.* 2024;28(2):e14739.
72. Halverson LP, Hachem RR. Antibody-mediated rejection: diagnosis and treatment. *Clin Chest Med.* 2023;44(1):95-103.
73. Grobman B, Diamond JM, Goldberg HJ, Courtwright AM. The impact of prelung transplant HLA antibodies on post-transplant outcomes in recipients with autoimmune lung disease. *Transplant Proc.* 2024;56(7):1646-1653.
74. Messika J, Belousova N, Parquin F, Roux A. Antibody-mediated rejection in lung transplantation: diagnosis and therapeutic armamentarium in a 21st century perspective. *Transpl Int.* 2024;37:12973.
75. Comins-Boo A, Mora-Fernández VM, Padrón-Aunceame P, et al. Non-HLA antibodies and the risk of antibody-mediated rejection without donor-specific anti-HLA antibodies after lung transplantation. *Transplant Proc.* 2025;57(1):73-76.
76. Wodajo A, Sarode R, De Simone N, Kaza V, Usmani A. Efficacy of a standardized regimen of therapeutic plasma exchange and IVIG for treatment of antibody-mediated rejection in lung transplant recipients. *J Clin Apher.* 2024;39(6):e22151.
77. Goldsby J, Beermann K, Frankel C, et al. Preemptive immune globulin therapy in sensitized lung transplant recipients. *Transpl Immunol.* 2023;80:101904.
78. Kleiboeker HL, Prom A, Paplaczyk K, Myers CN. A complement to traditional treatments for antibody-mediated rejection? Use of eculizumab in lung transplantation: a review and early center experience. *Ann Pharmacother.* 2024;58(9):947-955.
79. Mallet H, Razat L, Perrier Q, et al. Effectiveness of complement inhibitors against refractory antibody-mediated rejection of lung transplantation: Two clinical cases. *Transpl Immunol.* 2025;89:102174.
80. January SE, Fester KA, Halverson LP, et al. Tocilizumab for antibody-mediated rejection treatment in lung transplantation. *J Heart Lung Transplant.* 2023;42(10):1353-1357.
81. Abdulqawi R, Alawwami M, Aldosari O, et al. Intravenous immunoglobulins alone for the desensitization of lung transplant recipients with preformed donor specific antibodies and negative flow cytometry crossmatch. *Clin Transpl.* 2024;38(7):e15374.
82. Levin K, Westall G, Ennis S, Snell G. Clinical outcomes following cessation of parenteral immunoglobulin therapy following lung transplantation. *J Heart Lung Transplant.* 2023;42(12):1642-1646.

83. Keller MB, Tian X, Jang MK, et al. Organizing pneumonia is associated with molecular allograft injury and the development of antibody-mediated rejection. *J Heart Lung Transplant*. 2024;43(4):563-570.

84. Herman J, Lerut E, Damme-Lombaerts RV, Emonds MP, Damme BV. Capillary deposition of complement C4d and C3d in pediatric renal allograft biopsies. *Transplantation*. 2005;79(10):1435-1440.

85. Choi J, Cho YM, Yang WS, Park TJ, Chang JW, Park SK. Peritubular capillary C4d deposition and renal outcome in post-transplant IgA nephropathy. *Clin Transpl*. 2007;21(2):159-165.

86. Fedson SE, Daniel SS, Husain AN. Immunohistochemistry staining of C4d to diagnose antibody-mediated rejection in cardiac transplantation. *J Heart Lung Transplant*. 2008;27(4):372-379.

87. Magro CM, Harman AP, Klinger D, et al. Use of C4d as a diagnostic adjunct in lung allograft biopsies. *Am J Transplant*. 2003;3(9):1143-1154.

88. Roden AC, Maleszewski JJ, Yi ES, et al. Reproducibility of complement 4d deposition by immunofluorescence and immunohistochemistry in lung allograft biopsies. *J Heart Lung Transplant*. 2014;33(12):1223-1232.

89. Roberts JA, Barrios R, Cagle PT, et al. The presence of anti-HLA donor-specific antibodies in lung allograft recipients does not correlate with C4d immunofluorescence in transbronchial biopsy specimens. *Arch Pathol Lab Med*. 2014;138(8):1053-1058.

90. Ngo C, Danel C, Duong-Quy S, et al. C4d detection and histological patterns in the diagnosis of antibody-mediated rejection after lung transplantation: a single-centre study. *Histopathology*. 2019;74(7):988-996.

91. Lunardi F, Vedovelli L, Pezzuto F, et al. Assessing the role of phosphorylated S6 ribosomal protein in the pathological diagnosis of pulmonary antibody-mediated rejection. *J Heart Lung Transplant*. 2024;43(3):403-413.

92. Cone BD, Zhang JQ, Sosa RA, Calabrese F, Reed EF, Fishbein GA. Phosphorylated S6 ribosomal protein expression by immunohistochemistry correlates with de novo donor-specific HLA antibodies in lung allograft recipients. *J Heart Lung Transplant*. 2021;40(10):1164-1171.

93. Calabrese DR, Greenland JR. Theseus and the search for an antibody-mediated rejection molecular state in lung transplant biopsies. *Am J Transplant*. 2023;23(12):1826-1827.

94. Gauthier PT, Mackova M, Hirji A, et al. Defining a natural killer cell-enriched molecular rejection-like state in lung transplant transbronchial biopsies. *Am J Transplant*. 2023;23(12):1922-1938.

95. Kramer MR, Marshall SE, Starnes VA, Gamberg P, Amitai Z, Theodore J. Infectious complications in heart–lung transplantation. Analysis of 200 episodes. *Arch Intern Med*. 1993;153:2010-2016.

96. Heldman MR, Saullo JL, Menachem BM, et al. Epidemiology of infections in lung transplant recipients treated with belatacept. *Transpl Infect Dis*. 2025;27(1):e14403.

97. Martin-Gandul C, Mueller NJ, Pascual M, Manuel O. The impact of infection on chronic allograft dysfunction and allograft survival after solid organ transplantation. *Am J Transplant*. 2015;15(12):3024-3040.

98. Burguete SR, Maselli DJ, Fernandez JF, Levine SM. Lung transplant infection. *Respirology*. 2013;18(1):22-38.

99. Gould FK, Freeman R, Taylor CE, et al. Prophylaxis and management of cytomegalovirus pneumonitis after lung transplantation: a review of experience in one center. *J Heart Lung Transplant*. 1993;12:695-699.

100. Shah PD, McDyer JF. Viral infections in lung transplant recipients. *Semin Respir Crit Care Med*. 2010;31:243-254.

101. Almaghrabi RS, Omrani AS, Memish ZA. Cytomegalovirus infection in lung transplant recipients. *Expert Rev Respir Med*. 2017;11(5):377-383.

102. Potena L, Solidoro P, Patrucco F, Borgese L. Treatment and prevention of cytomegalovirus infection in heart and lung transplantation: an update. *Expert Opin Pharmacother*. 2016;17(12):1611-1622.
103. Fernández SGM, Laporta R, Fadul CG, et al. CMV infection risk factors and viral dynamics after valganciclovir prophylaxis: 10 years of experience in lung transplant recipients. *Microorganisms*. 2024;12(11):2360.
104. Patrucco F, Curtoni A, Sidoti F, et al. Herpes virus infection in lung transplantation: diagnosis, treatment and prevention strategies. *Viruses*. 2023;15(12):2326.
105. Cahill CB, Hibbs JR, Savik K, et al. *Aspergillus* airway colonization and invasive disease after lung transplantation. *Chest*. 1997;112:1160-1164.
106. Kanj SS, Welty-Wolf K, Madden J, et al. Fungal infections in lung and heart–lung transplant recipients. Report of 9 cases and review of the literature. *Medicine (Baltimore)*. 1996;75:142-156.
107. Pasupneti S, Manouvakhova O, Nicolls MR, Hsu JL. *Aspergillus*-related pulmonary diseases in lung transplantation. *Med Mycol*. 2017;55(1):96-102.
108. Gryzan S, Paradis IL, Zeevi A, et al. Unexpectedly high incidence of *Pneumocystis carinii* infection after lung–heart transplantation. Implications for lung defense and allograft survival. *Am Rev Respir Dis*. 1988;137:1268-1274.
109. Mah JK, Tam PCK, Chang YC, et al. Limited utility of Epstein-Barr virus (EBV) surveillance for predicting post-transplant lymphoproliferative disorders in adult EBV seropositive lung transplant recipients. *J Clin Virol*. 2025;176:105758.
110. Randhawa PS, Yousem S, Paradis IL, Dauber JA, Griffith BP, Locker J. The clinical spectrum, pathology, and clonal analysis of Epstein–Barr virus-associated lymphoproliferative disorders in heart–lung transplant recipients. *Am J Clin Pathol*. 1989;92:177-185.
111. Kremer B, Reshef R, Misleh J, et al. Post-transplant lymphoproliferative disorder after lung transplantation: a review of 35 cases. *J Heart Lung Transplant*. 2012;31(3):296-304.
112. Leclercq C, Sansen PY, Collinge E, et al. Late-onset hemophagocytic lymphohistiocytosis in a lung transplant patient: a case of T-cell post-transplant lymphoproliferative disorder. *Am J Case Rep*. 2024;25:e944761.
113. Caillard S, Lelong C, Pessione F, Moulin B. Post-transplant lymphoproliferative disorders occurring after renal transplantation in adults: report of 230 cases from the French Registry. *Am J Transplant*. 2006;6(11):2735-2742.
114. Morscio J, Dierickx D, Tousseyn T. Molecular pathogenesis of B-cell posttransplant lymphoproliferative disorder: what do we know so far? *Clin Dev Immunol*. 2013;2013:150835.
115. Nalesnik MA, Jaffe R, Starzl TE, et al. The pathology of posttransplant lymphoproliferative disorders occurring in the setting of cyclosporine A-prednisone immunosuppression. *Am J Pathol*. 1988;133:173-192.
116. Knowles DM, Cesarman E, Chadburn A, et al. Correlative morphologic and molecular genetic analysis demonstrates three distinct categories of posttransplant lymphoproliferative disorders. *Blood*. 1995;85:552-565.
117. Chadburn A, Chen JM, Hsu DT, et al. The morphologic and molecular genetic categories of posttransplantation lymphoproliferative disorders are clinically relevant. *Cancer*. 1998;82:1978-1987.
118. WHO Classification of Tumours Editorial Board. *Haematolymphoid Tumours*. WHO Classification of Tumours Series, 5th ed., Vol. 11. International Agency for Research on Cancer; 2024. https://publications.iarc.who.int/637
119. Campo E, Jaffe ES, Cook JR, et al. The International Consensus Classification of Mature Lymphoid Neoplasms: a report from the Clinical Advisory Committee. *Blood*. 2022;140(11):1229-1253.
120. Falini B, Martino G, Lazzi S. A comparison of the International Consensus and 5th World Health Organization classifications of mature B-cell lymphomas. *Leukemia*. 2023;37(1):18-34.

121. Swerdlow SH, Webber SA, Chaburn A, Ferry JA. Post-transplant lymphoproliferative disorders. In: Swerdlow SH, Campo E, Harris NL, eds. *WHO Classification of Tumours of Hematopoietic and Lymphoid Tissues*. IARC Press; 2017.
122. LaCasce AS. Post-transplant lymphoproliferative disorders. *Oncologist*. 2006;11(6): 674-680.
123. Djokic M, Le Beau MM, Swinnen LJ, et al. Post-transplant lymphoproliferative disorder subtypes correlate with different recurring chromosomal abnormalities. *Genes Chromosomes Cancer*. 2005;45:313-318.
124. Kampers J, Orjuela-Grimm M, Schober T, et al. Classical Hodgkin lymphoma-type PTLD after solid organ transplantation in children: a report on 17 patients treated according to subsequent GPOH-HD treatment schedules. *Leuk Lymphoma*. 2017;58(3):633-638.
125. Rosendale B, Yousem SA. Discrimination of Epstein–Barr virus-related posttransplant lymphoproliferations from acute rejection in lung allograft recipients. *Arch Pathol Lab Med*. 1995;119:418-423.
126. Leblond V, Dhedin N, Mamzer Bruneel MF, et al. Identification of prognostic factors in 61 patients with posttransplantation lymphoproliferative disorders. *J Clin Oncol*. 2001;19(3):772-778.
127. Ghobrial IM, Habermann TM, Maurer MJ, et al. Prognostic analysis for survival in adult solid organ transplant recipients with post-transplantation lymphoproliferative disorders. *J Clin Oncol*. 2005;23(30):7574-7582.
128. Zhang Y, Ruiz P. Solid organ transplant-associated acute graft-versus-host disease. *Arch Pathol Lab Med*. 2010;134(8):1220-1224.
129. Weinstein A, Dexter D, KuKuruga DL, Philosophe B, Hess J, Klassen D. Acute graft-versus-host disease in pancreas transplantation: a comparison of two case presentations and a review of the literature. *Transplantation*. 2006;82:127-131.
130. Smith DM, Agura E, Netto G, et al. Liver transplant-associated graft-versus-host disease. *Transplantation*. 2003;75:118-126.
131. Dai DW, Garber B, Weigt SS, et al. Pulmonary allograft versus host disease. *Transplant Direct*. 2017;3(12):e333.
132. Shulman HM, Kleiner D, Lee SJ, et al. Histopathologic diagnosis of chronic graft-versus-host disease: National Institutes of Health consensus development project on criteria for clinical trials in chronic graft-versus-host disease: II. Pathology working group report. *Biol Blood Marrow Transplant*. 2006;12(1):31-47.
133. Luckraz H, Zagolin M, McNeil K, Wallwork J. Graft-versus-host disease in lung transplantation: 4 case reports and literature review. *J Heart Lung Transplant*. 2003;22(6):691-769.
134. Xu L, Drachenberg C, Tavora F, Burke A. Histologic findings in lung biopsies in patients with suspected graft-versus-host disease. *Hum Pathol*. 2013;44(7):1233-1240.
135. Milman N, Andersen CB, Burton CM, Perch M, Carlsen J, Iversen M. Recurrent sarcoid granulomas in a transplanted lung derive from recipient immune cells. *Eur Respir J*. 2005;26(3):549-552.
136. Collins J, Hartman MJ, Warner TF, et al. Frequency and CT findings of recurrent disease after lung transplantation. *Radiology*. 2001;219:503-509.
137. Lu L, Wein AN, Villanueva A, et al. Clinical and histopathologic characteristics of recurrent sarcoidosis in posttransplant lungs: 25 years of experience. *Am J Surg Pathol*. 2023;47(9):1034-1038.
138. Parker LA, Novotny DB. Recurrent alveolar proteinosis following double lung transplantation. *Chest*. 1997;111(5):1457-1458.
139. Tarabichi Y, Saggar R, Wallace WD, Lynch JP III, Saggar R. Primary disease recurrence after single lung transplantation in a patient with prior hard metal exposure. *J Heart Lung Transplant*. 2015;34(9):1216-1218.

11

LYMPHOID LESIONS OF THE LUNG

Lymphoid lesions involving the lung are relatively rare and span the entire spectrum from benign to malignant processes. Significant changes in our understanding of these disorders have occurred during the past few decades owing to advances in the application of immunologic and molecular tools for diagnosis of this family of tumors. The modern evaluation of lymphoproliferative disorders relies heavily on immunophenotypic analysis of the cell type for correct and specific classification, as well as on characterization of immunoarchitecture to assess growth patterns, and detection of a clonal population to help separate reactive from neoplastic proliferations in edge cases. Given that the diagnosis of pulmonary lymphoma is often established on smaller biopsy specimens, these findings often need to be integrated with the results of molecular genetic analyses to arrive at a definitive diagnosis.[1,2] Immunohistochemistry, flow cytometry, and molecular genetic techniques now form a part of the routine armamentarium in the evaluation of lymphoproliferative disorders and play a critical role in their diagnosis.

The lung may be involved by various lymphoproliferative processes (Table 11.1). Benign lymphoid proliferations include follicular bronchiolitis (FB), nodular lymphoid hyperplasia (NLH), and diffuse lymphoid hyperplasia (DLH). Malignant conditions include extranodal marginal zone

TABLE 11.1 Pulmonary Lymphoid Lesions

Benign/Borderline	Malignant
Follicular bronchiolitis	Marginal zone lymphoma
Nodular lymphoid hyperplasia	Diffuse large B-cell lymphoma
Diffuse lymphoid hyperplasia	Anaplastic large cell lymphoma
	Lymphomatoid granulomatosis
	Hodgkin lymphoma
	Plasmacytoma
	Posttransplant lymphoproliferative disorder

lymphoma of mucosa-associated lymphoid tissue (MALT lymphoma), diffuse large B-cell lymphoma (DLBCL), anaplastic large cell lymphoma (ALCL), lymphomatoid granulomatosis (LYG), pulmonary classic Hodgkin lymphoma (CHL), plasmacytoma, and posttransplant lymphoproliferative disorder (PTLD). PTLD was discussed in detail in Chapter 10 dealing with transplant pathology and will not be further discussed in this chapter. The lung may also rarely be involved by other lymphoid and hematologic malignancies, including solid manifestations of leukemias, follicular lymphoma, chronic lymphocytic leukemia (CLL)/small lymphocytic lymphoma, Burkitt lymphoma, and lymphoplasmacytic lymphoma (LPL)[3-6]; however, these almost never occur as primary pulmonary disease and are more often encountered in patients with a prior history of a hematologic malignancy and thus will not be discussed in detail here.

Finally, as previously mentioned in Chapter 10, the 5th edition of the World Health Organization introduced some changes to the previously used terminology for many hematolymphoid tumors; a change that is at odds with the competing classification system of the International Consensus Classification (ICC).[7,8] These changes in nomenclature and classification primarily apply to PTLD in the context of pulmonary hematolymphoid pathology and are overall inconsequential to the material covered within this chapter. For the sake of simplicity, this book will use the traditional nomenclature and criteria established in the prior edition of the World Health Organization and continued forward in the current ICC scheme.

BENIGN/HYPERPLASTIC LYMPHOID PROCESSES

Our understanding of benign hyperplastic lymphoid proliferations of the lung has evolved significantly over the past 20 years. Historically, the process we now designate as DLH was regarded by Liebow[9] as a distinctive type of idiopathic interstitial pneumonia, which he designated as lymphoid interstitial pneumonia. Although some experts still propose that we continue to include DLH among the group of idiopathic interstitial pneumonias for historical reasons, it is now widely recognized that there may be a great deal of overlap between DLH and the "cellular" form of nonspecific interstitial pneumonia as well as with other lymphoid interstitial infiltrates observed in several specific autoimmune conditions, such as acute lupus pneumonitis. The term *DLH* or *diffuse bronchial-associated lymphoid tissue* (BALT) hyperplasia is therefore currently favored. The term *pseudolymphoma* was also used in the previous years to refer to some of these conditions, particularly for the process we now designate as NLH.[10] With the advent of modern immunohistochemical and molecular diagnostic testing, a more thorough understanding has been attained of these processes. It is now believed that some of these conditions may serve as precursor lesions to malignant lymphomas in the lung, although most cases will regress spontaneously or follow an indolent clinical course.

Follicular Bronchiolitis

FB refers to a process in which lymphoid aggregates are deposited around or in the vicinity of the small airways. The process is thought to be secondary to some form of antigenic stimulation with a reactive polyclonal lymphoid hyperplasia.[11] FB can occur at any age, is more common in males than in females, and usually involves the lungs bilaterally producing an interstitial pattern of involvement of lung parenchyma.[12] This process may be primary (idiopathic) or secondary, where it is most often seen in association with immunodeficiency states, collagen vascular diseases, infections, interstitial lung diseases, or in patients with inflammatory airway disease (chronic obstructive pulmonary disease, bronchiectasis, asthma).[11,13,14] Symptoms may include progressive dyspnea and cough, and chest X-rays will show bilateral reticular or reticulonodular infiltrates, which are lower lobe predominant.[15,16]

The histologic hallmark of FB is the accumulation of dense aggregates of mature small lymphocytes in the vicinity or at the periphery of bronchioles that may compress or distort the bronchiolar lumens (Fig. 11.1). The lymphoid aggregates are usually small and well delimited and do not extend into the surrounding alveolar septa, and they may or may not show well-developed germinal centers. The CD20+ small lymphocytes are

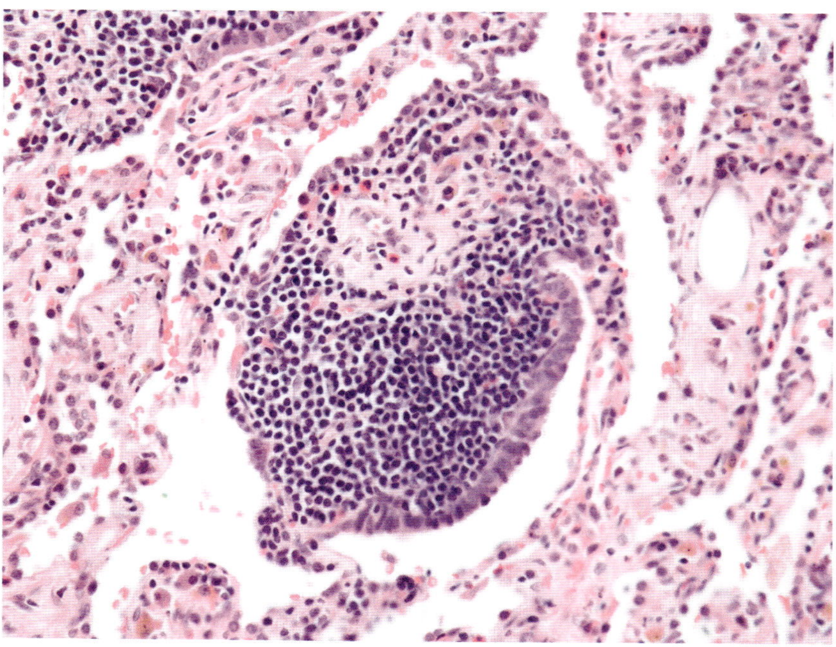

FIGURE 11.1 **Small lymphoid follicle is seen adjacent to the lining of a bronchiole in follicular bronchiolitis.** Notice that the lymphoid follicle is located in the alveolar wall and is compressing the lumen of the bronchiole.

polytypic and do not show evidence of light chain restriction. CD21 may highlight residual follicular dendritic cell (FDC) meshworks underlying the germinal centers. The germinal center B cells will additionally follow the expected reactive pattern of positivity for CD10 (may be weakly expressed in many laboratories) and BCL6 and negativity for BCL2 (though this is expressed both in the T cells and in the mantle zone naive B cells) The diagnosis of a reactive lymphoid infiltrate requires a lack of architectural effacement, as this is a consistent feature of malignant lymphomas, though assessment is more challenging in needle core biopsies and relies heavily on characterization of immunoarchitecture by at least CD20 and CD3 immunostains as a starting point.

FB is most often diagnosed in open lung biopsy or video-assisted thoracoscopic surgery (VATS) specimens, although occasionally they may be encountered in transbronchial lung biopsies. It must be emphasized that FB is not a distinct or discrete disease entity but a nonspecific reaction pattern of lung parenchyma to an underlying stimulus. Clinical correlation is always required to determine the underlying or associated conditions.

Nodular Lymphoid Hyperplasia

NLH, also known as nodular BALT hyperplasia, is a reactive process characterized by follicular lymphoid hyperplasia with interfollicular plasmacytosis and prominent reactive germinal centers. In the past, lesions with these features were termed *pseudolymphoma*, an outdated term that is no longer in use.[17] NLH occurs between 19 and 80 years of age (median, 65 years), is more common in females than in males, and may be associated with collagen vascular disorders or autoimmune diseases.[17-20] Chest X-rays and computed tomography (CT) will show a solitary nodule or, in some instances, multiple confluent nodules that can measure up to 5 cm in greatest diameter.[18,19] Histologically, the process is characterized by a well-demarcated area of the lung showing replacement of the parenchyma by a proliferation of multiple enlarged lymphoid follicles with reactive germinal centers. The germinal centers in the nodules display prominent polarization (which when in doubt can additionally be appreciated by Ki67 or PD1 immunostains), commonly have prominent tingible body macrophages, and are surrounded by a well-developed mantle zone (which is BCL2+). There is striking interfollicular lymphoplasmacytosis, which is polytypic, and atypical cells or transformed lymphocytes are not a feature of the process. The lesions are sharply demarcated from the surrounding lung parenchyma and do not extend along alveolar septa or into the alveolar walls.[21,22] Immunohistochemical analysis will stain the lymphocytes in the germinal centers positive for CD20 and negative for BCL2 (though the latter will label associated T cells, and B cells within the mantle cuffs, which can complicate assessment to the untrained eye). The interfollicular lymphocytes primarily comprise small T cells that are CD3 and CD5 positive. The B cells also show a polytypic pattern of expression for κ and λ light chains; rarely, germinal center B cells can demonstrate a slight κ or λ light chain excess in reactive conditions as a feature of somatic hypermutation, and this is best appreciated by flow cytometry.

Recently, studies have raised the possibility that NLH may be related to IgG4-related disease because of the finding of increased numbers of IgG4+ plasma cells[10]; however, other studies have contradicted these findings. It appears that although some cases of NLH may show increased staining with IgG4 immunohistochemistry, the majority of the lesions have low numbers of IgG4+ cells.[23] Elevated IgG4 staining alone should not be used for diagnosis of this condition in the absence of clinical evidence of IgG4-related disease (such as elevated serum levels of immunoglobulins [IGs]) and without the additional histologic features associated with the disease (storiform fibrosis, obliterative phlebitis, etc.).

The diagnosis of NLH is best made in open lung biopsy specimens (wedge resections or nodulectomy specimens). The nodular pattern of the lesion may not be appreciated in core biopsy specimens or transbronchial biopsies, and the best diagnostic offering under such circumstances is to indicate that the lymphoid infiltrate does not demonstrate evidence of monotypic light chain restriction by immunophenotypic studies or monoclonal *IGH* rearrangements by fluorescence in situ hybridization (FISH), polymerase chain reaction (PCR), or next generation sequencing (NGS). Surgical excision is associated with an excellent prognosis without recurrences.[24]

Diffuse Lymphoid Hyperplasia

DLH, also known as diffuse BALT hyperplasia and formerly designated as lymphoid interstitial pneumonia, is a reactive process characterized by a polyclonal proliferation of lymphocytes and plasma cells occupying the pulmonary interstitium and distending the alveolar walls.[12,21,25] DLH is a common manifestation in the lung of patients with a number of collagen vascular diseases (ie, Sjögren syndrome, rheumatoid arthritis, systemic lupus erythematosus), autoimmune disorders, and immunodeficiency conditions (such as acquired immunodeficiency syndrome [AIDS] and common variable immunodeficiency syndrome [CVID]). It is a common manifestation in children with AIDS.[26,27] It can also be associated with certain infections, such as *Pneumocystosis* and *Legionella* infection. Clinical symptoms include dyspnea and cough, and it is often accompanied by polyclonal gammopathy or hypergammaglobulinemia. Chest X-rays show patchy, bilateral reticulonodular infiltrates with predilection for the lower lobes. CT shows scattered ground-glass opacities with centrilobular and subpleural nodules. There can be scattered perivascular cystlike structures as well.[28,29] Between 30% and 50% of patients die within 5 years of the diagnosis, and a small percentage of cases (<5%) transform into lymphoma.[30]

The process is histologically characterized by a dense, predominantly interstitial proliferation of small lymphocytes that distend the alveolar walls (Fig. 11.2; eFig. 11.1). Small follicles with residual germinal centers

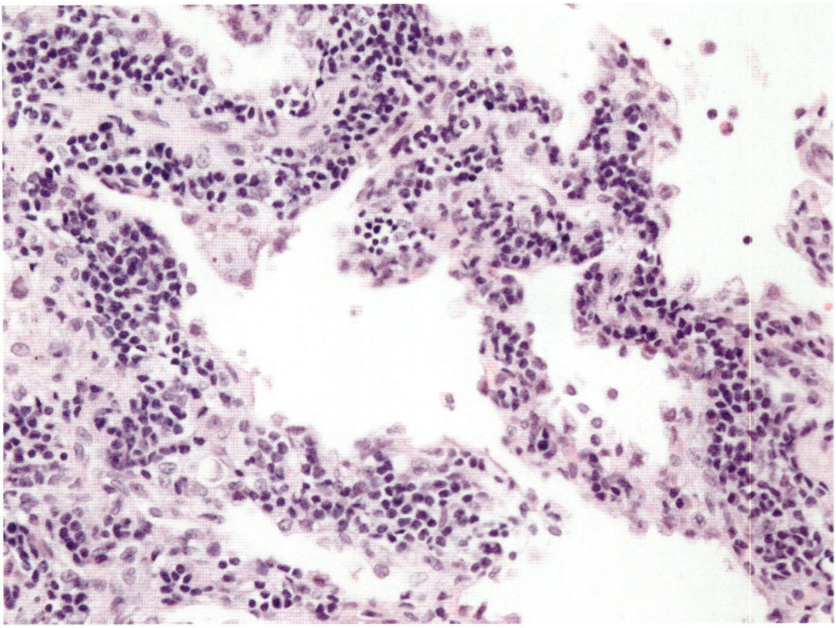

FIGURE 11.2 **Diffuse interstitial lymphoid infiltrate is seen distending the alveolar walls in diffuse lymphoid hyperplasia.** The lymphoid infiltrate is distinguished from a low-grade mucosa-associated lymphoid tissue lymphoma by the polyclonality of the lymphoid cells. Some authors still designate this process as "lymphoid interstitial pneumonia."

showing a distribution reminiscent of FB may be seen admixed with the diffuse lymphoid infiltrates. The interstitial infiltrate may also contain scattered plasma cells and histiocytes, but no atypical or transformed lymphocytes are present. Small, ill-defined granulomas or scattered giant cells have also been reported in a percentage of cases, raising the differential diagnosis with hypersensitivity pneumonitis.[31] Focal infiltration of bronchial epithelium by small lymphocytes may lead to the formation of lymphoepithelial lesions; these can be appreciated by keratin immunostains (Fig. 11.3). Immunohistochemical stains will demonstrate a predominant population of CD3+/CD5+ small T lymphocytes in the interstitium admixed with a polytypic lymphoplasmacytic small B-cell population.[32] Cases occurring in the context of AIDS will show immunoreactivity for the p21 protein of human immunodeficiency virus (HIV). IG heavy-chain gene rearrangement studies will yield a polyclonal pattern of expression.[33] In the small percentage of cases which develop lymphoma, it is thought that DLH is the precursor lesion. DLH may be very difficult to diagnose in small biopsy specimens (transbronchial or core biopsies) and will require immunohistochemical, flow cytometric, or other support to rule out monoclonality. Lung involvement by CLL may also be indistinguishable from DLH. The lymphoid cells in CLL, however, are clonal and coexpress CD5, LEF1, and usually CD23 and are negative for other T-cell markers.

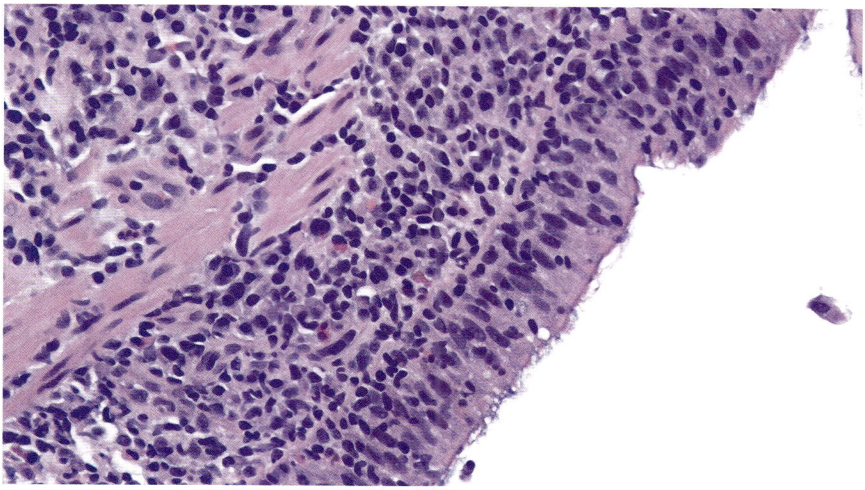

FIGURE 11.3 **Example of diffuse lymphoid hyperplasia with a prominent epithelial lesion involving a bronchiole.** Notice the dense subepithelial lymphocytic infiltrate with scattered intraepithelial lymphocytes.

The process may be impossible to separate morphologically from DLH in the absence of a clinical history, particularly in small biopsies, and short of careful immunophenotypic assessment.

MALIGNANT LYMPHOID PROCESSES

The lung is a common site for primary extranodal lymphomas and may be often involved secondarily in advanced systemic nodal-based disease. Primary lung lymphoma is diagnosed when the disease is confined or restricted to the lungs.[34,35] Malignant pulmonary lymphoid processes include extranodal marginal zone lymphoma of bronchial MALT, DLBCL, CHL, ALCL, LYG, plasmacytoma, PTLD (also known as: immune deficiency and dysregulation [IDD]-associated Epstein-Barr virus [EBV] positive lymphoproliferative disorders), and secondary involvement of the lung by systemic leukemias and lymphomas.

Adults are more commonly affected by primary lymphoma of the lung. Diagnosis is usually made by a combination of imaging studies and histologic examination of biopsy material or resection specimens. Application of immunohistochemical stains and molecular studies now form an integral and critical part of the evaluation of these tumors.[36] Flow cytometric immunophenotyping, when adequately preserved tissue with good cell viability is obtained and preserved in Roswell Park Memorial Institute (RPMI) medium, is an important tool for making a definitive and specific diagnosis. Endoscopic biopsies may yield variable results depending on the preservation of the tissue and amount of crush artifact but are often sufficient to formulate a differential diagnosis that will prompt an additional, more definitive diagnostic procedure. VATS or open biopsies are the most ideal vehicle for obtaining adequate and representative tissue and for maximizing the opportunity to render a specific diagnosis. Procurement of fresh frozen tissue for gene rearrangement studies and other molecular studies is always recommended when there is a suspicion of a malignant lymphoproliferative process.

Marginal Zone B-Cell Lymphoma

Marginal zone lymphoma of the lung or MALT lymphoma is an extranodal lymphoma of B lymphocytes derived from the marginal zones of lymphoid follicles. The tumors comprise sheets of small lymphocytes, which may range from mature small lymphocytes to small lymphocytes with abundant rims of cytoplasm resembling monocytoid B cells, to small lymphocytes with plasmacytoid features or with plasmacytic differentiation.[1] They are characterized on scanning magnification by numerous reactive appearing lymphoid follicles displaying a distinctive lymphangitic pattern of spread; in the past, many such lesions were regarded as examples of "pseudolymphoma" because of the prominence of lymphoid follicles with reactive germinal centers.[37] A confounding histologic feature and pitfall, however, is that of follicular colonization by MALT lymphoma, which can impart an abnormal morphology to the follicles, as discussed further below.

MALT lymphomas account for approximately 80% to 90% of all primary pulmonary lymphomas. The majority of patients are in their fifth or sixth decade of life, with a slight male predilection.[38] The disease can also be seen in younger patients who are immunosuppressed. The most common presentation is as a solitary parenchymatous nodule discovered incidentally on chest X-ray. The lesions can also be multiple and bilateral and present as well-defined masses or alveolar opacities associated with air bronchograms on high-resolution CT.[39] The diagnosis can often be made on transbronchial biopsy, although an open biopsy or wedge biopsy is the ideal vehicle for making a definitive diagnosis. Core needle biopsies can also yield a diagnosis of malignant lymphoma when supported by adequate ancillary studies and demonstration of monoclonality, but the lesions may be difficult to subtype into a specific lymphoma category (Fig. 11.4) or even to separate from a reactive infiltrate in the absence of a clonal population or aberrant CD43 expression. The prognosis for these tumors is excellent, and bilateral or diffuse lesions can be followed without treatment with a 5-year survival that often exceeds 90%.[1,40,41] Localized lesions respond well to surgical excision. A small percentage (<10%) of MALT lymphomas can progress to DLBCL.[38]

Histologically, pulmonary MALT lymphoma is characterized by a diffuse infiltrate of small B lymphocytes that surrounds reactive lymphoid follicles (eFigs. 11.2 and 11.3).[42] The infiltrate is centered in the marginal zone of the follicles and usually extends into and expands the interfollicular areas (Fig. 11.5; eFigs. 11.4 and 11.5). The follicles may be often obscured by overgrowth of the neoplastic small lymphocytes, a phenomenon described as "colonization" of the follicles. A prominent feature

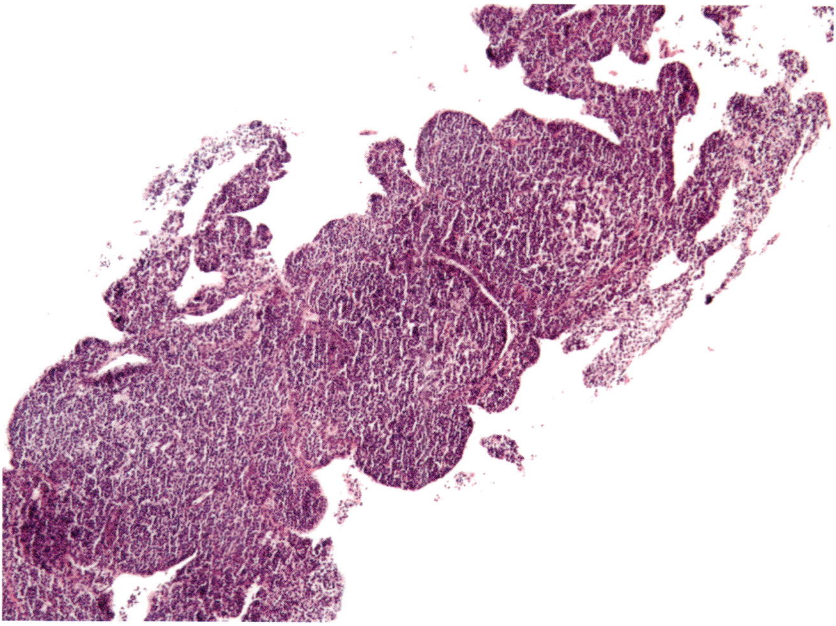

FIGURE 11.4 Percutaneous core biopsy of mucosa-associated lymphoid tissue lymphoma of the lung shows marked widening of alveolar septa by a monotonous population of small lymphoid cells with a few residual germinal centers.

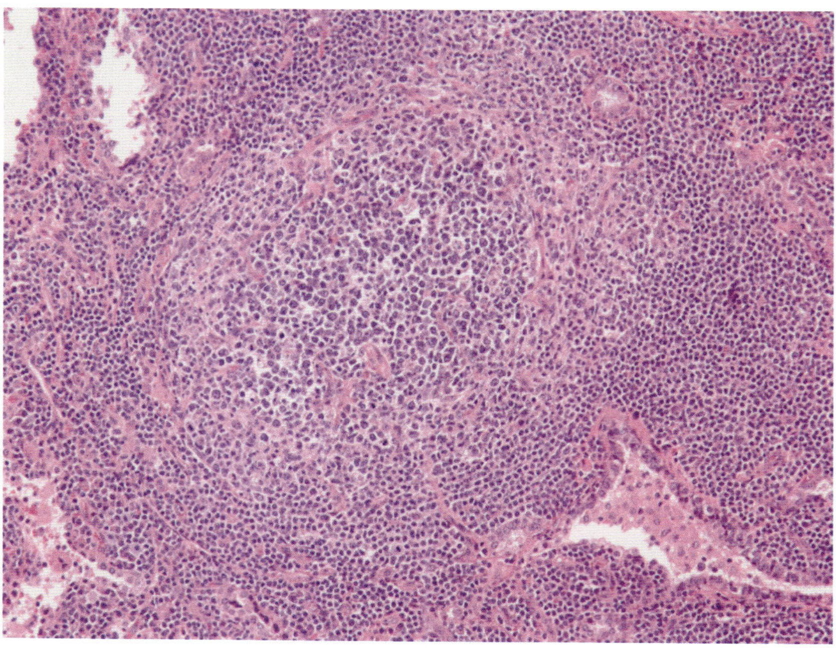

FIGURE 11.5 High magnification from an open biopsy of mucosa-associated lymphoid tissue lymphoma shows a lymphoid follicle with a reactive germinal center surrounded by a dense, monotonous population of small lymphoid cells expanding the marginal zone of the follicle.

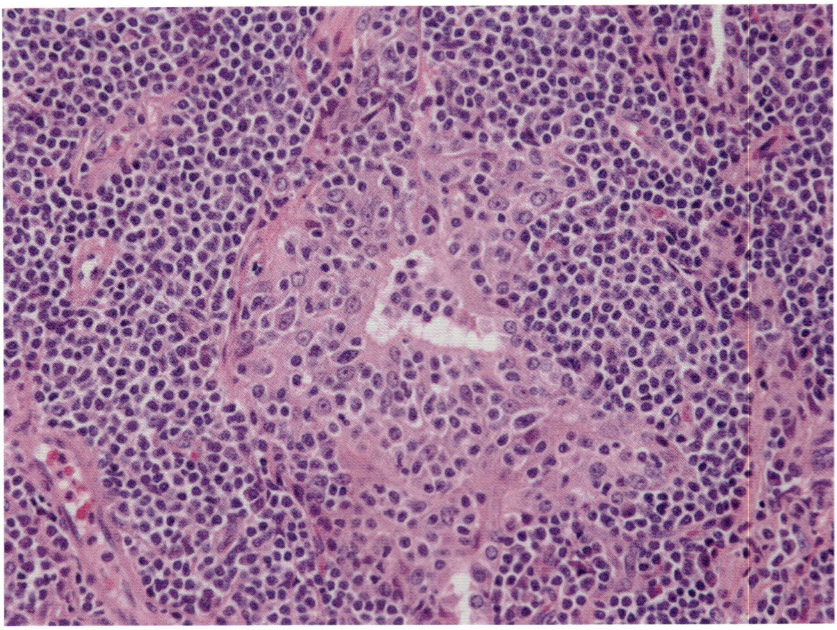

FIGURE 11.6 High magnification of mucosa-associated lymphoid tissue lymphoma shows a characteristic lymphoepithelial lesion displaying extensive infiltration and expansion of the wall of a bronchiole by atypical small lymphocytes.

in these tumors is infiltration by the small lymphocytes of bronchial, bronchiolar, or alveolar epithelium resulting in the formation of "lymphoepithelial lesions" (Fig. 11.6). The latter are quite distinctive but not pathognomonic and may be also seen occasionally in reactive processes. When the infiltrate becomes dense and confluent, it can consolidate and replace the lung parenchyma and may undergo prominent stromal sclerosis. Peripheral lesions may show pleural infiltration. Poorly formed epithelioid granulomas can also be occasionally found. The lesions rarely give rise to tumor necrosis or are associated with destruction of the airways. The neoplastic cell population in the interfollicular areas may comprise sheets of monotonous mature small lymphocytes with minimal nuclear irregularities, cells with prominent plasmacytoid features, and "monocytoid" cells characterized by small, round to indented nuclei surrounded by an ample rim of amphophilic to lightly eosinophilic cytoplasm forming a perinuclear halo. Cells containing prominent plasmacytic differentiation can be mistaken for plasmacytoma; ample sampling and identification of monocytoid cells or sheets of small lymphocytes forming lymphoepithelial lesions should permit correct identification of the process. The identification of a monotypic B-cell population, in addition to a monotypic plasma cell population, resolves the differential with a pure plasmacytoma (even one with aberrant CD20 expression). Demonstration of a B-cell lymphoma with plasmacytic differentiation generally implies either a MALT lymphoma or a LPL–distinction between these two relies on bone marrow involvement (almost universal in LPL) and demonstration of the *MYD88* L265P mutation (present in the vast majority of LPLs and highly uncommon in MALT lymphomas). Scattered larger cells resembling centroblasts or immunoblasts may also be present admixed with the small lymphocytes, but they are usually in the minority. The presence of sheets of large cytologically atypical lymphocytes heralds the transformation to DLBCL. Amyloid deposits associated with MALT lymphoma within the lung may be seen and may manifest as nodular pulmonary amyloidosis (Fig. 11.7).[43]

The neoplastic B-cell population is monoclonal, and light chain restriction can sometimes be demonstrated either on fresh tissue or paraffin sections, although light chain restriction is most reliably established by flow cytometry. Testing of the IG heavy chain can detect monoclonality in up to 60% of cases using PCR in paraffin sections,[36] though the test is imperfectly specific and false positives exist in reactive processes. In nearly all cases, the tumor cells are strongly positive for CD20, PAX5, and CD79a, and they may also express BCL2 (unlike reactive "monocytoid" B cells; Fig. 11.8; eFig. 11.5) and nuclear staining for BCL10. The cells are negative for CD5 (with rare exceptions), CD10, CD23, BCL1/cyclin D1, and BCL6, as well as the follicular derivation markers LMO2 and HGAL. Cases are frequently positive for MNDA and IRTA4, though these markers are nonspecific and not in widespread clinical use. The use of cytokeratin stains is again useful for highlighting lymphoepithelial lesions (Fig. 11.9). Stains for CD21, CD23, and CD35 may be helpful for highlighting FDC meshworks underlying residual germinal centers overrun/colonized by the tumor cells and in MALT lymphoma classically demonstrate an expanded or disrupted appearance (in contrast to the tight/intact FDC meshwork pattern in reactive follicles). Another marker in popular use is CD43, which ordinarily labels T cells and is commonly positive in MALT lymphoma B cells, though not nearly frequently enough to be a consistent and reliable diagnostic finding. Finally, the finding of large numbers of CD20+ B cells which greatly outnumber CD3+ T cells is a tipoff to a lymphoproliferative disorder and implies a low-grade B-cell lymphoma in an extranodal setting over a reactive infiltrate. This finding is particularly useful in small biopsies, when it becomes exponentially more difficult to demonstrate architectural effacement (the key diagnostic criterion for establishment of lymphoma over a reactive process).

The genetic abnormality of t(11;18)(q21;q21) is demonstrated in approximately 50% of marginal zone lymphomas.[44] The t(11;18) involves the *BIRC3 (API2)* and *MALT1* genes and will lead to the production of a fusion protein. Additional genetic aberrations described in these tumors include trisomy 3, t(14;18)(q32;q21) *IGH::BCL10*, and t(1;14)(p22;q32) *IGH::MALT1*.[45]

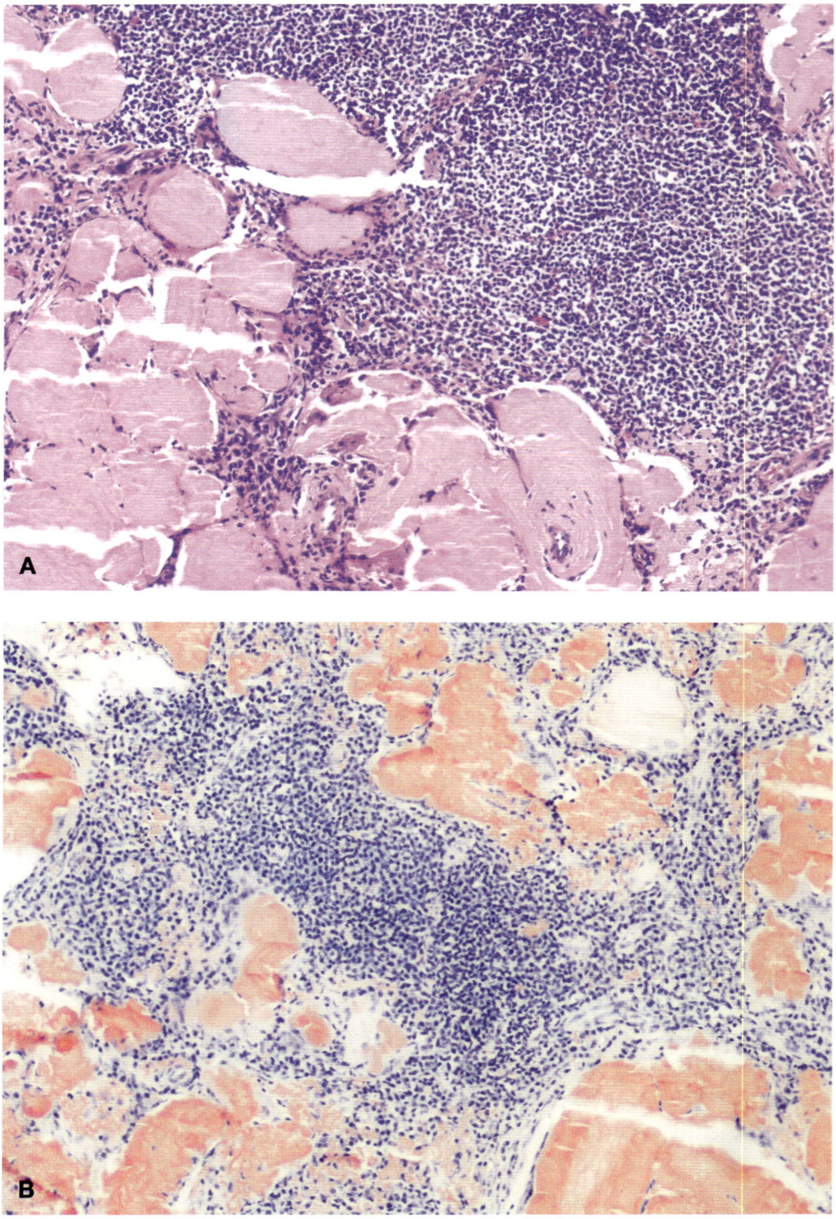

FIGURE 11.7 **A.** Wedge biopsy from a patient with a solitary nodule; there is a dense lymphoid infiltrate with associated deposition of amorphous eosinophilic material consistent with amyloid. **B.** Special stain for Congo Red highlights the amyloid deposits.

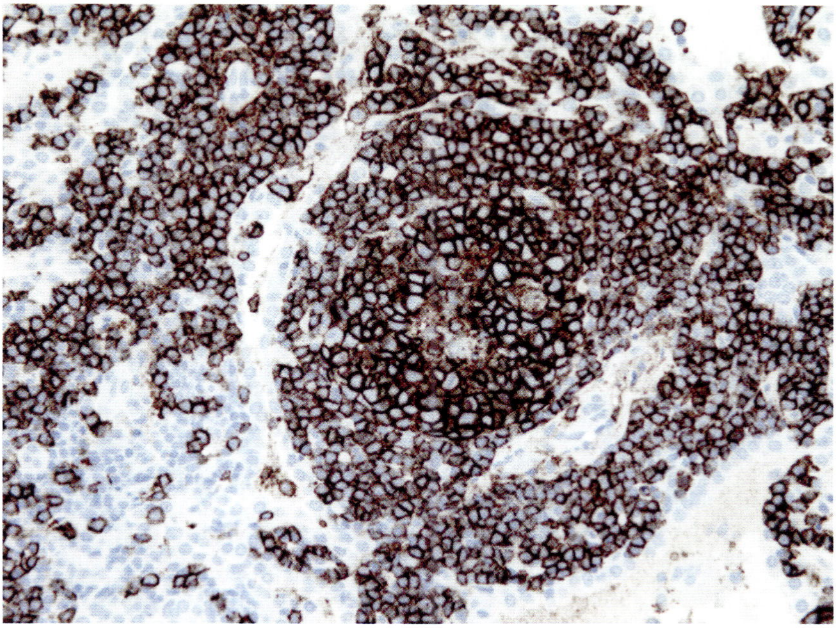

FIGURE 11.8 **Mucosa-associated lymphoid tissue lymphoma shows strong positivity of the small lymphoid cells for CD20 antibodies.**

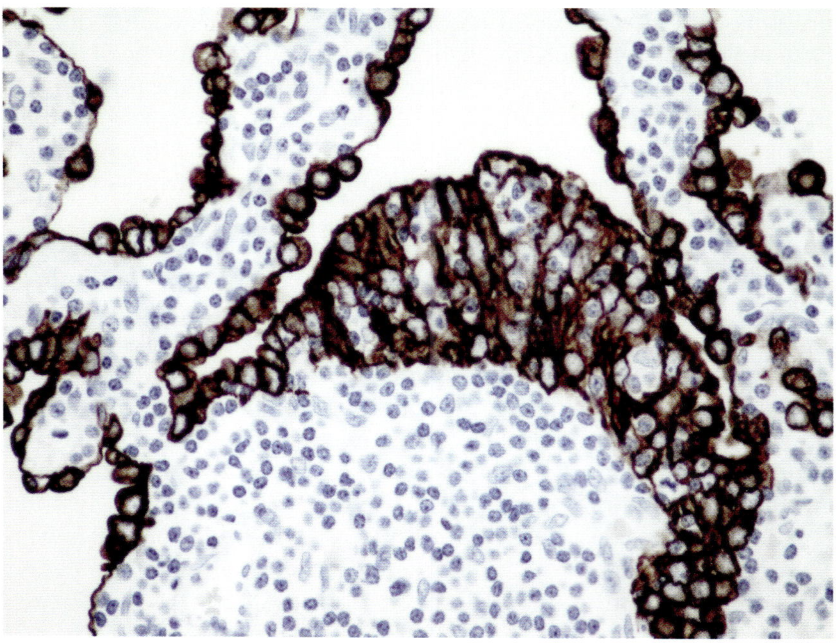

FIGURE 11.9 **Cytokeratin (AE1/AE3) stain in mucosa-associated lymphoid tissue lymphoma highlights epithelial elements in a lymphoepithelial lesion.** Notice the keratin-negative small lymphocytes percolating in-between the epithelial cells.

The diagnosis of MALT lymphoma of the lung can be established with confidence on transbronchial biopsies when sheets of the characteristic small lymphoid cells expanding the interfollicular areas are seen that show the appropriate phenotype (CD20/CD79a/BCL2+, CD5/CD10−) and demonstrate light chain restriction by immunohistochemistry or flow cytometry.

Diffuse Large B-Cell Lymphoma

DLBCL accounts for approximately 10% of all primary lymphomas of the lung and comprises a diffuse proliferation of large B cells that are more than twice the size of a normal lymphocyte. Pulmonary DLBCL has a nonspecific clinical presentation and imaging findings, making the lesions difficult to diagnose sans histology. The tumors show a tendency to arise in peripheral locations and are usually single but may present as multiple discrete nodules that are sharply delimited from the surrounding lung parenchyma. Hilar lymph nodes may also be involved in some cases. Rarely, the process may present as lung consolidation.[46] Patients are generally adults in their fifth or sixth decade of life, and the tumors occur more often in immunocompromised patients (HIV+, organ transplant patients) than in healthy individuals. Symptoms include cough, dyspnea, and hemoptysis, although the patients are more often asymptomatic. The genetic profile of DLBCL is highly variable with IG gene rearrangements and numerous described somatic mutations, copy number alterations, cellular pathway alterations, and chromosomal rearrangements.[1,47-50] A detailed discussion of the molecular genetics of DLBCL is beyond the scope of this text; however, it is worth noting that there is limited literature on the genetic landscape of primary pulmonary DLBCL. The prognosis for DLBCL of the lung is much worse than for MALT lymphoma with a median survival of 3 to 5 years in most instances, despite treatment with combination chemotherapy.[38]

Histologically, DLBCL of the lung comprises sheets of large, atypical lymphocytes displaying enlarged nuclei with coarse chromatin and prominent nucleoli and surrounded by a rim of amphophilic cytoplasm (Figs. 11.10 and 11.11; eFigs. 11.6-11.8). Mitoses can be easily identified in many cases, and there may be focal areas of necrosis with replacement and destruction of the underlying lung parenchyma (in contrast to low-grade lymphomas, in which necrosis is unusual). The tumors may invade the pleura or the bronchial walls and are usually sharply demarcated from the surrounding parenchyma without displaying the lymphangitic pattern of spread observed in MALT lymphoma. Foci of low-grade MALT lymphoma are sometimes identified in well-sampled cases. In some cases, particularly on needle core biopsies, the tumor cells may suffer artifactual distortion and adopt a spindled appearance (Fig. 11.12). Immunohistochemical stains are of help in such instances by demonstrating the lymphoid nature of the spindle cells. An immunoblastic variant of

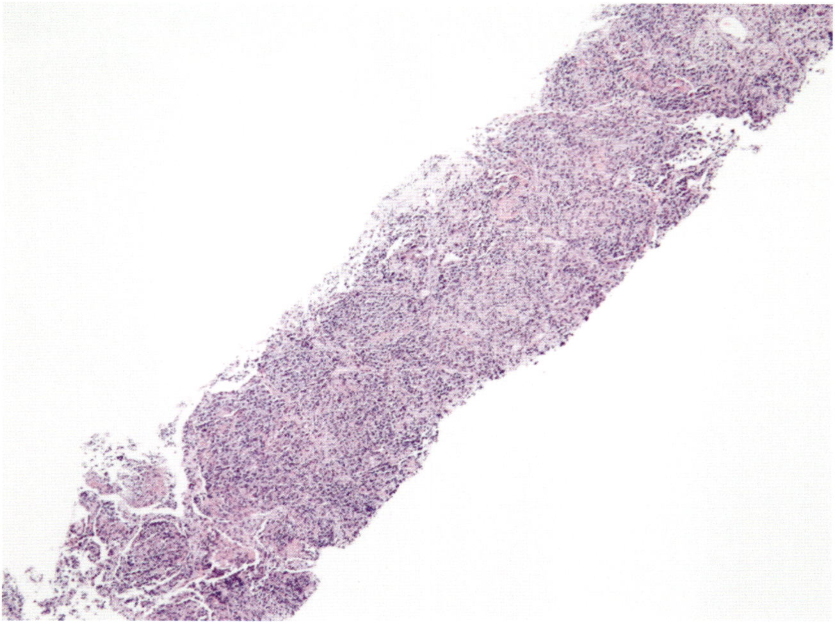

FIGURE 11.10 **Core needle biopsy of peripheral mass in the lung shows diffuse large B-cell lymphoma.** Notice complete effacement of the underlying lung architecture.

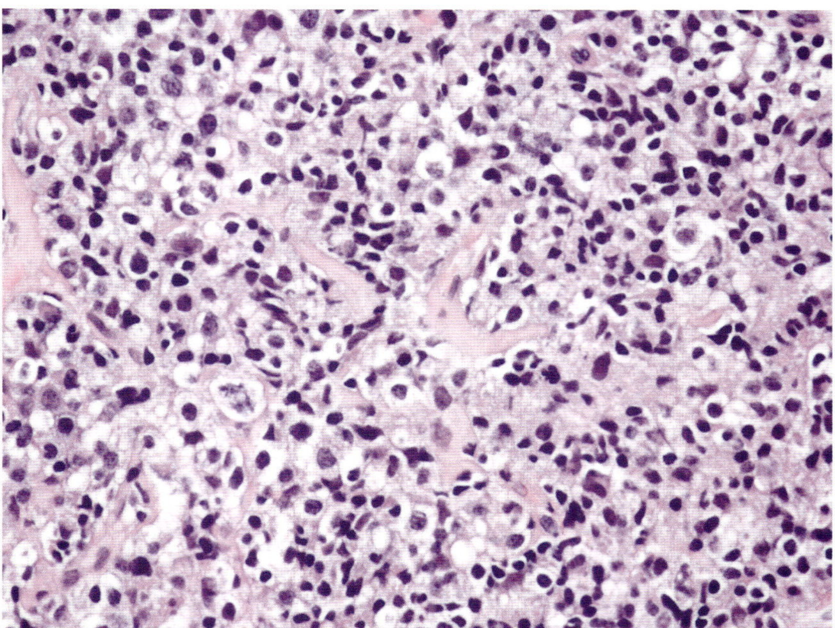

FIGURE 11.11 **Higher magnification from core needle biopsy of diffuse large cell lymphoma of the lung showing atypical lymphoid cells with large nuclei and prominent nucleoli.** The tumor cells showed strong CD20 positivity.

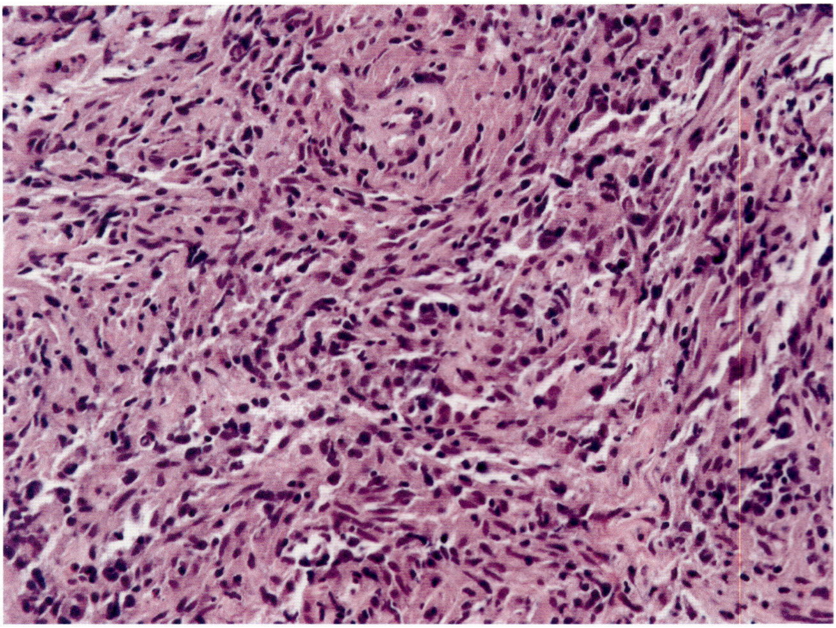

FIGURE 11.12 **Core needle biopsy of the lung in patient with diffuse large B-cell lymphoma shows artifactual distortion of the cells that adopt a vaguely spindled appearance.** It is important not to mistake such cases for a spindle cell sarcoma; immunohistochemical staining for CD20 will strongly label the spindle cells in such instances.

DLBCL can be observed that is characterized by large cells with vesicular nuclei, prominent eosinophilic nucleoli, and an abundant rim of eosinophilic, plasmacytoid cytoplasm (Fig. 11.13). Cases with such features are generally associated with a more aggressive course.[47]

Immunohistochemical studies of DLBCL will demonstrate strong positivity of the tumor cells for pan B-cell markers, including CD19, CD20, PAX5, and CD79a (Fig. 11.14). In addition, DLBCLs may show variable expression of CD10, BCL6, and MUM1, allowing them to be classified into prognostically important subtypes, either germinal center B-cell–like or activated B-cell–like (the most common algorithm for this in use is the Hans algorithm), and cell of origin classification is now mandatory in DLBCL.[48] Background CD3+ small lymphocytes may be sparse or brisk. Light chain restriction for κ or λ can sometimes be demonstrated by immunohistochemistry, in situ hybridization, or flow cytometry, though this is not required for the diagnosis of DLBCL, which is primarily made based on cytologic features (sheets of large cells) and immunophenotype.[36] PCR or NGS for the IG heavy-chain gene will demonstrate a clonal gene rearrangement in most cases.

In the lung, DLBCL is often diagnosed first on core needle biopsy specimens because of its predominantly peripheral location but can also

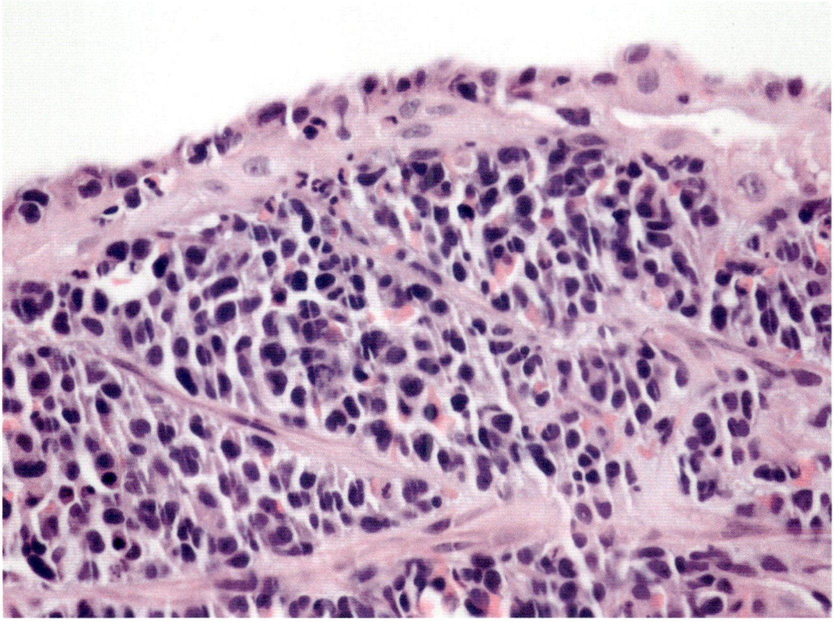

FIGURE 11.13 Higher magnification from endoscopic biopsy in patient with diffuse large B-cell lymphoma, immunoblastic type, shows large tumor cells with hyperchromatic nuclei and abundant rim of plasmacytoid cytoplasm.

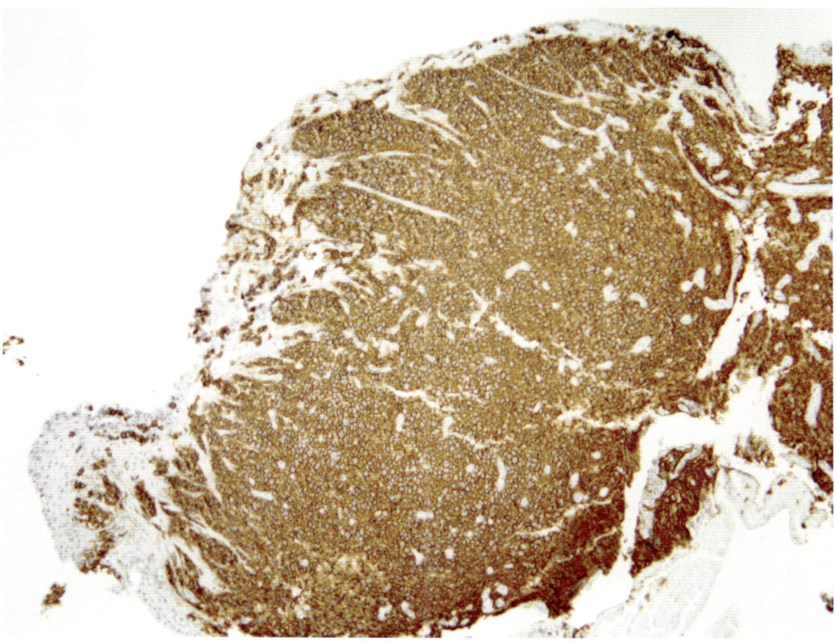

FIGURE 11.14 Immunohistochemical staining for CD20 shows strong cytoplasmic staining of the tumor cells in diffuse large B-cell lymphoma (endoscopic biopsy).

be diagnosed on endoscopic transbronchial biopsies when the tumor involves the bronchial wall. Sometimes, the distinction between DLBCL and MALT lymphoma with increased large cells (but not bona fide transformation to DLBCL) cannot be established with confidence on small endoscopic biopsies. Open or laparoscopic surgery with incisional biopsy, wedge resection, or lobectomy may be required for a more definitive diagnosis. DLBCL must be distinguished from poorly differentiated carcinoma, melanoma, undifferentiated round blue cell sarcomas, and large cell neuroendocrine carcinoma; the distinction can sometimes be problematic on small endoscopic biopsies, particularly when there is prominent crush artifact (Figs. 11.15 and 11.16). Immunohistochemical stains, in particular negative results for cytokeratins, melanocytic markers, and small round blue cell sarcoma–associated markers (CD99, BCOR, ETV4, WT1, etc.) combined with positive staining for leukocyte common antigen (LCA), and CD20 will be of help in this context. Distinction from high-grade LYG may also be quite difficult, particularly when the characteristic angiocentric pattern of involvement of LYG is not present in a small endoscopic biopsy. Demonstration of Epstein-Barr virus (EBV) in the atypical B cells will be of help to properly identify LYG, although EBV+ subtypes of DLBCL exist

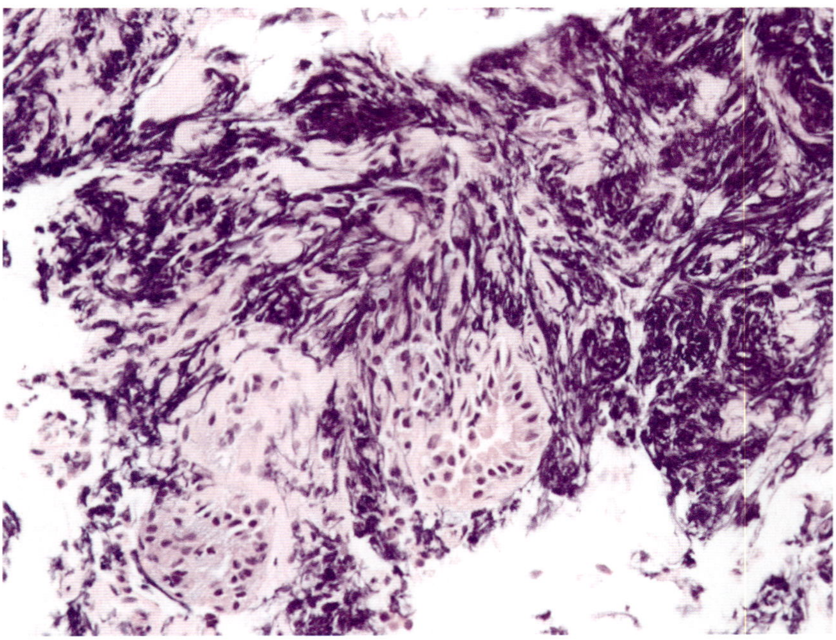

FIGURE 11.15 **Endoscopic biopsy in diffuse large B-cell lymphoma shows prominent crush artifact.** Such cases can be mistaken for small cell lung carcinoma. Use of special stains may be of aid in the correct diagnosis by highlighting the crushed lymphocytes with CD20 and CD45.

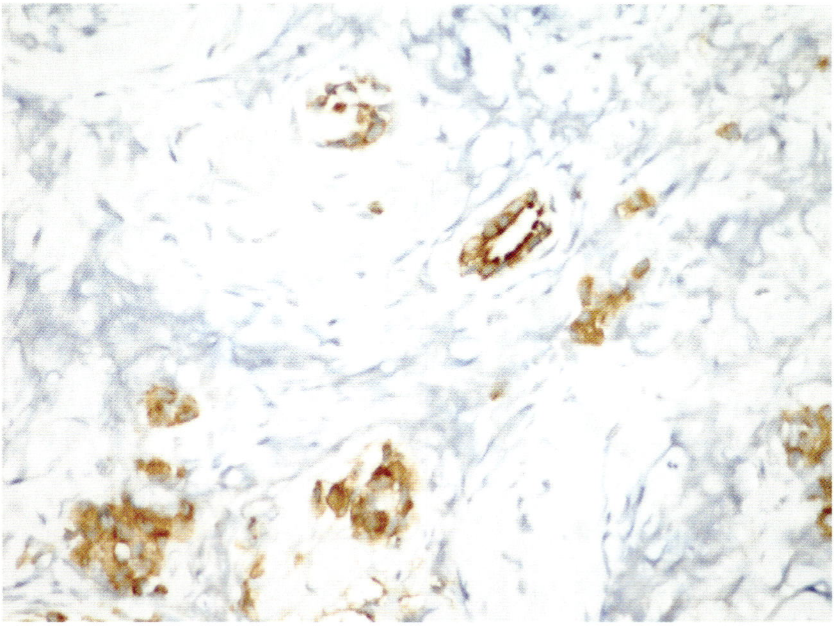

FIGURE 11.16 Immunohistochemical staining for cytokeratin is also of help in the diagnosis of diffuse large cell lymphoma with crush artifact by highlighting the entrapped residual bronchial glands, although the crushed cells that surround them are negative.

as well. Clinical correlation with patient history is important in rare cases of EBV+/CD30+ DLBCL where PTLD may enter the differential.

Additional entities that are important to separate from DLBCL are Burkitt lymphoma, blastoid mantle cell lymphoma, and B-lymphoblastic lymphoma. Helpful markers for Burkitt include BCL2 (negative in Burkitt) and CMYC (positive in the majority of Burkitt tumor cells, more variable expression patterns in many DLBCL cases), and Ki67 (>90% in Burkitt, more variable expression in DLBCL). Useful markers in blastoid mantle cell lymphoma include CD5 (positive in mantle, may be positive or negative in DLBCL), cyclin D1 (positive in majority of mantle cell lymphoma), and SOX11 (expressed in cyclin D1–negative mantle). Commonly requested markers in B-lymphoblastic lymphoma include CD34 and TdT, as these are virtually never expressed in DLBCL. Though as mentioned earlier, these hematologic malignancies rarely involve the lungs.[51,52]

Finally, the workup of DLBCL generally involves fluorescence in situ hybridization testing for *MYC*, *BCL2*, and *BCL6* rearrangements, assuming tissue is left over after exclusion of other large cell tumors and large cell lymphomas, and establishment of the cell of origin classification (by CD10, BCL6, and MUM1 immunohistochemistry). The presence of *MYC* and *BCL2* and/or *BCL6* rearrangements removes the tumor from the category of DLBCL and places it within a specific high-grade B-cell lymphoma with the requisite rearrangements (so-called double and triple hit lymphomas).

Anaplastic Large Cell Lymphoma

ALCL has become increasingly recognized in the lung.[53-58] The tumors may present as peripheral solitary nodules, although cases presenting as an endobronchial lesion have also been described.[59,60] The tumors can be single or multiple and generally present as well-circumscribed nodules. The clinical presentation is similar to that of DLBCL. ALCL can be divided into anaplastic lymphoma kinase (*ALK*)-positive and *ALK*-negative categories, an important distinction, as the *ALK*-negative tumors tend to have a worse prognosis.[1]

The *ALK* gene in ALCL can be involved in various chromosomal translocations that will lead to the formation of chimeric fusion proteins. The most frequent genetic alteration is a translocation between the *ALK* gene on chromosome 2 and the nucleophosmin (*NPM*) gene on chromosome 5, t(2;5)(p23;q35), but more than 10 variant forms have been identified.[61] ALK-negative cases have been shown to have numerous genetic findings, including activating mutations of *JAK1* and *STAT3*, copy number alterations, and chromosomal rearrangements; however, none of these have a role as diagnostic markers as of yet.[1,61,62] For this reason, immunohistochemistry may be more reliable, in the appropriate morphological context, for making a definitive diagnosis because molecular testing for the more common *ALK::NPM* translocation may be negative in a significant percentage of patients.[63,64] More than 90% of cases show clonal rearrangement of the T-cell receptor (*TCR*) genes irrespective of whether the cells express T-cell antigens.

Histologically, the tumors are characterized by sheets of large, anaplastic tumor cells with pleomorphic nuclei and abundant cytoplasm (Fig. 11.17). Multinucleated tumor cells with a wreathlike arrangement of nuclei and prominent eosinophilic nucleoli resembling Reed–Sternberg cells are often present. Cells with horseshoe- or kidney-shaped nuclei (so-called hallmark cells) are characteristic for this condition (Fig. 11.18). Cells showing invaginations of the nuclear membrane resembling nuclear inclusions can also be seen ("doughnut" cells). Occasional tumors can show a prominent component of background epithelioid histiocytes. The anaplastic tumor cells tend to display a cohesive growth pattern that can closely mimic carcinoma, or even a classic Hodgkin lymphoma. Mitotic figures, including abnormal mitoses, are frequently encountered. Eosinophils can sometimes be prominent. Rarely, signet-ring cell forms can also be seen. Some lesions may be accompanied by a prominent stromal response comprising fascicles of spindle cells adopting a vague storiform pattern that can resemble a sarcoma.

The tumors are characterized by the strong immunohistochemical expression of CD30, a mandatory diagnostic finding. The pattern of CD30

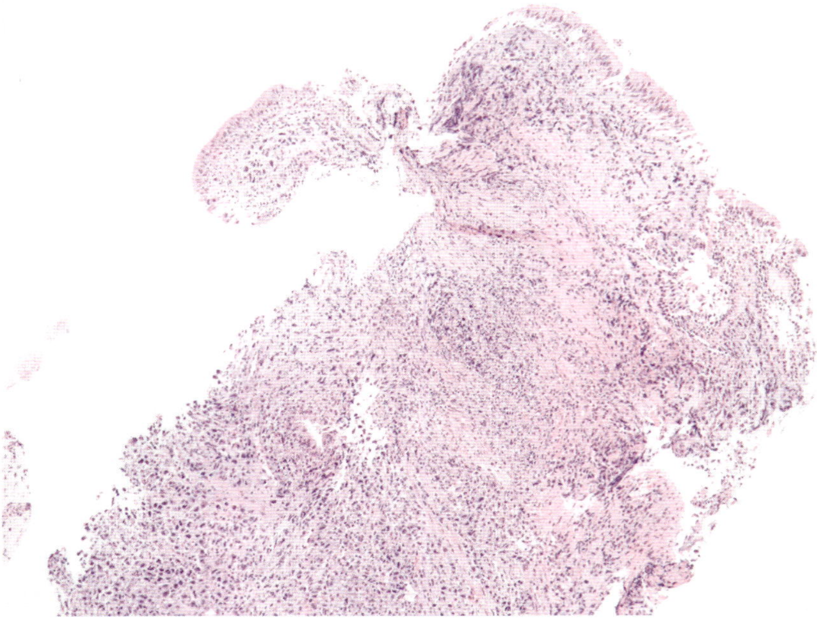

FIGURE 11.17 **Core needle biopsy of the lung in patient with anaplastic large cell lymphoma shows confluent sheets of large tumor cells underneath the bronchial epithelium.** Even at this low magnification, it is possible to appreciate the large size of many of the tumor cells.

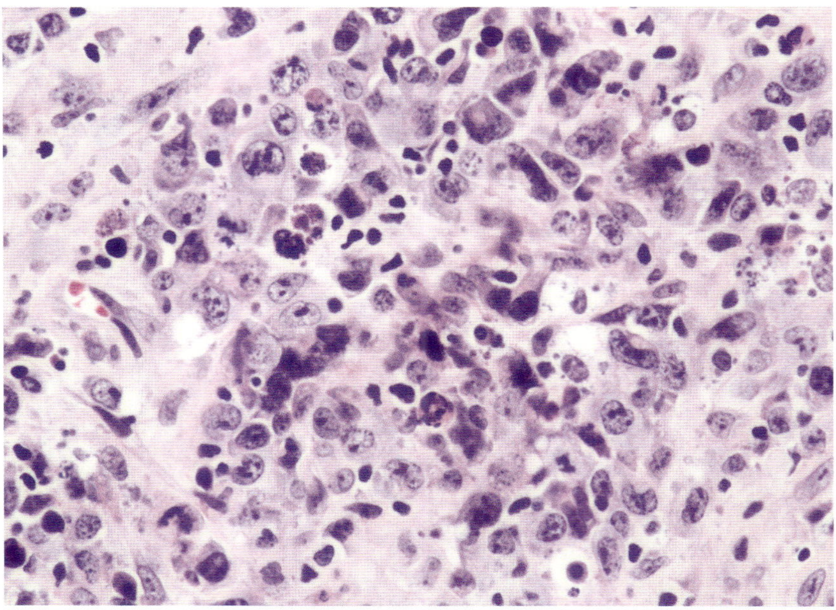

FIGURE 11.18 **Higher magnification of core biopsy in anaplastic large cell lymphoma shows pleomorphic population of cells containing large, irregular nuclei with prominent nucleoli.** Some of the cells show a horseshoe or kidney-shaped configuration (so-called hallmark cells).

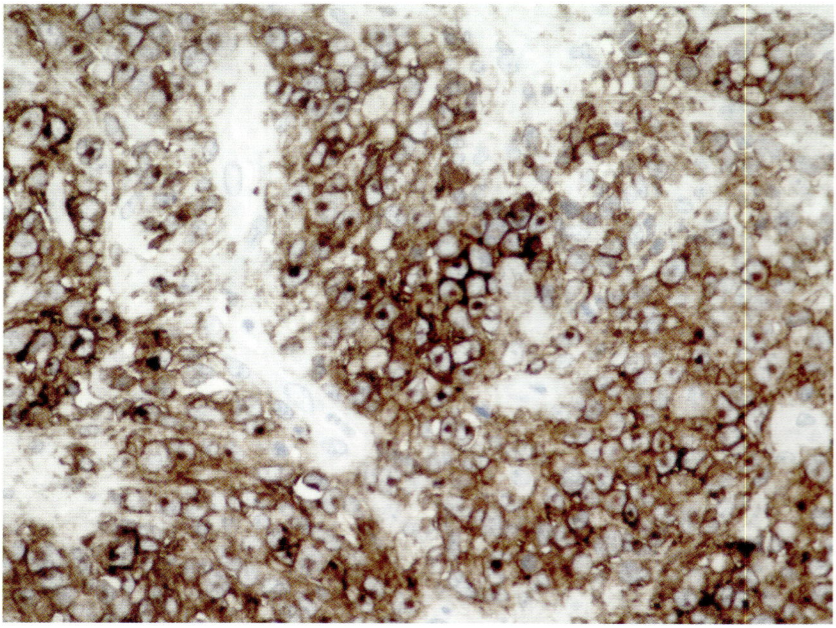

FIGURE 11.19 **Immunohistochemical staining for CD30 in anaplastic large cell lymphoma of the lung shows strong membrane and cytoplasmic staining for this marker.** Notice the dotlike paranuclear positivity in the golgi region in association with the membrane staining. CD15 and ALK-1 can show a similar pattern of staining in these lesions.

staining is membranous and cytoplasmic, with prominent paranuclear dotlike positivity in the Golgi zone (Fig. 11.19). The tumor cells usually express one or more T-cell markers, although some cases may display a "null" phenotype, and present a diagnostic challenge with classic Hodgkin lymphoma; in such cases, dim nuclear PAX5 expression and CD15 expression argue for classic Hodgkin lymphoma, and expression of EMA argues for ALCL. CD3, the most common pan–T-cell marker, and CD8 are often negative in the tumor cells, but stains for CD2, CD4, and CD5 are usually positive in a significant number of cases (>70%). Most cases also show positivity for cytotoxicity-associated antigens such as TIA1, granzyme B, and perforin. The tumor cells are usually positive for CD43.

ALCL can express the ALK1 nuclear and cytoplasmic protein in *ALK*-positive by immunohistochemistry. The ALK1-positive cases are usually also positive for epithelial membrane antigen (EMA).[65] Gene rearrangement studies can be of value in cases that are negative for all T-cell markers tested, particularly in separating classic Hodgkin lymphoma and ALCL that may be difficult to diagnose on small endoscopic biopsies. Immunostaining for CD30 should always be considered in small biopsy samples showing a mixed population containing pleomorphic tumor cells. In situ hybridization for Epstein-Barr virus (EBV) is also useful, as a positive result excludes ALCL. Open lung wedge biopsy or VATS biopsies are the most reliable way for establishing a definitive diagnosis. Peripheral tumors are amenable to diagnosis through percutaneous core biopsies.

Lymphomatoid Granulomatosis

LYG represents a neoplastic clonal proliferation of EBV-infected B cells that are associated with a heavy population of reactive T lymphocytes. The condition was initially described by Liebow et al.[66] More recently, the term "angiocentric immunoproliferative lesion" has been proposed for this condition.[1] It most often affects patients in the sixth decade of life with a small male predominance. Most cases have been associated with immunodeficiency states, including AIDS, organ transplant, and the Wiskott-Aldrich syndrome.[67] The process can involve several organs, including skin, central nervous system, and kidney, but pulmonary involvement is seen in nearly 100% of patients.[68] Patients will show bilateral lung nodules that can measure more than 6 cm in diameter and frequently undergo cavitation.[69,70] The patients can also present with diffuse reticulonodular infiltrates or a solitary lesion.[71] The higher-grade lesions may show IG heavy-chain gene rearrangements.

Histologically, the lesions are characterized by a mixed lymphoid infiltrate predominantly comprising small lymphocytes together with variable numbers of larger, atypical mononuclear lymphoid cells that can be admixed with histiocytes and plasma cells. The large cells can resemble immunoblasts; some of the large cells can also display double-nuclei reminiscent of Reed-Sternberg cells. The term *granulomatosis* is misleading; epithelioid granulomas and multinucleated giant cells are not a feature of these lesions. A hallmark of the process is that the lymphoid infiltrate characteristically shows prominent angiocentrism. The lymphoid cells will tend to surround the wall of pulmonary arteries and veins in a concentric distribution (Fig. 11.20; eFigs. 11.9 and 11.10). Necrosis is a common feature in LYG and can range from focal and minimal to extensive and diffuse. A histologic grading system has been established that is based on the proportion of the atypical large cells to the background T lymphocytes.[72] Grade 1 lesions are polymorphous and contain few EBV-infected B cells (<5 per 10 high-power fields); grade 2 lesions contain an increased number of EBV-infected atypical B cells as well as foci of necrosis and still show marked cellular polymorphism; and grade 3 lesions contain sheets of large, atypical EBV-infected B cells with abundant necrosis, essentially resembling DLBCL.

By immunohistochemistry, LYG shows an abundance of polyclonal CD3+ small T lymphocytes against a background of scattered larger CD20+ B cells (Fig. 11.21). The enlarged, atypical B cells will show strong positivity for EBV by in situ hybridization (ie, EBV-encoded RNA [EBER]; Fig. 11.22).[73] The atypical cells can also react with CD30. The diagnosis of

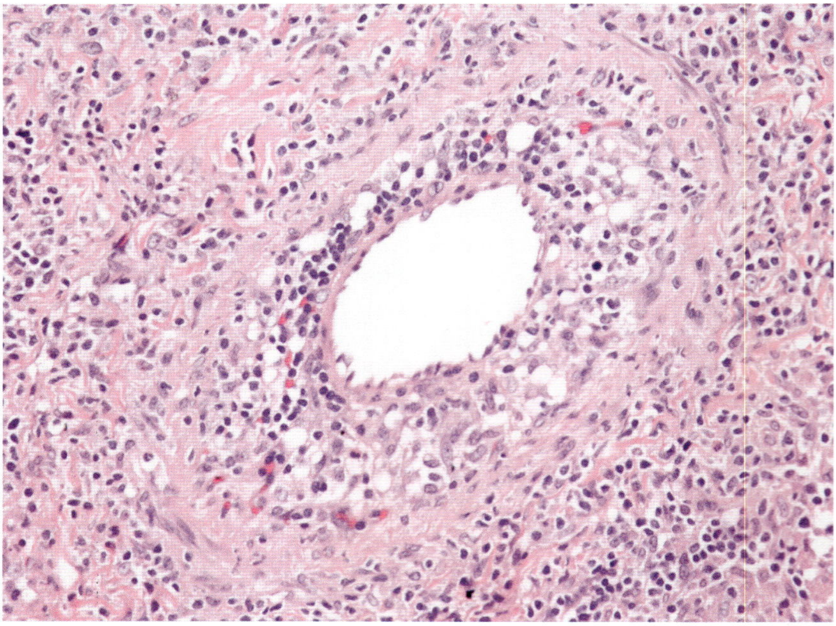

FIGURE 11.20 **Lung biopsy in lymphomatoid granulomatosis shows a polymorphous lymphoid cell infiltrate surrounding a midcaliber vessel.** Notice the extensive infiltration of the vessel wall by atypical lymphoid cells in a concentric distribution.

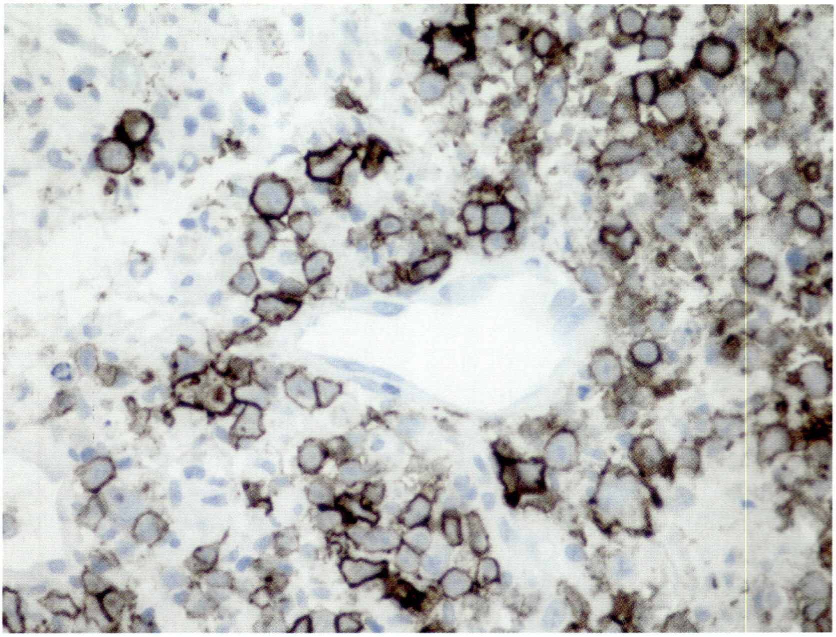

FIGURE 11.21 **Immunohistochemical staining for CD20 highlights enlarged, atypical lymphocytes surrounding the wall of a vessel in lymphomatoid granulomatosis.**

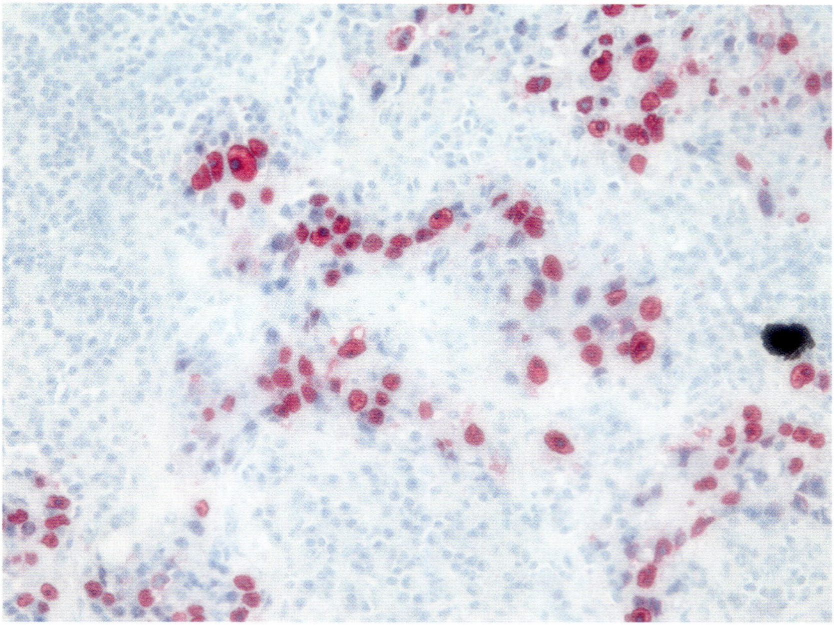

FIGURE 11.22 DNA in situ hybridization shows strong positivity (red signal) for Epstein-Barr virus (EBV-encoded RNA) in the enlarged lymphocytes surrounding a vessel wall in pulmonary lymphomatoid granulomatosis.

LYG may be very difficult on small transbronchial biopsies. Less than 30% of cases are successfully diagnosed on endoscopic biopsies. Sometimes the biopsy will yield only necrotic debris, or the cellular infiltrate in grade 1 lesions may appear quite banal disguising the underlying process. Because of the heavy small T-cell component, it may also be quite difficult to distinguish this process from a T-cell–rich large B-cell lymphoma. Identification of the characteristic angiocentric pattern of involvement of large and midcaliber vessels can be very helpful, although a similar finding can be observed rarely in pulmonary involvement by peripheral T-cell lymphoma. The clinical presentation of multiple, necrotizing nodules in an immunosuppressed patient should also raise the index of suspicion when confronted with a negative yield on an endoscopic biopsy. Open lung biopsy is the most reliable method for making a definitive diagnosis.

Hodgkin Lymphoma

Most cases of HL involving the lung represent secondary involvement of regional or systemic disease, and the diagnosis is generally established on lymph node biopsy. In rare instances, however, HL can be localized to the lung and presents as a primary lesion.[74-78] Presenting symptoms in such cases include fever, night sweats, weight loss, and cough. The disease has a bimodal age distribution, with peaks between 20 to 30 and 60 to 80 years of age, although it can also occur in children.[78] Chest X-rays or CT typically reveal single or multiple or sometimes bilateral nodules that may occasionally show cavitation secondary to necrosis. The tumors may also present as endobronchial lesions.[79]

In lymph nodes, Hodgkin lymphomas occur as classic Hodgkin lymphoma (CHL, of which four subtypes are recognized) and nodular lymphocyte predominant Hodgkin lymphoma (NLPHL or nodular lymphocyte predominant B-cell lymphoma in the terminology of the ICC). NLPHL exists on a morphologic continuum with T-cell/histiocyte–rich large B-cell lymphoma and DLBCL and has a distinct immunophenotype from CHL. As only exceedingly rare case reports of pulmonary lymphocyte-predominant HL exist,[80] this section will focus on CHL.

Histologically, classic Hodgkin lymphoma is characterized by a mixed lymphoid infiltrate that is remarkable for the presence of multinucleated Reed-Sternberg cells and mononuclear Hodgkin cells (collectively known as Hodgkin-Reed-Sternberg or HRS cells) (Figs. 11.23 and 11.24). The background infiltrate can comprise a population of small, bland-appearing small T lymphocytes or a mixture of small lymphocytes with plasma cells, histiocytes, eosinophils, and neutrophils. Four histologic subtypes have been identified: nodular sclerosis, mixed cellularity, lymphocyte rich, and lymphocyte-depleted subtypes (Table 11.2). The nodular sclerosis

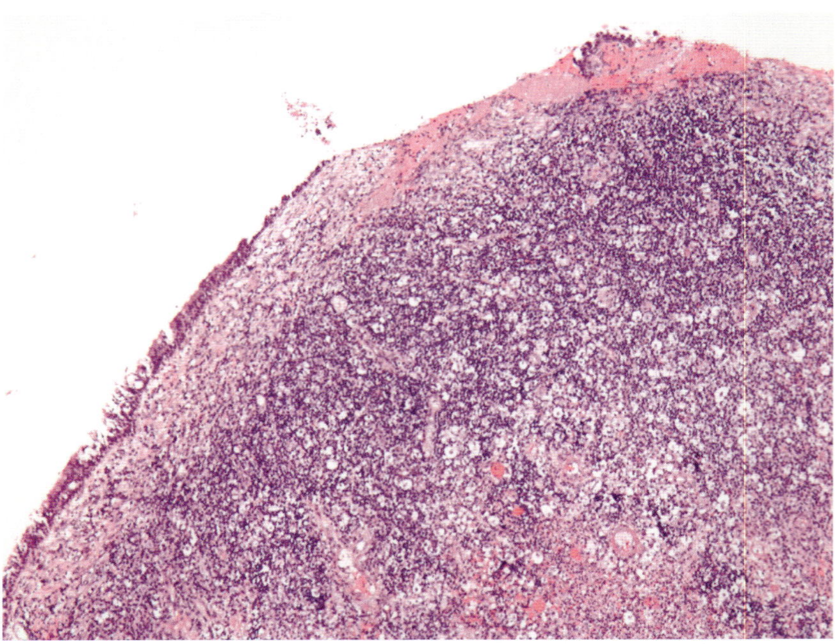

FIGURE 11.23 **Endobronchial biopsy in patient with pulmonary Hodgkin lymphoma shows dense lymphoid cell population underlying the bronchial mucosa.** Endobronchial cases of pulmonary HL are extremely rare, and the diagnosis may be extremely difficult to establish on endoscopic biopsies.

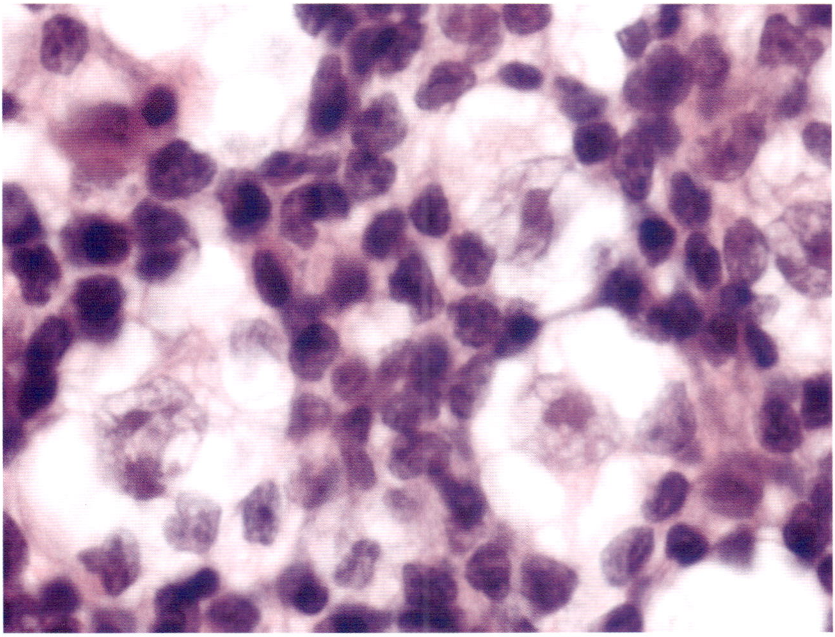

FIGURE 11.24 Higher magnification from endobronchial Hodgkin lymphoma shows multiple lacunar Reed-Sternberg cells displaying large, vesicular nuclei with prominent eosinophilic nucleoli and marked retraction artifact from the surrounding stroma.

and mixed cellularity subtypes are the ones most commonly encountered in the lung (Figs. 11.25 and 11.26).[74]

The classical or diagnostic Reed-Sternberg cell is usually large, with abundant slightly basophilic cytoplasm and at least two nuclear lobes or nuclei (Fig. 11.27). The nuclei are large and contain prominent eosinophilic nucleoli. The cells may contain multiple nuclei and adopt bizarre forms similar to the tumor cells in ALCL. The prototype of the Reed-Sternberg cell is characterized by an "owl-eyed" configuration, where two large nuclei sit in parallel next to each other, each displaying a prominent eosinophilic nucleolus. Mononuclear variants are designated Hodgkin cells and show identical features to the multinucleated types. HRS cells in the nodular sclerosis subtype are characterized by a retraction artifact and are termed *lacunar* cells. HRS cells can undergo apoptosis and appear as a dense, hyperchromatic body ("mummy" cells). Except for the rare lymphocyte-depleted variant, HRS cells are usually few and widely scattered and generally overshadowed by the reactive mixed infiltrate in the background. Pulmonary lesions of HL may undergo extensive necrosis and cavitation. Some cases will form noninfectious epithelioid granulomas; the granulomas can sometimes be observed surrounding the areas of necrosis. The tumors can invade the bronchial wall with destruction of the

TABLE 11.2 Comparison of Types of Hodgkin Lymphomas

Histologic Type	Histology	Type of HRS Cells	Immunophenotype
Nodular lymphocyte-predominant HL (nonclassical)	Nodular or nodular and diffuse Background: small lymphocytes and epithelioid histiocytes	LP cells (“popcorn” cells) (mononuclear cells with folded or multilobated nuclei and small nucleoli)	CD20+, CD45+, BCL-6+, CD79a+, OCT-2+, BOB-1+, EMA+ (in up to 50%) CD15/CD30–
Classic lymphocyte-rich HL	Nodular (or rarely) diffuse Background: small lymphocytes; no eosinophils or neutrophils Small regressed germinal centers	Classical HRS cells (the cells are found within the nodules but not in the germinal centers)	CD30+, CD15+, PAX-5+ CD20/CD45– CD21 highlights regressed germinal centers
Classic nodular sclerosis HL	Nodules separated by dense collagen bands Background: eosinophils, histiocytes, and neutrophils	Lacunar cells (classical HRS with retraction artifact)	CD30+, CD15+, PAX-5+ EBER/LMP EBV+ (10%-40%) CD20/CD45–
Classic mixed cellularity HL	Diffuse growth pattern Background: eosinophils, plasma cells, histiocytes, and neutrophils, may have small granulomas	Classical HRS cells	CD30+, CD15+, PAX-5+ EBER/LMP EBV+ (75%) CD20/CD45–
Classic lymphocyte-depleted HL	Diffuse with predominance of HRS cells over the other elements	Classical HRS cells	CD30+, CD15+ CD20/CD45– T-cell markers negative

EBER, EBV-encoded RNA; EBV, Epstein-Barr virus; EMA, epithelial membrane antigen; HL, Hodgkin lymphoma; HRS, Hodgkin-Reed-Sternberg cells; LMP, latent membrane protein; LP, lymphocyte-predominant.

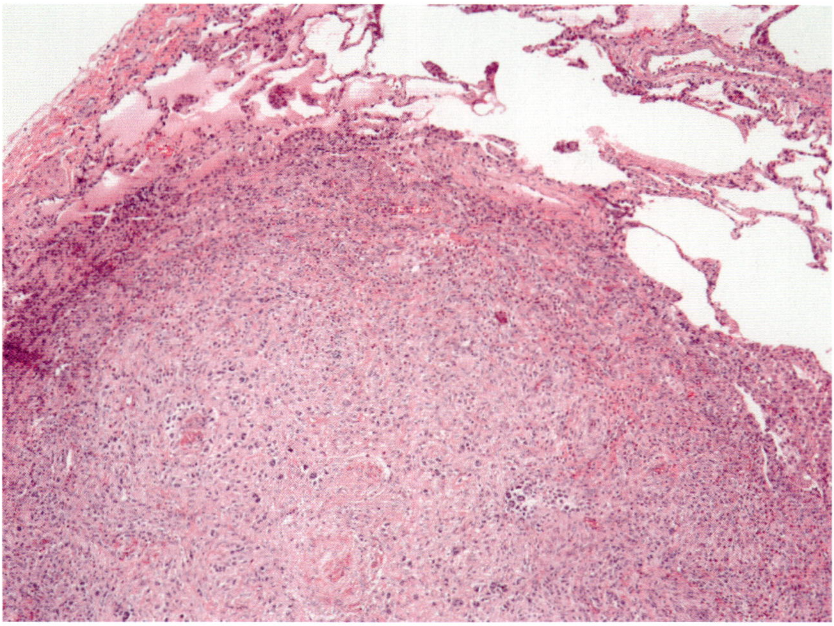

FIGURE 11.25 Wedge biopsy of pulmonary nodule with Hodgkin lymphoma, nodular sclerosis type, shows a well-circumscribed subpleural nodule containing a large cell population admixed with fibrotic stroma.

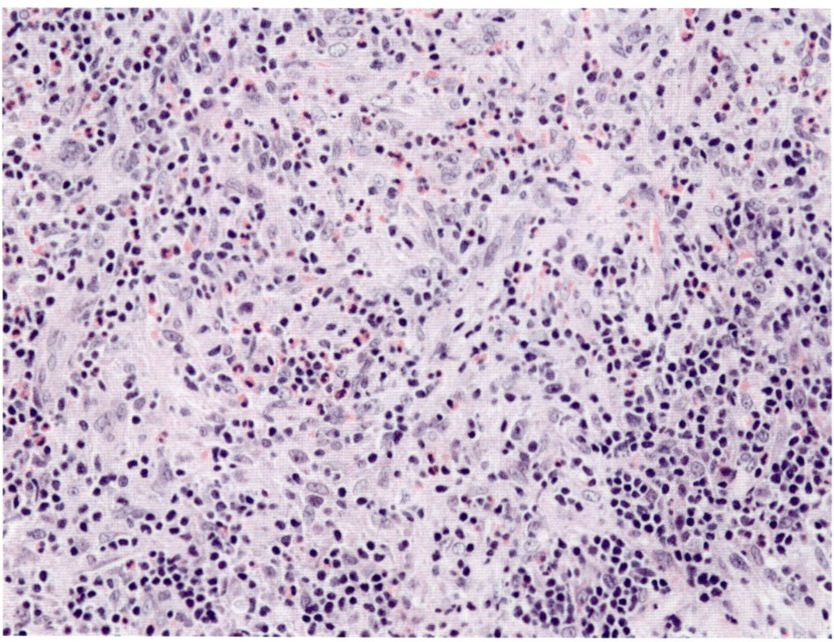

FIGURE 11.26 Hodgkin lymphoma of the lung, mixed cellularity, shows a mixed population of cells comprising small lymphocytes, plasma cells, eosinophils, and scattered larger, atypical mononuclear, and multinucleated Reed-Sternberg cells. The presence of a predominant mixed cellular background is an important clue to the diagnosis in these cases.

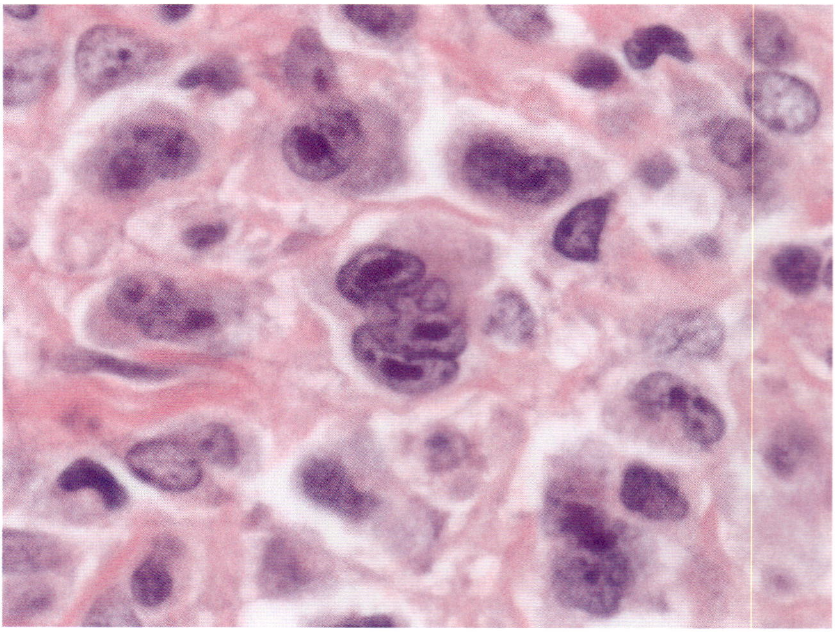

FIGURE 11.27 Classical Hodgkin-Reed-Sternberg cell in pulmonary Hodgkin lymphoma shows three large nuclei with prominent eosinophilic nucleoli surrounded by clear perinuclear halos.

cartilaginous plate or can infiltrate the pleura. The cellular infiltrate can also involve the walls of arteries and pulmonary veins.

Classic HL has been shown to represent a monoclonal B-cell neoplasm derived from B cells.[81] HRS cells are characterized by a distinctive immunophenotype; the cells are positive for CD30 (Fig. 11.28), PAX5 (weak to moderate nuclear expression as discussed below), and CD15 (most cases) and are negative for CD45 and, in the majority of instances, for CD20 (though weak or subset CD20 expression does not preclude the diagnosis).[1] They also do not stain for the transcription factor OCT-2 and its coactivator BOB-1 (these are characteristic features of NLPHL). It is postulated that HRS cells are derived from germinal center B cells that have lost the B-cell–specific expression program and have acquired inappropriate gene products. A strong association between EBV infections has also been demonstrated for classic Hodgkin lymphoma (CHL), particularly in cases of mixed cellularity and, to a lesser extent, nodular sclerosis subtypes. The HRS cells in such cases strongly express EBV-encoded latent membrane protein (LMP) by immunohistochemistry and strongly label for the EBER by in situ hybridization. EBV can also be detected in the plasma in some cases with molecular techniques.[82]

Clonal IG gene rearrangements can be demonstrated in the majority of microdissected HRS cells, supporting the germinal center derivation. Another

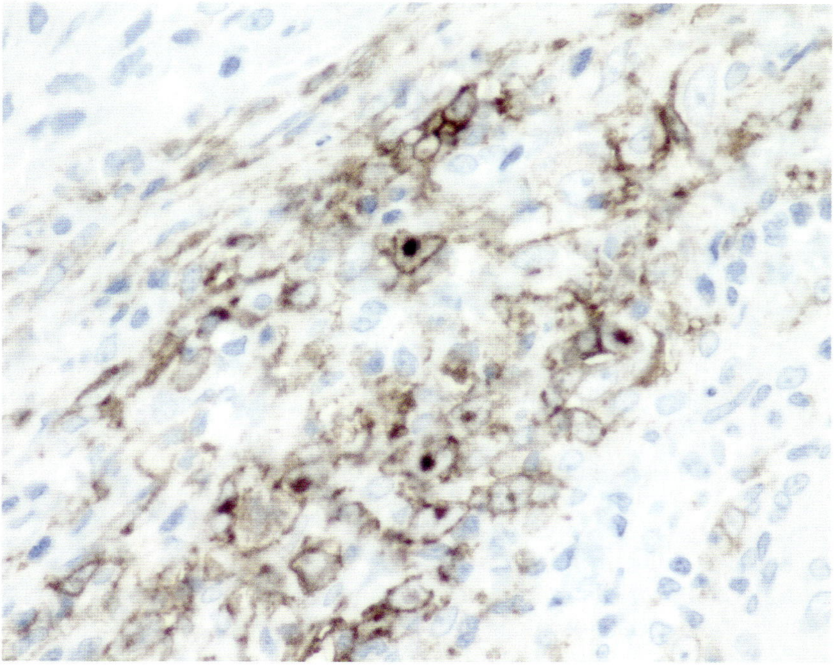

FIGURE 11.28 **Immunohistochemical staining for CD30 in Hodgkin lymphoma shows scattered positive cells admixed with nonreactive lymphocytes and other elements.** Notice the strong cytoplasmic and dotlike paranuclear positivity in the Hodgkin-Reed-Sternberg cells.

marker that can also be of aid for the diagnosis is PAX-5, a B-cell–specific activator protein. The immunostaining of HRS cells in CHL is usually weaker than in reactive B cells, a feature that makes the PAX-5+ HRS cells more easily identifiable. HRS cells typically display a peculiar "rosetting" effect owing to their being surrounded by a peripheral ring of small T lymphocytes. Both CD30 and CD15 are characterized by membrane and paranuclear (dotlike Golgi zone) cytoplasmic positivity. CD30 strongly stains the majority of HRS cells, but CD15 may stain only a few tumor cells or may be absent altogether in some cases. EMA and ALK are usually negative in the HRS cells, though T-cell markers may be expressed and are thought to confer an adverse prognosis.[1]

The main differential diagnosis for pulmonary CHL is with ALCL and CD30+ DLBCL. Because the identification of HRS cells necessary for the diagnosis of CHL can be difficult in small biopsy samples, definitive diagnosis may not be possible in endoscopic or transthoracic core biopsies of the lung. Furthermore, because HRS-like cells may be observed in other conditions, such as small lymphocytic lymphoma/CLL and acute infectious mononucleosis, care must be taken in not overinterpreting such cells out of context. Attention to the background will be indispensable for appropriate interpretation. Small biopsies in which the background infiltrates cannot be adequately assessed may require deferral of the diagnosis to an open biopsy.

Plasmacytoma

Secondary involvement of the lung in multiple myeloma is an infrequent occurrence; primary pulmonary plasmacytoma in the absence of systemic plasma cell dyscrasia is even rarer.[83-85] The tumors affect adult patients between the fifth and the seventh decades. Symptoms include cough, dyspnea, and hemoptysis. The tumors most often present as well-circumscribed, solitary intraparenchymal masses but can also occur in the hilum, as multiple masses, or associated with a prominent endobronchial component.[85,86] Tumors that harbor a peribronchial component or involve at least partially a major bronchus are amenable to endoscopic biopsy diagnosis. Serum monoclonal gammopathy can be identified in some cases; however, approximately 50% of patients with pulmonary plasmacytoma present with nonsecretory tumors.[83]

Histologically, the tumors are characterized by monotonous sheets of plasma cells with few other intervening cellular elements (Fig. 11.29). Germinal centers are usually absent, a feature that facilitates differentiation from MALT lymphoma with plasmacytic differentiation. The plasma

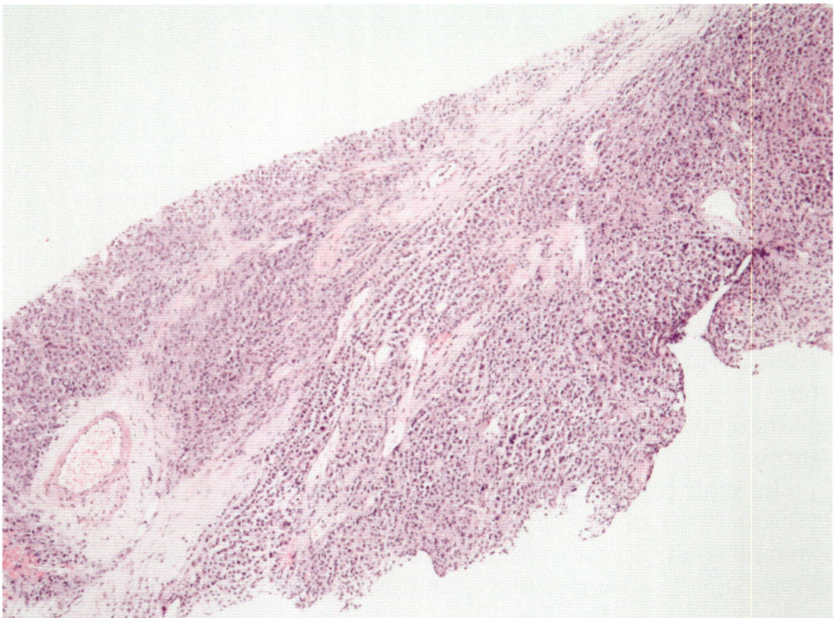

FIGURE 11.29 Needle core biopsy of pulmonary plasmacytoma shows sheets of monotonous small plasmacytoid cells without any intervening lymphoid follicles or germinal centers.

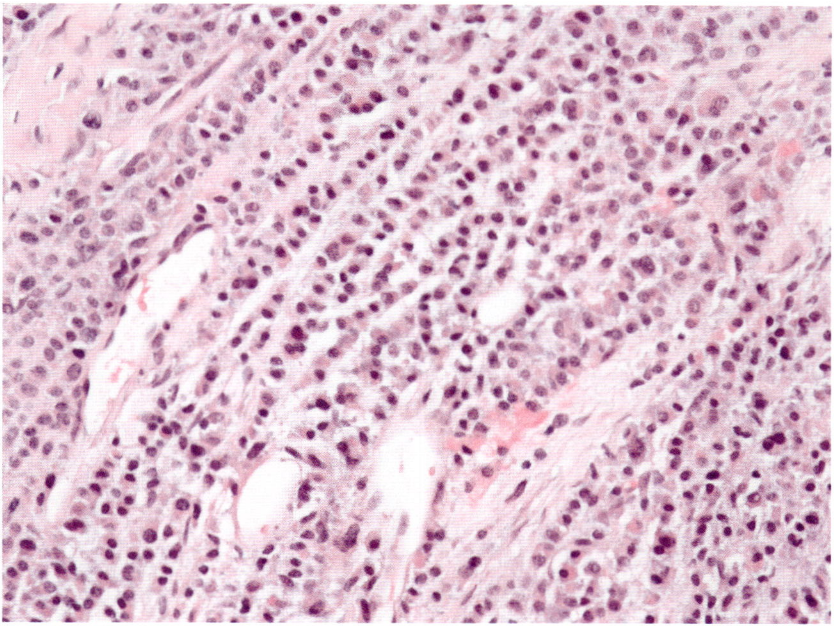

FIGURE 11.30 Higher magnification from a core biopsy of pulmonary plasmacytoma shows sheets of small, mature plasma cells adopting a linear configuration.

cells are usually mature and indistinguishable from benign plasma cells (Fig. 11.30); some cases, however, may show progressive cytologic atypia and loss of plasmacytic differentiation resembling plasmablastic lymphoma or an immunoblastic variant of DLBCL.

Mature plasma cells will generally display uniform, round, eccentrically located nuclei with dispersed chromatin. The cytoplasm is brightly eosinophilic and abundant. Stromal amyloid deposits may be seen in some cases, and rare cases have been reported in association with epithelioid granulomas. Russell bodies can also be frequently observed. Well-differentiated plasmacytomas comprise terminally differentiated B-cells and, as such, will usually be negative for B-cell markers such as CD45 (LCA), CD19, CD20, and PAX5. In the majority of instances, however, they will demonstrate cytoplasmic light chain restriction for κ or λ by paraffin section immunohistochemistry or by in situ hybridization (Fig. 11.31). CD138 (syndecan-1) and MUM1 are other useful markers that will help identify plasma cells on routine immunohistochemistry. Plasma cells may also be positive for EMA, CD56, and CD117. IG light- and heavy-chain genes will show clonal rearrangements.

The diagnosis is usually straightforward on wedge resection or open lung biopsy specimens but may be occasionally difficult in small endoscopic biopsies. Differentiating between MALT lymphoma with plasmacytic differentiation and LPL can be challenging; a descriptive diagnosis and

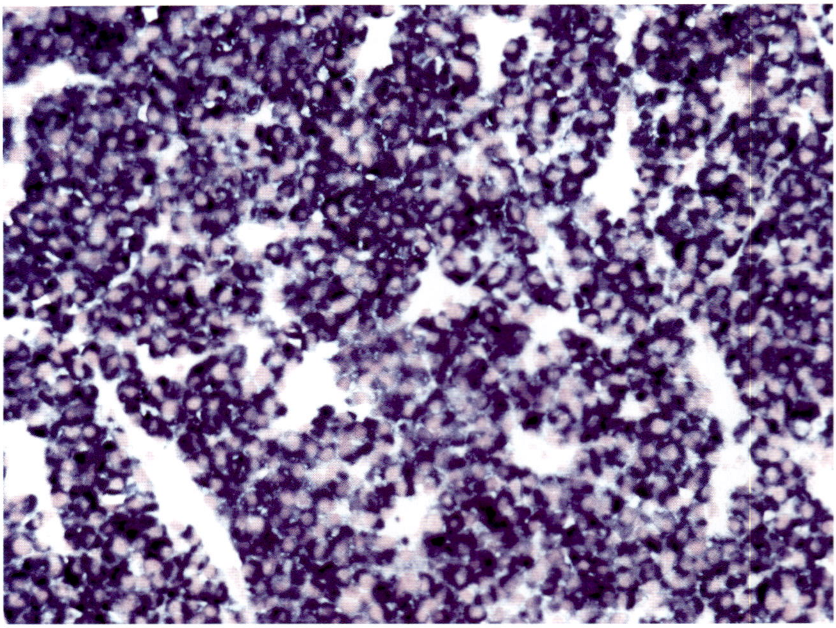

FIGURE 11.31 **DNA in situ hybridization of pulmonary plasmacytoma shows κ light chain restriction.** Notice the intense signal (*blue*) is present in virtually every cell.

differential may be necessary in some cases. The presence of more than 20% of nonplasmacytic lymphocytes in the biopsy sample should raise the possibility of these alternative diagnoses.

Immunohistochemical analysis showing strong positivity for multiple B-cell markers and negativity for CD138 will support a diagnosis of lymphoma over plasmacytoma. Inflammatory myofibroblastic tumor may also pose difficulty because of increased numbers of plasma cells but is differentiated by a polytypic pattern of light chain expression, a significant stromal fibroblastic cell population, and *ALK* (and other less common) gene rearrangements in approximately 50% to 60% of cases.[87] Another condition that deserves consideration in the differential diagnosis is IgG4-related disease. The sheets of plasma cells in IgG4-related disease, however, are polyclonal, and the process is characterized by an increased number of IgG4+ plasma cells, in addition to displaying significant stromal sclerosis.[88]

REFERENCES

1. Swerdlow SH, Campo E, Harris NL, et al. *World Health Organization Classification of Tumours of Hematopoietic and Lymphoid Tissues*. IARC; 2017.
2. Pina-Oviedo S, Roggli VL, Sporn TA, et al. Diagnostic approach to pulmonary B-cell lymphomas in small biopsies, with practical recommendations to avoid misinterpretation. *Diagnostics (Basel)*. 2023;13:3321.

3. Trisolini R, Agli LL, Poletti V. Bronchiolocentric pulmonary involvement due to chronic lymphocytic leukemia. *Haematologica*. 2000;85:1097.
4. Kyrtsonis MC, Angelopoulou MK, Kontopidou FN, et al. Primary lung involvement in Waldenstrom's macroglobulinaemia: report of two cases and review of the literature. *Acta Haematol*. 2001;105:92-96.
5. Kobayashi T, Hyodo M, Honda N. Primary endobronchial Burkitt's lymphoma in a child: a case report. *Int J Pediatr Otorhinolaryngol*. 2013;77:875-878.
6. Thawani R, Chichra A, Mahajan A, Jadhav L. Granulocytic sarcoma of the lung in acute myeloid leukemia. *Indian Pediatr*. 2014;51(2):145-146.
7. WHO Classification of Tumours Editorial Board. *Haematolymphoid Tumours. World Health Organization Classification of Tumours of Hematopoietic and Lymphoid Tissues*. 5th ed. IARC; 2024.
8. Campo E, Jaffe ES, Cook JR, et al. The International Consensus Classification of Mature Lymphoid Neoplasms: a report from the Clinical Advisory Committee. *Blood*. 2022;140:1229-1253.
9. Liebow AA. Definition and classification of interstitial pneumonias in human pathology. *Prog Resp Dis*. 1975;8:1-33.
10. Guinee DG, Franks TJ, Gerbino AJ, Murakami SS, Acree SC, Koss MN. Pulmonary nodular lymphoid hyperplasia (pulmonary pseudolymphoma): the significance of increased numbers of IgG4-positive plasma cells. *Am J Surg Pathol*. 2013;37(5):699-709.
11. Tashtoush B, Okafor NC, Ramirez JF, Smolley L. Follicular bronchiolitis: a literature review. *J Clin Diagn Res*. 2015;9(9):OE01-OE05.
12. Nicholson AG, Wotherspoon AC, Diss TC, et al. Reactive pulmonary lymphoid disorders. *Histopathology*. 1995;26:405-412.
13. Yousem SA, Colby TV, Carrington CB. Follicular bronchitis–bronchiolitis. *Hum Pathol*. 1990;16:700-706.
14. Kinnane BT, Mansell AL, Zwerdling RG, Lapey A, Shannon DC. Follicular bronchitis in the pediatric population. *Chest*. 1993;104:1183-1186.
15. Weinman JP, Manning DA, Liptzin DR, Krausert AJ, Browne LP. HRCT findings of childhood follicular bronchiolitis. *Pediatr Radiol*. 2017;47(13):1759-1765.
16. Pipavath SJ, Lynch DA, Cool C, Brown KK, Newell JD. Radiologic and pathologic features of bronchiolitis. *AJR Am J Roentgenol*. 2005;185(2):354-363.
17. Kobzik L. Benign pulmonary lesions that may be misdiagnosed as malignant. *Semin Diagn Pathol*. 1990;7:129-138.
18. Yell M, Rosado FG. Pulmonary nodular lymphoid hyperplasia. *Arch Pathol Lab Med*. 2019;143(9):1149-1153.
19. Sirajuddin A, Raparia K, Lewis VA, et al. Primary pulmonary lymphoid lesions: radiologic and pathologic findings. *Radiographics*. 2016;36(1):53-70.
20. Koss M, Hochholzer L, Nichols PW, Wehunt WD, Lazarus AA. Primary non-Hodgkin's lymphoma and pseudolymphoma of the lung: a study of 161 patients. *Hum Pathol*. 1983;14:1024-1038.
21. Abbondanzo SL, Rush W, Bijwaard KE, Koss MN. Nodular lymphoid hyperplasia of the lung: a clinicopathologic study of 14 cases. *Am J Surg Pathol*. 2000;24:587-597.
22. Sim J, Koh HH, Choi S, et al. Pulmonary nodular lymphoid hyperplasia with mass-formation: clinicopathologic characteristics of nine cases and review of the literature. *J Pathol Transl Med*. 2018;52(4):211-218.
23. Bois MC, Sekiguchi H, Ryu JH, Yi ES. No definite clinical features of immunoglobulin G4-related disease in patients with pulmonary nodular lymphoid hyperplasia. *Hum Pathol*. 2017;59:80-86.
24. Fang L, Xu J, Wang L, He Z, Lv W, Hu J. Pulmonary nodular lymphoid hyperplasia: a rare benign disease with malignant mask. *Ann Transl Med*. 2019;7(3):43.

25. Arcadu A, Moua T, Yi ES, Ryu JH. Lymphoid interstitial pneumonia and other benign lymphoid disorders. *Semin Respir Crit Care Med.* 2016;37(3):406-420.
26. Marchevsky A, Rosen MJ, Crystal G, Kleinerman J. Pulmonary complications of the acquired immunodeficiency syndrome: a clinicopathologic study of 70 cases. *Hum Pathol.* 1985;16:659-670.
27. Joshi VV, Oleske JM, Minnefor AB, et al. Pathologic pulmonary findings in children with the acquired immunodeficiency syndrome: a study of 10 cases. *Hum Pathol.* 1985;16:241-246.
28. Lynch DA, Travis WD, Müller NL, et al. Idiopathic interstitial pneumonias: CT features. *Radiology.* 2005;236(1):10-21.
29. Panchabhai TS, Farver C, Highland KB. Lymphocytic interstitial pneumonia. *Clin Chest Med.* 2016;37(3):463-474.
30. Swigris JJ, Berry GJ, Raffin TA, Kuschner WG. Lymphoid interstitial pneumonia: a narrative review. *Chest.* 2002;122(6):2150-2164.
31. Koss MN, Hochholzer L, Langloss JM, Wehunt WD, Lazarus AA. Lymphoid interstitial pneumonia: clinicopathological and immunopathological findings in 18 cases. *Pathology.* 1987;19(2):178-185.
32. Nicholson AG, Kim H, Corrin B, et al. The value of classifying interstitial pneumonitis in childhood according to defined histological patterns. *Histopathology.* 1998;33:203-211.
33. Shiota T, Chiba W, Ikeda S, Ikei N. Gene analysis of pulmonary pseudolymphoma. *Chest.* 1993;103(2):335-338.
34. Fiche M, Capron F, Berger F, et al. Primary pulmonary non-Hodgkin's lymphomas. *Histopathology.* 1995;26:529-537.
35. Habermann TM, Ryu JH, Inwards DJ, Kurtin PJ. Primary pulmonary lymphoma. *Semin Oncol.* 1999;26:307-315.
36. Nicholson AG, Wotherspoon AC, Diss TC, et al. Pulmonary B-cell non-Hodgkin's lymphomas. The value of immunohistochemistry and gene analysis in diagnosis. *Histopathology.* 1995;26:395-403.
37. Adis BJ, Hyjek E, Isaacson PG. Primary pulmonary lymphoma: a reappraisal of its histogenesis and its relationship to pseudolymphoma and lymphoid interstitial pneumonia. *Histopathology.* 1998;13:1-17.
38. Li G, Hansmann ML, Zwingers T, Lennert K. Primary lymphomas of the lung: morphological, immunohistochemical and clinical features. *Histopathology.* 1990;16:519-531.
39. Du C, Zhang J, Wei Y, et al. Retrospective analysis of 9 cases of primary pulmonary mucosa-associated lymphoid tissue lymphoma and literature review. *Med Sci Monit Basic Res.* 2018;25:233-240.
40. Boric R, Wislez G, Antoine M, et al. Clinical characteristics and prognostic factors of pulmonary MALT lymphoma. *Eur Respir J.* 2009;34:1408-1416.
41. Stefanovic A, Morgenstern D, Fong T, Lossos IS. Pulmonary marginal zone lymphoma: a single center experience and review of SEER database. *Leuk Lymphoma.* 2008;49:1311-1320.
42. Kurtin RJ, Myers JL, Adlakha H, et al. Pathologic and clinical features of primary pulmonary extranodal marginal zone B-cell lymphoma of MALT type. *Am J Surg Pathol.* 2001;25:997-1008.
43. Upadhaya S, Baig M, Towfiq B, Hadidi SA. Nodular pulmonary amyloidosis with primary pulmonary MALT lymphoma masquerading as metastatic lung disease. *J Community Hosp Intern Med Perspect.* 2017;7(3):185-189.
44. Okabe M, Inagaki H, Oshima K, et al. API2-MALT1 fusion defines a distinctive clinicopathologic subtype in pulmonary extranodal marginal zone lymphoma of mucosa-associated lymphoid tissue. *Am J Surg Pathol.* 2003;162:1113-1122.

45. Schreuder MI, van den Brand M, Hebeda KM, Groenen PJTA, van Krieken JH, Scheijen B. Novel developments in the pathogenesis and diagnosis of extranodal marginal zone lymphoma. *J Hematop*. 2017;10(3-4):91-107.
46. Jandial A, Mishra K, Dey P, et al. Diffuse large B-cell lymphoma: a rare cause of lung consolidation. *Indian J Hematol Blood Transfus*. 2018;34(4):768-771.
47. Horn H, Staiger AM, Vöhringer M, et al. Diffuse large B-cell lymphomas of immunoblastic type are a major reservoir for MYC-IGH translocations. *Am J Surg Pathol*. 2015;39(1):61-66.
48. Hans CP, Weisenburger DD, Greiner TC, et al. Confirmation of the molecular classification of diffuse large B-cell lymphoma by immunohistochemistry using a tissue microarray. *Blood*. 2004;103(1):275-282.
49. Monti S, Savage KJ, Kutok JL, et al. Molecular profiling of diffuse large B-cell lymphoma identifies robust subtypes including one characterized by host inflammatory response. *Blood*. 2005;105(5):1851-1861.
50. Dubois S, Viailly PJ, Mareschal S, et al. Next-generation sequencing in diffuse large B-cell lymphoma highlights molecular divergence and therapeutic opportunities: a LYSA study. *Clin Cancer Res*. 2016;22(12):2919-2928.
51. Chuah KL, Ng SB, Poon L, Yap WM. Plasmablastic lymphoma affecting the lung and bone marrow with CD10 expression and t(8,14)(q24;q32) translocation. *Int J Surg Pathol*. 2009;17:163-166.
52. Gong JZ, Stenzel TT, Bennett ER, et al. Burkitt lymphoma arising in organ transplant recipients: a clinicopathologic study of five cases. *Am J Surg Pathol*. 2003;27:818-827.
53. Yang HB, Li J, Shen T. Primary anaplastic large cell lymphoma of the lung: report of two cases and review of the literature. *Acta Haematol*. 2007;118:188-191.
54. Rush WL, Andriko JA, Taubenberger JK, et al. Primary anaplastic large cell lymphoma of the lung: a clinicopathologic study of five patients. *Mod Pathol*. 2000;13:1285-1292.
55. Xu X. ALK-negative anaplastic large cell lymphoma primarily involving the bronchus: a case report and literature review. *Int J Clin Exp Pathol*. 2014;7:460-463.
56. Von Ende E, Kauffman T, Munoz PA, Martinez-Jiménez S. Primary pulmonary anaplastic large cell lymphoma: a rare malignancy and rare cause of the Luftsichel sign. *Case Rep Radiol*. 2018;2018:8574642.
57. Wang LJ, Wu HB, Zhang Y, Zhou WL, Wang QS. A rare case of neutrophil-rich, ALK-negative anaplastic large cell lymphoma in the lung mimicking a pulmonary abscess on 18F-FDG PET/CT. *Clin Nucl Med*. 2019;44(3):234-237.
58. Han SH, Maeng YH, Kim YS, et al. Primary anaplastic large cell lymphoma of the lung presenting with acute atelectasis. *Thorac Cancer*. 2014;5(1):78-81.
59. Chott A, Kaserer K, Augustin I, et al. Ki-1-positive large cell lymphoma: a clinicopathologic study of 41 cases. *Am J Surg Pathol*. 1998;14:439-448.
60. Guerra J, Echeverria M, Barrio N, Velez-Rosario R. Primary endobronchial anaplastic large cell lymphoma in a pediatric patient. *P R Health Sci J*. 2006;25:159-161.
61. Crescenzo R, Abate F, Lasorsa E, et al. Convergent mutations and kinase fusions lead to oncogenic STAT3 activation in anaplastic large cell lymphoma. *Cancer Cell*. 2015;27(4):516-532.
62. Castellar ERP, Jaffe ES, Said JW, et al. ALK-negative anaplastic large cell lymphoma is a genetically heterogeneous disease with widely disparate clinical outcomes. *Blood*. 2014;124(9):1473-1480.
63. Lamant L, Maggetto F, al Saati T, et al. High incidence of the t(2,5)(p23;q35) translocation in anaplastic large cell lymphoma and its lack of detection in Hodgkin's disease. *Blood*. 1996;87:284-291.
64. Morris SW, Kirstein MN, Valentine MB, et al. Fusion of a kinase gene, ALK, to a nucleolar protein gene, NPM, in non-Hodgkin's lymphoma. *Science*. 1994;263:1281-1284.

65. Delsol G, Al Saati T, Gatter KC, et al. Coexpression of epithelial membrane antigen (EMA), Ki-1, and interleukin-2 receptor by anaplastic large cell lymphomas. Diagnostic value in so-called malignant histiocytosis. *Am J Pathol.* 1988;130(1):59-70.
66. Liebow A, Carrington CR, Friedman PJ. Lymphomatoid granulomatosis. *Hum Pathol.* 1972;3:457-558.
67. Haque AK, Myers JL, Hudnall SD, et al. Pulmonary lymphomatoid granulomatosis in acquired immunodeficiency syndrome: lesions with Epstein–Barr virus infection. *Mod Pathol.* 1998;11:347-356.
68. Song JY, Pittaluga S, Dunkleavy K, et al. Lymphomatoid granulomatosis, a single institute experience: pathologic findings and clinical correlations. *Am J Surg Pathol.* 2015;39:141-156.
69. Koss MN, Hocholzer L, Nichols PW, Wehunt WD, Lazarus AA, Nichols PW. Lymphomatoid granulomatosis: a clinicopathologic study of 42 patients. *Pathology.* 1986;18:283-288.
70. Katzenstein AL, Carrington CB, Liebow AA. Lymphomatoid granulomatosis: a clinicopathologic study of 152 cases. *Cancer.* 1979;43:360-373.
71. Yamanouchi T, Kawanami S, Kamitani T, et al. Lymphomatoid granulomatosis: two different phenotypes of computed tomography findings. *J Thorac Imaging.* 2016;31(6):W80-W82.
72. Lipford EH Jr, Margolick JB, Longo DL, Fauci AS, Jaffe ES. Angiocentric immunoproliferative lesions: a clinicopathologic spectrum of post-thymic T-cell proliferations. *Blood.* 1988;72:1674-1681.
73. Guinee D Jr, Jafee ES, Kingma D, et al. Pulmonary lymphomatoid granulomatosis: evidence for a proliferation of Epstein–Barr virus infected B-lymphocytes with a prominent T-cell component and vasculitis. *Am J Surg Pathol.* 1994;18:753-764.
74. Yousem SA, Weiss LM, Colby TV. Primary pulmonary Hodgkin's disease: a clinicopathologic study of 15 cases. *Cancer.* 1986;57:1217-1224.
75. Lowenthal BM, Xu X, Subash M, Jih LJ. Hodgkin's lymphoma with unusual pulmonary presentations: reporting two cases. *Indian J Pathol Microbiol.* 2017;60(2):272-274.
76. Foderaro AE, Reagan JL. Hodgkin lymphoma mimicking lung abscess. *Blood.* 2016;128(25):3011.
77. Rodriguez J, Tirabosco R, Pizzolitto S, Rocco M, Falconieri G. Hodgkin lymphoma presenting with exclusive or preponderant pulmonary involvement: a clinicopathologic study of 5 new cases. *Ann Diagn Pathol.* 2006;10(2):83-88.
78. Urasinski T, Kamienska E, Gawlikowska-Sroka A, et al. Pediatric pulmonary Hodgkin lymphoma: analysis of 10 years data from a single center. *Eur J Med Res.* 2010;15(suppl 2):206-210.
79. Harper PG, Fisher C, McLennan K, Souhami RL. Presentation of Hodgkin's disease as an endobronchial lesion. *Cancer.* 1984;53:147-150.
80. Soliman M, Neemuchwala F, Sankar A, et al. Multiple cavitary lung lesions in an adolescent: case report of a rare presentation of nodular lymphocyte predominant Hodgkin lymphoma. *J Pediatr Hematol Oncol.* 2018;40(7):e454-e457.
81. Marafioti T, Hummel M, Foss HD, et al. Hodgkin and Reed–Sternberg cells represent an expansion of a single clone originating from a germinal center B-cell with functional immunoglobulin gene rearrangements but defective immunoglobulin transcription. *Blood.* 2000;95:1443-1450.
82. Meyer RM. EBV DNA: a Hodgkin lymphoma biomarker? *Blood.* 2013;121(18):3541-3542.
83. Koss MN, Hochholzer L, Moran CA, Frizzera G. Pulmonary plasmacytomas: a clinicopathologic and immunohistochemical study of five cases. *Ann Diagn Pathol.* 1998;2:1-11.

84. Morinaga S, Watanabe H, Gemma A, et al. Plasmacytoma of the lung associated with nodular deposits of immunoglobulins. *Am J Surg Pathol.* 1987;11:989-995.
85. Etienne G, Grenouillet M, Ghiringhelli C, et al. Plasmocytome pulmonaire: à propos de deux nouvelles observations et revue de la literature [in French]. *Rev Méd Interne.* 2004;25(8):591-595.
86. Edelstein E, Gal AA, Mann KP, Miller JI Jr, Mansour KA. Primary solitary endobronchial plasmacytoma. *Ann Thorac Surg.* 2004;78:1448-1449.
87. Antonescu CR, Suurmeijer AJ, Zhang L, et al. Molecular characterization of inflammatory myofibroblastic tumors with frequent ALK and ROS1 fusions and rare novel RET gene rearrangement. *Am J Surg Pathol.* 2015;39(7):957-967.
88. Zen Y, Inoue D, Kitao A, et al. IgG4-related lung and pleural disease: a clinicopathologic study of 21 cases. *Am J Surg Pathol.* 2009;33:1886-1893.

12

EPITHELIAL LUNG NEOPLASMS

Epithelial lung neoplasms are the most common type of lung cancer and are amenable to sampling by several techniques. Lung cancer in general remains the leading cause of cancer-related death in the world, with the World Health Organization (WHO) and International Agency for Research on Cancer estimating approximately 2.5 million new lung cancer diagnoses and over 1.8 million deaths from the disease in 2022.[1-5] It goes to follow that pulmonary pathologists will see many endoscopic and core needle biopsies for lung carcinoma in routine practice. Core needle and open biopsies are indicated for peripheral tumors located away from the main bronchi; endoscopic biopsies will usually yield adequate diagnostic material for the majority of central lesions. Because many lung tumors are found in advanced stages precluding surgical removal, the initial biopsy is sometimes the only diagnostic tissue available and the one on which all future management of the patient will rest, particularly if a patient is not amenable to rebiopsy to procure additional tissue. This is a particularly important consideration in the era of molecular diagnostics, where proper triaging of the tissue may be critical for the diagnosis and management of the patient. Carcinoma of the lung can arise from the squamous epithelium lining the main bronchi, from respiratory epithelium, including the lining of the alveoli and bronchial adnexa, and from specialized cells within the walls of the bronchial tree such as neuroendocrine cells. The most common and widely accepted classification system for lung carcinoma is the 2021 WHO classification of tumors of the lung, pleura, thymus, and heart; though it is expected that some modifications will be introduced in the upcoming 2026-2027 update of the WHO.[6] This system was partially adopted from the International Association for the Study of Lung Cancer/American Thoracic Society/European Respiratory Society (IASLC/ATS/ERS) international multidisciplinary classification of lung adenocarcinoma,[7] with additional revisions to the classification of squamous cell carcinoma (SCC) (Table 12.1). The WHO and IASLC/ATS/ERS have also outlined an updated criterion for the reporting of lung biopsy terminology (Table 12.2).[6,7] It is also worth noting that a new system specifically designed for reporting lung cytopathology has also been created, though evaluation of cytologic specimens is not covered

TABLE 12.1 2021 WHO Classification of Epithelial Lung Neoplasms Excluding Neuroendocrine Tumors

Classification of Lung Adenocarcinoma in Resection Specimens
Preinvasive lesions:
Atypical adenomatous hyperplasia (<0.5 cm)
Adenocarcinoma in situ (<3 cm, noninvasive)
Mucinous
Nonmucinous
Minimally invasive adenocarcinoma (<3 cm overall, lepidic-predominant tumor with <5 mm invasion)
Mucinous
Nonmucinous
Invasive nonmucinous adenocarcinoma:
Lepidic predominant adenocarcinoma
Acinar predominant adenocarcinoma
Papillary predominant adenocarcinoma
Micropapillary predominant adenocarcinoma
Solid predominant adenocarcinoma
Variants of invasive adenocarcinoma:
Invasive mucinous adenocarcinoma
Colloid adenocarcinoma
Fetal adenocarcinoma
Enteric adenocarcinoma
Classification of Lung Squamous Cell Carcinoma in Resection Specimens
Preinvasive lesions:
Squamous dysplasia
Squamous cell carcinoma in situ
Squamous cell carcinoma:
Keratinizing squamous cell carcinoma
Nonkeratinizing squamous cell carcinoma
Basaloid (small cell variant) squamous cell carcinoma
Lymphoepithelial carcinoma
NUT carcinoma (listed in "other epithelial tumors" category in WHO)
Classification of Other Lung Tumors in Resection Specimens
Adenosquamous carcinoma (listed as own category in WHO)
Large cell carcinoma (listed as own category in WHO)

(continued)

TABLE 12.1 2021 WHO Classification of Epithelial Lung Neoplasms Excluding Neuroendocrine Tumors (*continued*)
Sarcomatoid carcinomas:
Pleomorphic carcinoma
Spindle cell carcinoma
Giant cell carcinoma
Carcinosarcoma
Pulmonary blastoma
Salivary gland tumors:
Mucoepidermoid carcinoma
Adenoid cystic carcinoma
Epithelial-myoepithelial carcinoma
Pleomorphic adenoma/myoepithelioma
Hyalinizing clear cell carcinoma
Myoepithelioma and myoepithelial carcinoma

NOTE: The WHO lung epithelial tumor classification may change based on modifications to the forthcoming 2026-2027 WHO edition of thoracic tumors.

WHO, World Health Organization.

Reprinted from Nicholson AG, Tsao MS, Beasley MB, et al. The 2021 WHO Classification of Lung Tumors: impact of advances since 2015. *J Thorac Oncol*. 2022;17(3):362-387, with permission from Elsevier.

TABLE 12.2 Consensus Recommendations for Small Biopsies
Classification of Lung Carcinoma in Small Biopsy Specimens
Morphologic adenocarcinoma patterns clearly present:
Adenocarcinoma: describe identifiable patterns present (including micropapillary)
Adenocarcinoma with lepidic pattern (if pure, add note that invasive component cannot be excluded)
Mucinous adenocarcinoma
Adenocarcinoma with fetal pattern
Adenocarcinoma with colloid pattern
Adenocarcinoma with (describe pattern) and signet ring cell features
Adenocarcinoma with (describe pattern) and clear cell features
Morphologic adenocarcinoma patterns not present but supported by special stains:
Non–small cell carcinoma, favor adenocarcinoma

TABLE 12.2 Consensus Recommendations for Small Biopsies (*continued*)
Morphologic squamous cell patterns clearly present: Squamous cell carcinoma
Morphologic squamous cell patterns not present but supported by special stains: Non–small cell carcinoma, favor squamous cell carcinoma
Morphologic squamous cell and adenocarcinoma patterns present: Non–small cell carcinoma, with squamous cell and adenocarcinoma patterns. Comment: this could represent adenosquamous carcinoma
No morphologic or immunohistochemical evidence of adenocarcinoma or squamous cell carcinoma (or other) lineage present: Non–small cell carcinoma, not otherwise specified
Morphologic squamous cell and adenocarcinoma patterns not present but immunostains favor separate glandular and squamous components: Non–small cell carcinoma, not otherwise specified (specify results of the immunohistochemistry and the interpretation). Comment: this could represent adenosquamous carcinoma
Sarcomatoid carcinoma: Poorly differentiated non–small cell lung carcinoma with spindle and/or giant cell features (mention if conventional adenocarcinoma or squamous cell carcinoma is present)

WHO, World Health Organization.

in this book.[8] Finally, although we recognize neuroendocrine carcinomas are derived from neuroepithelial elements and, as such, belong in the family of epithelial neoplasms, they will be dealt with separately in Chapter 13 owing to the highly specialized nature of their particular line of differentiation.[9,10]

Although the classification of epithelial neoplasms on lung resection specimens has become relatively standardized, evaluation of neoplastic processes on biopsy material presents numerous challenges for proper interpretation. The diagnosis of lung carcinoma, in particular for tumors that are not very well differentiated, can be fraught with difficulties in small biopsy samples. For several decades, the diagnosis of non–small cell lung carcinoma (NSCLC) versus small cell lung carcinoma was all that the physician submitting the biopsy sample may have been interested in. This approach was acceptable in the prepersonalized medicine era where patients were stratified for treatment based solely on this distinction. In the past, as many as 10% to 30% of cases were diagnosed generically as

NSCLC, not otherwise specified (NOS).[11-13] This has changed in the last few decades with the advent of more robust immunohistochemical stains and molecular diagnostics that have allowed pathologists to increase the number of cases classified as adenocarcinoma or SCC. Currently, the appropriate classification of lung carcinoma has become highly significant for clinical decision making as targeted therapies are now available for many different tumor types.[14]

Some basic principles need to be acknowledged when dealing with limited biopsy sample material for the diagnosis of lung cancer: **(1)** The diagnosis rendered on a limited biopsy sample cannot accurately predict what the remainder of the tumor will look like or its exact cellular composition; variations in degrees of differentiation or tumors with mixed histology cannot be predicted from the findings in a small biopsy; **(2)** lung cancer, in particular NSCLC, is notorious for its heterogeneity and a precise and definitive diagnosis may not be possible on a limited small biopsy sample; **(3)** poorly differentiated malignancies may be difficult to precisely categorize on small tissue samples, even with special techniques; **(4)** tumors of mixed histogenesis containing combined elements (ie, carcinosarcoma, biphasic pulmonary blastoma, adenosquamous carcinoma) may not show all of their components in a small biopsy and a higher-grade or more aggressive component could be missed; **(5)** endoscopic and core biopsies may be prone to artifactual distortion that can be extensive and preclude a definitive diagnosis; **(6)** small biopsy samples may not be adequate for counting mitoses per 10 high-power fields, thus limiting the use of such criterion for precise subclassification of certain types of neoplasms based on current diagnostic standards (ie, neuroendocrine tumors). **(7)** Tissue conservation is of utmost importance in lung biopsies because of the need for multiple types of testing modalities (light microscopy, immunohistochemistry [IHC], targeted polymerase chain reaction assays, and next-generation sequencing); whenever possible, at the time of tissue procurement, it is always prudent to separate the samples into separate tissue blocks if multiple cores are available (Fig. 12.1); **(8)** appropriate laboratory protocols should be instituted for optimized processing of lung tissue biopsy specimens; for example, two glass slides with one to three profiles per glass slide is generally adequate for H&E diagnosis; three glass slides with six or more tissue profiles per slide may exhaust the entire core needle biopsy before any ancillary testing may be performed (Fig. 12.2).

IMMUNOHISTOCHEMISTRY TESTING IN LUNG CARCINOMA BIOPSIES

IHC is an indispensable tool for tumor classification and evaluation of diagnostic and predictive biomarkers in lung carcinoma. Several immunohistochemical panels have been proposed for the evaluation of small biopsies and for making the distinction between adenocarcinoma and SCC.[15,16] The search for the elusive optimal panel is made more difficult by the

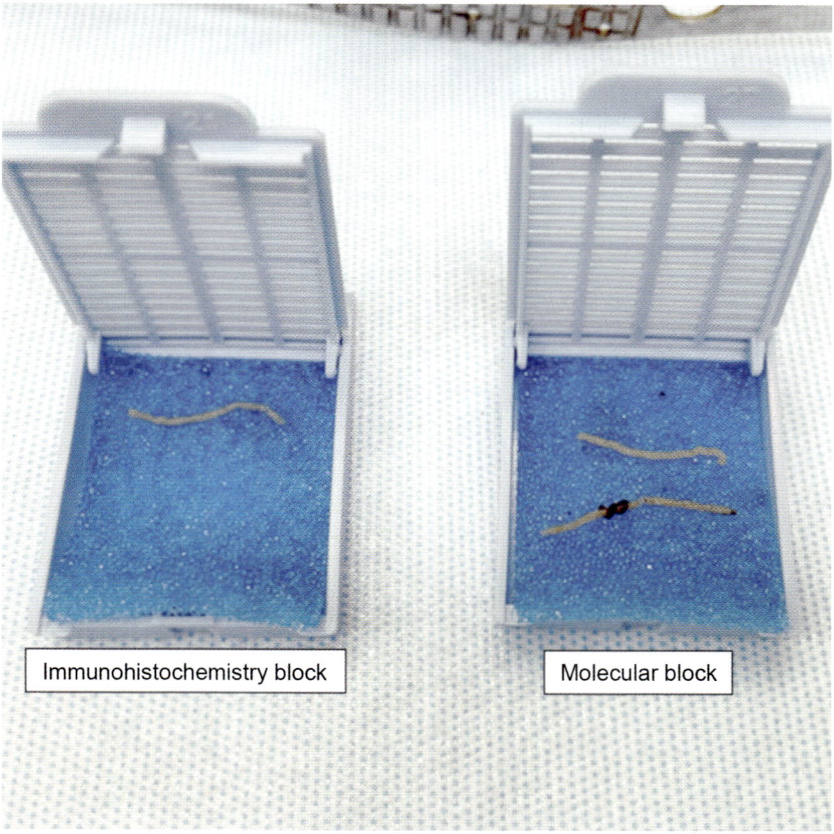

FIGURE 12.1 **Diagram depicting appropriate triage of core needle biopsy specimens into processing cassettes.** In this case, one core is separated into a cassette to create a tissue block for microscopic evaluation and immunohistochemistry, while the other two cores are separated into a second cassette to create a tissue block for molecular testing. If the first tissue block is nondiagnostic and does not contain tumor, the second block may be used.

lack of strict specificity of most of the markers currently in use for either lines of differentiation or for their capability for distinguishing between a primary tumor of lung origin and a metastasis from an extrapulmonary carcinoma. Most studies recommend a mixture of p63/p40 and CK5/6 as markers of squamous differentiation and thyroid transcription factor-1 (TTF-1) and napsin A as adenocarcinoma markers. It goes without saying that these markers must be evaluated in the context of appropriate laboratory protocols and controls.[15-19]

It is important to point out a few caveats with regard to these IHC markers. P63 has been shown to react with lung adenocarcinoma in a significant percentage of cases.[20] Another limitation of p63 is its strong expression in large cell lymphomas, a finding observed in approximately

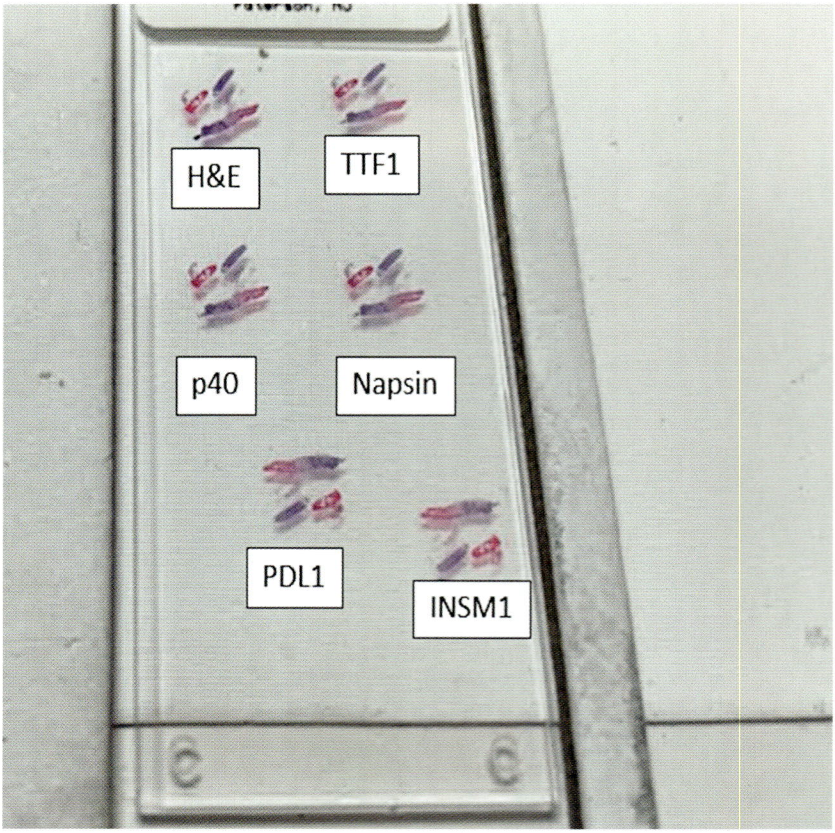

FIGURE 12.2 **Example of a glass slide with six total tissue profiles.** In this particular case, the tumor was evident on the initial tissue profile. The labels beneath each tissue profile indicate what the ideal workup of this case would have been instead of one slide with six tissue profiles.

50% of pulmonary lymphoma cases that can be confused morphologically for anaplastic or poorly differentiated NSCLC.[21] More recent studies have shown that a p63 isoform–p40 (ΔNp63)–shows much higher specificity and sensitivity for SCC and does not appear to react with adenocarcinoma cells and other tumors, thus representing a much better choice for immunohistochemical evaluation of squamous differentiation in lung cancer biopsies.[22-25] TTF-1–a transcription factor expressed in lung epithelial cells and thyroid follicular epithelium–has been acknowledged as a helpful and sensitive marker for the diagnosis of lung adenocarcinoma. However, its specificity is not restricted to primary lung adenocarcinoma, and a few studies have reported reactivity in SCCs and other tumor types such as lymphomas with some antibodies.[18,26] This may be related to the fact that multiple different antibody clones exist for TTF-1 with much variability in the antibodies used by different labs; clones SPT24 and SP141 are more sensitive but overall less specific for lung adenocarcinoma, while clone 8G7G3/1 is less sensitive but more specific for lung adenocarcinoma.[27] Likewise, napsin A–an epithelial marker commonly expressed in up to 80% of lung adenocarcinomas–has also been shown to be positive in lung SCC as well as in the epithelial cells in numerous other organ systems.[19,28-32] Caution, therefore, should be exercised in making purely "immunohistochemical" diagnoses based on the results of these stains in isolation of the morphologic and clinical context.

IHC for predictive pulmonary biomarkers has also become important in recent years and is now accepted as a screening tool for identifying underlying molecular alterations. For the sake of simplicity, we will restrict the discussion to the use of IHC for the most commonly tested biomarkers, PD-L1, anaplastic lymphoma kinase (ALK), and ROS1. However, it is important to note that other biomarkers are also available, including immunostains for epidermal growth factor receptor (EGFR) (no longer recommended for routine use); serine/threonine-protein kinase B-Raf (BRAF), and neurotrophic tyrosine receptor kinase (NTRK), which may also be requested by clinicians from time to time. These IHC stains generally serve as a low-cost screening test for particular genetic abnormalities that are targetable with specific therapies or, in the case of PD-L1, that can help predict tumor response to immunotherapies. The use of these markers is heavily dependent on pre- and postanalytic variables (such as specimen fixation or the particular antibody used), and pathologists should become familiar with the specific antibodies and performance characteristics of the assays used in their laboratories.[33]

ALK IHC is used to detect genomic rearrangements of the *ALK* gene, which occur in 1% to 5% of NSCLCs.[34] ALK IHC is generally scored using a +1/+2/+3 system.[33] Tumors with *ALK* rearrangements will generally show positivity for ALK IHC within all the tumor cells. In general, cases that display strong staining intensity have shown *ALK* rearrangements by confirmatory fluorescence in situ hybridization (FISH) testing or molecular testing.[34] One particular pitfall related to ALK IHC is that *ALK*-rearranged tumors may display signet ring cell morphology in which the intracytoplasmic mucin droplets can obscure the ALK staining; a similar pitfall occurs with ROS1 IHC.[34,35]

ROS1 IHC is used to detect genomic rearrangements of the *ROS1* gene that occur in 1% to 2% of NSCLCs.[36] Similar to ALK IHC, ROS1 IHC is generally scored using a +1/+2/+3 system, and tumors with rearrangements should show staining within all of the tumor cells.[33] Tumors displaying strong staining will usually show positive results by confirmatory molecular tests. In addition, it shares the same pitfalls with ALK; tumors with *ROS1* rearrangements will often display signet ring cell morphology that can obscure positive staining.[37]

NTRK IHC may be potentially used to screen NSCLC for fusions involving the *NTRK* gene. *NTRK* gene fusions are extremely rare in NSCLC and occur almost exclusively in adenocarcinoma histology, occurring at a rate of 0.1% to 3% of NSCLC.[38] Targeted treatments are available so the *NTRK* fusion status is of particular interest in tumors that do not display any of the more common genetic alterations found in NSCLC. However, it should be noted that NTRK immunohistochemical positivity and protein expression has been documented in the absence of underlying NTRK fusions casting some doubt on the utility of NTRK IHC.[38]

PD-L1 IHC is used to predict tumoral response to immunotherapy agents including pembrolizumab, nivolumab, and atezolizumab, among others.[39] In general, scoring of PD-L1 IHC is based on different cutoffs of positive overall tumor cell staining (tumor proportion score of 1%, 5%, and 50%) based on numerous different clinical trials that examined tumor response in relation to these values.[40-43] Cells with complete membranous or partial membranous staining at any intensity should be counted as positive (Fig. 12.3A and B).[39] It is important to note that multiple different antibodies with slightly different performance characteristics exist for PD-L1, which are associated with specific assays (i.e., the 22C3 mouse antibody and pembrolizumab IHC assay).[44] In addition, there are numerous pitfalls with scoring PD-L1 staining in biopsy samples; PD-L1 immunostaining may be positive in endothelial cells, lymphocytes, macrophages, and other inflammatory cells (Fig. 12.3C). These can sometimes be intimately admixed with tumor cells, falsely increasing the apparent percentage of positive tumor cells.[45,46] Sampling is also an issue on biopsy material as

A

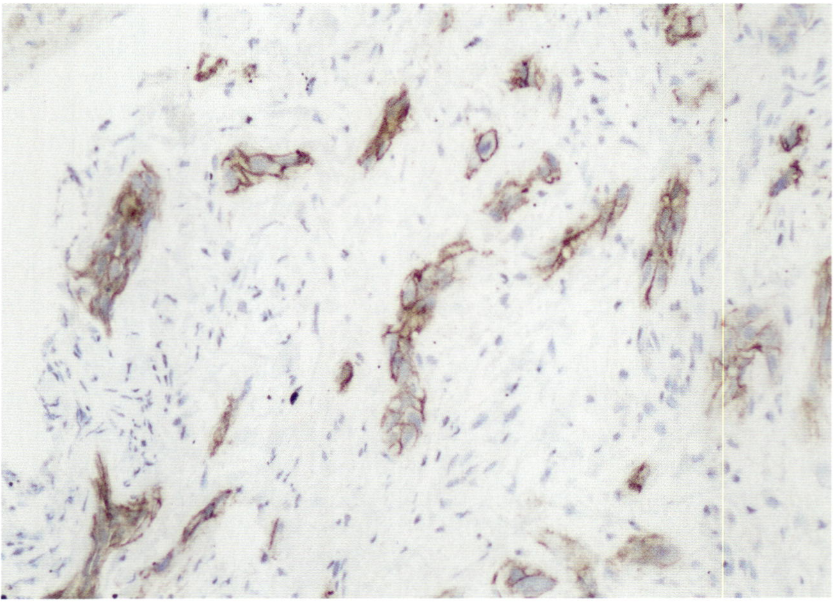

FIGURE 12.3 **A.** PD-L1 immunostaining in squamous cell carcinoma shows strong membranous staining of the majority of tumor cells. A stain such as this would be reported as having a tumor proportion score of >50%.

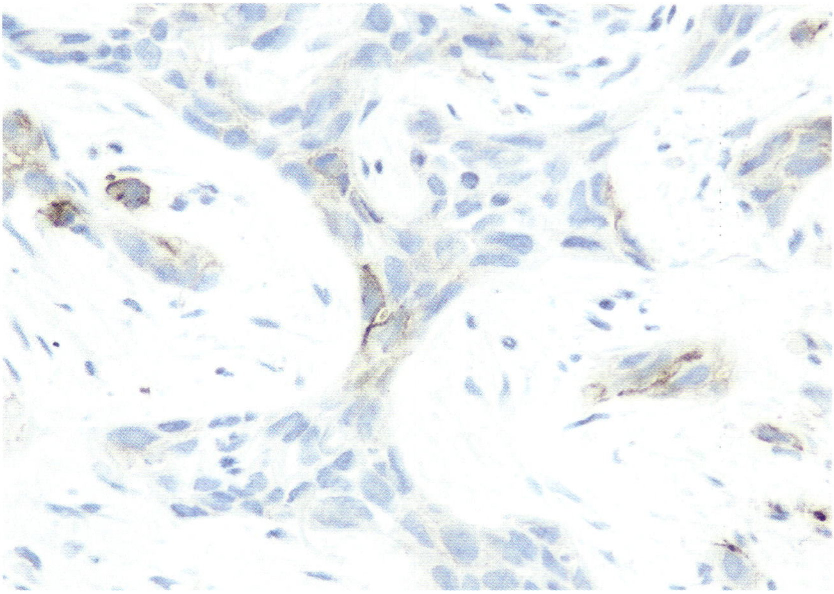

B

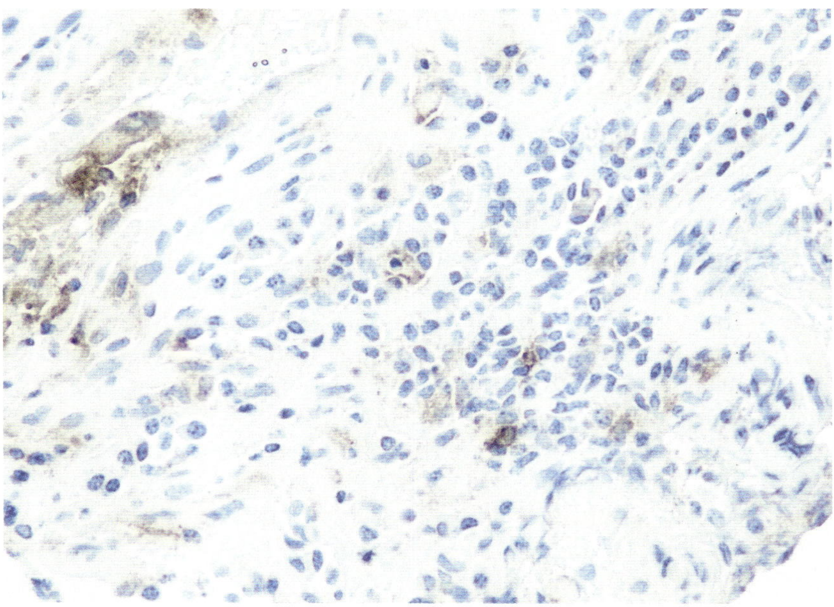

C

FIGURE 12.3 (*continued*) **B.** PD-L1 immunostaining in squamous cell carcinoma shows variably positive membranous staining; note however, that even in cases such as this, all cells with partial membranous staining of strong or weak intensity should be counted toward the percent score. **C.** PD-L1 immunostaining within a lymphoid aggregate shows nonspecific cytoplasmic and membranous staining of inflammatory cells.

PD-L1 expression has been shown to be heterogeneous and as many as 10% of patients with negative PD-L1 IHC results will still respond to immunotherapy.[47,48] Despite these pitfalls, following the established guidelines should allow the pathologist to appropriately score PD-L1 IHC and provide the clinical team with as much information as possible.[39]

IHC for predictive biomarkers should play a secondary role in lung biopsies to IHC for primary diagnosis. If sufficient tissue is available or if clinicians request specific biomarkers, the IHC may be added on, although there should be an attempt to conserve tissue for molecular studies as well. A suggested algorithm for handling of lung biopsy specimens and subsequent diagnostic procedures including light microscopy, IHC, and molecular testing for lung biopsies is provided (Fig. 12.4).

MOLECULAR GENETIC TESTING OF LUNG CARCINOMA

Advances in molecular pathology have opened multiple new avenues for diagnosis and treatment in patients with NSCLC. Genomic profiling has given us new insights into the molecular landscape of lung cancer and identified numerous oncogenic driver mutations and alterations, many of which are amenable to targeted therapy.[49-51] Currently, the majority of targeted therapies are aimed at the treatment of NSCLC. As NSCLC comprises approximately 85% of new lung cancer diagnosis, it follows that comprehensive molecular testing to guide clinical management is rapidly becoming the standard of care for patients with lung carcinoma and will one day be commonplace as molecular diagnostic technologies evolve and continue to decline in cost.[52] As most of the targetable therapies are indicated for mutations identified in lung adenocarcinoma, the majority of testing revolves around that tumor subtype; however, ongoing clinical trials may one day add additional tumors to the list with approved targeted therapy. In 2013, the College of American Pathologists, the International Association for the Study of Lung Cancer (IASLC), and the Association for Molecular Pathology created a set of guidelines for the molecular testing of lung carcinoma specimens.[53] These guidelines were subsequently updated in 2018 and endorsed by the American Society of Clinical Oncology.[54,55] In short, the guidelines recommend the following: *EGFR*, *ALK*, and *ROS1*, at a minimum, should be tested on all lung cancers. A second group of genes including *BRAF*, *MET*, *RET*, *ERBB2 (HER2)*, and *KRAS* should be offered as an expanded panel if sufficient diagnostic material is available.[54] In general, this can be accomplished either by comprehensive molecular panels or with smaller sequential panels. In addition, the committee recommended the use of ALK1 IHC as a screening test, and discouraged the use of EGFR IHC as a screening test. These guidelines were based around testing for patients with "advanced" NSCLC (ie, stage III and IV cancers). A revised version of these guidelines is expected shortly with changes in the testing recommendations and will likely move some genes from the second-line category, such as *BRAF* to the recommended first-line category.

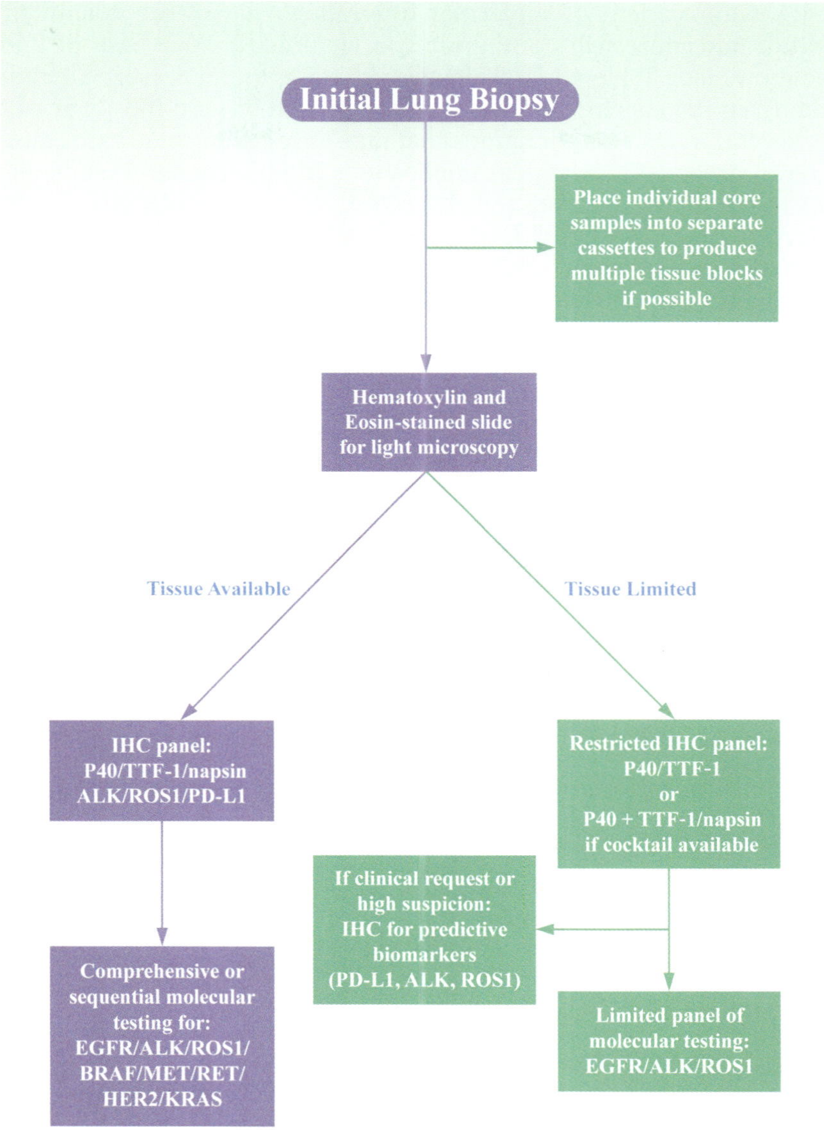

FIGURE 12.4 **A simple schematic for triage and diagnosis of lung biopsy specimens.** ALK, anaplastic lymphoma kinase; BRAF, serine/threonine-protein kinase B-Raf; EGFR, epidermal growth factor receptor; HER2, human epidermal growth factor receptor 2; IHC, immunohistochemistry; KRAS, Kirsten rat sarcoma viral oncogene homolog; MET, MET proto-oncogene receptor tyrosine kinase; RET, RET proto-oncogene tyrosine-protein kinase receptor; ROS1, ROS1 proto-oncogene receptor tyrosine kinase; TTF-1, thyroid transcription factor-1.

A wide variety of molecular aberrations have been identified in NSCLC, and more will continue to be identified as our base of knowledge grows (see Table 12.3 for details regarding the molecular alterations included in the current guidelines).[54-69] Although beyond the scope of this text, several molecular alterations that may have (or in some cases already do have) prognostic/treatment implications in lung cancer include alterations in the following genes: *KRAS*, *NTRK*, *ERBB2*, *FGFR*, *MEK*, *NRG1*, *NF1*, *KIT*, *NRAS*, *MTOR*, *TSC1/2*, and *PDGFRA*, among others.[54] Current National Cancer Center guidelines are more comprehensive and recommend many of these genes as first-line tests and advocate that they should be conducted as part of a broad molecular profiling panel.[70] Finally, it is important to note that patients who receive targeted therapies tend to develop resistance mutations or alterations, which must then be treated with alternative therapies; testing for some of these resistance mutations, such as the classic *EGFR* T790M resistance mutation, is incorporated into the current molecular testing guidelines.[68,69] In centers where molecular testing is available, these patients will commonly be rebiopsied not for diagnosis, but specifically for updated molecular testing; the pathologist should be aware of this possibility when receiving additional biopsies from a patient with a prior lung cancer diagnosis and triage the diagnostic material appropriately.

BRONCHOGENIC CARCINOMA

The term "bronchogenic carcinoma" is understood generically as any tumor that arises from the bronchial tree and its branches, including the terminal respiratory unit (alveolar ducts and alveoli) and epithelial cells located along the walls of the entire bronchial tree. Bronchogenic carcinoma generally refers to adenocarcinoma and SCC and represents the most common form of lung cancer.

Lung Adenocarcinoma

Adenocarcinoma of the lung represents a malignant glandular proliferation that most commonly originates in the peripheral airways. Lung adenocarcinoma is the most common form of epithelial malignancy of this organ. Its peripheral location makes this tumor less likely to be diagnosed through endoscopic biopsy. Nonetheless, large tumors may invade extensively and be present in the vicinity of large airways where they will be accessible to endoscopic biopsies. Molecularly, these tumors are characterized by mutations in numerous genes including *TP53*, *STK11*, *KEAP1*, *EGFR*, *KRAS*, *ROS1*, and *ALK*, among others, the most important of which are those with targetable therapies discussed in the section above. Lung adenocarcinoma is subclassified by the WHO[6] into five basic histologic subtypes: lepidic, acinar, papillary, solid, and micropapillary. It has been increasingly acknowledged that lung adenocarcinoma is characterized by

TABLE 12.3 Common Molecular Driver Alterations in Non–Small Cell Lung Adenocarcinoma

Gene	Molecular Alterations	Incidence of Known Mutations	Resistance Mechanisms	Available Therapies
Kirsten rat sarcoma viral oncogene homolog (*KRAS*)	• G12C mutation • G12V mutation • G12D mutation	25%-30%		Sotorasib (G12C only) Adagrasib (G12C only)
Epidermal growth factor receptor (*EGFR*)	• L858R mutation exon 21 • Exon 19 deletions	15%-20%	• *EGFR* T790M mutation exon 20 • *EGFR* C797S mutation • Various other *EGFR* mutations • *Met* amplification • *HER2* amplification • Small cell transformation	Erlotinib Afatinib Gefitinib Osimertinib Durvalumab Dacomitinib
Anaplastic lymphoma kinase (*ALK*)	• *ALK*::*EML4* fusion • Multiple fusion partners	5%-10%	• *ALK* L1196M mutation • *ALK* G1202R mutation • Various other mutations in *ALK*	Crizotinib Alectinib Ceritinib Lorlatinib Brigatinib
ROS1 proto-oncogene receptor tyrosine kinase (*ROS1*)	• *ROS1*::*EZR* fusion • Multiple fusion partners	1%-2%	• *ROS1* G2032R mutation • Various other mutations	Crizotinib Entrectinib Repotrectinib

(*continued*)

TABLE 12.3 **Common Molecular Driver Alterations in Non–Small Cell Lung Adenocarcinoma (*continued*)**

Gene	Molecular Alterations	Incidence of Known Mutations	Resistance Mechanisms	Available Therapies
MET proto-oncogene receptor tyrosine kinase (*MET*)	• Exon 14 skipping mutations	4%	• *MET* Y1230C mutation • *MET* D1228N mutation	Crizotinib Capmatinib Tepotinib
Human epidermal growth factor receptor 2 (*HER2*)	• Exon 20 insertions and duplications	2%	• *HER2* C805S mutation • *PIK3CA* mutations • *HER2* copy number gain	Trastuzumab
RET proto-oncogene tyrosine-protein kinase receptor (*RET*)	• *MET*::*KIF5B* fusion	1%-2%	• *RET* V804L mutation • *RET* G810A mutation • *EGFR*, AXL bypass signaling	Selpercatinib Pralsetinib Cabozantinib
Serine/threonine-protein kinase B-Raf (*BRAF*)	• V600E mutation • Non-V600E mutations	1%-2%	• MAPK signaling reactivation • *EGFR* signaling • Elevated *YAP1* expression	Vemurafenib Dabrafenib Encorafenib
Neurotrophic tyrosine receptor kinase (*NTRK 1/2/3*)	• *NTRK1/2/3* with various fusion partners	0.2%-<1%		Larotrectinib
Fibroblast growth factor receptor (FGFR)	• *FGFR* mutations • *FGFRx::TACC3 fusions*	0.2%-2%		Entrectinib Erdafitinib

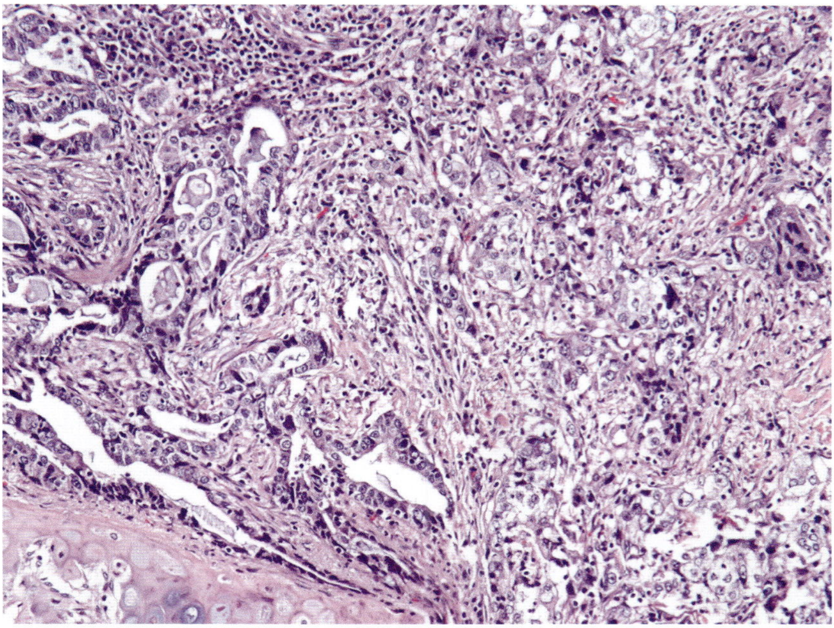

FIGURE 12.5 Transbronchial biopsy showing mixed adenocarcinoma, with areas containing well to moderately differentiated adenocarcinoma with acinar pattern (*left*) and areas containing a more poorly differentiated, solid adenocarcinoma pattern (*right*).

marked morphologic heterogeneity and that a large proportion of these tumors (>90%) display a mixed histologic pattern (Fig. 12.5).[71,72] It has also been demonstrated that some histologic patterns, specifically solid and micropapillary, may be associated with a worse prognosis.[73,74] Recently, the high-grade patterns have been incorporated into a formal grading system for adenocarcinomas of the lung. This grading system stratifies invasive lung adenocarcinomas into well-differentiated, moderately differentiated, and poorly differentiated tumors based on predominant histology of the tumor and whether there is a significant component of any of the high-grade patterns that include micropapillary, solid, and complex glandular (cribriform) architecture in the tumor. This system has been validated as an independent prognostic factor.[75] The system of course is not applicable to small biopsy material; however, larger wedge biopsies that remove an entire tumor can still be used for grading purposes. On smaller biopsies, the specific pattern identified within a lung biopsy should be reported; however, the pathologist should be aware that sampling bias may be masking the predominant pattern or other secondary patterns (Table 12.4).

The 2021 WHO classification also contains the categories of atypical adenomatous hyperplasia, adenocarcinoma in situ, and minimally invasive adenocarcinoma[6]; these categories pertain primarily to resection specimens and should not be diagnosed on biopsy material. Atypical

TABLE 12.4 Grading System for Invasive Pulmonary Adenocarcinoma Proposed by the International Association for the Study of Lung Cancer.

Grade	Differentiation	Patterns
1	Well-differentiated	Lepidic predominant with no or <20% high-grade[a] pattern (any or combination)
2	Moderately differentiated	Acinar or papillary predominant with no or <20% high-grade[a] pattern (any or combination)
3	Poorly differentiated	Any tumor with 20% or more of a high-grade[a] pattern (any combination)

[a]High-grade patterns = micropapillary architecture, solid architecture, complex glandular (cribriform) architecture.

adenomatous hyperplasia, a premalignant lesion that is histologically indistinguishable from lepidic pattern adenocarcinoma, can be separated from the latter based only on its size (<0.5 cm). Adenocarcinoma in situ is defined as a well-differentiated tumor with a lepidic growth pattern that is less than 3 cm in greatest diameter and does not show evidence of invasion. Minimally invasive adenocarcinoma is defined as a tumor with predominantly lepidic growth pattern that measures less than 3 cm and shows areas of invasion that are less than 5 mm. Because these features cannot be demonstrated in small endoscopic biopsies, the diagnosis of "lepidic adenocarcinoma," "atypical adenomatous hyperplasia," "in situ adenocarcinoma," or "minimally invasive adenocarcinoma" cannot be rendered on endoscopic or core biopsy material.[6] This was the reasoning behind the IASLC/ATS/ERS panel recommendation that the interpretation of small biopsies harboring adenocarcinoma be reported as: **(1)** "adenocarcinoma," followed by the description of the specific growth patterns identified; **(2)** "adenocarcinoma with lepidic growth pattern admixed with other growth pattern," and **(3)** "adenocarcinoma with pure lepidic growth pattern," in which case a disclaimer to the effect that an invasive component cannot be excluded should be appended.[7] This recommendation was subsequently adopted by the WHO in 2015.[6] Although a biopsy may show only lepidic pattern, it should still be reported as "adenocarcinoma with lepidic pattern" as many mixed-type adenocarcinomas will often show a lepidic growth pattern in part of the tumor, whereas other areas may harbor acinar, papillary, micropapillary, or solid features. The same rationale applies to large cell carcinoma and adenosquamous carcinoma. It is also important to point out that metastases to the lung from adenocarcinoma from other organs can also display a prominent lepidic growth pattern. It should be noted that the old terminology of "bronchioloalveolar cell carcinoma" is no longer a valid diagnostic category, and the term should no longer be used when interpreting endoscopic lung biopsies (eFigs. 12.1 and 12.2).

Features that can introduce difficulties for the diagnosis in small endoscopic biopsies include artifactual distortion of the cells owing to mechanical crushing by the forceps or secondary to prominent desmoplastic reaction, obscuring of the tumor cells by heavy inflammatory stromal infiltrates, and subtle infiltration by cancer cells underneath an intact respiratory mucosa. Artifactual distortion of tumor cells owing to a prominent desmoplastic reaction is a common source of diagnostic difficulty; the desmoplastic stroma can almost completely obliterate the underlying tumor cells, making them very difficult to recognize as such (Fig. 12.6A and B). Mechanical distortion from the forceps can also damage the tumor cells to a degree that it may be very difficult to recognize them or make a proper histologic characterization of the tumor (Fig. 12.7). Some tumors may be accompanied by a very heavy lymphoplasmacytic inflammatory stromal infiltrate; the tumor cells in such instances may be overshadowed by the inflammation. Attention to the irregular architecture of the glands and the increased cytologic atypia may be of help in identifying an underlying adenocarcinoma (Fig. 12.8A and B). Endoscopic biopsies may often display a normal intact mucosa lining the bronchus but will contain cancerous elements in the submucosa that sometimes may be quite subtle (Fig. 12.9). A careful search for atypical cells or abnormal glands should always be undertaken in small endoscopic biopsies; deeper sections and special stains for cytokeratin may be helpful in cases with a strong clinical suspicion of malignancy.

In clinical practice, identification of adenocarcinoma on a biopsy sample is not usually difficult, except when dealing with poorly differentiated tumors, adenocarcinoma with solid pattern, or when the biopsy is inadequate and does not contain sufficient viable tumor. More problematic is making a distinction between a primary adenocarcinoma of the lung and a metastasis to the lung from another organ. Metastases to the lung from adenocarcinomas originating from other organs are a frequent occurrence. Although most metastatic adenocarcinomas to the lung present as multiple lesions with a history of a primary tumor elsewhere, solitary metastases can be observed in up to 10% of cases.[9,10] Furthermore, an appropriate clinical history may have not been provided at the time of histologic examination that would allow the pathologist to properly identify the tumor as primary versus metastatic. Clinical correlation is therefore an indispensable step when evaluating a small lung biopsy containing adenocarcinoma. When in doubt, immunohistochemical stains are helpful. Most lung adenocarcinomas (~80%) express nuclear positivity for TTF-1 and cytoplasmic reactivity for napsin A (Fig. 12.10).[16] Although these markers display high sensitivity for the diagnosis of pulmonary adenocarcinoma, they lack specificity and may also be expressed in other types of tumors.[76,77] Napsin A, a proteinase involved in the maturation of surfactant protein B, has paradoxically been found to be strongly expressed in a

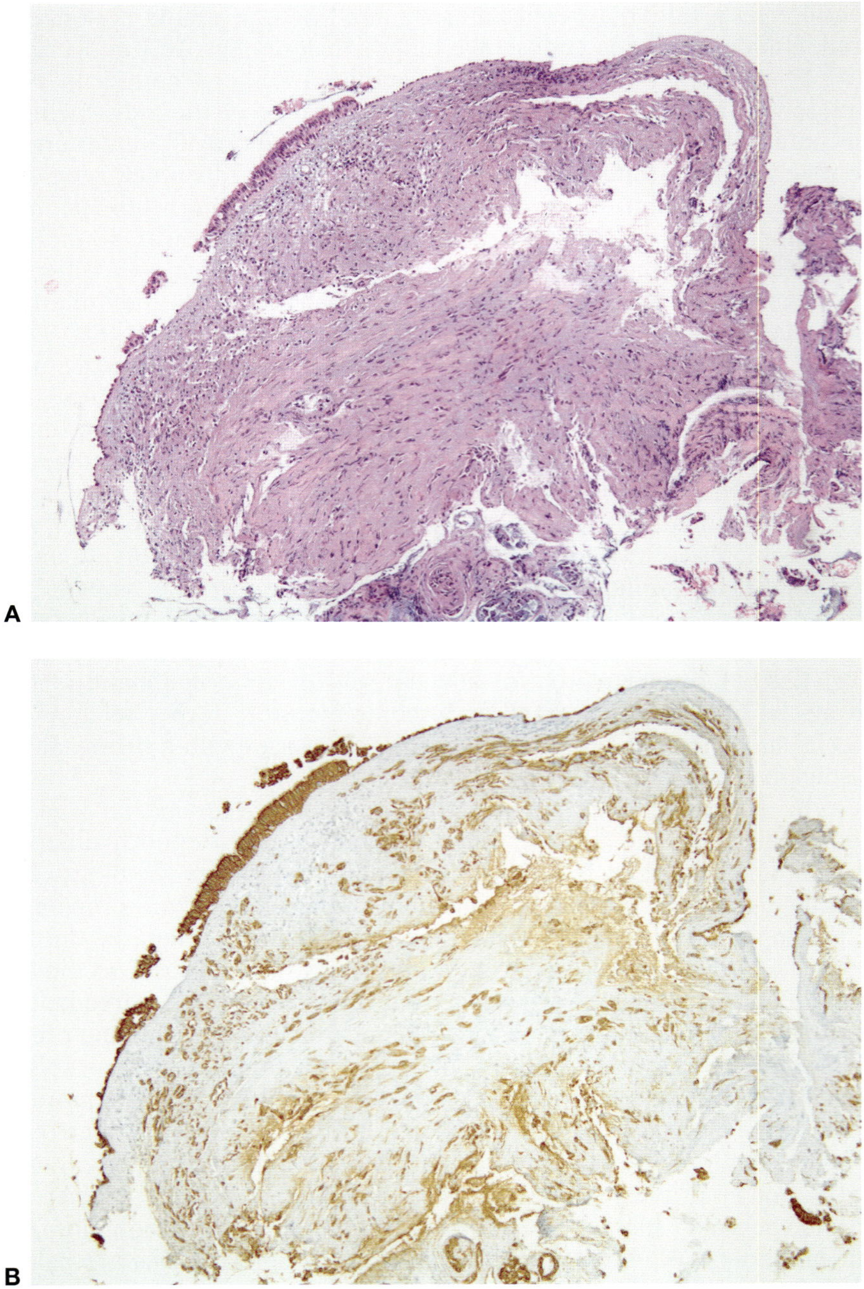

FIGURE 12.6 **A.** Transbronchial biopsy showing an intact layer of bronchial mucosa with thickening of the submucosa by dense fibrous connective tissue. Scattered cells are seen embedded in the connective tissue. **B.** Broad-spectrum cytokeratin stain highlights entrapped tumor cells within the connective tissue.

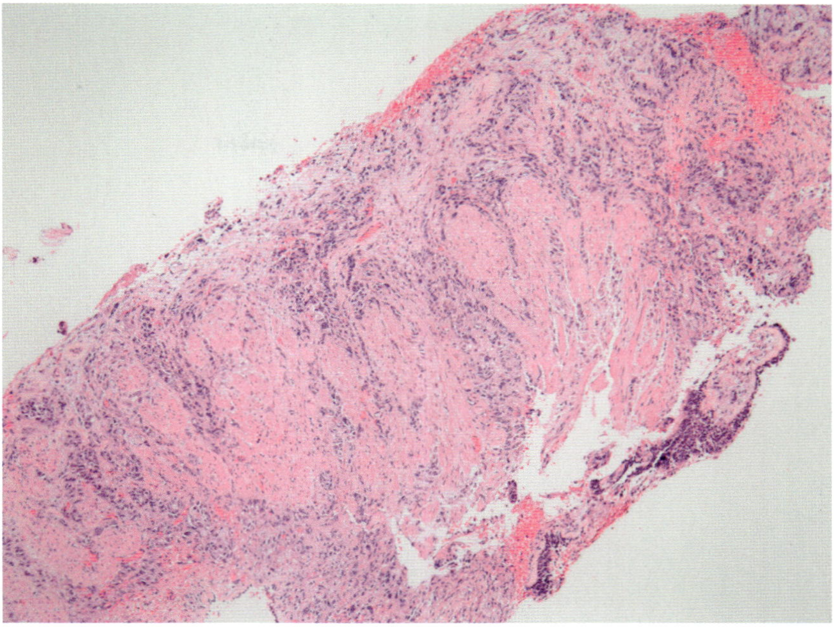

FIGURE 12.7 **Transbronchial biopsy shows extensive mechanical distortion of tumor cells in the submucosa by compression because of the forceps.** It may be difficult in such instances to determine the exact type of tumor contained in this biopsy without the aid of special stains.

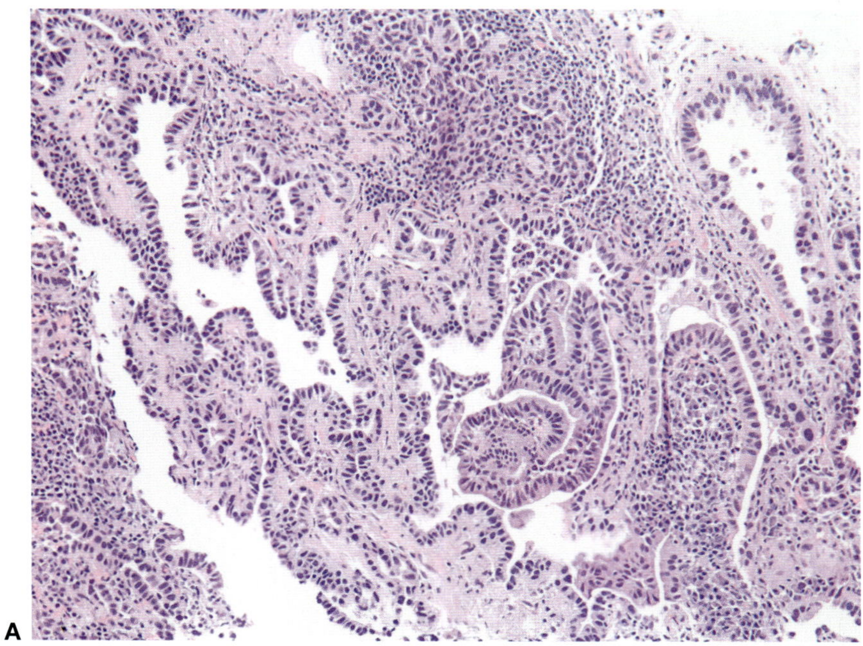

FIGURE 12.8 **A.** Core needle biopsy of peripheral lung mass shows dense lymphoid stromal infiltrates overshadowing the glandular elements. The tortuous character of the glands, complex branching, and atypia of the tumor cells serve to distinguish them from entrapped normal alveolar structures.

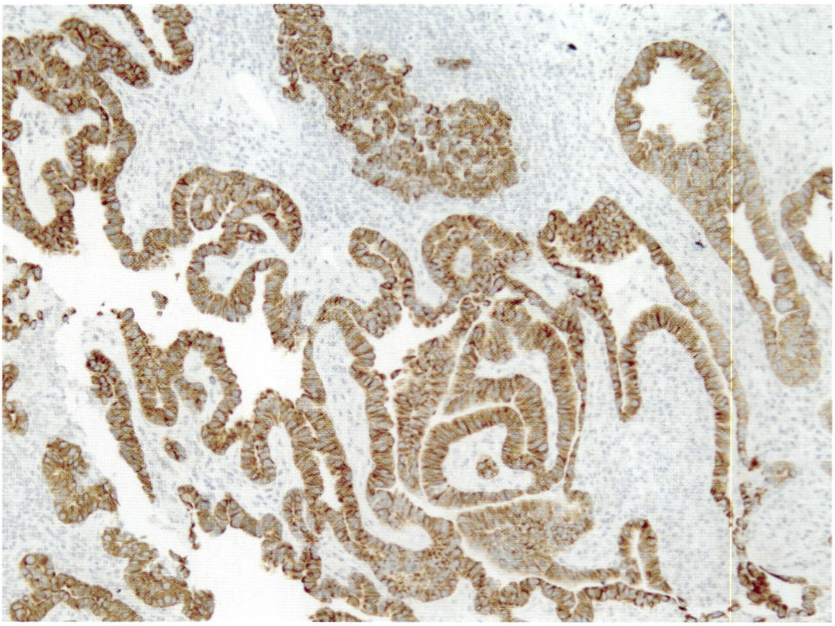

B

FIGURE 12.8 (*continued*) **B.** Cytokeratin stain (CK7) serves to highlight the complex glandular component in this biopsy.

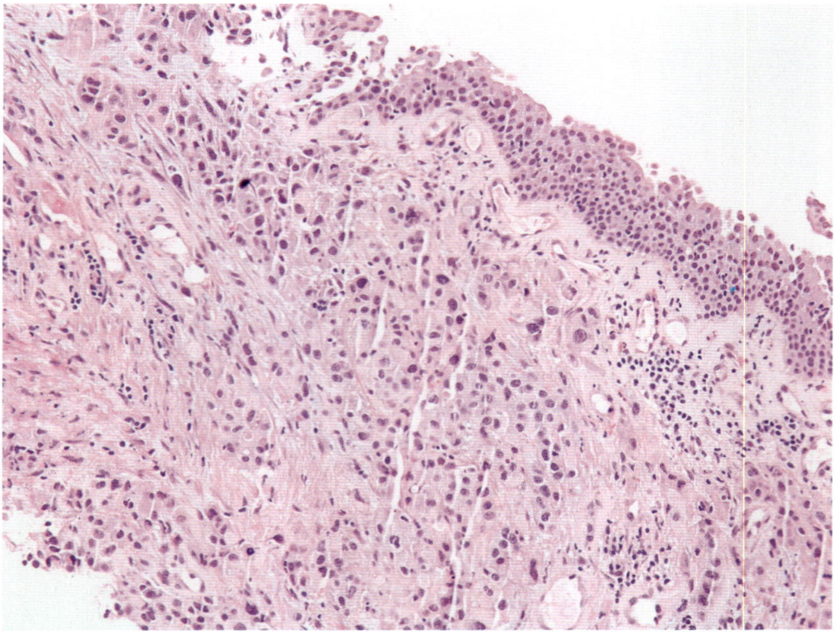

FIGURE 12.9 **Transbronchial biopsy shows unremarkable bronchial mucosa lining the lumen; notice, however, scattered atypical cells in the submucosa with subtle, abortive gland formation in this poorly differentiated adenocarcinoma of the lung.**

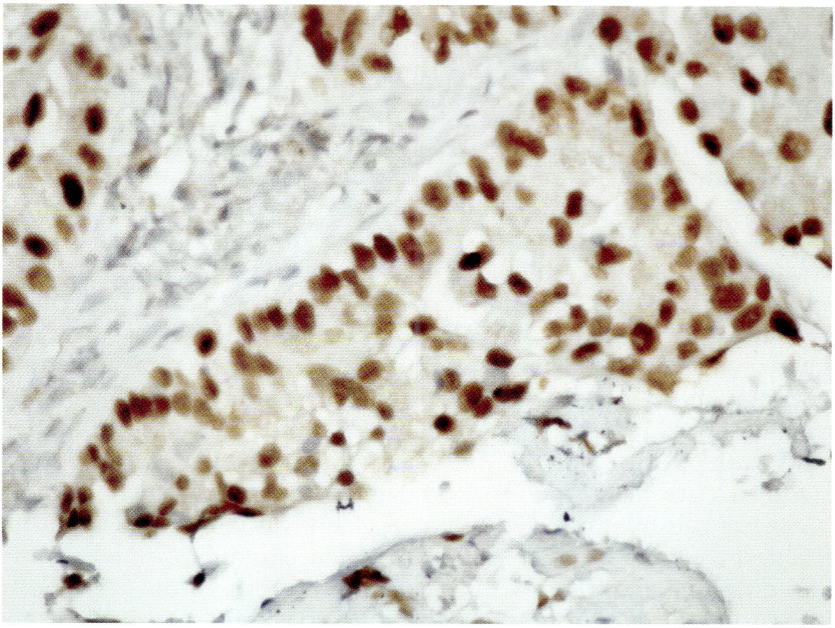

FIGURE 12.10 Immunohistochemical staining shows strong nuclear positivity for thyroid transcription factor-1 in the tumor cells of lung adenocarcinoma.

significant number of cases of renal cell carcinoma of both papillary and clear cell types, as well as in other malignancies.[28-32] TTF-1, a transcription factor expressed in thyroid and lung epithelial cells, on the other hand, has been consistently absent in renal cell carcinomas. TTF-1, however, is not entirely specific for lung adenocarcinoma and is strongly expressed in most types of thyroid cancer and has shown variable expression in a number of other tumors, such as breast carcinoma,[78] colorectal adenocarcinoma,[79] and endometrial and endocervical adenocarcinomas.[80] For this reason, it has been postulated that double labeling of napsin A and TTF-1 can increase the specificity for the diagnosis of lung adenocarcinoma, which has led to the proposal that the combination of both stains should be utilized when evaluating lung biopsies of adenocarcinoma to increase the yield for an accurate diagnosis. It should also be kept in mind that the results of immunostaining for TTF-1 in adenocarcinoma with lepidic pattern may yield different results depending on its subtype. One study found that more than 90% of nonmucinous lung adenocarcinomas of lepidic type were positive for TTF-1, whereas only 20% of cases of the mucinous variant showed weak and focal positivity.[81] TTF-1 may, therefore, not be an entirely reliable or sensitive marker for evaluating lung biopsies of adenocarcinoma with mucinous features. Conventional histochemical stains for mucin, in particular mucicarmine, also play a role in the diagnosis of adenocarcinoma, particularly of the solid type or in poorly differentiated cases. Care must be taken, however, not to overinterpret focal positive staining for mucin in poorly differentiated tumors because SCCs can also harbor occasional foci of aberrant mucin-secreting cells as an expression of tumor heterogeneity.

Once a diagnosis of primary lung adenocarcinoma has been established, it may also be of importance to specify the degree of differentiation, cytologic grade of the tumor, and any other specific morphologic features pertinent for the prognosis or treatment of the patient. Formal grading of adenocarcinoma may be performed as per the aforementioned newly established grading system that stratifies tumors into well-differentiated, moderately differentiated, and poorly differentiated categories based on the percentage of so called high-grade patterns.[75] From a more generalized, conceptual, morphologic/cytologic perspective; well-differentiated adenocarcinoma is characterized by well-formed glands with mild to moderate cytologic atypia that may or may not be accompanied by a prominent desmoplastic stromal response. Moderately differentiated adenocarcinoma is characterized by imperfectly formed glands, usually displaying a more marked degree of cytologic atypia and often containing small or imperfectly formed lumens. Poorly differentiated adenocarcinoma is characterized by solid clusters of tumor cells with very minimal gland formation, often growing in sheets without readily identifiable lumens and displaying marked cytologic atypia (Fig. 12.11A; eFigs. 12.3 and 12.4). Poorly differentiated adenocarcinoma may be distinguished from large cell carcinoma and other subtypes of poorly differentiated carcinoma with the help of IHC or special stains. The diagnosis can sometimes be confirmed using mucicarmine or other stains for mucin (Fig. 12.11B). Unusual patterns of growth that are less frequently observed in primary lung adenocarcinoma include cribriform (now referred to as "complex glandular pattern"), signet ring cell, mucinous ("colloid"), clear cell, fetal type (previously referred to as monophasic pulmonary blastoma), endometrioid-like, and hepatoid. The current recommendation by the WHO/IASLC/ATS/ERS[6,7] for small biopsy sample reporting is that when an adenocarcinoma pattern is identified, any specific or unusual pattern of growth observed also be recorded in the diagnosis.

Lepidic adenocarcinoma of the lung is characterized by a neoplastic proliferation of cells with low-grade cytology that grows along preexisting alveolar septa (Fig. 12.12). Tumors with this morphology usually correlate with ground-glass opacities on imaging and for the most part represent low-grade lesions.[82] Of note, studies have shown that lepidic adenocarcinomas tend to be more commonly associated with *EGFR* mutations than other subtypes.[83] By definition, these tumors should not contain an invasive component; however, on biopsy, sometimes only a lepidic noninvasive component may be sampled. This lepidic pattern may be seen in atypical adenomatous hyperplasia, adenocarcinoma in situ, and minimally invasive adenocarcinoma. However, as mentioned above, these entities should not be diagnosed on biopsy material, and when a purely

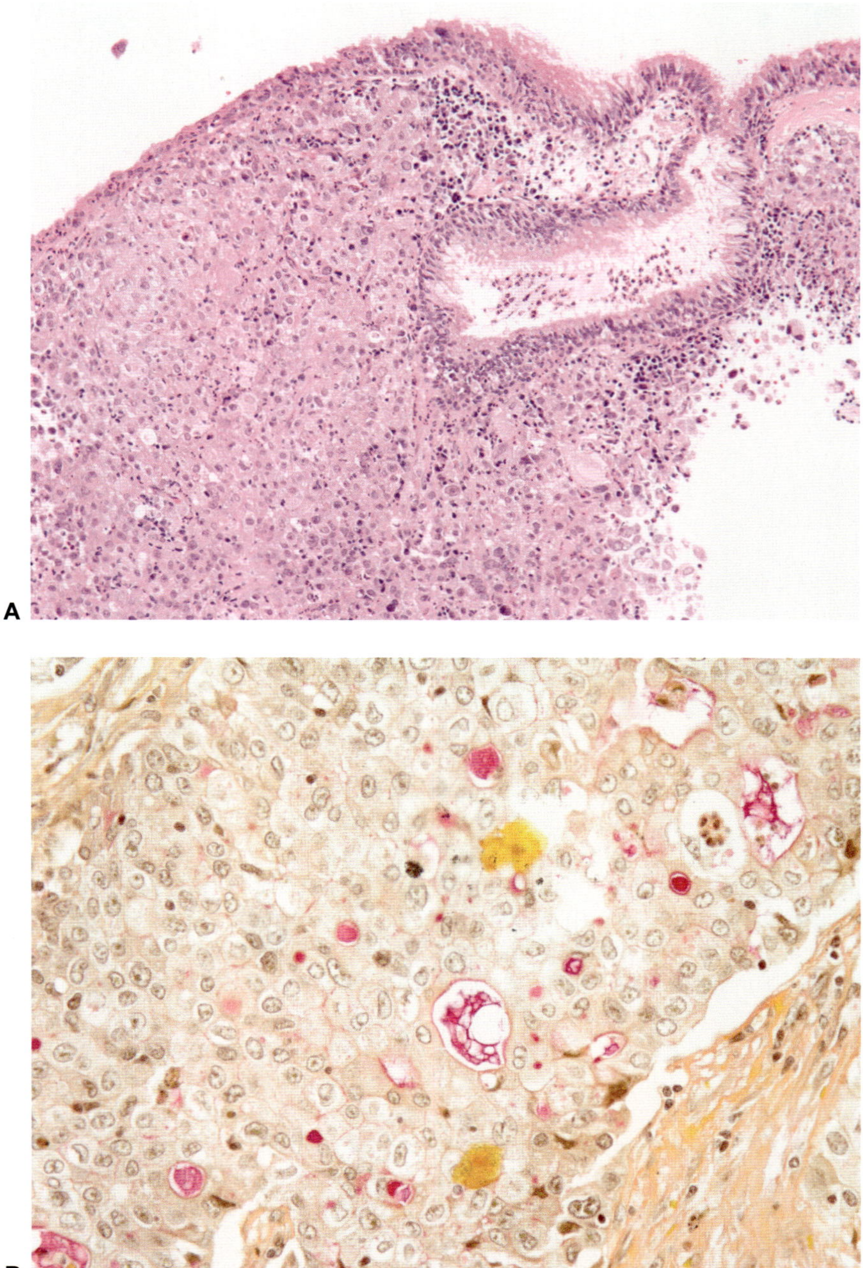

FIGURE 12.11 **A.** Endoscopic biopsy of the lung shows a solid sheet of tumor cells replacing the submucosa without any gland formation. **B.** Mucicarmine stains highlight scattered single cells containing intracellular mucin, establishing a diagnosis of adenocarcinoma, solid pattern with mucin.

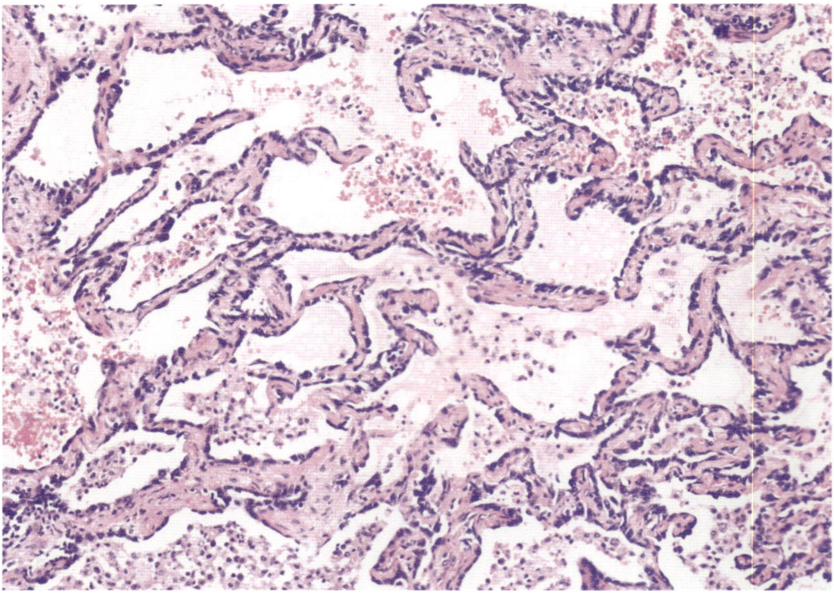

FIGURE 12.12 **Wedge biopsy of pulmonary adenocarcinoma with lepidic growth pattern.** Notice growth of atypical cells lining alveolar spaces. In the past, these biopsies were diagnosed as "bronchioloalveolar carcinoma."

lepidic pattern is encountered, it should be diagnosed as "adenocarcinoma with lepidic pattern" with a note indicating that other patterns or areas of definitive invasion must be assessed on resection. An unusual pattern of growth sometimes seen in lepidic adenocarcinoma is one characterized by papillary tufting of the lining cells into the lumen, imparting the lesion with a papillolepidic architecture (Fig. 12.13A).[9] This can pose a pitfall for diagnosis and may be confused on small biopsy samples for papillary adenocarcinoma, which is a higher-grade tumor and generally displays higher-grade cytologic features. The distinction is made by paying attention to the cytology, which is nearly always low-grade in lepidic adenocarcinomas and shows the characteristic hobnail cells, and to the fact that the papillary tufts are in continuity with the characteristic lepidic growth lining the rest of the alveolar spaces (Fig. 12.13B). Occasionally, lepidic adenocarcinoma may display prominent intranuclear cytoplasmic inclusions, creating a resemblance with metastases from papillary thyroid carcinoma (Fig. 12.14A). Stains for CK7/TTF-1 will not be of assistance in such instances as both lung and thyroid adenocarcinomas will be positive for these markers; use of thyroglobulin or a surfactant protein–associated marker (such as napsin A) will aid in the distinction between the two (Fig. 12.14B).

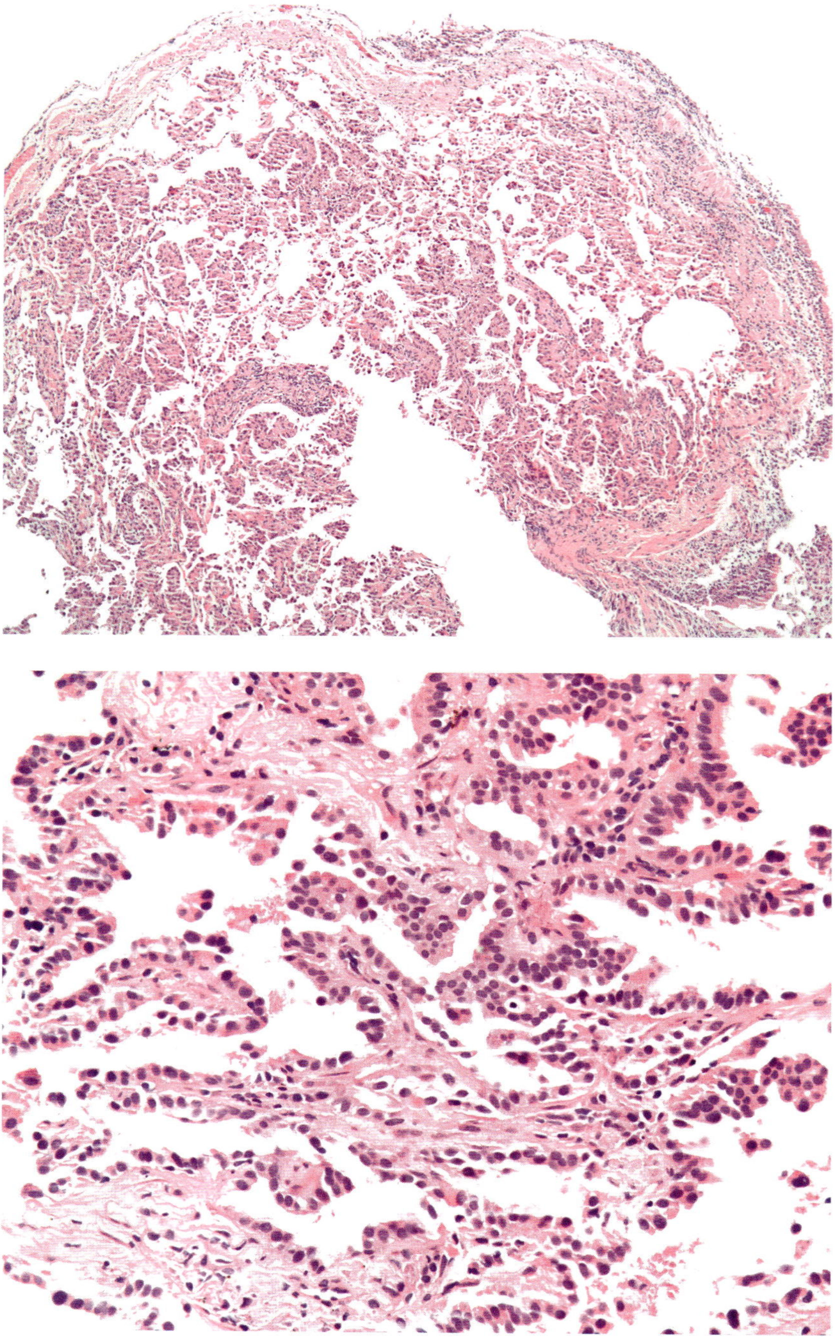

A

B

FIGURE 12.13 **A.** Endoscopic biopsy of lepidic-type adenocarcinoma that displays intra-alveolar papillary projections. **B.** Higher magnification shows that the papillary structures are connected with the alveolar septa, and the tumor cells show bland cytologic features.

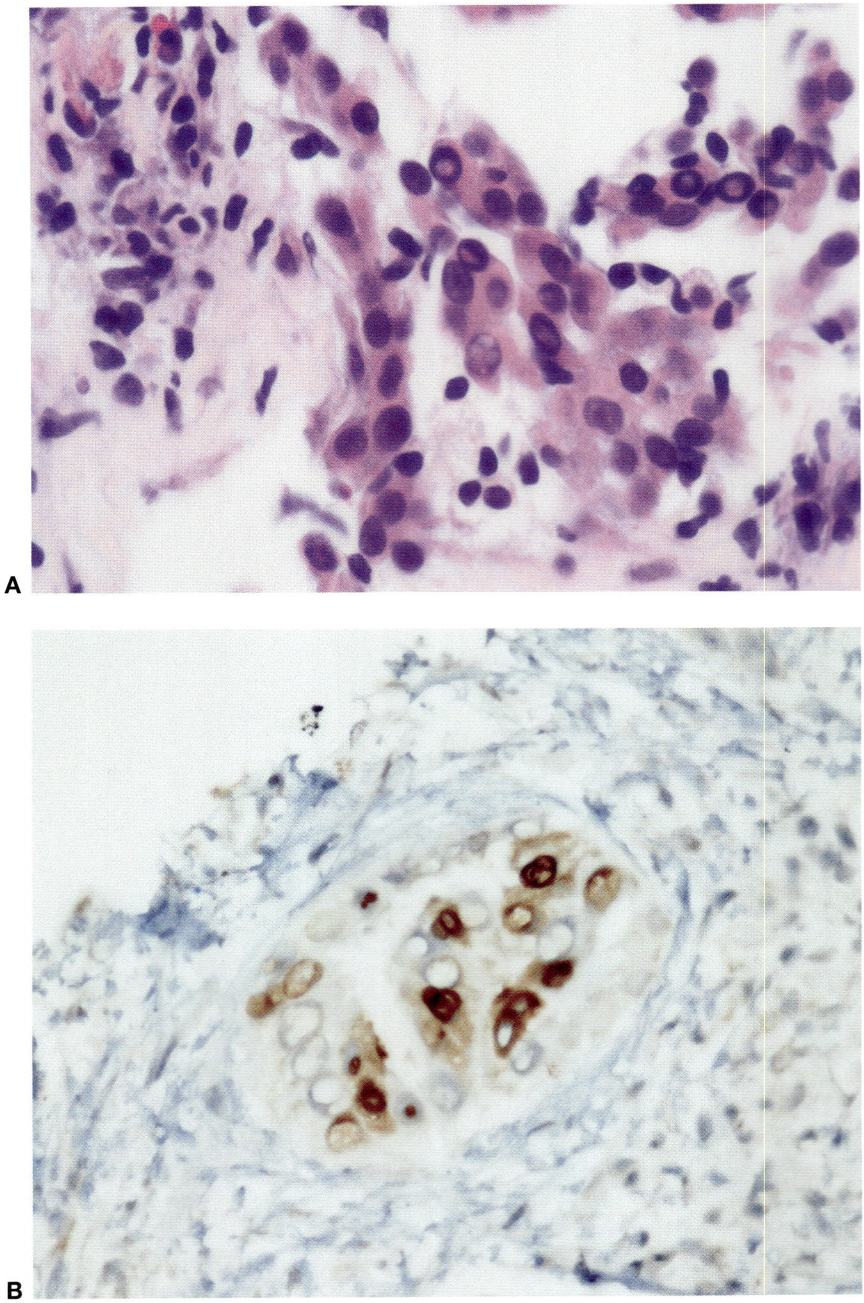

FIGURE 12.14 **A.** Transbronchial biopsy shows a lepidic-type adenocarcinoma displaying prominent intranuclear cytoplasmic inclusions mimicking metastatic papillary thyroid carcinoma. **B.** Immunohistochemical stain for napsin A shows strong cytoplasmic reactivity in the tumor cells, indicating a primary lung origin.

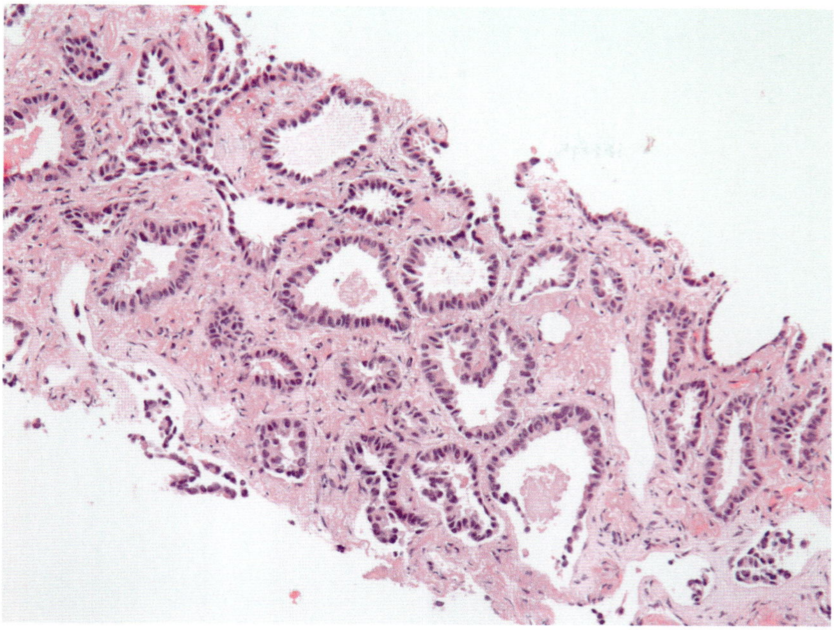

FIGURE 12.15 Endoscopic biopsy of well-differentiated pulmonary acinar adenocarcinoma showing irregular, evenly distributed glands separated by a desmoplastic stroma.

Acinar adenocarcinoma of the lung is the most common pattern of lung adenocarcinoma and is characterized by glandular formation that displays evidence of invasion (Fig. 12.15). Generally, the invasive nature of the glands can be identified because of reactive stromal patterns. The tumors may be associated with mucin production. A potential diagnostic pitfall is with lepidic-predominant adenocarcinoma in which glandlike structures are formed because of collapse of the interstitium or secondary to interstitial fibrosis that may compress preexisting alveolar structures (Fig. 12.16). In some cases, this process may mimic papillary-type architecture as well. This may be difficult to assess on biopsy material and is better interpreted on resection specimens where the overall architecture of the tumor can be evaluated. In some cases, elastic stains to evaluate the underlying elastic framework of the alveoli may be useful because in the lepidic pattern, the elastic network tends to remain relatively intact.[84]

Cribriform adenocarcinoma of the lung is an unusual histologic variant of lung cancer that is characterized by glandular structures with regular, punched-out luminal spaces that resemble in situ ductal carcinoma of the breast or high-grade cribriform adenocarcinoma of the prostate (Fig. 12.17). The cribriform pattern has been commonly observed in primary lung adenocarcinoma of enteric type (or with enteric differentiation) but may also be seen in tumors that more closely resemble metastases from

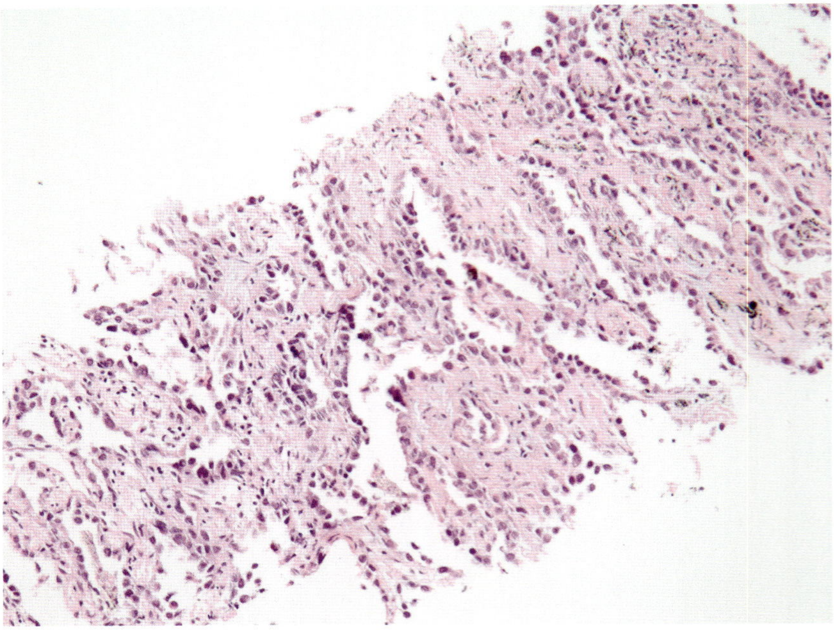

FIGURE 12.16 **In some cases, collapse of the surrounding lung parenchyma in lepidic-type adenocarcinomas can cause small glandlike spaces to form, leading to confusion with acinar adenocarcinoma.**

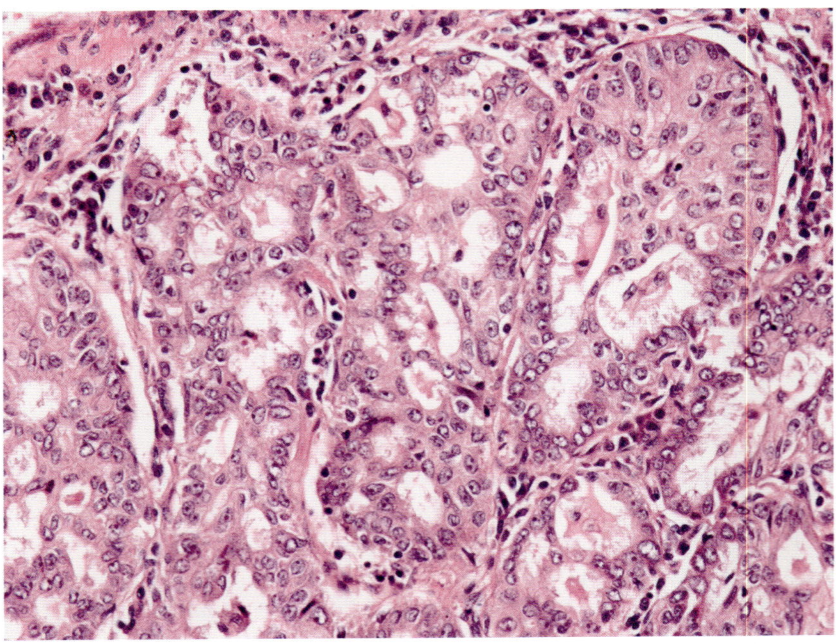

FIGURE 12.17 **Cribriform adenocarcinoma of the lung is characterized by a glandular proliferation containing regular, evenly spaced punched out lumens; these tumors can resemble metastases of breast or prostate carcinoma.** The tumors are characterized by strong cytokeratin 7/thyroid transcription factor-1 positivity and are negative for breast- or prostate-associated markers.

the breast, prostate, uterus, ovaries, and salivary glands.[85] Tumors with these features are classified as having the "complex glandular pattern" introduced in the new grading system established for invasive pulmonary adenocarcinoma.[75] Although currently classified as simply a histologic subtype of acinar adenocarcinoma in the WHO, cribriform adenocarcinomas were initially proposed to be a distinct clinicopathologic entity based on overall worse prognosis compared to conventional acinar adenocarcinoma.[86] Although the cribriform architecture most often suggests the possibility of a metastasis, primary lung adenocarcinomas with cribriform pattern are strongly positive for CK7 and TTF-1 and will be negative for other specific differentiation markers.

Papillary adenocarcinoma of the lung is characterized by a complex proliferation of papillary structures with secondary and tertiary branches that contain well-developed fibrovascular cores (Fig. 12.18A and B).[6] The cytology in such tumors is usually high grade, with frequent mitotic figures and foci of necrosis. In small biopsies, the tumors need to be distinguished from metastases from papillary thyroid carcinoma as well as other metastatic tumors that may display papillary morphology such as serous adenocarcinoma of the uterus and ovaries. IHC for napsin A or PE-10 (surfactant protein) and thyroglobulin may be of help in separating papillary lung tumors from papillary thyroid tumors, whereas IHC for PAX8 and WT1 may be helpful for separating papillary lung tumors from papillary tumors of the gynecologic tract.

Micropapillary adenocarcinoma of the lung is characterized by small, abortive papillae devoid of fibrovascular cores that appear to be lying within an empty space caused by retraction artifact simulating lymphatics plugged by tumor or aerogenous tumor spread through the air sacs (Fig. 12.19A and B).[87] The micropapillary growth pattern has been associated with more aggressive behavior in early-stage adenocarcinoma.[73] These tumors have been associated with a higher incidence of regional lymph node and distant metastases. Micropapillary lesions need to be differentiated from metastases of breast micropapillary adenocarcinoma and from metastases from other tumors that can display micropapillary structures, such as endometrial and ovarian serous carcinoma. Generally, the use of IHC for various nuclear transcription factors can help differentiate the cell of origin.

Solid adenocarcinoma of the lung is characterized by solid nests of tumor cells that do not have immediately recognizable features of adenocarcinoma (Fig. 12.20A).[6] The differential diagnosis for these tumors is with nonkeratinizing SCCs, as well as metastasis from other tumors that display a solid pattern of growth. Usually, inspection of the tumor will reveal focal features suggestive of adenocarcinoma such as focal gland formation or intracellular mucin production (Fig. 12.20B). This pattern, like micropapillary, has been associated with a worse prognosis.[82] Of note, rare cases of solid adenocarcinoma may develop prominent squamoid features including cytoplasmic keratinlike hyaline globular inclusions, large

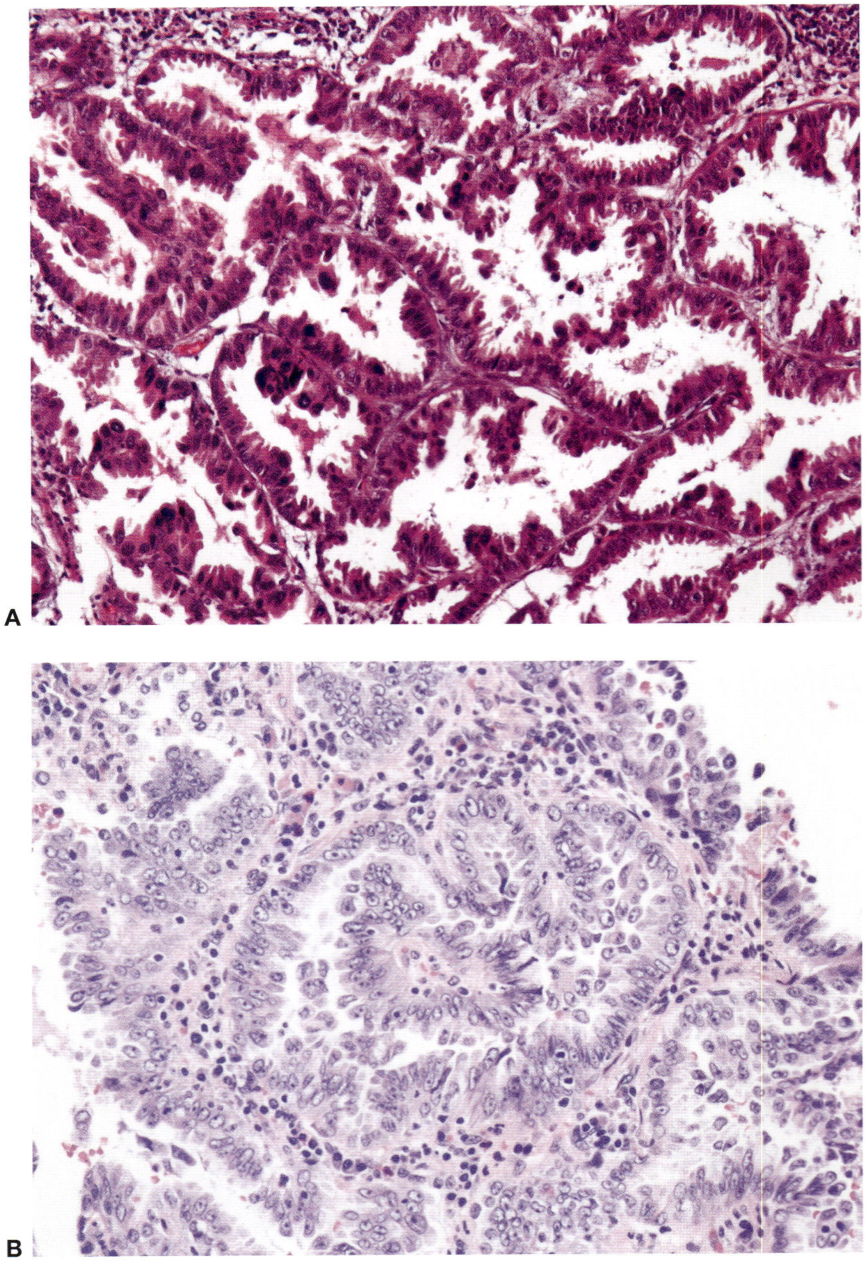

FIGURE 12.18 **A.** Papillary carcinoma of the lung shows complex branching of papillary structures lined by cells with marked cytologic atypia (differentiating it from the lower-grade cytology seen in Fig. 12.13B). **B.** Core needle biopsy of a papillary adenocarcinoma of the lung demonstrating a tumor with increased cytologic atypia and a well-formed papillary structure with a true fibrovascular core.

A

B

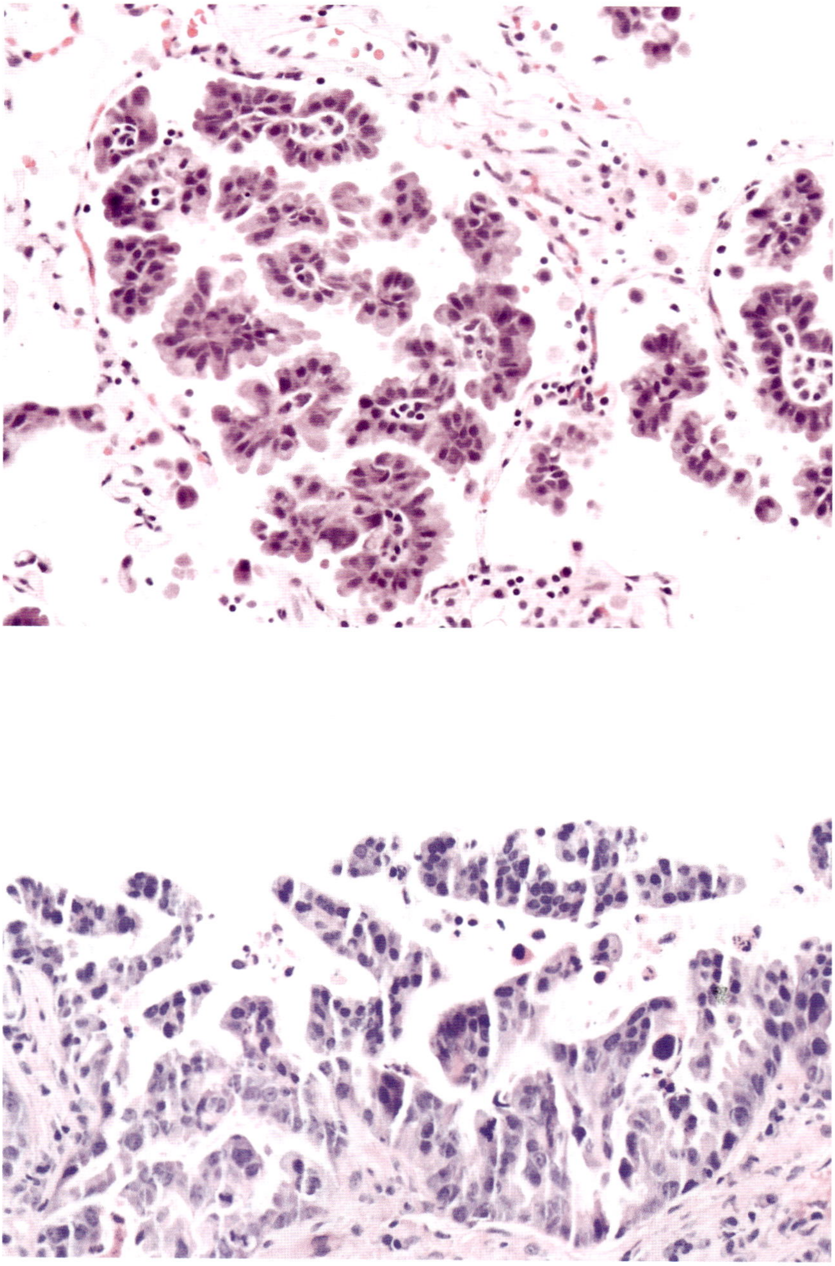

FIGURE 12.19 **A.** Micropapillary carcinoma of the lung is characterized by small papillary structures floating within the alveolar lumen. The cells lining the papillae have a hobnail appearance. **B.** Endoscopic biopsy of micropapillary adenocarcinoma shows small detached papillary structures and increased mitotic activity with cytologic atypia.

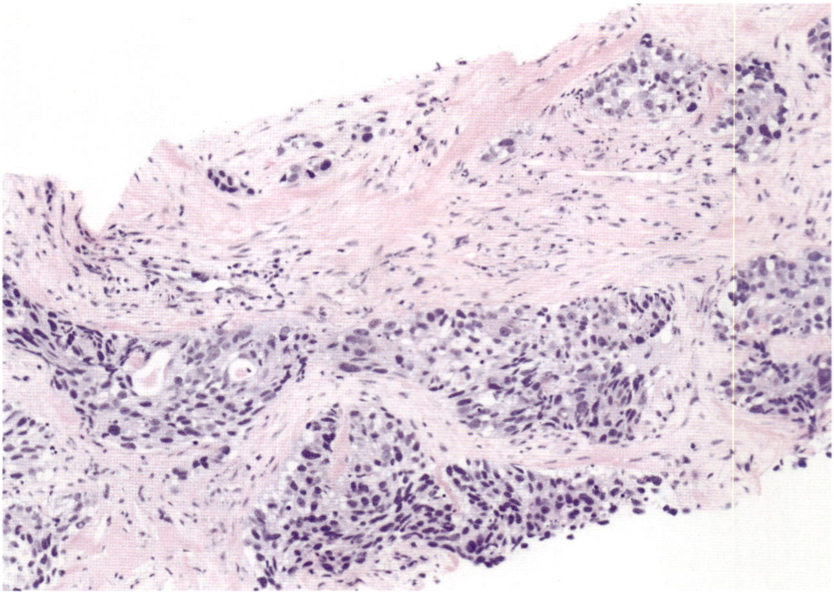

A

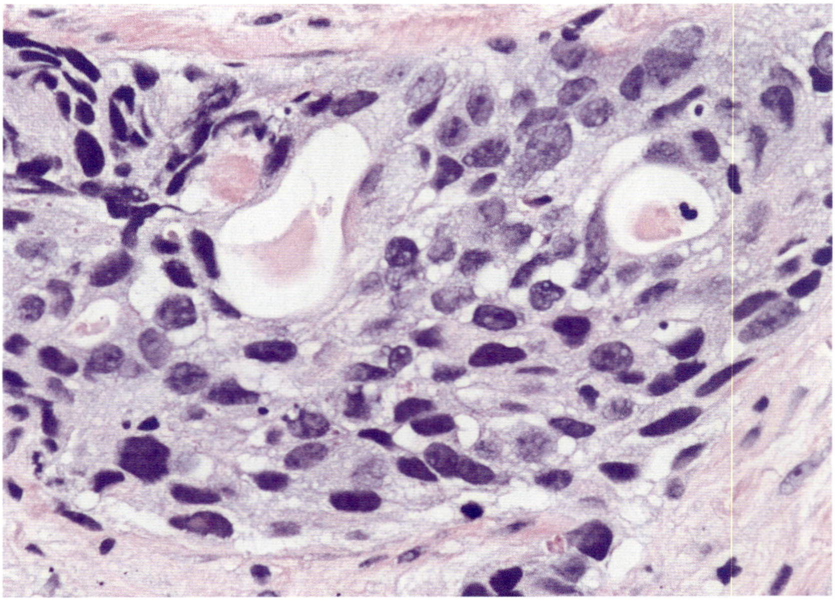

B

FIGURE 12.20 **A.** Core needle biopsy of solid pattern adenocarcinoma of the lung. The majority of the tumor shows cohesive nests of tumor cells that may be confused for poorly differentiated squamous cell carcinoma or neuroendocrine carcinoma. **B.** Higher-power magnification shows focal areas of glandular formation giving away its adenocarcinomatous nature.

polygonal cells with sharp cell borders, and pavementlike architecture.[88] We term these tumors "pseudosquamous adenocarcinomas"; this histologic variant of adenocarcinoma represents a diagnostic pitfall with SCC, particularly if IHC is not performed (Figs. 12.21-12.24). These tumors may also occasionally be encountered in small biopsy material leading to further confusion (Fig. 12.25-12.27). IHC for TTF-1, napsin A, and P40 are critical in these lesions because solid pattern adenocarcinoma will be negative for squamous markers and positive for adenocarcinoma markers.

Colloid adenocarcinoma of the lung is a tumor characterized by pools of extracellular mucin containing small clusters or single mucin-secreting tumor cells floating in the mucin.[89] The tumor cells are usually of goblet cell type but may be simple mucin-secreting cells. These tumors can often undergo cystic changes, in which case they are designated as mucinous cystadenocarcinoma. They can be identified in endoscopic biopsies by the presence of single atypical cells or small clusters of cells floating in pools of mucin (Fig. 12.28). The tumors are most often TTF-1/CK7+ but may also show a TTF-1/CK7−, CDX2/CK20+ immunophenotype. It may be very difficult to distinguish the latter cases from metastases from a colorectal or pancreaticobiliary tumor (see Chapter 15 for a more detailed discussion);

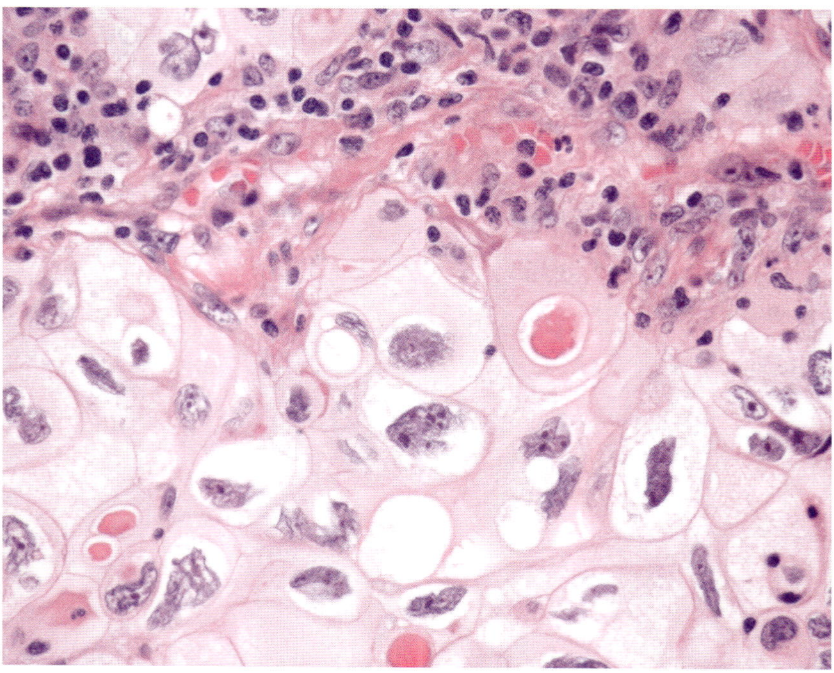

FIGURE 12.21 **Pseudosquamous adenocarcinoma of the lung shows a strong resemblance to squamous cell carcinoma.** In this image, there are large epithelioid cells with sharp cell borders and intracytoplasmic eosinophilic hyaline globules that may be confused for abortive foci of keratinization.

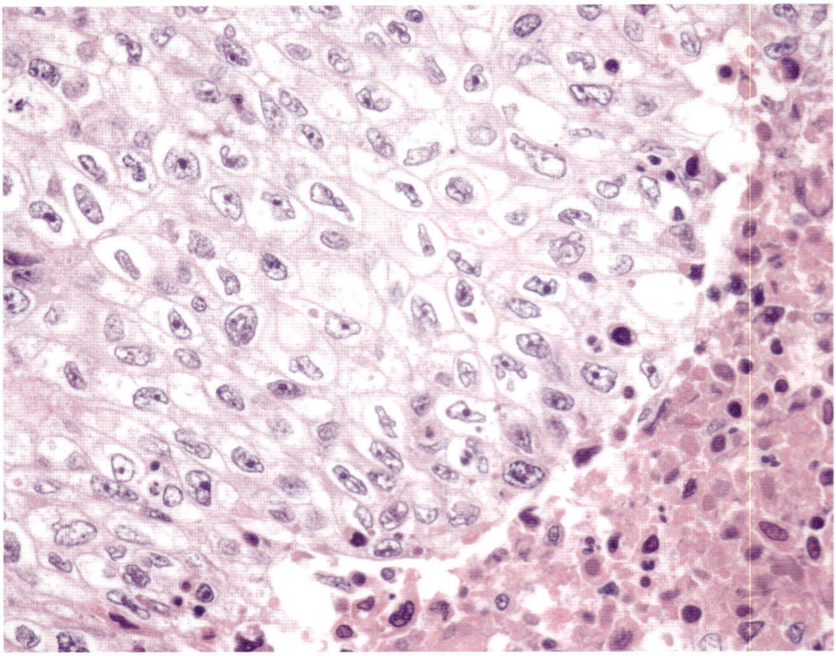

FIGURE 12.22 Pseudosquamous adenocarcinoma of the lung demonstrates squamoid morphology with pavementlike architecture and numerous irregularly shaped nucleoli that are reminiscent of koilocytes as seen in cervical squamous dysplasia.

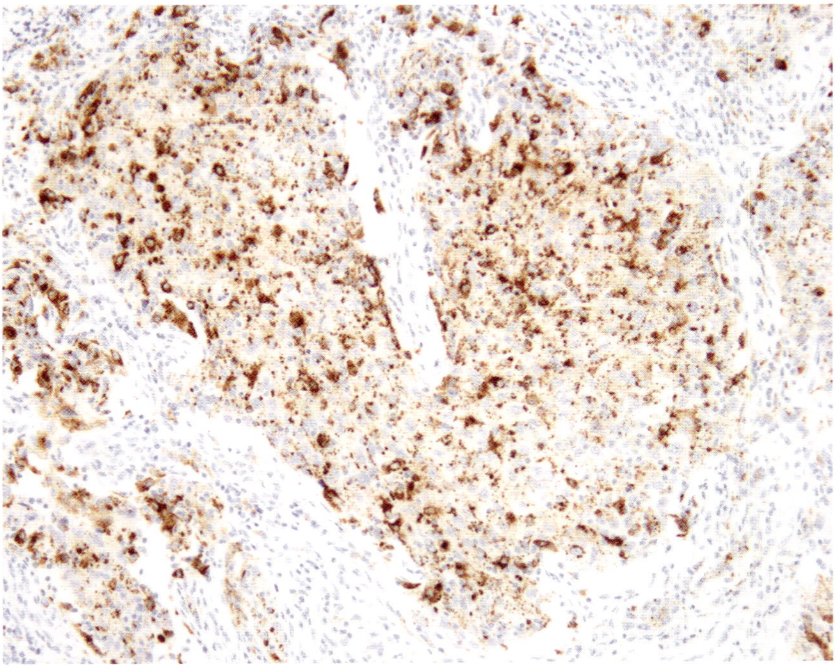

FIGURE 12.23 Pseudosquamous adenocarcinoma of the lung showing strong napsin A positivity.

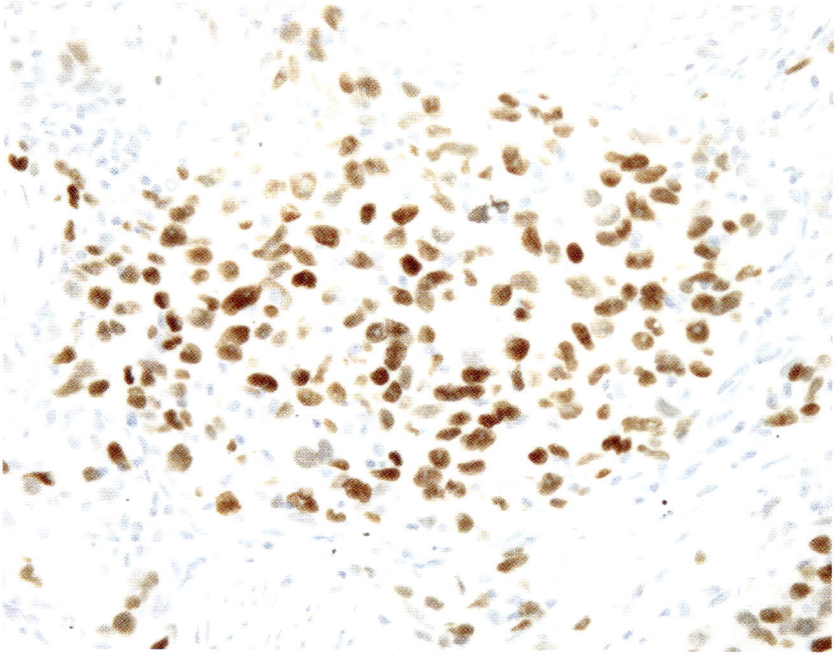

FIGURE 12.24 Pseudosquamous adenocarcinoma of the lung showing strong thyroid transcription factor-1 positivity.

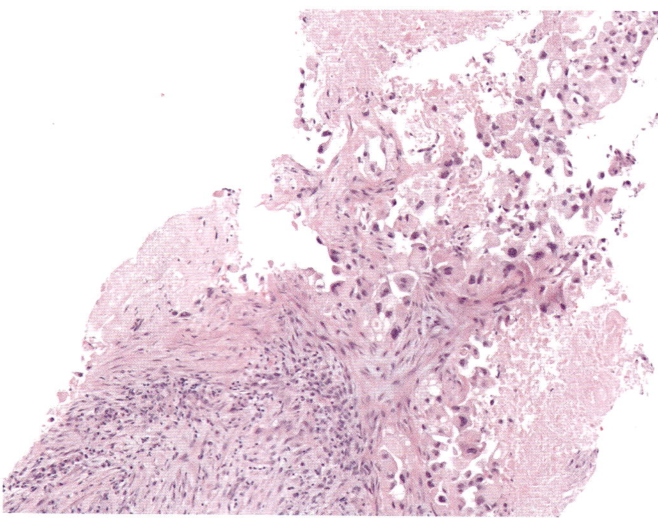

FIGURE 12.25 Core needle biopsy of pseudosquamous adenocarcinoma of the lung showing solid nests of cells with ample eosinophilic cytoplasm, some of which demonstrate sharp cell borders.

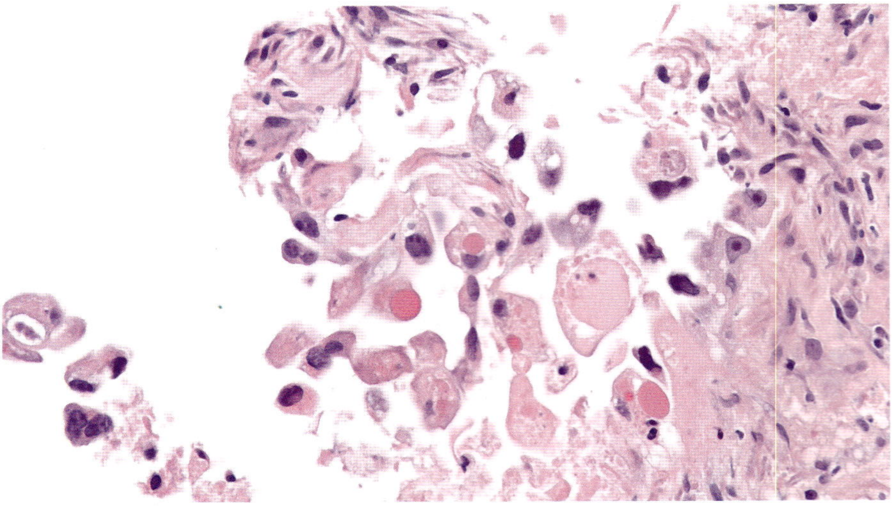

FIGURE 12.26 Higher-power magnification shows large epithelioid cells with intracytoplasmic hyaline globules initially confused for possible abortive keratinization.

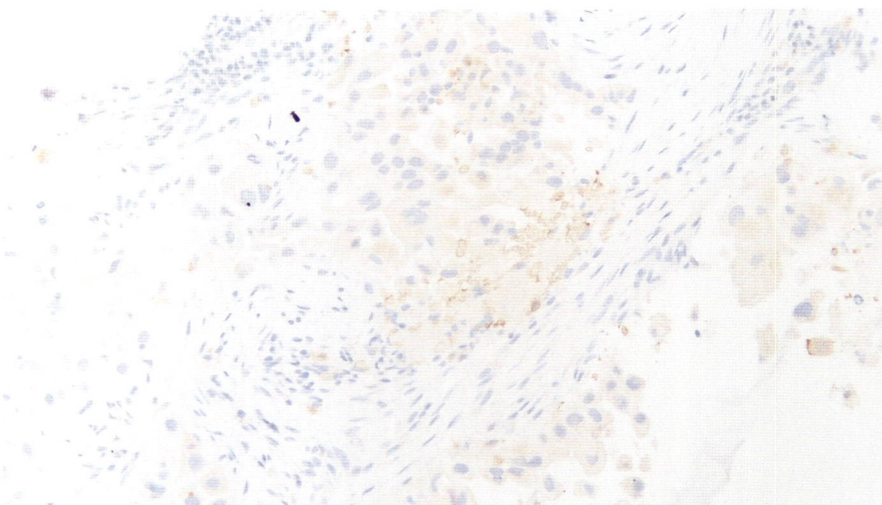

FIGURE 12.27 P40 immunostain in the prior biopsy specimen shows complete absence of staining excluding a squamous cell carcinoma. The tumor cells in this case displayed strong positivity for TTF1 and Napsin A.

clinicopathologic correlation is always necessary for establishing the correct diagnosis. It is also important to distinguish colloid carcinoma from mucinous carcinoma displaying a lepidic growth pattern.

Invasive mucinous adenocarcinoma includes adenocarcinomas that have tumor cells that show goblet cell morphology or columnar cells with abundant intracytoplasmic mucin (Figs. 12.29-12.31).[6] They tend to be

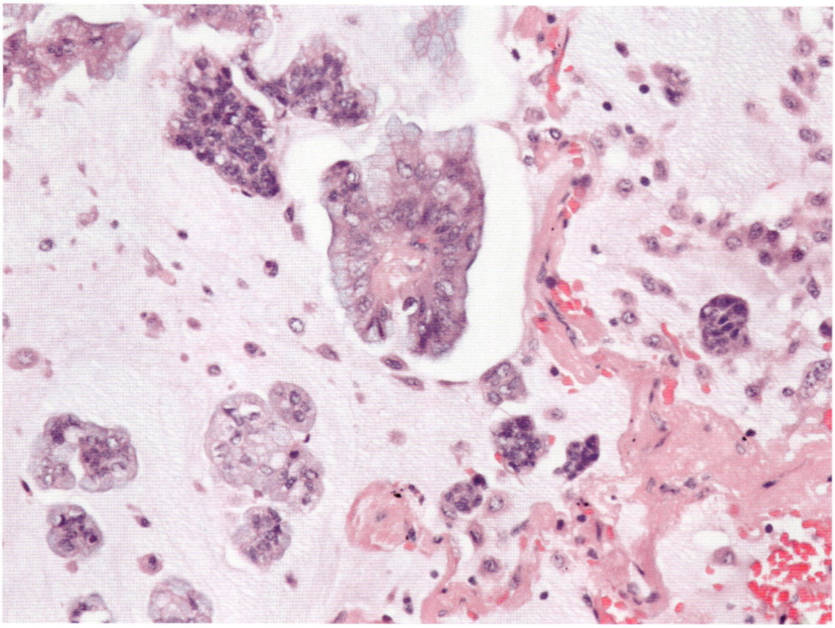

FIGURE 12.28 Colloid carcinoma of the lung showing clusters of mucinous epithelium as well as single atypical cells floating in mucin within the distended alveolar spaces.

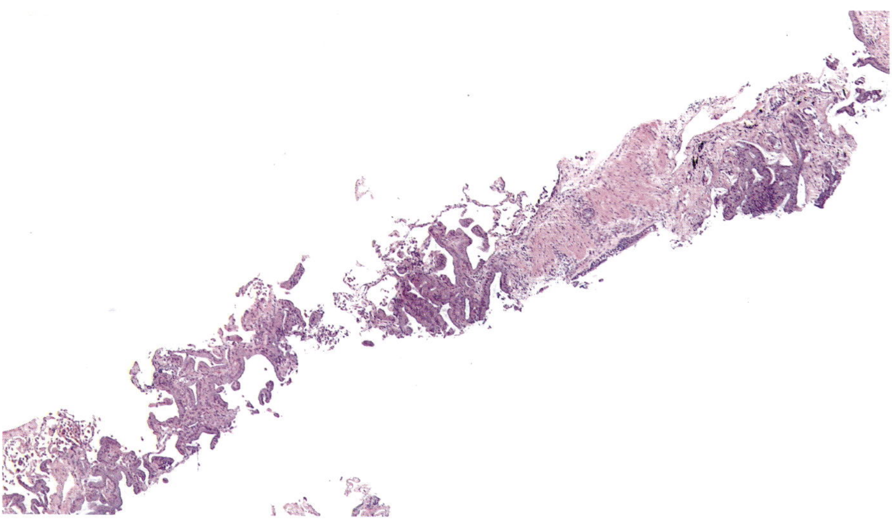

FIGURE 12.29 Core needle biopsy of an invasive mucinous adenocarcinoma of the lung shows an infiltrative tumor growing in a mostly lepidic pattern with focal glandular formation.

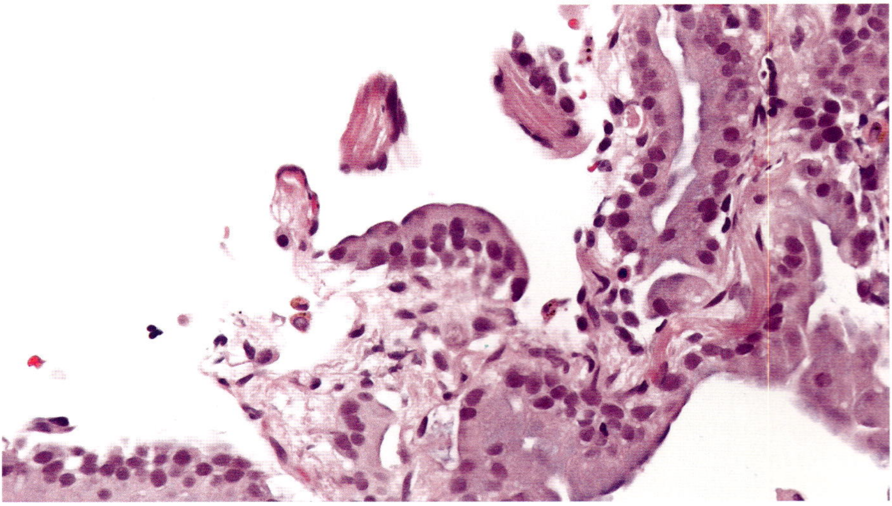

FIGURE 12.30 **Higher-power magnification shows a small tuft of cells (so-called fan sign).** Notice the mucinous characteristic of the epithelial cells with areas of gray coloration in the cytoplasm.

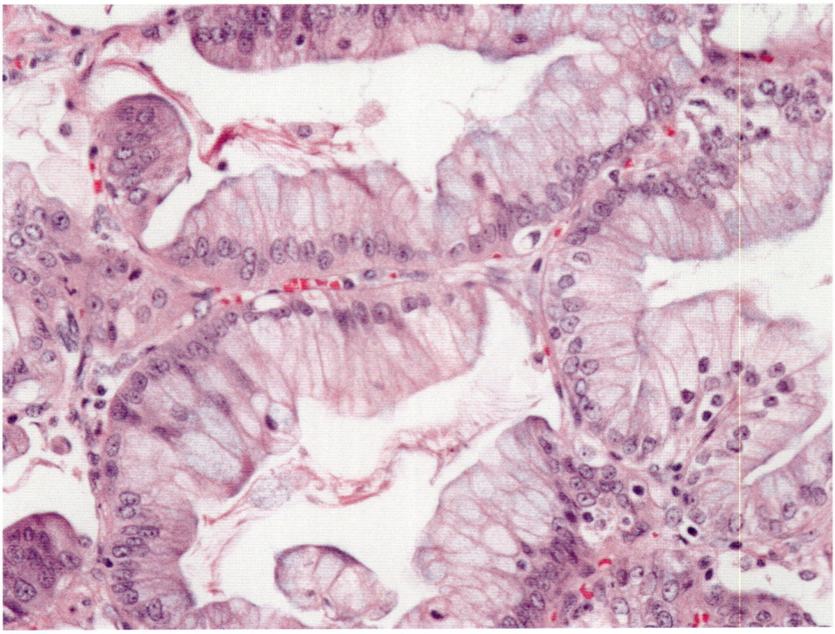

FIGURE 12.31 **Invasive mucinous adenocarcinoma shows replacement of the lining of the alveoli by tall columnar, mucin-secreting cells admixed with occasional goblet cells.**

low-grade lesions and are characterized molecularly by frequent *KRAS* mutations.[83] Up to 25% of cases demonstrate *NKX2-1* mutations or *NRG1* fusions.[90,91] The mucinous morphology will sometimes show an abrupt transition with normal pneumocytes, with small tufts or rows of mucinous cells that can sometimes protrude into the alveolar spaces (a feature we term the "fan-sign"). These tumors tend to grow in a multifocal fashion and may be difficult to diagnose on biopsy material as conventional adenocarcinomas may also produce mucin and have focal areas that resemble invasive mucinous adenocarcinoma. The tumors can display confounding immunohistochemical profiles including negative staining for TTF-1 and napsin A, with positivity for CK20 and CDX2, owing to its "enteric" phenotype (Figs. 12.32 and 12.33). The current WHO classification separates them into mucinous adenocarcinoma in situ, minimally invasive mucinous adenocarcinoma, or invasive mucinous adenocarcinoma.[6] These distinctions, however, cannot be made on small endoscopic biopsies; a generic diagnosis of mucinous adenocarcinoma should be rendered on small biopsy samples with a note indicating that the findings need to be correlated with the imaging studies, that an invasive component cannot be ruled out, and that metastasis from mucinous tumors of various other organs must be excluded clinically.

Signet ring cell adenocarcinoma of the lung is another rare histologic variant that is characterized by the presence of signet ring cells; these may be only focally identified and mixed with other growth patterns (Fig. 12.34). The tumor cells are negative for CK20 and strongly positive for TTF-1, an important feature that distinguishes them from metastatic signet ring cell adenocarcinoma from the gastrointestinal tract.[92] As mentioned earlier,

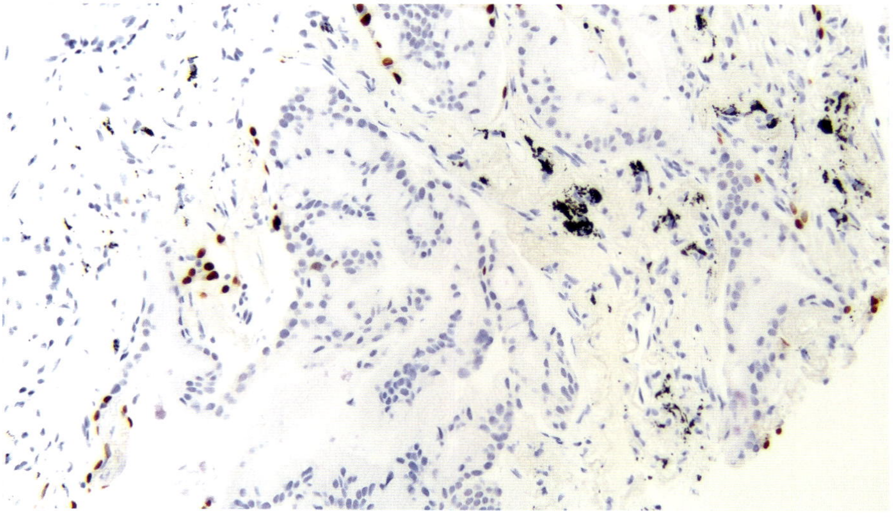

FIGURE 12.32 Thyroid transcription factor-1 immunostain in invasive mucinous carcinoma shows nearly complete absence of staining.

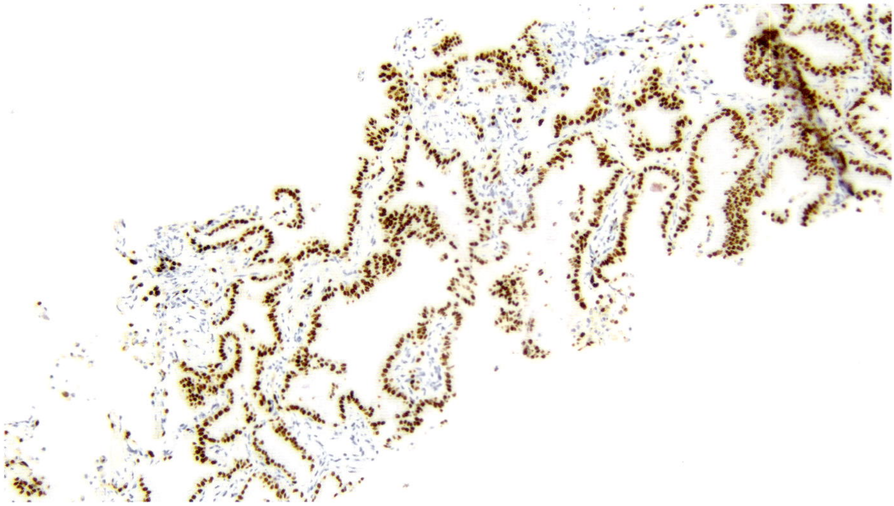

FIGURE 12.33 CDX2 immunostain in invasive mucinous carcinoma shows strongly nuclear positivity; notice the basal distribution of the nuclei highlighted by the stain.

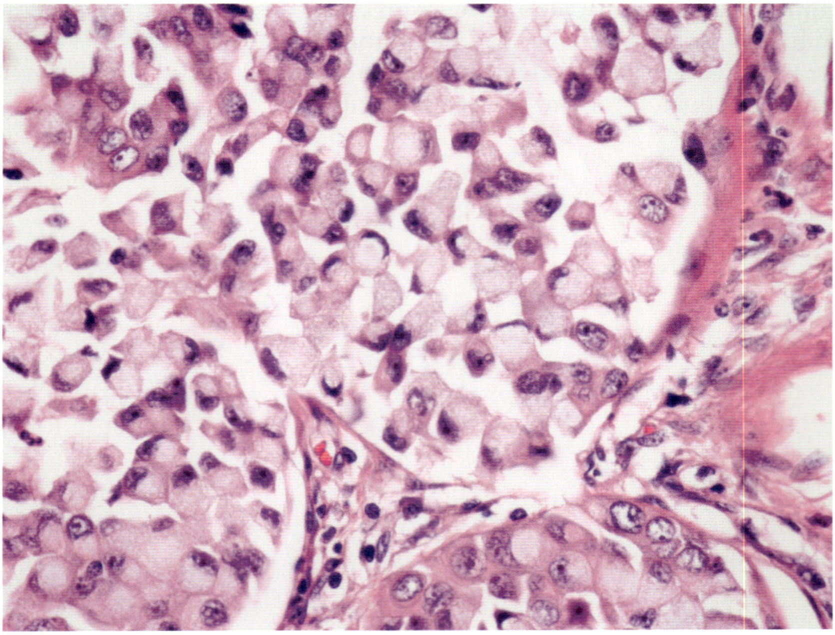

FIGURE 12.34 Signet ring cell adenocarcinoma of the lung is characterized by cells displaying abundant intracytoplasmic mucin displacing the nuclei toward the periphery.

tumors with signet cell morphology may be associated with *ALK* and *ROS1* rearrangements and warrant IHC stains for ALK and ROS1 if sufficient tissue is available.[33,37]

Secretory endometrioid-like adenocarcinoma of the lung is another morphologic variant of adenocarcinoma that is characterized by complex glandular structures that are lined by columnar cells with clear cytoplasm resembling secretory endometrium.[93] The tumor cells are positive for CK7 and TTF-1 but do not stain with CK20, WT1, chromogranin, and estrogen and progesterone receptors, helping to facilitate the distinction between a metastasis from the uterus, ovary, or fetal-type adenocarcinoma (monophasic pulmonary blastoma), which it may closely resemble.

Fetal adenocarcinoma of the lung is a rare tumor, regarded by some as a monophasic variant of pulmonary blastoma, characterized by glandular structures with a striking cribriform appearance that are lined by columnar cells containing abundant clear vacuoles in the cytoplasm and basally oriented nuclei resembling fetal lung tubules (Fig. 12.35A and B). A common finding is the presence of squamoid "morules" at the base of the glands (Fig. 12.36A and B). The tumor cells contain abundant diastase-resistant periodic acid-Schiff material in the cytoplasm and are positive for TTF-1 and CK7. Low- and high-grade variants have been described in the literature.[94-96] A distinctive feature of the low-grade tumors is the presence of *CTNNB1* mutations, a feature shared with biphasic pulmonary blastoma. IHC will show reactivity for β-catenin in both nuclear and cytoplasmic distribution within tumor cells.[97] The lesions can also be positive for chromogranin and other neuroendocrine markers. The cribriform architecture may cause confusion with cribriform adenocarcinoma of the lung, a tumor with a more aggressive behavior. Identification of glandlike structures with basally oriented nuclei, clear cytoplasm, and the presence of squamous morules in any lung biopsy should prompt IHC and molecular testing for β-catenin.

Hepatoid adenocarcinoma of the lung is a rare variant of lung adenocarcinoma characterized by sheets of monotonous round to polygonal tumor cells with abundant eosinophilic cytoplasm admixed with scattered small empty vacuoles resembling hepatic parenchyma. The tumor cells show cytoplasmic positivity for α-fetoprotein.[98,99] Of note, these tumors can also be positive for HepPar1 leading to confusion with metastatic hepatocellular carcinoma of the lung (Figs. 12.37 and 12.38).[99] One study reported that epithelial cell adhesion molecule (EpCAM) markers (HEA125 and MOC31) are useful in distinguishing hepatoid lung adenocarcinoma from metastatic hepatocellular carcinoma as these markers are negative in the latter; however, the study only examined five cases.[99] Of note, it is likely that tumors previously classified as hepatoid adenocarcinomas of the lung actually represent poorly differentiated SMARCA4-deficient adenocarcinomas.[100] IHC and close clinical and radiologic correlation is recommended in these cases to help identify the primary site.

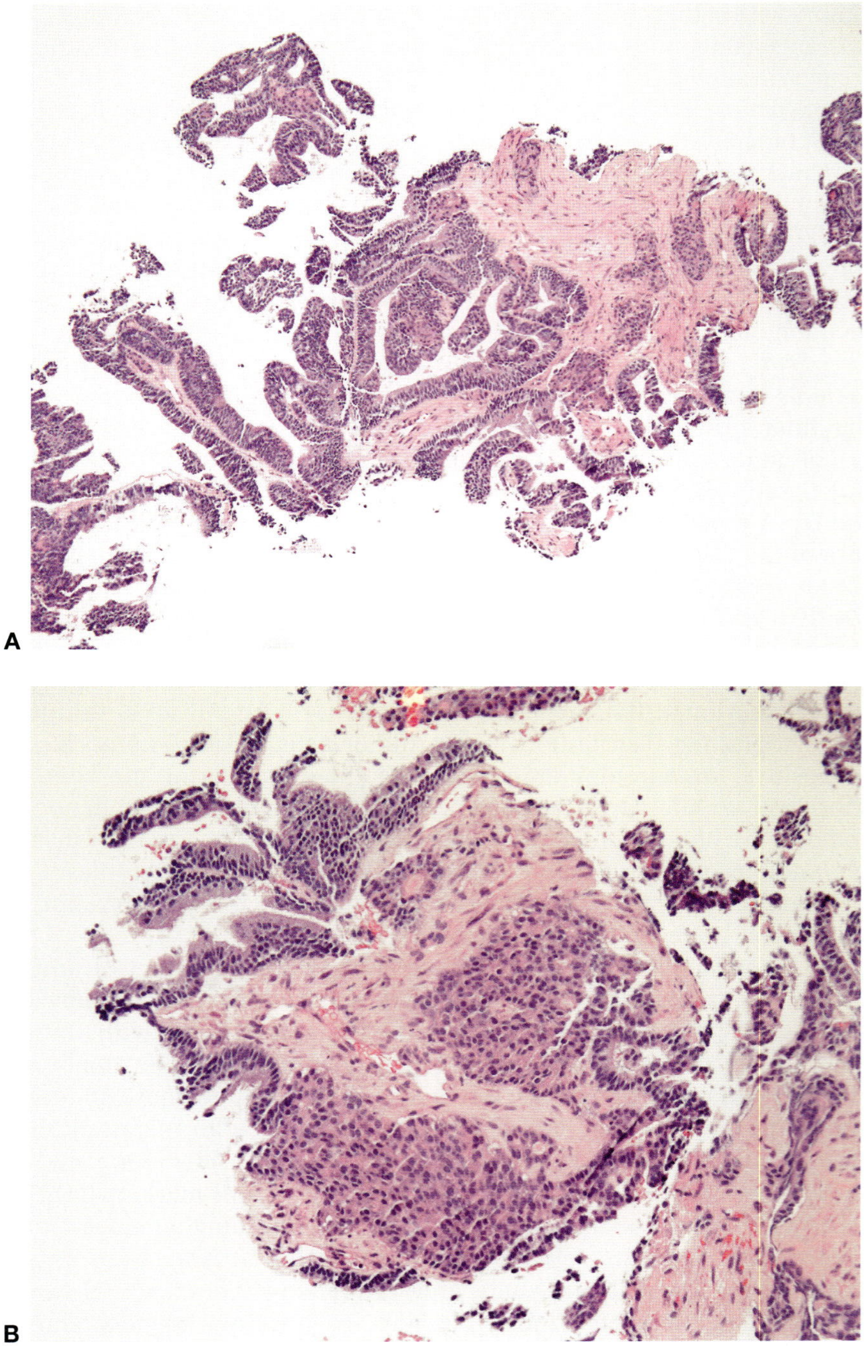

FIGURE 12.35 **A.** Core needle biopsy of fetal adenocarcinoma is characterized by glandular structures with a cribriform architecture that are lined by columnar cells with basally oriented nuclei that resemble fetal lung. Although absent in this small biopsy, the clear cell features were identified in the subsequent resection specimen. **B.** Higher-power magnification of the glandular structures may show a solid proliferation of vaguely squamoid appearing cells located at the base of the glands ("morules").

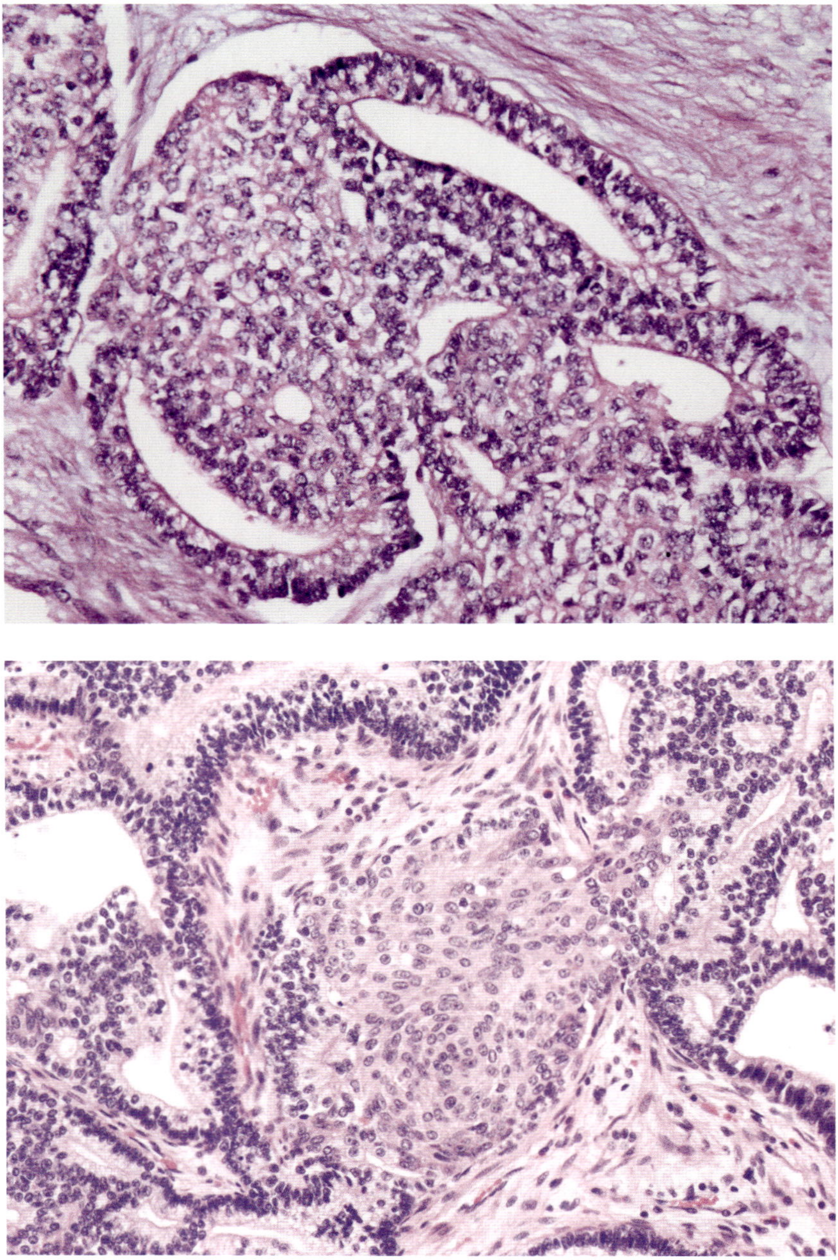

A

B

FIGURE 12.36 **A.** Wedge biopsy of fetal adenocarcinoma showing cribriform architecture lined by columnar cells with the characteristic clearing of the cytoplasm and with basally oriented nuclei. **B.** Some of the glandular formations will show well-formed squamous morules (as compared to the less well-formed morules seen in Fig. 12.35B).

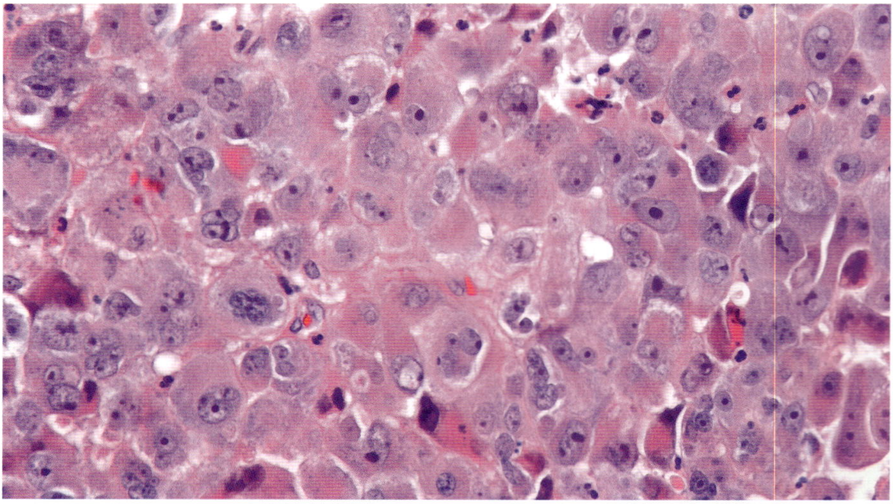

FIGURE 12.37 Hepatoid adenocarcinoma of the lung is characterized by very large epithelioid cells with an ample amount of eosinophilic cytoplasm.

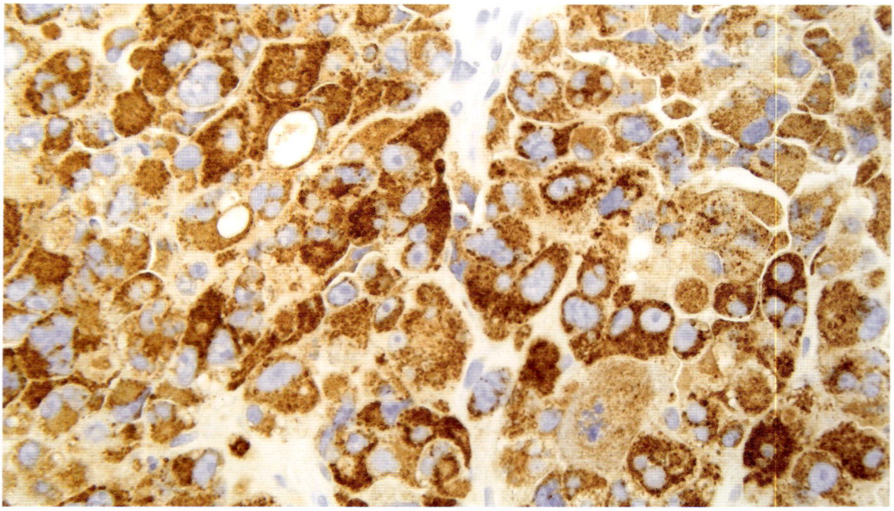

FIGURE 12.38 Immunostaining for HepPar1 shows strong positivity within the tumor cells. In tumors like this, BRG1/BRM immunostaining should be performed to exclude SMARCA4-deficient tumors.

Sarcomatoid or spindle cell adenocarcinoma is an unusual histologic variant that shows extensive overlap with large cell carcinoma and SCC with spindle cell features (sarcomatoid SCC) and falls under the broader category of *sarcomatoid carcinomas* of the lung in the WHO classification. Sarcomatoid adenocarcinoma can be appropriately diagnosed only on resection specimens in which ample sampling may allow proper identification of the better-differentiated areas and where the sarcomatoid component comprises at least 10% of the total tumor volume. According to the latest WHO classification, the category of sarcomatoid carcinoma includes pleomorphic carcinoma, pulmonary blastoma, and carcinosarcoma. The category of pleomorphic carcinoma incorporates spindle cell carcinomas and giant cell carcinomas (Fig. 12.39A-C).[6] In advanced tumors that are entirely sarcomatoid, molecular testing may be invaluable as it can identify adenocarcinoma-associated mutations that support the tumor as being derived from a preexisting adenocarcinoma even in the absence of a conventional adenocarcinoma component.[101] Carcinosarcoma and biphasic pulmonary blastoma are discussed in later sections of this chapter (see "Biphasic Pulmonary Blastoma" and "Carcinosarcoma"). In small endoscopic biopsies, it may not be possible to state more than "spindle cell carcinoma" based on results of immunohistochemical stains (cytokeratin positivity), but further subcategorization may be impossible. It is also important to distinguish these tumors from monophasic synovial sarcoma, which is also cytokeratin positive but will show a more uniform and monotonous cell population devoid of nuclear pleomorphism. Synovial sarcoma can be distinguished from sarcomatoid adenocarcinoma because it will strongly react with antibodies to SS18-SSX, SSX c-terminus, and TLE-1.

SMARCA4-deficient undifferentiated thoracic tumors are a recently described group of tumors characterized by rhabdoid or undifferentiated

A

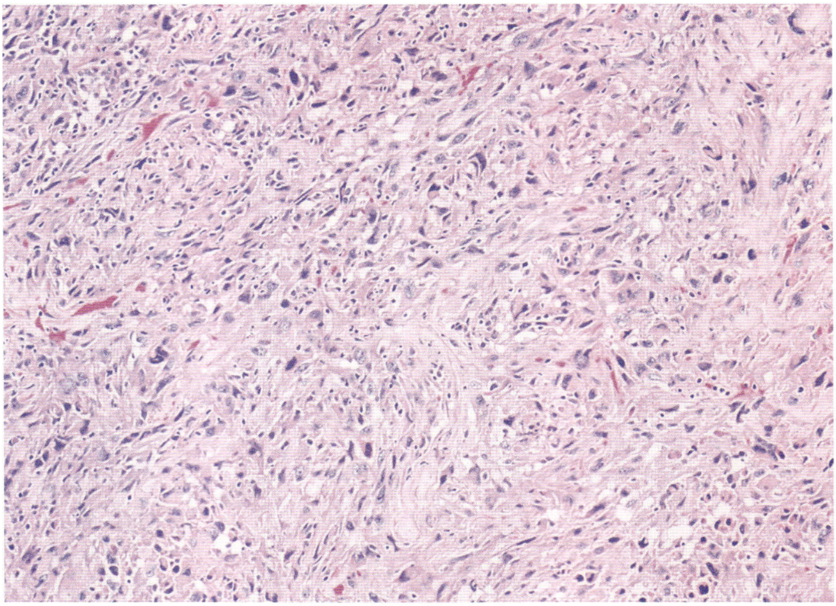

FIGURE 12.39 **A.** Sarcomatoid carcinoma showing a poorly differentiated neoplasm with large pleomorphic cells with a disordered growth pattern and vague fascicular growth.

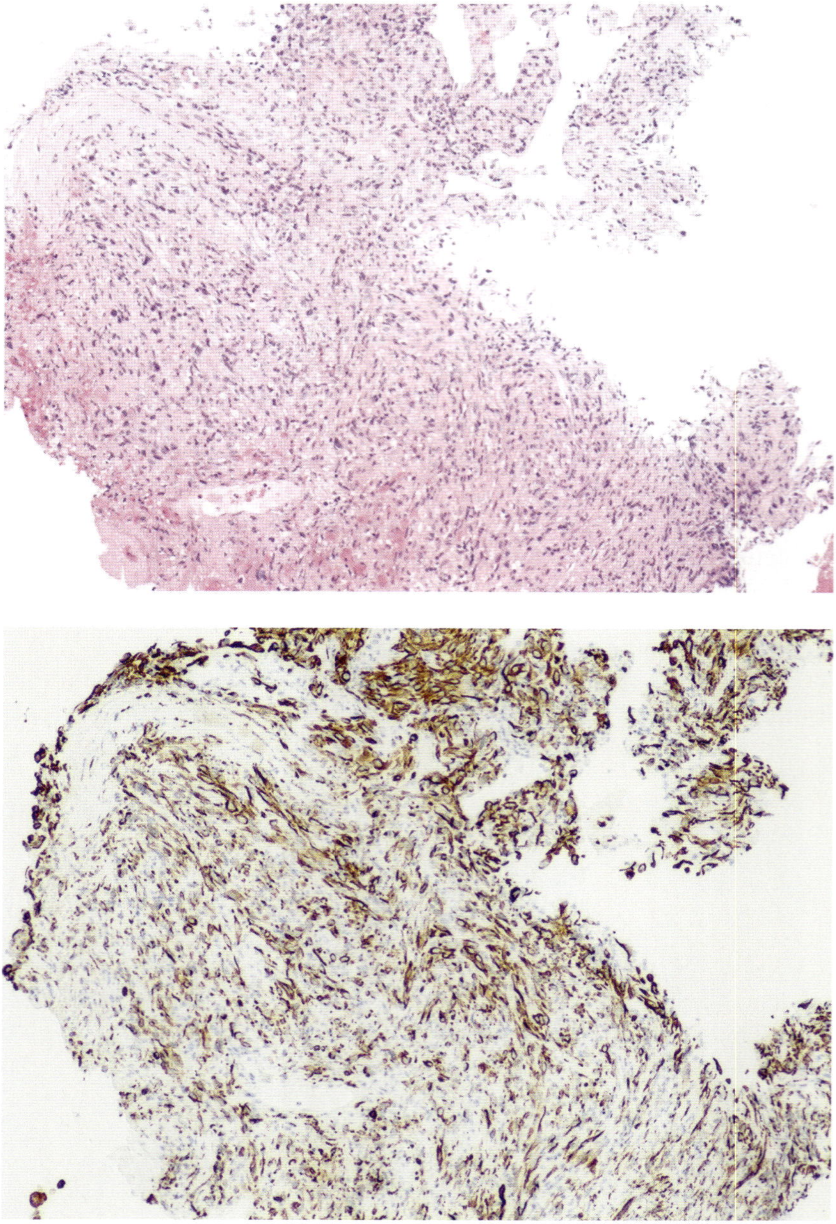

B

C

FIGURE 12.39 (*continued*) **B.** Core needle biopsy shows a poorly differentiated spindle cell neoplasm with no obvious adeno- or squamous cell carcinoma components. **C.** A keratin stain highlights the epithelial nature of the tumor cells.

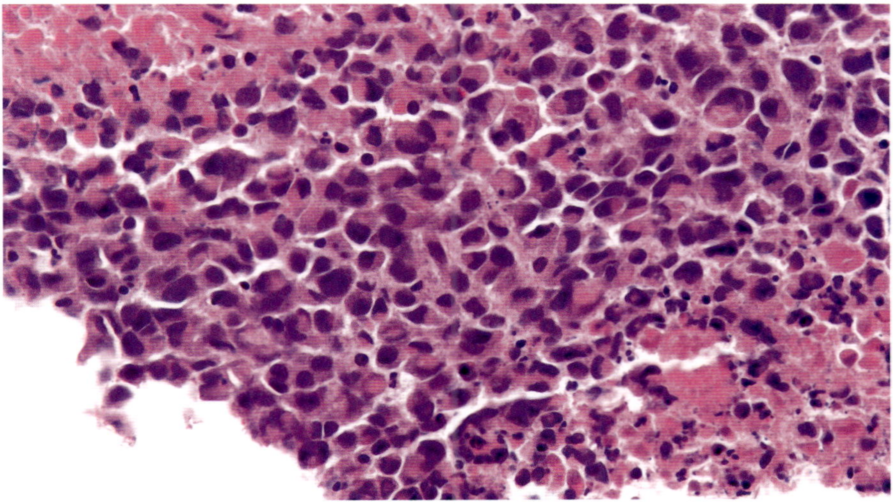

FIGURE 12.40 Example of a SMARCA4-deficient undifferentiated thoracic tumor shows sheets of anaplastic appearing cells with necrosis and prominent rhabdoid morphology.

morphology that demonstrate highly aggressive behavior (Fig. 12.40). The tumors were initially believed to represent undifferentiated thoracic sarcomas; however, subsequent studies have identified transitions from preexisting conventional NSCLC and smoking-related genetic signatures in these tumors that strongly suggest that they actually represent very poorly differentiated or undifferentiated carcinomas of the lung and thorax.[102-105] It should be noted that a small subset (~10%) lack pulmonary involvement and do not harbor the smoking-related signatures identified in many of these tumors, suggesting that some of these may represent true *SMARCA4*-deficient sarcomas of the thorax. The tumors are molecularly characterized by loss of the *SMARCA4* gene. Immunohistochemically, the tumors often show loss of nuclear expression of BRG1 (SMARCA4) and BRM (SMARCA2) (Fig. 12.41).[105] Given their undifferentiated histology, these tumors can be conceptualized as falling under the category of sarcomatoid carcinomas when harboring NSCLC-associated mutations and smoking-related genetic signatures. It is recommended that any lung or thoracic tumor showing rhabdoid morphology undergo immunohistochemical testing for BRG1 and BRM.

Adenocarcinoma with clear cells is currently considered to be a histologic variant of lung adenocarcinoma[6] and is characterized by cells with abundant clear cytoplasm; the tumors need to be distinguished from metastases to the lung from renal cell carcinoma, adrenal carcinoma, and other clear cell tumors. Special stains and close clinicopathologic correlation are indispensable in such cases. Rarely, this pattern may be confused for fetal-type adenocarcinoma, which can also show clearing of the

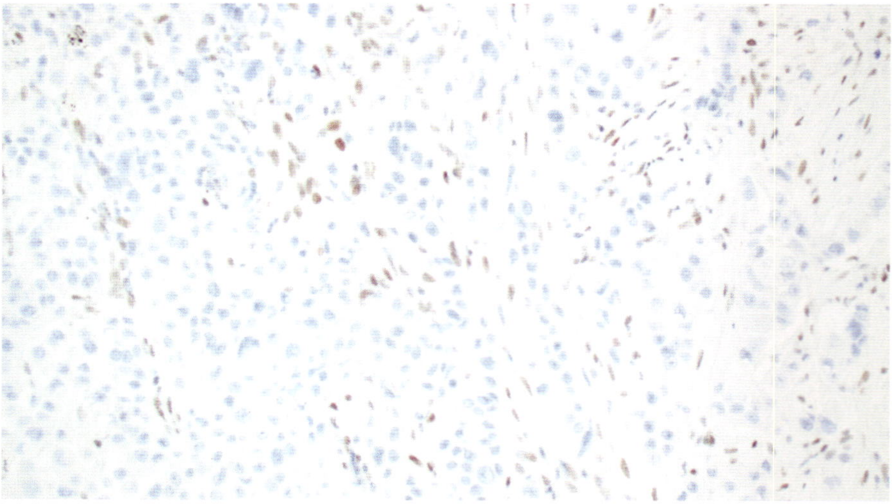

FIGURE 12.41 **BRG1 immunohistochemistry in a SMARCA4-deficient tumor shows loss of nuclear staining in the tumor cells.** Notice the retained internal controls.

cytoplasm. Some studies have suggested that clear cell carcinomas of the lung tend to show mostly solid architecture and behave in a more aggressive fashion as compared to conventional NSCLC (Fig. 12.42).[106] A small subset of these tumors with clear cell histology have been demonstrated to show recurrent *FGFR3::TACC3* fusions, an important observation as emerging literature suggests tumors with *FGFRx* alterations may be amenable to targeted therapy with tyrosine kinase inhibitors.[107]

Large cell basaloid adenocarcinoma is a recently described entity that superficially resembles large cell neuroendocrine carcinoma of the lung but is characterized by uniformly negative neuroendocrine markers and positivity for TTF1 and napsin A antibodies.[108] The histology is characterized by large nests, cords, and trabeculae of large epithelioid tumor cells with frequent comedolike areas of necrosis and prominent peripheral palisading of nuclei (Fig. 12.43-12.46). The importance of recognizing these tumors lies in separating them from large cell neuroendocrine carcinomas of the lung, which are treated with different regimens as compared to adenocarcinomas.

Squamous Cell Carcinoma

SCC is a malignant neoplasm that arises from bronchial epithelium and can show varying degrees of squamous differentiation. The most recent WHO classification has divided SCC into two categories: conventional (with numerous morphologic patterns possible) and basaloid SCC.[6] More than 90% of SCCs of the lung are associated with a history of cigarette smoking.[109] Molecularly, these tumors are characterized by mutations in

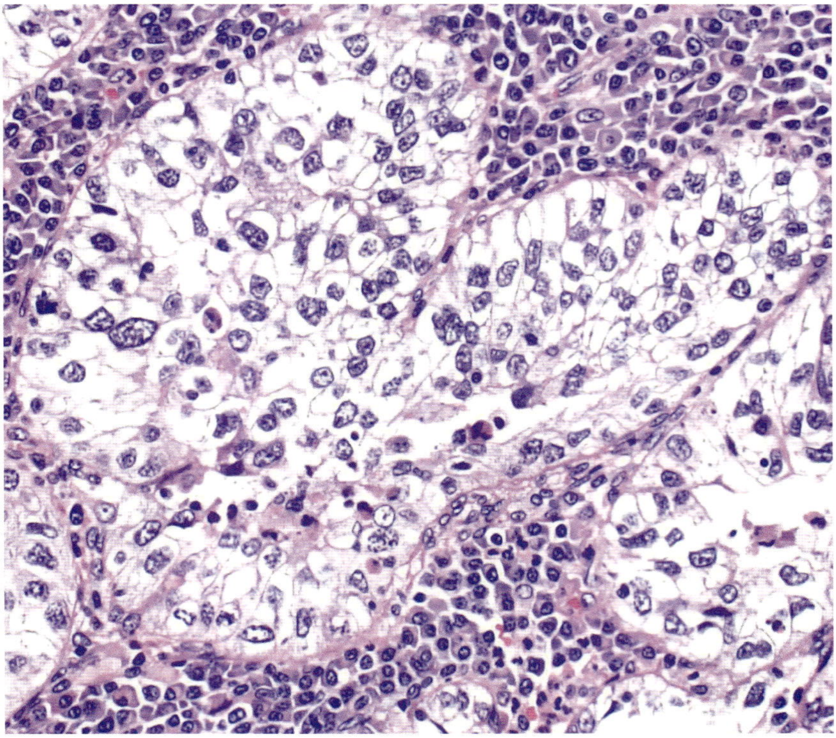

FIGURE 12.42 **Solid pattern adenocarcinoma of the lung with prominent clear cell changes.** Note a hint of possible gland formation (best seen on **right side** of image, central part of tumor nest).

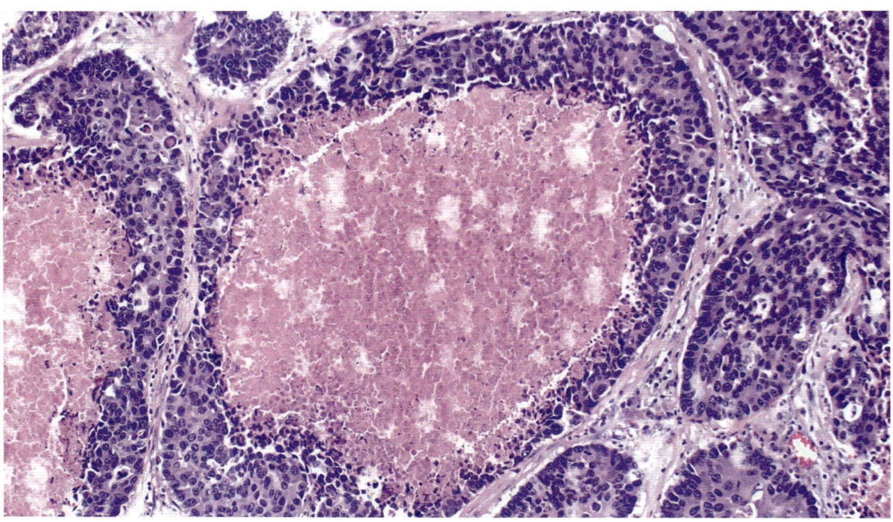

FIGURE 12.43 **Large cell basaloid adenocarcinoma of the lung shows a tumor growing in large nests with prominent central comedolike necrosis.** Notice the hint of peripheral palisading and large cell morphology that is very reminiscent of large cell neuroendocrine carcinoma.

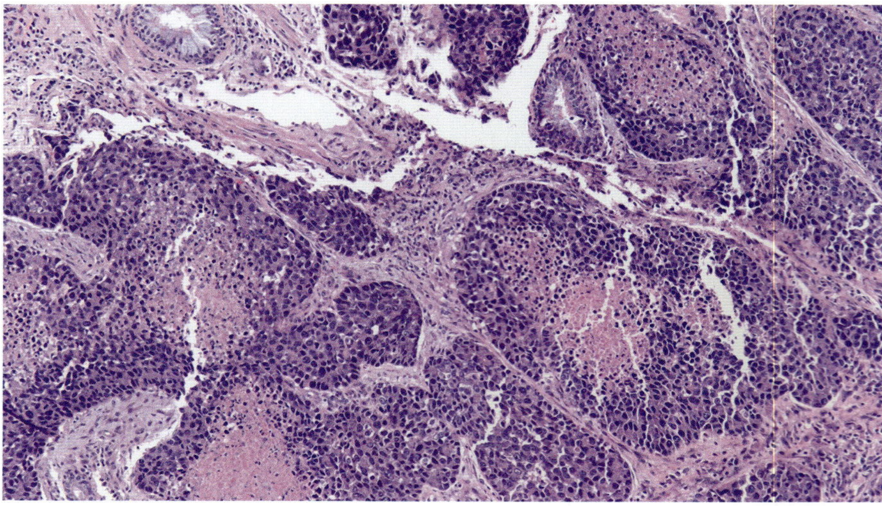

FIGURE 12.44 Another example of a large cell basaloid adenocarcinoma of the lung with areas of central comedolike necrosis.

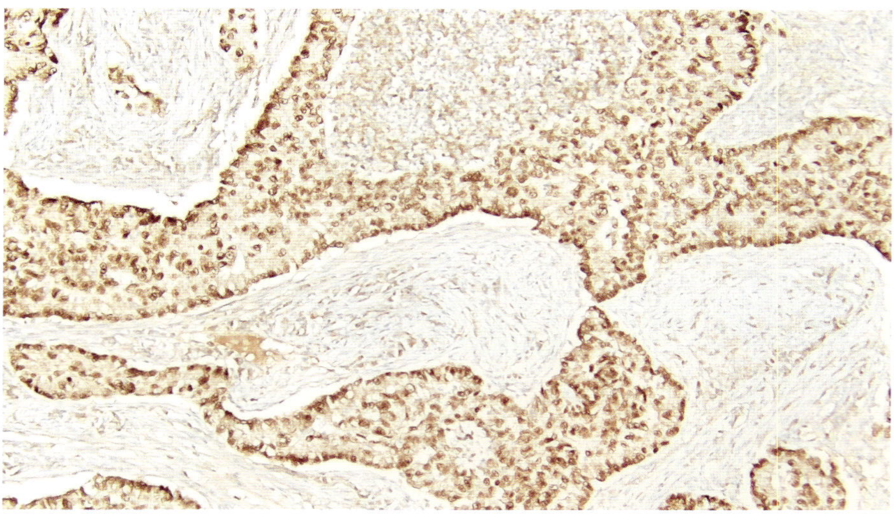

FIGURE 12.45 Thyroid transcription factor-1 immunohistochemistry shows strong nuclear staining and highlights the peripheral palisading in large cell basaloid adenocarcinoma of the lung.

TP53, *CDKN2A*, *PTEN*, *AKT1*, *PIK3CA*, *KEAP1*, *MLL2*, and *NOTCH1*, as well as numerous other genetic aberrations.[110] Of note, unlike adenocarcinoma, the targeted therapies available for SCC are extremely limited, although new clinical trials are currently underway. SCC, more often than adenocarcinoma, is treated with immunotherapy for PD-L1. The majority

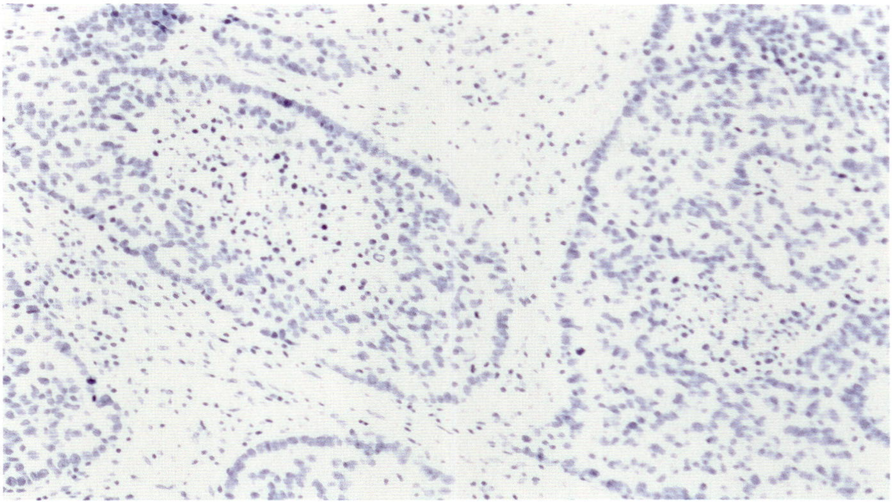

FIGURE 12.46 An immunostain for INSM1 shows complete absence of nuclear staining in large cell basaloid adenocarcinoma of the lung.

of pulmonary SCCs arise from the mainstem bronchi or segmental bronchi and are readily accessible to biopsy on endoscopy. SCC is thus the most frequently diagnosed cancer in endobronchial biopsy material. SCC may also arise in the periphery of the lung and form an expansile nodule that can secondarily infiltrate the pleura and chest wall. Some tumors may be cavitated and show extensive central areas of necrosis. Occasionally, the tumor can show an endobronchial polypoid, exophytic growth pattern; such tumors can display a papillary architecture. SCC is often associated with an in situ or high-grade dysplastic component. The dysplastic, in situ lesion is often seen in continuity with normal respiratory epithelium and will display lack of maturation, nucleomegaly, cytologic atypia, and abnormal mitotic figures (Fig. 12.47). It may or may not show evidence of an endophytic or superficially invasive component.[6] Occasionally, the in-situ component may extend into and replace the bronchial glands resembling invasive carcinoma. It may also be difficult to confirm the presence of an invasive component in a small endoscopic biopsy, thus requiring a disclaimer in the report that an invasive component cannot be ruled out. The presence of an in-situ carcinoma component in any endoscopic biopsy sample from a patient with an abnormal lung imaging study will require strict clinicopathologic correlation. In clinically equivocal cases, it will most likely represent an indication for surgical excision as it invariably heralds the existence of an invasive component. Smaller lesions can be managed with alternative therapies such as cryotherapy and argon plasma coagulation.[111]

Histologically, SCC of the lung may be well, moderately, or poorly differentiated and can be keratinizing or nonkeratinizing. SCC is not

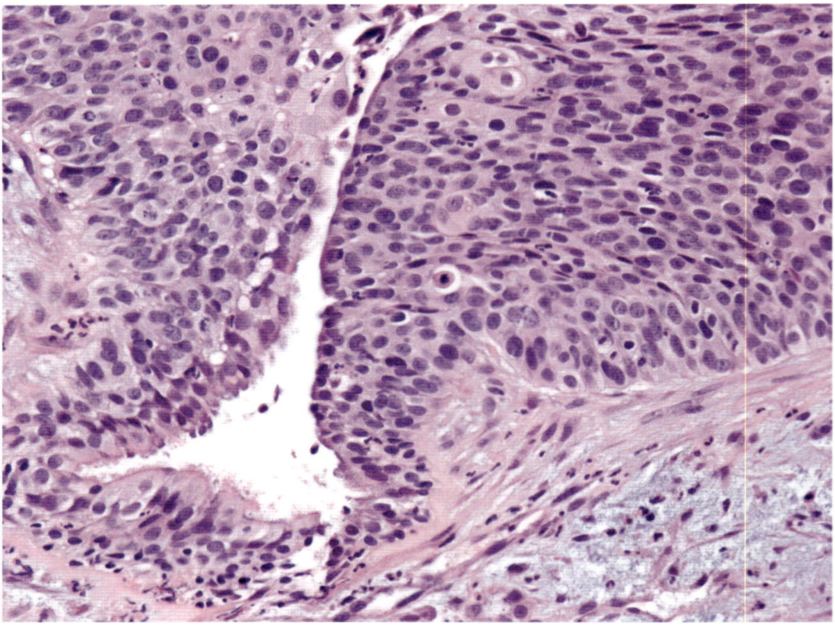

FIGURE 12.47 **Endobronchial squamous cell carcinoma in situ.** There is full-thickness atypia with lack of maturation, nucleomegaly, and scattered mitoses in the in situ component. Notice a focus of residual normal respiratory mucosa showing tall ciliated columnar cells (**lower left**) in continuity with the in-situ carcinoma.

currently routinely graded; though grading system for this tumor type is currently being finalized. The most distinctive features of well-differentiated squamous cell carcinoma are keratinization with keratin pearl formation and intercellular bridges. The tumor cells show enlarged nuclei and are surrounded by abundant eosinophilic cytoplasm displaying sharp cell borders (eFigs. 12.5 and 12.6). The nuclei will show increased chromatin and one or multiple nucleoli. Mitotic figures can be easily identified. The cells usually have a tendency to form small, cohesive groups that adopt a pavementlike architecture and are attached to each other by intercellular bridges. Foci of central keratinization with concentric islands of keratin "pearl" formation are frequently identified (Fig. 12.48A and B). Moderately differentiated neoplasms show a tendency to display a less obvious pavementlike architecture, with only occasional or no intercellular bridges, increased size of the nuclei with more prominent nucleoli, and foci of single-cell keratinization. Poorly differentiated tumors show more pronounced loss of keratinization; the cells may adopt bizarre shapes with nucleomegaly and nucleolar prominence and abundant, often abnormal mitoses. Extensive tumor cell necrosis is often a prominent feature in these tumors (Fig. 12.49A and B). Islands of poorly differentiated SCC will show a tendency to display central, comedolike areas of necrosis with prominent peripheral palisading of the tumor cells (eFig. 12.7).

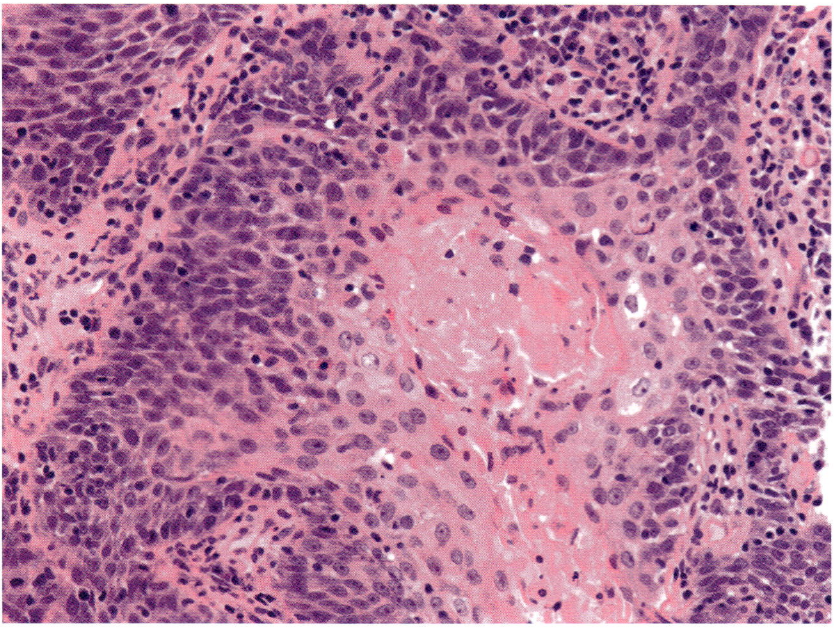

A

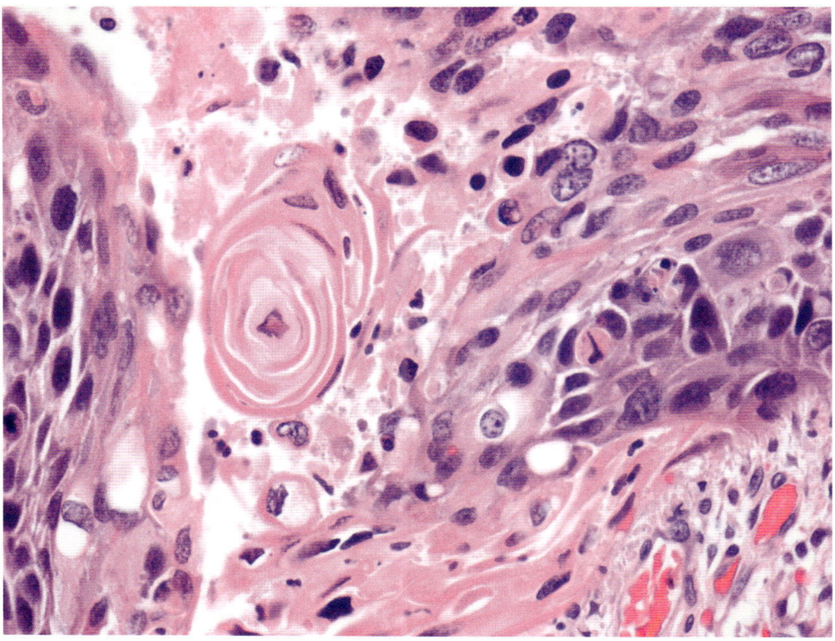

B

FIGURE 12.48 **A.** Well-differentiated squamous cell carcinoma (SCC) shows cohesive tumor cells with pavementlike architecture and central areas of keratinization. **B.** Higher magnification of well-differentiated SCC shows atypical tumor cells and a focus of keratin pearl formation.

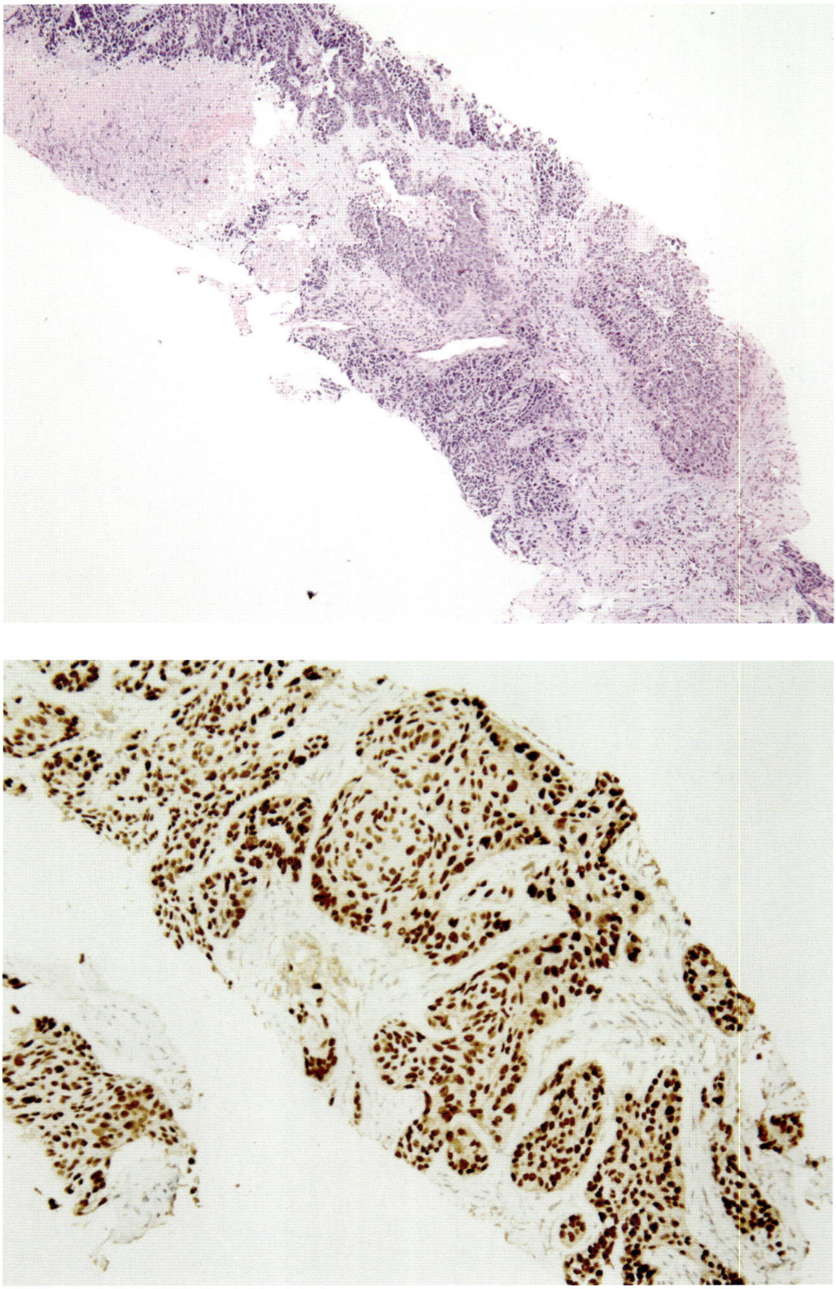

A

B

FIGURE 12.49 **A.** Core biopsy shows poorly differentiated squamous cell carcinoma (SCC) with clusters of large cells with pleomorphic and hyperchromatic nuclei and areas of necrosis. **B.** P63 stain in poorly differentiated SCC shows strong nuclear positivity in the tumor cells.

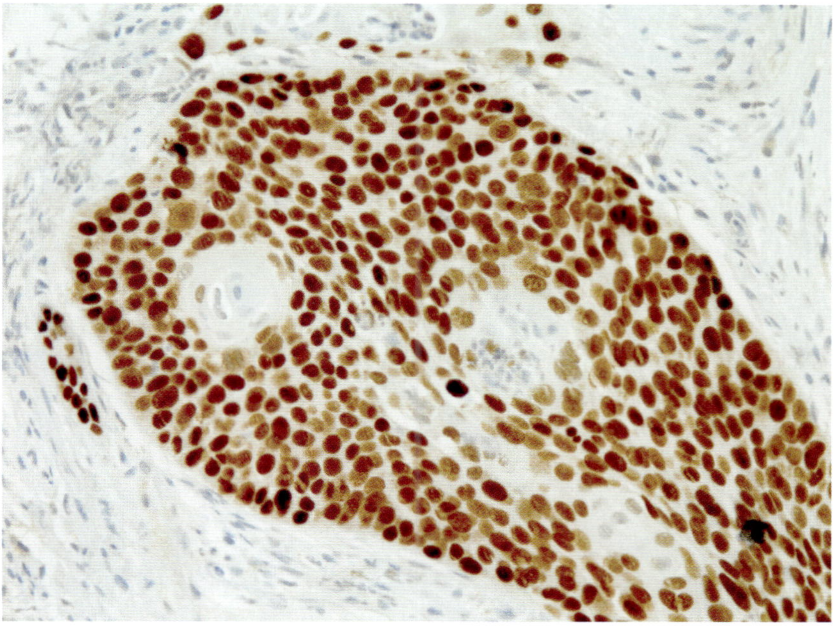

FIGURE 12.50 A small island of squamous cell carcinoma of the lung shows strong nuclear staining for p40.

IHC can be successfully applied in some cases to support a diagnosis of SCC on small endoscopic biopsies of the lung that contain poorly differentiated tumors. In general, CK5/6 and p63/p40 are strongly positive in most SCCs (Fig. 12.50). Expression of p63, however, may be lost or significantly diminished in poorly differentiated examples of SCC, and some cases may express only low molecular weight cytokeratins and vimentin. P40, an isoform of p63, is more specific as a marker of squamous differentiation but can show diminished expression in poorly differentiated tumors as well, thus limiting its utility for distinguishing poorly differentiated SCC from other poorly differentiated tumors.[22-24] P63 expression can also occur in up to one-third of adenocarcinomas, although the pattern is usually more heterogeneous.[112] Exact categorization of poorly differentiated SCC in small biopsy samples may not always be feasible, and a noncommittal diagnosis of "poorly differentiated, non–small cell carcinoma" may be more appropriate in such instances than attempting to categorize the tumor based on equivocal or potentially misleading results of IHC. It has been stated that excluding squamous differentiation in poorly differentiated tumors is of importance to determine eligibility of patients for treatment with pemetrexed (because of increased efficacy)[113] or bevacizumab (because of increased toxicity).[114] Additional studies are needed, however, to determine whether this also applies to poorly differentiated tumors or only to those that can be readily identified as squamous by routine histology alone.

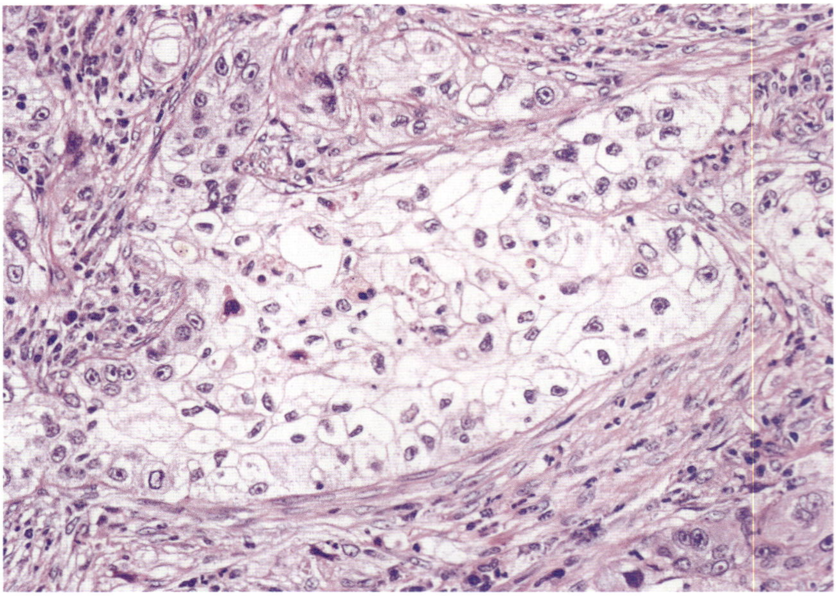

FIGURE 12.51 Squamous cell carcinoma of the lung can show prominent clear cell changes; care must be taken not to confuse these changes for metastases from other clear cell lesions.

Unusual morphologic appearances in SCC of the lung include tumors displaying clear cell features with abundant, optically clear cytoplasm filled with glycogen (Fig. 12.51), tumors with prominent spindling of the cells that can closely resemble a spindle cell sarcoma, and tumors comprising relatively small cells with scant cytoplasm that may resemble small cell neuroendocrine carcinoma (the so-called basaloid or small cell variant of poorly differentiated SCC). Such cases may be extremely difficult to diagnose with confidence on small endoscopic biopsies unless more conventional, better-differentiated areas are present in the sample. Tumors with ample clear cytoplasm may be confused with metastases of clear cell carcinoma, such as metastatic renal cell carcinoma. Spindle (sarcomatoid) SCC may be confused with various spindle cell sarcomas, in particular monophasic synovial sarcoma, which can also express cytokeratin positivity. Molecular testing for the *SS18* fusion product of the X;18 translocation associated with synovial sarcoma may be of assistance in such instances for making that distinction.

A "basaloid" variant of SCC has also been described, which may show some morphologic overlap with several entities, including neuroendocrine carcinomas. It is likely that basaloid carcinoma corresponds to the same entity as the small cell variant of SCC (Fig. 12.52).[115-118] It has been proposed that these lesions behave in a more aggressive manner compared to conventional SCC.[115] On biopsy material, the most important

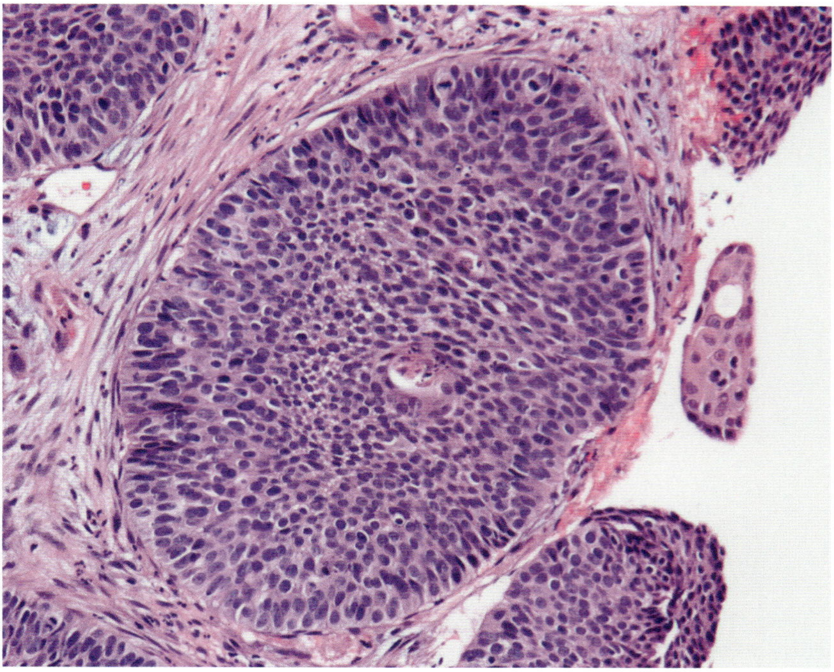

FIGURE 12.52 Small cell variant/basaloid variant of squamous cell carcinoma is characterized by the relatively smaller size of the tumor cells, which are monotonous, contain scant cytoplasm, and show striking peripheral palisading of nuclei.

distinction to make is from large cell neuroendocrine carcinoma or an intermediate-grade neuroendocrine tumor (atypical carcinoid). In cases of the small cell/basaloid variant of SCC, absence of reactivity for chromogranin, synaptophysin, INSM1 and CD56 coupled with nuclear positivity for p63/p40 will generally help with this distinction.

Finally, two unusual types of lung tumors that may bear some relationship to SCC are lymphoepithelial carcinoma (LECA) of the lung and NUT carcinoma. *LECA* essentially corresponds to a nonkeratinizing, poorly differentiated SCC containing a heavy lymphoplasmacytic cell infiltrate in the stroma (Fig. 12.53). The tumors resemble poorly differentiated nasopharyngeal carcinomas and "LECA" carcinomas at other locations and are associated with an aggressive behavior.[119,120] Some of these tumors have been found to be related to Epstein-Barr virus (EBV) infection and may contain Epstein-Barr virus latent membrane protein.[120] The cells in these tumors are large, round to oval, with vesicular nuclei and prominent, usually centrally placed nucleoli, and are surrounded by a scant rim of amphophilic cytoplasm with indistinct cell borders. The tumors are invariably strongly positive for p40/p63 and negative for markers of lung adenocarcinoma. The differential diagnosis includes primarily metastases of LECAs from other sites and differentiating these lesions requires strict

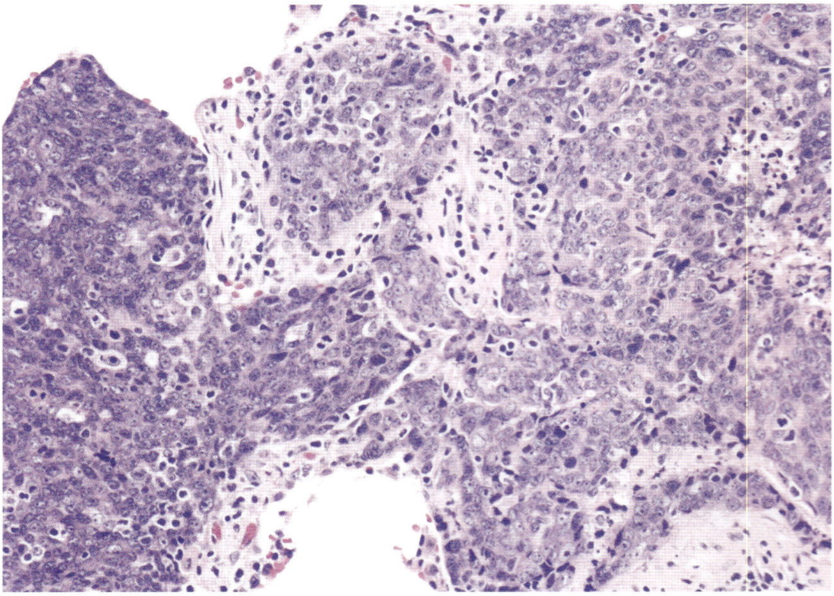

FIGURE 12.53 **Core needle biopsy of lymphoepithelial carcinoma of the lung shows a poorly differentiated neoplasm with large, atypical sheets of cells growing in cohesive nests with prominent nucleoli.** Scattered lymphocytes and plasma cells are seen within the interstitium.

clinical correlation. *NUT carcinoma* corresponds to a poorly differentiated carcinoma that is characterized by a t(15;19) translocation that produces a *NUTM1*::*BRD4* rearrangement, although some variant rearrangements have been described as well.[121] These lesions were originally described within midline structures but have now been described in various other locations. They are highly aggressive lesions with short survival times from diagnosis.[122,123] Histologically, they are characterized by sheets of poorly differentiated atypical cells with abrupt foci of keratinization. These foci of keratinization may be missed on small biopsy material. They will often stain with p40 and p63 by IHC. The differential diagnosis for these lesions includes other poorly differentiated carcinomas, melanoma, round blue cell sarcomas, and poorly differentiated mesotheliomas. These lesions can be separated from other tumors in the differential by the use of an available NUT IHC antibody,[124] as well as by FISH and molecular methods for identification of the rearrangement.

ADENOSQUAMOUS CARCINOMA

Adenosquamous carcinoma is characterized by showing components of both SCC and adenocarcinoma (Fig. 12.54).[125] By the current WHO definition, each component must comprise at a minimum 10% of the tumor[6]

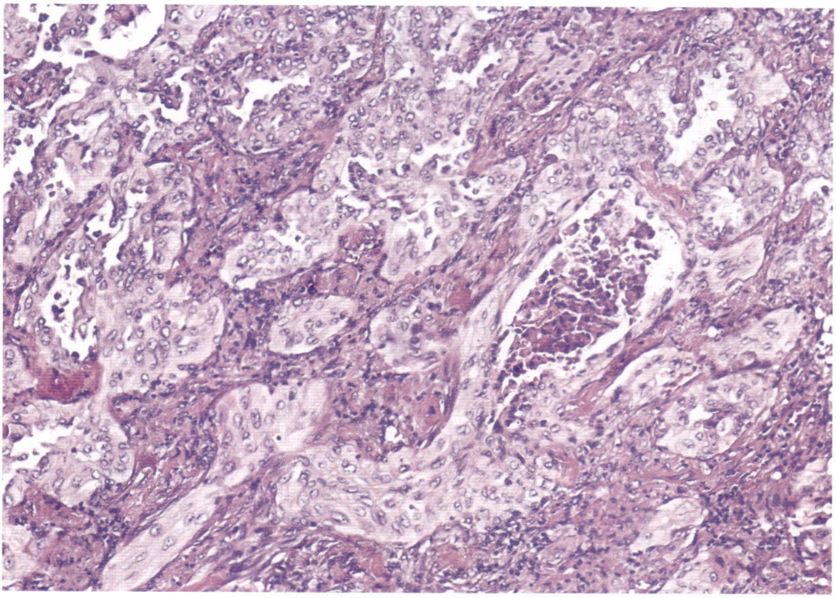

FIGURE 12.54 Adenosquamous carcinoma of the lung; the lesion is composed of solid squamous components (*bottom*) admixed with glandular elements (*top*).

Adenosquamous carcinoma is an aggressive neoplasm with increased metastatic potential.[126] Interestingly, enough mutational profiling has identified that many of these tumors harbor mutations seen in adenocarcinoma or SCC and that in some cases, they occur concurrently. High rates of *EGFR* gene alterations have been identified as well, suggesting that these tumors may be amenable to targeted therapies with tyrosine-kinase inhibitors.[127] Definitive diagnosis of adenosquamous carcinoma requires a resection specimen to determine the exact composition of the different components; however, the diagnosis may be suggested on biopsy material showing morphologic features of both SCC and adenocarcinoma (see Table 12.2).

Large Cell Carcinoma

Large cell carcinoma has traditionally been defined as a malignant epithelial neoplasm of the lung characterized by undifferentiated large cell morphology lacking features of squamous or glandular differentiation (Fig. 12.55A and B). The term essentially overlaps with poorly differentiated NSCLC and essentially represents a catch-all category for lesions that cannot fit into other categories of lung carcinoma.[128] A large number of carcinoma subtypes have been described under the umbrella of the "large cell" category, including clear cell, pleomorphic, anaplastic, and giant cell carcinoma, though many of these are now reclassified as sarcomatoid carcinomas. A distinctive subtype of poorly differentiated carcinoma encountered in the lung, that has recently been reclassified as a sarcomatoid carcinoma, is the anaplastic

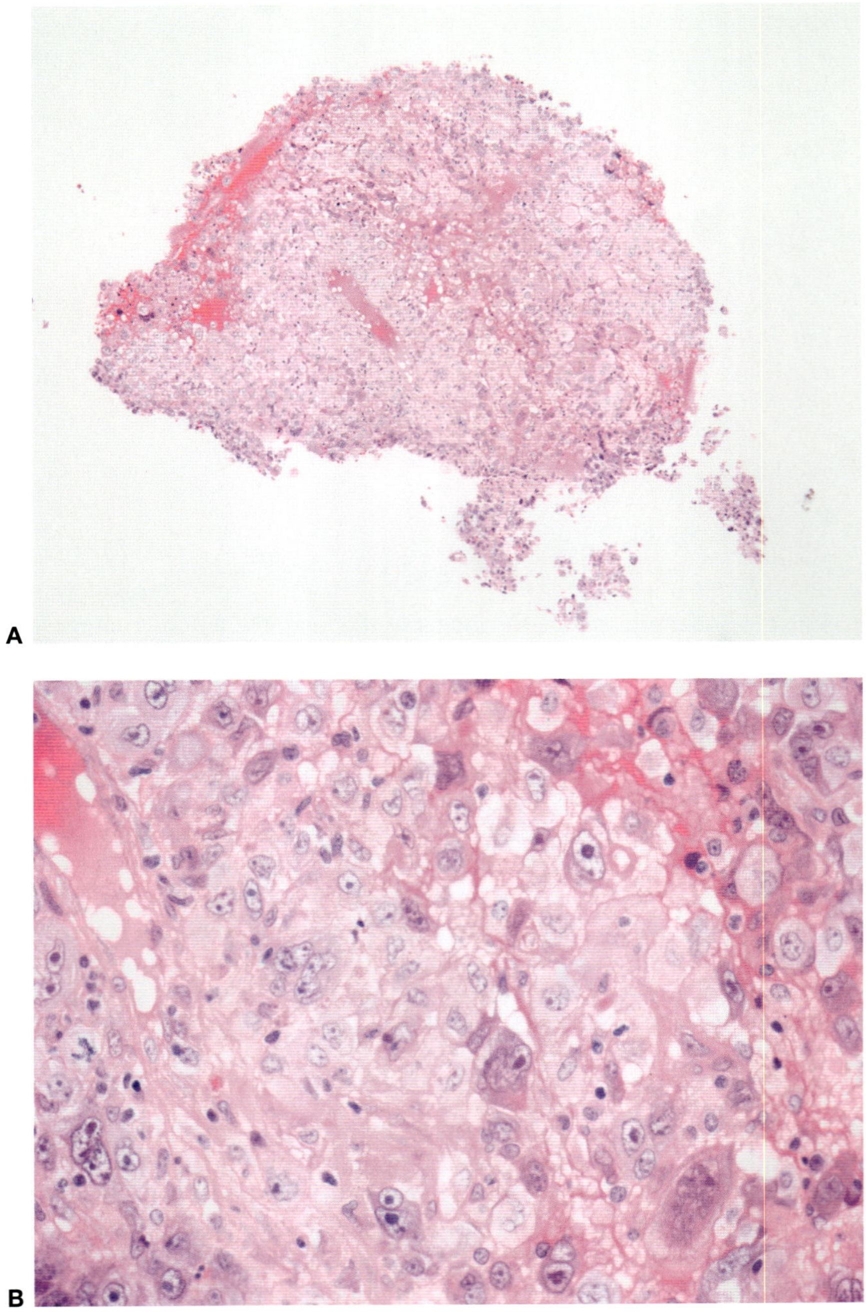

FIGURE 12.55 **A.** Endobronchial biopsy shows replacement of the wall of the bronchus by sheets of large, atypical cells without evidence of gland formation or keratinization. **B.** Higher magnification of large cell carcinoma of the lung shows large tumor cells with pleomorphic nuclei containing prominent eosinophilic nucleoli.

carcinoma variant containing a prominent inflammatory component, (also known as inflammatory giant cell carcinoma of the lung).[101] These tumors are currently placed under the umbrella of sarcomatoid (pleomorphic) carcinomas of the lung by the WHO. Such tumors are characterized by discohesive sheets of large, anaplastic tumor cells admixed with prominent inflammatory elements, including small lymphocytes, neutrophils, eosinophils, plasma cells, and histiocytes (Fig. 12.56A and B). Another histologic variant that can be seen is one characterized by cells containing prominent "rhabdoid" cytoplasmic inclusions that displace the nuclei toward the periphery (Fig. 12.57); although many of such tumors previously classified as large cell carcinoma are now known to represent *SMARCA4*-deficient tumors.[129] Large cell carcinoma of the lung in general is characterized by large, pleomorphic, and bizarre cells with enlarged nuclei containing very large and prominent eosinophilic nucleoli (eFigs. 12.8-12.10). Multinucleated, trophoblastic-type giant cells can also be seen, and in some cases, they may stain positive for human chorionic gonadotrophic hormone.[130] What all these tumors have in common is the absence of features of either squamous or glandular differentiation at the light microscopic level, non–small cell morphology (ie, large size of the tumor cells), and absence of immunohistochemical markers of conventional NSCLC or other lung carcinoma types.

The current guidelines for reporting of these tumors on small biopsy samples is that the term "large cell carcinoma" should be avoided in small biopsy or cytology specimens because of the possibility that better-differentiated areas might be present in a resected specimen.[6,7] A directed immunohistochemical panel on such tumors is recommended to attempt to define whether there is evidence of squamous or glandular differentiation, including TTF-1 for the diagnosis of adenocarcinoma and p63, p40, or CK5/6 for SCC. Mucin stains (such as mucicarmine) for the identification of intracellular mucin may also be applied. To conserve tissue for molecular studies, the use of cocktails of nuclear and cytoplasmic antigens, such as TTF-1/CK5/6 or p40/napsin A, may be used if available. If available, BRG1 (SMARCA4) should be tested in all large cell carcinomas to exclude the possibility of a SMARCA4-deficient tumor. It is recommended that cases positive for an adenocarcinoma marker and/or mucin stains with a negative squamous marker be classified as "NSCLC, favor adenocarcinoma," and those positive for a squamous marker and a negative adenocarcinoma and/or mucin marker be classified as "NSCLC, favor SCC." Unfortunately, this formula is not foolproof, and there exists some overlap in the expression patterns of these antibodies as well as aberrant expression of markers that may lead to incorrect assumptions by clinicians. In some cases, it may be impossible and impractical to attempt to force a given sample into a defined diagnostic category. Such cases are best reported as NSCLC, NOS; poorly differentiated NSCLC; or NSCLC, large cell type. This is particularly true when equivocal or conflicting results are obtained using immunohistochemical markers (ie, positivity for both adenocarcinoma and SCC-associated markers; or negative staining for both).

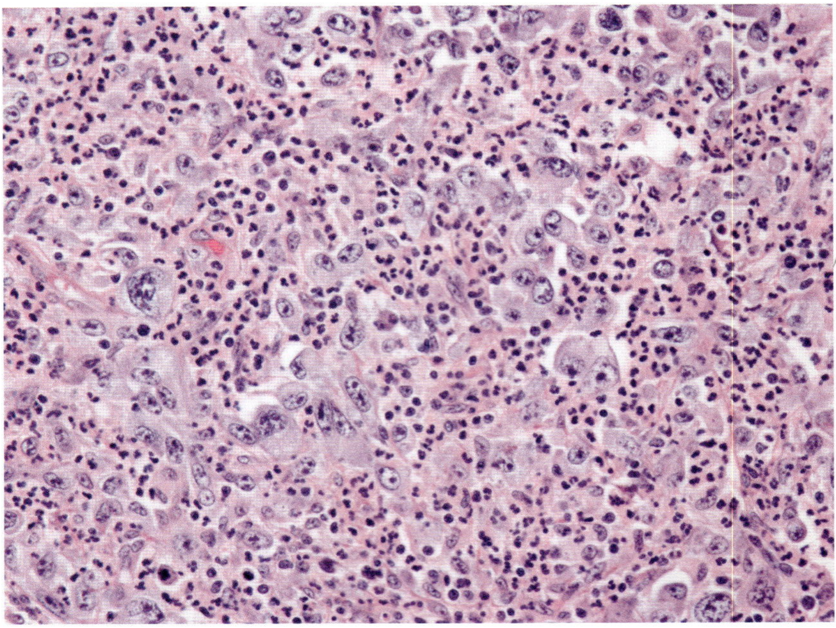

A

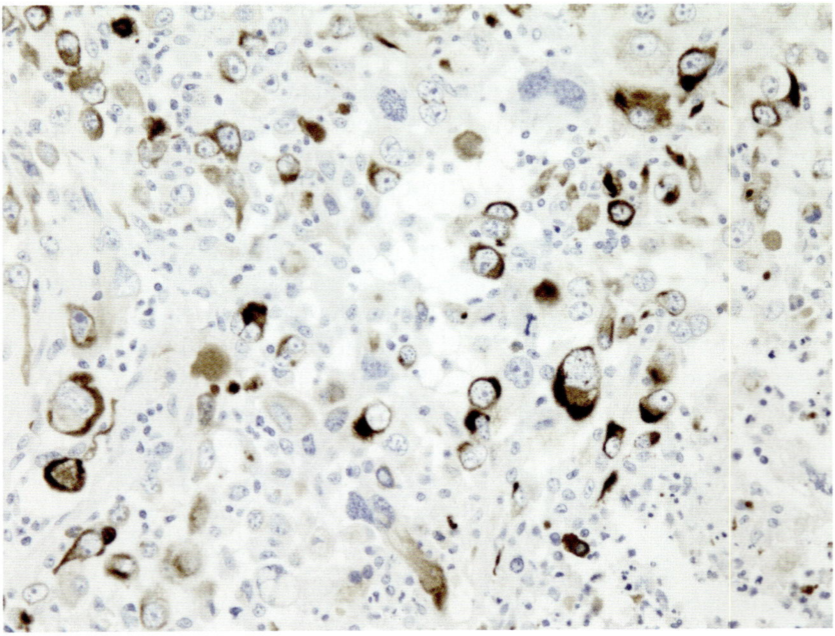

B

FIGURE 12.56 **A.** Giant cell carcinoma of the lung, "inflammatory" type (also known as "inflammatory giant cell carcinoma"), shows abundant singly scattered, large, pleomorphic tumor cells with bizarre nuclei and prominent nucleoli, surrounded by dense inflammatory infiltrate. **B.** Low molecular weight cytokeratin (CAM5.2) shows positivity in the scattered atypical epithelial cells.

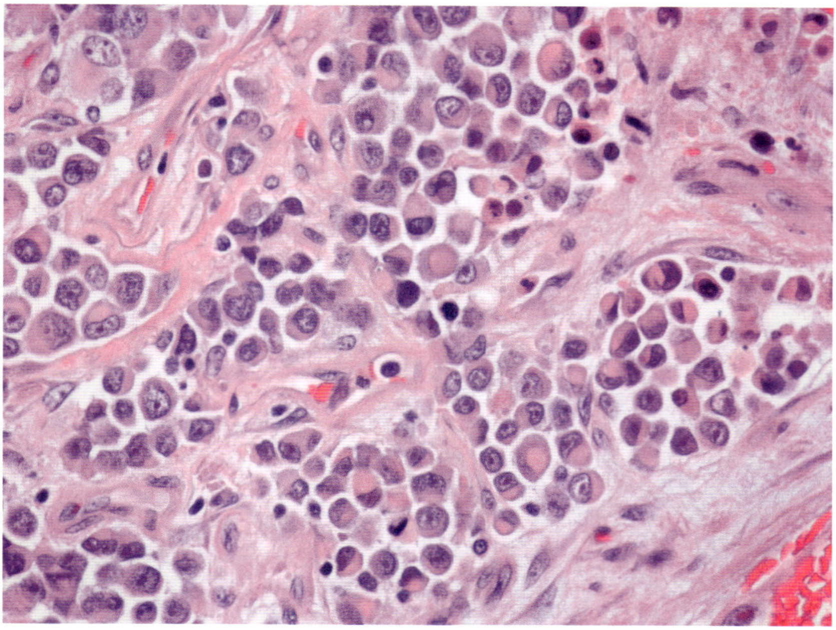

FIGURE 12.57 Anaplastic carcinoma of the lung with "rhabdoid" features shows a population of cells with large, atypical nuclei that are displaced to the periphery by densely eosinophilic cytoplasmic inclusions containing intermediate filaments.

Perhaps a more important issue is to separate poorly differentiated, large cell carcinoma (NSCLC, NOS) from other large cell malignancies of nonepithelial origin, such as epithelioid or pleomorphic sarcomas, melanomas, large cell lymphomas, and metastases from germ cell tumors or other poorly differentiated large cell neoplasms. A short battery of immunohistochemical stains may be of value in such instances to verify that the tumor is, indeed, of epithelial origin. In particular, a combination of broad-spectrum cytokeratin and low molecular weight cytokeratins (such as AE1/AE3 and CAM5.2) at a minimum is indicated to demonstrate epithelial origin. Undifferentiated pleomorphic sarcoma, epithelioid sarcoma, epithelioid variants of angiosarcoma, malignant peripheral nerve sheath tumors, and leiomyosarcoma as well as various other nonepithelial neoplasms with large cell morphology may arise as primary tumors in the lung or can metastasize to the lung from other primary sites. Use of appropriate immunohistochemical stains and molecular testing is indicated in such instances to better define the phenotype and genotype; clinicopathologic correlation is required in all cases of poorly differentiated large cell malignancies in the lung to rule out the possibility of a metastasis from another source. Diffuse large cell lymphoma, as mentioned previously, may also express p63 in a significant number of cases[21]; use of appropriate lymphoid markers such as CD3, CD20, CD30, CD45, and ALK-1 is indicated if there is a suspicion of lymphoma. Large cell or anaplastic carcinomas arising from other organs, including the thyroid, breast, gastrointestinal tract, pancreas, biliary tract, and urinary bladder, may also metastasize to the lung; clinicopathologic correlation and a proper history are indispensable for arriving at a correct diagnosis. In addition, as is always the case when dealing with a poorly differentiated neoplasm, melanoma should be ruled out by the use of melanocytic markers such as S100, HMB45, Melan A, and SOX10.

SALIVARY GLAND–TYPE TUMORS OF THE LUNG

Tumors recapitulating the features of salivary gland neoplasms can infrequently arise in the lung. Such tumors are felt to originate from bronchial glands located along the bronchial tree and because of their close relationship to the bronchus will often present as endobronchial masses, leading to early symptoms of bronchial obstruction. Some cases can also rarely present as well-circumscribed, peripheral lung nodules. Because of their predilection for the central airways, they are easily amenable to diagnosis through endoscopic biopsies. Clinicopathologic correlation and careful clinical history are indispensable to rule out a late or occult metastasis from a primary lesion in the salivary glands.

Mucoepidermoid Carcinoma

Mucoepidermoid carcinoma is one of the most frequent endobronchial tumors to occur in the pediatric age population, although they can also affect older individuals.[131] Histologically, they resemble their salivary gland counterpart and are characterized by a proliferation of squamous cells admixed with mucin-secreting cells and cells showing intermediate features. The tumors can be either of low- or high-grade histology, based on the degree of cytologic atypia, mitotic activity, necrosis, and degree of differentiation of the tumor cells.[132] Low-grade tumors often display cystic changes and contain sheets of epidermoid cells with intercellular bridges and foci of keratinization alongside "intermediate" cells with less-developed squamous features. Admixed with the squamoid elements are small glands, tubules, and cysts lined by cytologically bland goblet or columnar cells showing secretion of abundant mucin into the lumens (Fig. 12.58). Low-grade mucoepidermoid carcinoma of the bronchus is associated with an overall better prognosis and lower rate of metastases to regional lymph nodes than its high-grade counterpart.[133,134] Children have a particularly indolent clinical course. The high-grade tumors are associated with aggressive behavior and in general are treated as other NSCLC, depending on their clinical stage at the time of diagnosis.[134] High-grade tumors show sheets and islands of less well-differentiated squamous cells with an inconspicuous mucinous component. The cells usually display more pronounced nuclear atypia with high mitotic activity, foci of necrosis, and extensive infiltration of surrounding pulmonary parenchyma. Overall, the immunohistochemical profile is nonspecific; the squamoid

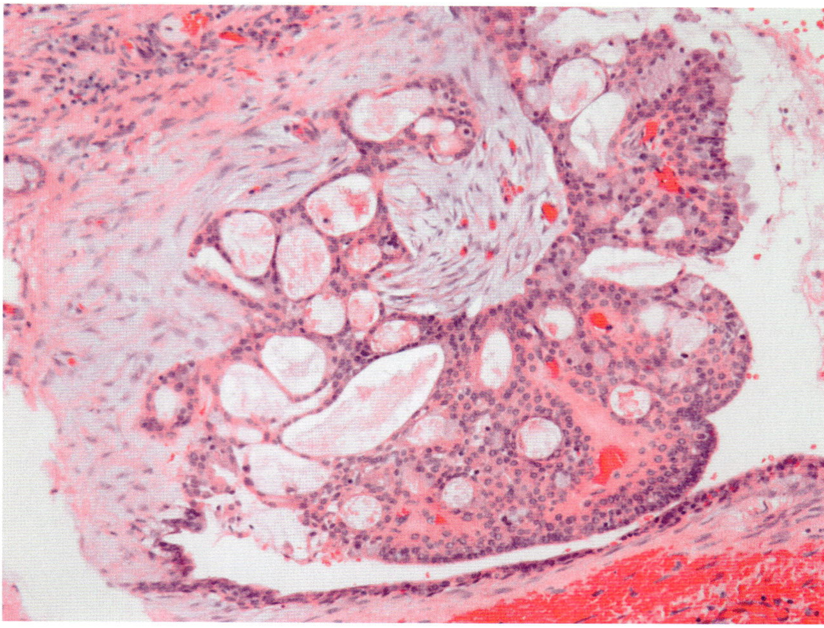

FIGURE 12.58 Mucoepidermoid carcinoma of bronchus shows sheets of monotonous squamoid cells admixed with luminal spaces containing periodic acid-Schiff/mucicarmine-positive mucinous secretions.

components will stain for p40/p63; however, the tumors can also be positive for TTF-1 and napsin A, as well as numerous other markers.[133] Mucicarmine stains are helpful for highlighting the isolated mucocytes admixed with the squamous elements. Rare cases may present with clear cell changes similar to that seen in SCC.[135] Distinction between high-grade mucoepidermoid carcinoma and adenosquamous carcinoma is not possible on endoscopic biopsies based on morphology alone. If FISH or next-generation sequencing panels for gene rearrangements are available, the detection of the characteristic *MECT1::MAML2* rearrangement may aid in the diagnosis, especially for low-grade lesions.[136,137] Distinction from adenosquamous carcinoma is of importance because of the different prognosis and treatment. In general, an intimate admixture of the squamous and mucinous elements favors mucoepidermoid carcinoma, as opposed to areas that clearly comprise only squamous elements alongside areas that purely comprise mucinous elements that are distinctive of adenosquamous carcinoma. Cases showing high-grade features in small biopsy samples can be reported as "high-grade NSCLC with predominantly squamous differentiation and foci of adenocarcinomatous differentiation," with a comment that the tumor is consistent with a high-grade mucoepidermoid carcinoma and that an adenosquamous carcinoma cannot be ruled out from the limited biopsy sample (Fig. 12.59).

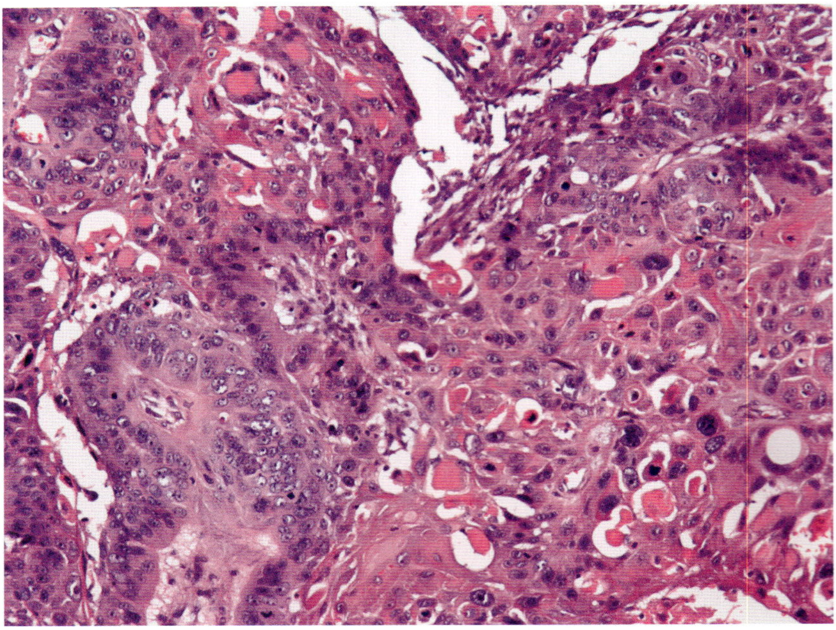

FIGURE 12.59 Endobronchial biopsy of tumor showing mixed features of squamous and glandular differentiation. It may not be possible on such limited material to distinguish a poorly differentiated mucoepidermoid carcinoma from an adenosquamous carcinoma.

Adenoid Cystic Carcinoma

Adenoid cystic carcinoma of the bronchus is a distinctive tumor comprising tubular structures with a prominent cribriform architecture that is surrounded by abundant deposits of extracellular eosinophilic basement membrane material along the periphery as well as in the lumens of the tubular structures.[138] The tubular structures are usually embedded in a hyalinized or myxoid matrix and are surrounded by a layer of myoepithelial cells that stain positive for myoepithelial markers (ie, a combination of smooth muscle actin/calponin/smooth muscle myosin with various epithelium-associated markers, including cytokeratins and p63/p40) (Fig. 12.60). In some cases, the tumors can adopt a solid configuration leading to confusion with basaloid SCC or other basaloid lesions, although this variant has not been well characterized in the pulmonary literature.[139] The myoepithelial cells can also be immunoreactive for S-100 protein, CD117, and GFAP. The cells lining the tubules are usually small, with scant cytoplasm and hyperchromatic nuclei with rare mitotic figures. The tumors can sometimes show a tubular growth pattern devoid of a cribriform architecture comprising single, discrete tubular structures surrounded by basement membrane material or may adopt a solid growth pattern characterized by sheets or islands of monotonous small tumor cells that will contain

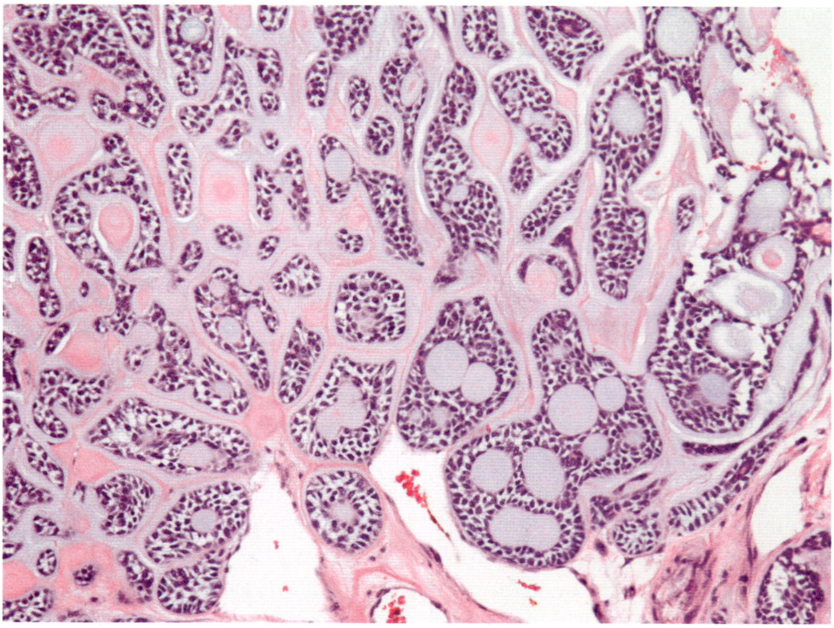

FIGURE 12.60 Adenoid cystic carcinoma of the bronchus shows tumor islands with cribriform architecture as well as individual acinar structures lined by a double layer of cells and displaying deposits of dense, eosinophilic hyaline material within the lumens and surrounding the tubules.

focally small abortive tubular structures. Adenoid cystic carcinoma of the bronchus almost always grows as an endobronchial, polypoid tumor that occludes the bronchial lumen. Perineural invasion is a common feature, and the tumor frequently extends along the bronchi and bronchioles as well as along lymphatics at the edges of the lesion, accounting for the high incidence of recurrence owing to incomplete excision. The tumors have a predilection for men in their fifth decade. They are, for the most part, slow-growing malignancies that may give rise to multiple recurrences and late metastases. Clinical stage at the time of initial diagnosis is the best predictor of prognosis.[138] Tumors within the salivary gland have been shown to harbor recurrent *MYB*::*NFIB* rearrangements in approximately 80% of cases; however, this molecular alteration appears to occur less frequently in pulmonary adenoid cystic carcinomas.[140,141]

Other Types of Salivary Gland–Type Tumors of the Lung

Other types of salivary gland–type tumors of the lung include acinic cell carcinoma, mixed tumor (pleomorphic adenoma), epimyoepithelial carcinoma, and oncocytoma. *Acinic cell carcinoma (Fechner tumor)* is rare and can present either as a central or as a peripheral lung lesion.[142-144] It is histologically characterized by islands of monotonous cells that can sometimes grow forming cords or acinar structures or may adopt a papillocystic architecture. The tumor cells are large and contain abundant granular eosinophilic cytoplasm with small nuclei. They can sometimes adopt a signet ring cell appearance with the nuclei displaced toward the periphery. The tumor cells can be positive for amylase and α-1-antichymotrypsin, but a negative reaction does not exclude the diagnosis. Periodic acid-Schiff histochemical stain will strongly stain the cytoplasm of the tumor cells; the reaction will not be abolished by treatment with diastase. The tumors are also characterized by positivity for DOG-1 IHC.[144] The most distinctive and sensitive marker for diagnosis is the demonstration of dense zymogen granules at the ultrastructural level. The tumors generally behave as low-grade neoplasms and are often cured by simple excision. Diagnosis of acinic cell carcinoma may be difficult to make on small endoscopic biopsies when the signet ring cell features predominate as it may not be possible to distinguish this tumor from a signet ring cell adenocarcinoma. *Mixed tumor (pleomorphic adenoma)* of the lung is another rare salivary gland–type tumor that occurs predominantly in adults without any gender predilection and can present in central or peripheral locations. Central lesions generally grow as endobronchial polypoid masses filling the bronchial lumen and causing obstruction. Histologically, the tumors are indistinguishable from mixed tumors of salivary glands and comprise an admixture of epithelial and mesenchymal elements (Fig. 12.61).[145,146] The epithelial component comprises tubular or cystic structures lined by a double layer of cells, with the luminal cells showing low cuboidal epithelium and the peripheral cells comprising a layer of myoepithelial cells. The intervening stroma is dense and collagenous and shows a prominent myxoid matrix. Cartilaginous differentiation, a common occurrence in the salivary gland tumors, is seldom a feature seen in the bronchial lesions.[145] Malignant forms have also been described, in which the malignant component is widely invasive, shows marked cytologic atypia with high mitotic activity, and may show transitions with preexisting areas of conventional mixed tumor.[145] Because of the myoepithelial cell component, the outer layer of tumor cells will stain for conventional myoepithelium-associated markers (see Adenoid Cystic Carcinoma). The tumors, including tumors of the lung, are known to harbor a recurrent gene rearrangement involving the *PLAG1* gene and can show positivity for PLAG1 IHC.[147] However, in small biopsy samples, it may be impossible to distinguish a mixed tumor from some of the tubular variants of adenoid cystic carcinoma or from an epimyoepithelial carcinoma. *Epimyoepithelial carcinoma* is one of the most unusual salivary gland–type lung tumors. The majority of the reported cases have occurred in adults in central locations. The tumors are usually endobronchial and well circumscribed and present with symptoms of bronchial obstruction; they are histologically characterized by a proliferation of small acinar structures containing a dual cell population.[148-150] There is an inner cell population surrounding the lumen comprising small,

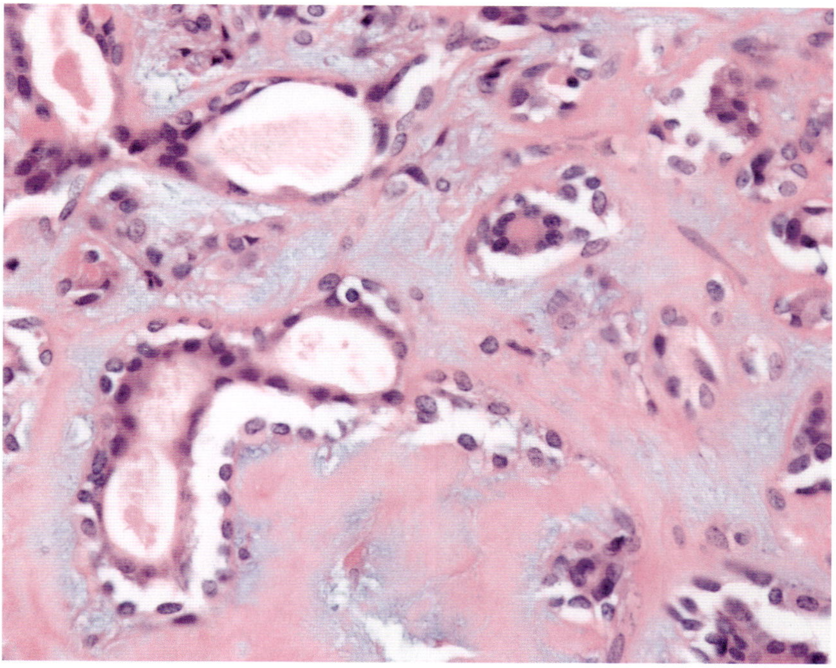

FIGURE 12.61 Endobronchial biopsy shows tubular structures lined by bland-appearing epithelial cells surrounded by abundant connective tissue comprising hyaline matrix with myxoid changes, characteristic of salivary gland–type mixed tumor of the lung.

basaloid cells with hyperchromatic nuclei and scant cytoplasm, surrounded by a peripheral cell layer of myoepithelial cells with abundant clear cytoplasm (Fig. 12.62). As with mixed tumors and adenoid cystic carcinoma, the myoepithelial component will stain with myoepithelium-associated markers. In a small endoscopic biopsy, it may be extremely difficult to distinguish an epimyoepithelial carcinoma of the lung from a mixed tumor or an adenoid cystic carcinoma. *Oncocytoma* is a rare lung tumor, with only a handful of case reports in the literature. The tumors are characterized by a monotonous population of large cells with abundant granular eosinophilic cytoplasm and small centrally placed nuclei. Their histologic appearance is indistinguishable from that of oncocytomas arising in other locations. These tumors need to be distinguished from other primary lung tumors showing oncocytic features, including oncocytic neuroendocrine tumors of the lung, adenocarcinoma with oncocytic changes, and metastases from oncocytic tumors from other organs to the lung. Finally, a few other salivary gland-type tumors including cases of hyalinizing clear cell carcinoma and myoepithelioma/myoepithelial carcinoma have been very rarely reported in the lung.[151-154]

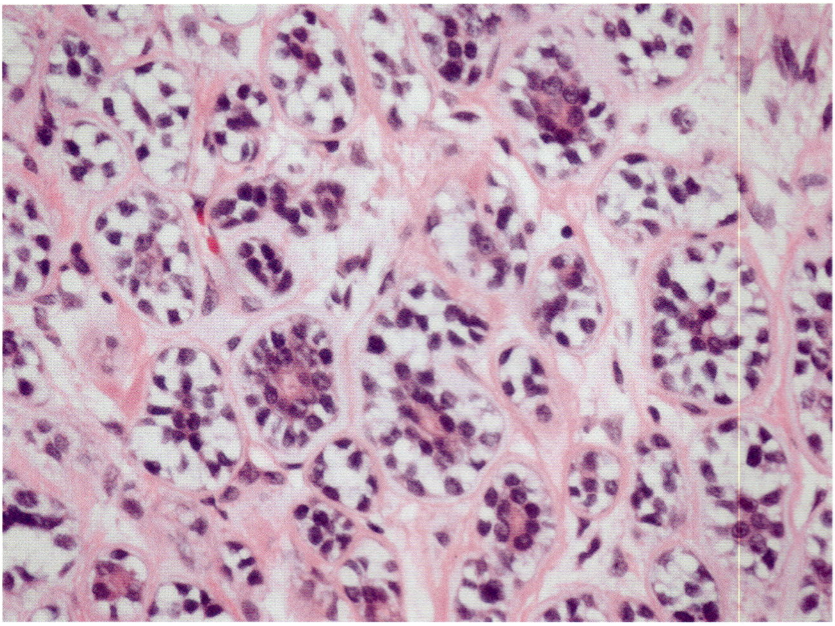

FIGURE 12.62 Epithelial-myoepithelial carcinoma of the lung is characterized by small ductular structures lined by a double layer of cells: an inner layer comprising small cuboidal epithelium and an outer layer comprising myoepithelial cells with prominent clearing of the cytoplasm.

BIPHASIC EPITHELIAL/MESENCHYMAL NEOPLASMS

Rare tumors showing a combination of both mesenchymal and epithelial neoplastic components within the same tumor mass have been described in the lung. These include mainly biphasic pulmonary blastoma and carcinosarcoma. Because of the variability in cellular composition of these tumors, it may not be possible to render a reliable and definitive diagnosis on small endoscopic or core needle biopsies except under very specific conditions. Such tumors, therefore, require a completely excised surgical specimen with adequate sampling for definitive diagnosis. A specific diagnosis can be suggested in cases where the features fulfill some of the requirements for this diagnosis. Synovial sarcoma is also worth mentioning here as it demonstrates both epithelial and mesenchymal lines of differentiation; however, this entity is generally regarded as a mesenchymal neoplasm and is covered in Chapter 14.

Pulmonary Blastoma

Pulmonary blastoma (previously called "biphasic pulmonary blastoma") is characterized by a primitive epithelial component that can be very similar to that observed in fetal adenocarcinoma (previously called "monophasic pulmonary blastoma"), admixed with a malignant mesenchymal component characterized by primitive atypical spindle cells that may harbor heterologous differentiation including osteosarcomatous, chondrosarcomatous, or rhabdomyosarcomatous elements.[155] Pulmonary blastoma is a highly aggressive tumor associated with a poor prognosis.[156,157] Similar to its monophasic counterpart (aka fetal adenocarcinoma), recurrent *β-catenin* mutations have been identified in these lesions.[158] In addition, somatic mutations in the *DICER1* gene are seen in a high number of cases.[159,160] The primitive spindle cell component in pulmonary blastoma often resembles the primitive blastemalike spindle cells seen in Wilms tumor (Fig. 12.63). The epithelial elements comprise glandular structures or tubules that are lined by glycogen-rich, tall cylindrical cells with basally oriented nuclei and abundant clear cytoplasm that resemble fetal lung at the pseudoglandular stage of development (between 10 and 16 weeks of gestation). The glandular structures can also be lined by pseudostratified, nonciliated columnar cells with large oval, hyperchromatic nuclei displaying brisk mitotic activity. The glandular structures sometimes contain solid aggregates of squamoid cells ("morules") at the base of the glands. The tumor cells will stain positively for neuroendocrine markers and β-catenin (see description of "fetal adenocarcinoma" above). As mentioned earlier, it may be extremely difficult to establish a definitive diagnosis of biphasic pulmonary blastoma on a small biopsy sample, unless both the epithelial

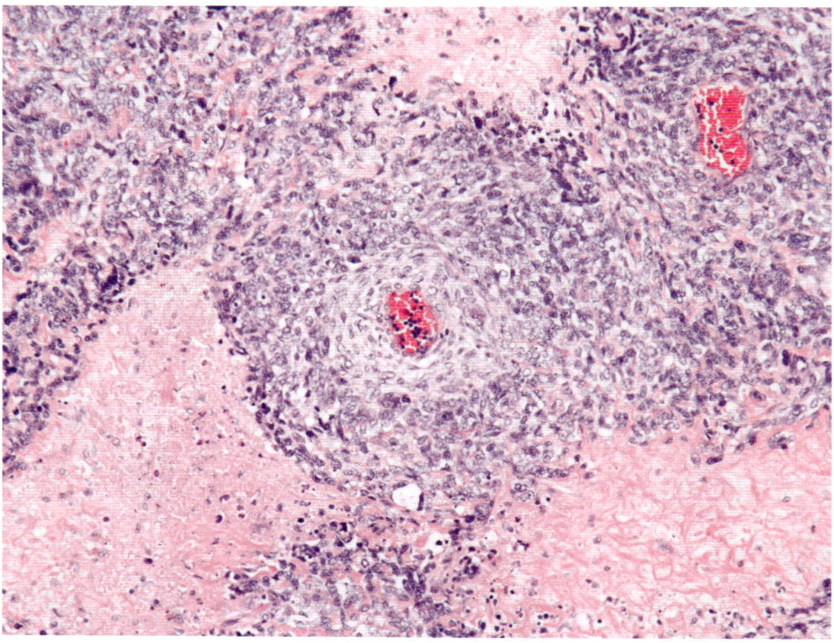

FIGURE 12.63 Mesenchymal component in a biphasic pulmonary blastoma shows a primitive population of atypical spindle cells embedded in a lightly myxoid stroma reminiscent of blastemal elements in Wilms tumor.

and mesenchymal components are clearly present in the biopsy. Cases in which only the mesenchymal component is present may be confused for spindle cell carcinoma or for different types of spindle cell sarcomas, including monophasic synovial sarcoma, fibrosarcoma, and solitary fibrous tumor. Cases in which only the epithelial component is present may be confused for metastasis of endometrial carcinoma or for a fetal adenocarcinoma. The latter, in particular, is an extremely important distinction with significant prognostic connotations because fetal adenocarcinoma is associated with a much better prognosis than pulmonary blastoma.

Carcinosarcoma

Carcinosarcoma represents an extremely rare lung tumor that is defined as a biphasic lung neoplasm comprising intimately admixed and clearly identifiable malignant epithelial and malignant mesenchymal elements within the same tumor mass (Fig. 12.64).[155,161-163] The epithelial component in carcinosarcoma may be made up of adenocarcinoma, SCC, large cell carcinoma, and neuroendocrine carcinoma. The mesenchymal component is generally made up of a well-defined and clearly recognizable sarcoma such as rhabdomyosarcoma, leiomyosarcoma, chondrosarcoma, angiosarcoma, or osteosarcoma. In some instances, the mesenchymal component will only consist of a primitive atypical spindle cell proliferation without any

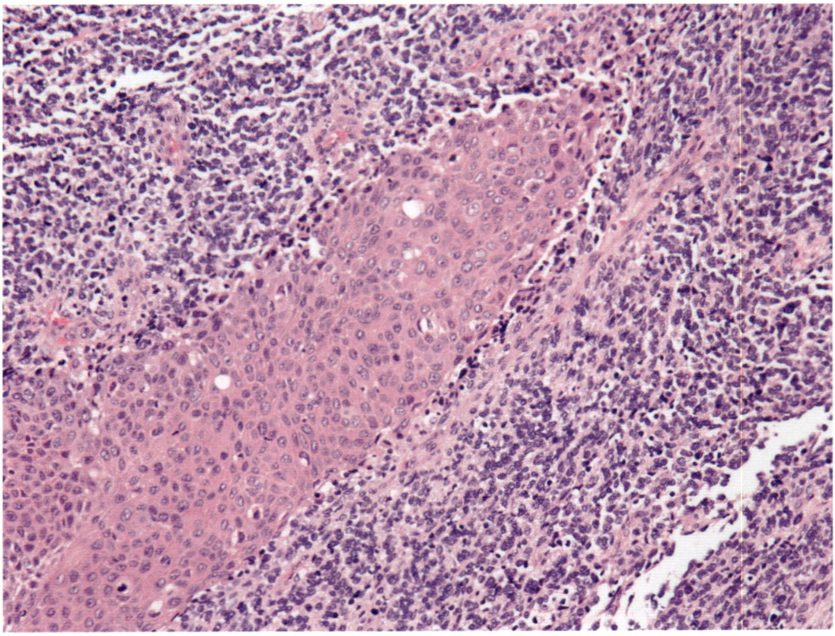

FIGURE 12.64 **Pulmonary carcinosarcoma shows an island of squamous cell carcinoma surrounded by primitive spindle cell sarcomatous elements.** Immunohistochemical stains in this case did not identify any epithelial markers within the spindle cell component.

particular line of differentiation, though tumors with a purely spindle cell or fibroblastic appearing component are classified under "pleomorphic carcinomas" by the WHO. Immunohistochemical stains may be of help in identifying the line of differentiation in the malignant mesenchymal component. The malignant epithelial component is usually quite evident and straightforward, although cytokeratin stains may highlight small, poorly differentiated epithelial elements entrapped within the sarcomatous components. The malignant epithelial component is often overshadowed by the sarcomatous elements in these lesions. Tumors showing small cell neuroendocrine carcinoma components tend to be endobronchial and polypoid and may be amenable to adequate sampling by endoscopy. Attention must be placed in such instances not to miss the atypical spindle stromal component so that the diagnosis of carcinosarcoma can be raised. The main differential diagnosis for these tumors is with spindle cell (sarcomatoid) carcinoma. In the latter, both the well-differentiated (squamous or adenocarcinomatous) epithelial elements and the atypical spindle (sarcomatoid) cells in the stroma should be positive for epithelial markers (cytokeratins, in particular low molecular weight cytokeratin); a subtle difference with carcinosarcoma, in which the atypical spindle cells should be negative for epithelium-associated markers and show instead staining for mesenchymal markers, depending on their specific line of differentiation. In small biopsies in which both components are not clearly evident, a noncommittal descriptive diagnosis of "high-grade spindle cell sarcomatoid neoplasm" or "high-grade spindle cell malignant neoplasm" may be warranted with a comment that carcinosarcoma or a high-grade NSCLC cannot be ruled out.

REFERENCES

1. World Health Organization. *Lung Cancer*. 2018. Accessed October 15, 2019. https://gco.iarc.fr/today/data/factsheets/cancers/15-Lung-fact-sheet.pdf
2. World Health Organization. *Lung Cancer*. 2023. Accessed March 3, 2025. https://www.who.int/news-room/fact-sheets/detail/lung-cancer
3. International Agency for Research on Cancer. *Lung Cancer*. 2025. Accessed March 3, 2025. https://www.iarc.who.int/cancer-type/lung-cancer/
4. Schwartz AG, Cote ML. Epidemiology of lung cancer. *Adv Exp Med Biol*. 2016;893:21-41.
5. Mao Y, Yang D, He J, Krasna MJ. Epidemiology of lung cancer. *Surg Oncol Clin N Am*. 2016;25(3):439-445.
6. WHO Classification of Tumors Editorial Board. *WHO Classification of Tumors*. 5th ed. IARC; 2021.
7. Travis WD, Brambilla E, Noguchi M, et al. International Association for the Study of Lung Cancer/American Thoracic Society/European Respiratory Society international multidisciplinary classification of lung adenocarcinoma. *J Thorac Oncol*. 2011;6:244-285.
8. International Academy of Cytology; International Agency for Research on Cancer; World Health Organization Joint Editorial Board. *WHO Reporting System for Lung Cytopathology*. IARC; 2022.

9. Suster S, Moran CA. The lung. In: Weidner N, Cote R, Suster S, Weiss LM, eds. *Modern Pathology*. Vol. I. 2nd ed. WB Saunders; 2009:365-433.
10. Suster S, Moran CA. Tumors of the lung and pleura. In: Fletcher CDM, ed. *Diagnostic Histopathology of Tumors*. 4th ed. Churchill-Livingstone; 2013:207-245.
11. Edwards SI, Roberts C, McKean ME, Cockburn JS, Jeffrey RR, Kerr KM. Preoperative histological classification of primary lung cancer: accuracy of diagnosis and use of the non-small cell category. *J Clin Pathol*. 2000;53:537-540.
12. Cataluna JJ, Perpina M, Greses JV, Calvo V, Padilla JD, París F. Cell type accuracy of bronchial biopsy specimens in primary lung cancer. *Chest*. 1996;109:1199-1203.
13. Travis WD, Rekhtman N, Riley GJ, et al. Pathologic diagnosis of advanced lung cancer based on small biopsies and cytology: a paradigm shift. *J Thorac Oncol*. 2010;5:411-414.
14. Moran CA. Importance of molecular features of non-small cell lung cancer for choice of treatment. *Am J Pathol*. 2011;178:1940-1948.
15. Mukhopadhyay S, Katzenstein AL. Subclassification of non-small cell lung carcinomas lacking morphologic differentiation on biopsy specimens: utility of an immunohistochemical panel containing TTF1, napsin A, p63, and CK5/6. *Am J Surg Pathol*. 2011;35:15-25.
16. Terry J, Leung S, Laskin J, Leslie KO, Gown AM, Ionescu DN. Optimal immunohistochemical markers for distinguishing lung adenocarcinomas from squamous cell carcinomas in small tumor samples. *Am J Surg Pathol*. 2010;34:1805-1811.
17. Rhigi L, Graziano P, Fornari A, et al. Immunohistochemical subtyping of nonsmall cell lung cancer not otherwise specified in fine needle aspiration cytology: a retrospective study of 103 cases with surgical correlation. *Cancer*. 2011;117:3416-3423.
18. Matoso A, Singh K, Jacob R, et al. Comparison of thyroid transcription factor 1 expression by 2 monoclonal antibodies in pulmonary and nonpulmonary primary tumors. *Appl Immunohistochem Mol Morphol*. 2010;18:142-149.
19. Loo PS, Thomas SC, Nicolson MC, Fyfe MN, Kerr KM. Subtyping of undifferentiated non-small cell carcinomas in bronchial biopsy specimens. *J Thorac Oncol*. 2010;5:436-441.
20. Yoshida A, Tsuta K, Watanabe S, et al. Frequent ALK rearrangement and TTF1/p63 coexpression in lung adenocarcinoma with signet ring cell component. *Lung Cancer*. 2011;72:309-315.
21. Hallack Neto AE, Siqueira SA, Dulley FL, Ruiz MA, Chamone DAF, Pereira J. p63 protein expression in high risk diffuse large B-cell lymphoma. *J Clin Pathol*. 2009;62:77-79.
22. Affandi KA, Tizen NMS, Mustangin M, Md Zin RRMR. p40 Immunohistochemistry is an excellent marker in primary lung squamous cell carcinoma. *J Pathol Transl Med*. 2018;52(5):283-289.
23. Walia R, Jain D, Madan K, et al. p40 & thyroid transcription factor-1 immunohistochemistry: a useful panel to characterize non-small cell lung carcinoma-not otherwise specified (NSCLC-NOS) category. *Indian J Med Res*. 2017;146(1):42-48.
24. Bishop JA, Teruya-Feldstein J, Westra WH, Pelosi G, Travis WD, Rekhtman N. p40 (ΔNp63) is superior to p63 for the diagnosis of pulmonary squamous cell carcinoma. *Mod Pathol*. 2012;25(3):405-415.
25. Pereira TC, Share SM, Magalhaes AV, Silverman JF. Can we tell the site of origin of metastatic squamous cell carcinoma? An immunohistochemical tissue microarray study of 194 cases. *Appl Immunohistochem Mol Morphol*. 2011;19:10-14.
26. Chang ST, Chen SW, Chen BJ, Pan ST, Karube K, Chuang SS. Aberrant TTF-1 expression in peripheral T-cell lymphomas: a diagnostic pitfall. *Int J Surg Pathol*. 2021;29:165-168.
27. Vidarsdottir H, Tran L, Nodin B, et al. Comparison of three different TTF-1 clones in resected primary lung cancer and epithelial pulmonary metastases. *Am J Clin Pathol*. 2018;150(6):533-544.

28. Yamashita Y, Nagasaka T, Naiki-Ito A, et al. Napsin A is a specific marker for ovarian clear cell adenocarcinoma. *Mod Pathol*. 2015;28(1):111-117.
29. Al-Maghrabi JA, Butt NS, Anfinan N, et al. Infrequent immunohistochemical expression of napsin A in endometrial carcinomas. *Appl Immunohistochem Mol Morphol*. 2017;25(9):632-638.
30. Nam SJ, Kim S, Kim JE, et al. Aberrant expression of napsin A in a subset of malignant lymphomas. *Histol Histopathol*. 2016;31(2):213-221.
31. Zhu B, Rohan SM, Lin X. Immunoexpression of napsin A in renal neoplasms. *Diagn Pathol*. 2015;10:4.
32. Vitkovski T, Chaudhary S, Sison C, Nasim M, Esposito MJ, Bhuiya T. Aberrant expression of napsin A in breast carcinoma with apocrine features. *Int J Surg Pathol*. 2016;24(5):377-381.
33. Thunnissen E, Allen TC, Adam J, et al. Immunohistochemistry of pulmonary biomarkers: a perspective from members of the Pulmonary Pathology Society. *Arch Pathol Lab Med*. 2018;142(3):408-419.
34. Dietel M, Bubendorf L, Dingemans A, et al. Diagnostic procedures for non-small-cell lung cancer (NSCLC): recommendations of the European Expert Group. *Thorax*. 2016;71(2):177-184.
35. Bubendorf L, Büttner R, Al-Dayel F, et al. Testing for ROS1 in non-small cell lung cancer: a review with recommendations. *Virchows Arch*. 2016;469(5):489-503.
36. Sholl LM, Sun H, Butaney M, et al. ROS1 immunohistochemistry for detection of lung adenocarcinomas. *Am J Surg Pathol*. 2013;37(9):1441-1449.
37. Yoshida A, Tsuta K, Wakai S, et al. Immunohistochemical detection of ROS1 is useful for identifying ROS1 rearrangements in lung cancers. *Mod Pathol*. 2014;27(5): 711-720.
38. Elfving H, Broström E, Moens LNJ, et al. Evaluation of NTRK immunohistochemistry as a screening method for NTRK gene fusion detection in non-small cell lung cancer. *Lung Cancer*. 2021;151:53-59. doi:10.1016/j.lungcan.2020.11.023
39. Sholl LM, Aisner DL, Allen TC, et al. Programmed death ligand 1 immunohistochemistry: a new challenge for pathologists: a perspective from members of the Pulmonary Pathology Society. *Arch Pathol Lab Med*. 2016;140(4):341-344.
40. Hamid O, Robert C, Daud A, et al. Safety and tumor responses with lambrolizumab (anti-PD-1) in melanoma. *N Engl J Med*. 2013;369(2):134-144.
41. Topalian SL, Hodi FS, Brahmer JR, et al. Safety, activity, and immune correlates of anti-PD-1 antibody in cancer. *N Engl J Med*. 2012;366(26):2443-2454.
42. Herbst RS, Soria JC, Kowanetz M, et al. Predictive correlates of response to the anti-PD-L1 antibody MPDL3280A in cancer patients. *Nature*. 2014;515(7528):563-567.
43. Sundar R, Soong R, Cho BC, Brahmer JR, Soo RA. Immunotherapy in the treatment of non-small cell lung cancer. *Lung Cancer*. 2014;85(2):101-109.
44. Gaule P, Smithy JW, Toki M, et al. A quantitative comparison of antibodies to programmed cell death 1 ligand 1. *JAMA Oncol*. 2017;3(2):256.
45. Yu H, Boyle TA, Zhou C, Rimm DL, Hirsch FR. PD-L1 expression in lung cancer. *J Thorac Oncol*. 2016;11(7):964-975.
46. Velcheti V, Schalper KA, Carvajal DE, et al. Programmed death ligand-1 expression in non-small cell lung cancer. *Lab Investig*. 2013;94(1):107-116.
47. Borghaei H, Paz-Ares L, Horn L, et al. Nivolumab versus docetaxel in advanced nonsquamous non-small-cell lung cancer. *N Engl J Med*. 2015;373(17):1627-1639.
48. Rittmeyer A, Barlesi F, Waterkamp D, et al. Atezolizumab versus docetaxel in patients with previously treated non-small-cell lung cancer (OAK): a phase 3, open-label, multicentre randomised controlled trial. *Lancet*. 2017;389(10066):255-265.

49. Lam VK, Tran HT, Banks KC, et al. Targeted tissue and cell-free tumor DNA sequencing of advanced lung squamous-cell carcinoma reveals clinically significant prevalence of actionable alterations. *Clin Lung Cancer*. 2019;20(1):30-36.e3.
50. Dacic S, Nikiforova MN. Present and future molecular testing of lung carcinoma. *Adv Anat Pathol*. 2014;21(2):94-99.
51. Hensing T, Chawla A, Batra R, Salgia R. A personalized treatment for lung cancer: molecular pathways, targeted therapies, and genomic characterization. *Adv Exp Med Biol*. 2014;799:85-117.
52. Tan O, Shrestha R, Cunich M, Schofield DJ. Application of next-generation sequencing to improve cancer management: a review of the clinical effectiveness and cost-effectiveness. *Clin Genet*. 2018;93(3):533-544.
53. Lindeman NI, Cagle PT, Beasley MB, et al. Molecular testing guideline for selection of lung cancer patients for EGFR and ALK tyrosine kinase inhibitors: guideline from the College of American Pathologists, International Association for the Study of Lung Cancer, and Association for Molecular Pathology. *J Thorac Oncol*. 2013;8(7):823-859.
54. Lindeman NI, Cagle PT, Aisner DL, et al. Updated molecular testing guideline for the selection of lung cancer patients for treatment with targeted tyrosine kinase inhibitors: guideline from the College of American Pathologists, the International Association for the Study of Lung Cancer, and the Association for Molecular Pathology. *J Thorac Oncol*. 2018;13(3):323-358.
55. Kalemkerian GP, Narula N, Kennedy EB, et al. Molecular testing guideline for the selection of patients with lung cancer for treatment with targeted tyrosine kinase inhibitors: American Society of Clinical Oncology Endorsement of the College of American Pathologists/International Association for the Study of Lung Cancer/Association for Molecular Pathology clinical practice guideline update. *J Clin Oncol*. 2018;36(9):911-919.
56. Griffin R, Ramirez RA. Molecular targets in non–small cell lung cancer. *Ochsner J*. 2017;17(4):388-392.
57. Li AR, Chitale D, Riely GJ, et al. EGFR mutations in lung adenocarcinomas. *J Mol Diagn*. 2008;10(3):242-248.
58. Boolell V, Alamgeer M, Watkins DN, Ganju V. The evolution of therapies in non-small cell lung cancer. *Cancers (Basel)*. 2015;7(3):1815-1846.
59. Collisson E, Campbell J, Brooks A, et al. Comprehensive molecular profiling of lung adenocarcinoma. *Nature*. 2014;511(7511):543-550.
60. Yu HA, Tian SK, Drilon AE, et al. Acquired resistance of EGFR-mutant lung cancer to a T790M-specific EGFR inhibitor: emergence of a third mutation (C797S) in the EGFR tyrosine kinase domain. *JAMA Oncol*. 2015;1:982-984.
61. Piotrowska Z, Thress KS, Mooradian M, et al. MET amplification (amp) as a resistance mechanism to osimertinib. *J Clin Oncol*. 2017;35:9020.
62. Niederst MJ, Hu H, Mulvey HE, et al. The allelic context of the C797S mutation acquired upon treatment with third-generation EGFR inhibitors impacts sensitivity to subsequent treatment strategies. *Clin Cancer Res*. 2015;21:3924-3933.
63. Wu SG, Shih JY. Management of acquired resistance to EGFR TKI-targeted therapy in advanced non-small cell lung cancer. *Mol Cancer*. 2018;17(1):38.
64. Ferrer I, Zugazagoitia J, Herbertz S, John W, Paz-Ares L, Schmid-Bindert G. KRAS-mutant non-small cell lung cancer: from biology to therapy. *Lung Cancer*. 2018;124:53-64.
65. Chin LP, Soo RA, Soong R, Ou SHI. Targeting ROS1 with anaplastic lymphoma kinase inhibitors. A promising therapeutic strategy for a newly defined molecular subset of non–small-cell lung cancer. *J Thorac Oncol*. 2012;7:1625-1630.

66. Bergethon K, Shaw AT, Ou SHI, et al. ROS1 rearrangements define a unique molecular class of lung cancers. *J Clin Oncol.* 2012;30:863-870.
67. Sgambato A, Casaluce F, Maione P, Gridelli C. Targeted therapies in non-small cell lung cancer: a focus on ALK/ROS1 tyrosine kinase inhibitors. *Expert Rev Anticancer Ther.* 2018;18(1):71-80.
68. Gainor JF, Dardaei L, Yoda S, et al. Molecular mechanisms of resistance to first- and second-generation ALK inhibitors in ALK-rearranged lung cancer. *Cancer Discov.* 2016;6(10):1118-1133.
69. Rotow J, Bivona TG. Understanding and targeting resistance mechanisms in NSCLC. *Nat Rev Cancer.* 2017;17(11):637-658.
70. National Comprehensive Cancer Network. *Non-Small Cell Lung Cancer Guidelines Version 3.* 2025. Accessed March 13, 2025. https://www.nccn.org/professionals/physician_gls/pdf/nscl.pdf
71. Kerr KM. Pulmonary adenocarcinomas: classification and reporting. *Histopathology.* 2009;54:12-27.
72. Motoi N, Szoke J, Riley GJ, et al. Lung adenocarcinoma: modification of the 2004 WHO mixed subtype to include the major histologic subtype suggests correlations between papillary and micropapillary adenocarcinoma subtypes, *EGFR* mutations and gene expression analysis. *Am J Surg Pathol.* 2008;32:810-827.
73. Cao Y, Zhu LZ, Jiang MJ, Yuan Y. Clinical impacts of a micropapillary pattern in lung adenocarcinoma: a review. *Onco Targets Ther.* 2015;9:149-158.
74. Solis LM, Behrens C, Raso MG, et al. Histologic patterns and molecular characteristics of lung adenocarcinoma associated with clinical outcome. *Cancer.* 2012;118(11):2889-2899.
75. Moreira AL, Ocampo PSS, Xia Y, et al. A grading system for invasive pulmonary adenocarcinoma: a proposal from the International Association for the Study of Lung Cancer Pathology Committee. *J Thorac Oncol.* 2020;15(10):1599-1610. doi:10.1016/j.jtho.2020.06.001
76. Bishop JA, Sharma R, Illei PB. Napsin A and thyroid transcription factor-1 expression in carcinomas of the lung, breast, pancreas, colon, kidney, thyroid, and malignant mesothelioma. *Hum Pathol.* 2010;41:20-25.
77. Ye J, Findeis-Hossey JJ, Yang Q, et al. Combination of napsin-A and TTF-1 immunohistochemistry help in differentiating primary lung adenocarcinoma from metastatic carcinoma in the lung. *Appl Immunohistochem Mol Morphol.* 2011;19:313-317.
78. Robens J, Goldstein L, Gown AM, Schnitt SJ. Thyroid transcription factor-1 expression in breast carcinoma. *Am J Surg Pathol.* 2010;34:1881-1885.
79. Comperat E, Zhang F, Perrotin C, et al. Variable sensitivity and specificity of TTF1 antibodies in lung metastatic adenocarcinoma of colorectal origin. *Mod Pathol.* 2005;18:1371-1376.
80. Siami K, McCluggage WG, Ordoñez NG, et al. Thyroid transcription factor-1 expression in endometrial and endocervical adenocarcinoma. *Am J Surg Pathol.* 2007;31:1759-1763.
81. Goldstein NS, Thomas M. Mucinous and nonmucinous bronchioloalveolar adenocarcinomas have distinct staining patterns with thyroid transcription factor and cytokeratin 20 antibodies. *Am J Clin Pathol.* 2001;116:319-325.
82. Kim M, Chung YS, Kim KA, Shim HS. Prognostic factors of acinar-or papillary-predominant adenocarcinoma of the lung. *Lung Cancer.* 2019;137:129-135.
83. Jiang L, Mino-Kenudson M, Roden AC, et al. Association between the novel classification of lung adenocarcinoma subtypes and EGFR/KRAS mutation status: a systematic literature review and pooled-data analysis. *Eur J Surg Oncol.* 2019;45(5):870-876.

84. Shih AR, Uruga H, Bozkurtlar E, et al. Problems in the reproducibility of classification of small lung adenocarcinoma: an international interobserver study. *Histopathology*. 2019;75:649-659.
85. MacKinnon A, Luevano A, de Araujo LC, Rao N, Le M, Suster S. Cribriform adenocarcinoma of the lung: clinicopathologic, immunohistochemical and molecular study of 15 cases of a distinctive morphologic subtype of lung adenocarcinoma. *Mod Pathol*. 2014;27:1063.
86. Kadota K, Yeh YC, Sima CS, et al. The cribriform pattern identifies a subset of acinar predominant tumors with poor prognosis in patients with stage I lung adenocarcinoma: a conceptual proposal to classify cribriform predominant tumors as a distinct histologic subtype. *Mod Pathol*. 2014;27(5):690-700.
87. Kamiya K, Hayashi Y, Douguchi J, et al. Histopathological features and prognostic significance of the micropapillary pattern in lung adenocarcinoma. *Mod Pathol*. 2008;21:992-1001.
88. Suster DI, Ronen N, Suster S. Pseudosquamous adenocarcinoma of the lung: clinicopathologic and immunohistochemical study of 10 cases. *Am J Surg Pathol*. 2024;48(7):901-908. doi:10.1097/PAS.0000000000002242
89. Moran CA, Hochholzer L, Fishback N, Travis WD, Koss MN. Mucinous (so-called colloid) carcinomas of the lung. *Mod Pathol*. 1992;5:634-638.
90. Hwang DH, Sholl LM, Rojas-Rudilla V, et al. KRAS and NKX2-1 mutations in invasive mucinous adenocarcinoma of the lung. *J Thorac Oncol*. 2016;11(4):496-503. doi:10.1016/j.jtho.2016.01.010
91. Chang JC, Offin M, Falcon C, et al. Comprehensive molecular and clinicopathologic analysis of 200 pulmonary invasive mucinous adenocarcinomas identifies distinct characteristics of molecular subtypes. *Clin Cancer Res*. 2021;27(14):4066-4076. doi:10.1158/1078-0432.CCR-21-0423
92. Castro CY, Moran CA, Flieder DG, Suster S. Primary signet ring cell adenocarcinoma of the lung: a clinicopathologic study of 15 cases. *Histopathology*. 2001;39:397-401.
93. Steinhauer JR, Moran CA, Suster S. "Secretory endometrioid-like" adenocarcinoma of the lung. *Histopathology*. 2005;47:219-220.
94. Morita S, Yoshida A, Goto A, et al. High-grade lung adenocarcinoma with fetal lung-like morphology: clinicopathologic, immunohistochemical, and molecular analyses of 17 cases. *Am J Surg Pathol*. 2013;37(6):924-932.
95. Ricaurte LM, Arrieta O, Zatarain-BarrÓn ZL, Cardona AF. Comprehensive review of fetal adenocarcinoma of the lung. *Lung Cancer (Auckl)*. 2018;9:57-63.
96. Zhang J, Sun J, Liang XL, Lu JL, Luo YF, Liang ZY. Differences between low and high grade fetal adenocarcinoma of the lung: a clinicopathological and molecular study. *J Thorac Dis*. 2017;9(7):2071-2018.
97. Sekine S, Shibata T, Matsuno Y, et al. Beta-catenin mutations in pulmonary blastomas: association with morule formation. *J Pathol*. 2003;200:214-221.
98. Terracciano LM, Glatz K, Mhawech P, et al. Hepatoid adenocarcinoma with liver metastases mimicking hepatocellular carcinoma: an immunohistochemical and molecular study of eight cases. *Am J Surg Pathol*. 2003;27:1302-1312.
99. Haninger DM, Kloecker GH, Bousamra Ii M, Nowacki MR, Slone SP. Hepatoid adenocarcinoma of the lung: report of five cases and review of the literature. *Mod Pathol*. 2014;27(4):535-542.
100. Agaimy A, Fuchs F, Moskalev EA, Sirbu H, Hartmann A, Haller F. SMARCA4-deficient pulmonary adenocarcinoma: clinicopathological, immunohistochemical, and molecular characteristics of a novel aggressive neoplasm with a consistent TTF1^{neg}/CK7^{pos}/HepPar-1^{pos} immunophenotype. *Virchows Arch*. 2017;471(5):599-609. doi:10.1007/s00428-017-2148-5
101. Suster DI, Mackinnon AC, Ronen N, et al. Inflammatory giant cell carcinoma of the lung: clinicopathologic, immunohistochemical, and next-generation sequencing study of 14

cases. *Am J Surg Pathol.* 2024;48(10):1215-1223. doi:10.1097/PAS.0000000000002285. PMID: 38989701.

102. Yoshida A, Kobayashi E, Kubo T, et al. Clinicopathological and molecular characterization of SMARCA4-deficient thoracic sarcomas with comparison to potentially related entities. *Mod Pathol.* 2017;30(6):797-809. doi:10.1038/modpathol.2017.11. PMID: 28256572.
103. Sauter JL, Graham RP, Larsen BT, Jenkins SM, Roden AC, Boland JM. SMARCA4-deficient thoracic sarcoma: a distinctive clinicopathological entity with undifferentiated rhabdoid morphology and aggressive behavior. *Mod Pathol.* 2017;30(10):1422-1432. doi:10.1038/modpathol.2017.61. PMID: 28643792.
104. Crombé A, Alberti N, Villard N, et al. Imaging features of SMARCA4-deficient thoracic sarcomas: a multi-centric study of 21 patients. *Eur Radiol.* 2019;29(9):4730-4741. doi:10.1007/s00330-019-06017-x. PMID: 30762113.
105. Rekhtman N, Montecalvo J, Chang JC, et al. SMARCA4-deficient thoracic sarcomatoid tumors represent primarily smoking-related undifferentiated carcinomas rather than primary thoracic sarcomas. *J Thorac Oncol.* 2020;15(2):231-247. doi:10.1016/j.jtho.2019.10.023. PMID: 31751681; PMCID: PMC7556987.
106. Suster D, Mackinnon AC, Ronen N, Mejbel HA, Harada S, Suster S. Non-small cell lung carcinoma with clear cell features and FGFR3::TACC3 gene rearrangement: clinicopathologic and next generation sequencing study of 7 cases. *Am J Surg Pathol.* 2024;48(3):284-291. doi:10.1097/PAS.0000000000002167. PMID: 38084010.
107. Suster DI, Ronen N, Mejbel HA, Harada S, Mackinnon AC, Suster S. Non-small cell lung carcinoma with clear cell features: a clinicopathologic, immunohistochemical, and molecular study of 31 cases. *Virchows Arch.* 2024;485(1):83-96. doi:10.1007/s00428-024-03833-5. PMID: 38814477.
108. Suster D, Mejbel HA, Mackinnon AC, Suster S. Large-cell basaloid adenocarcinoma of the lung: a clinicopathologic study of 12 cases of a distinctive form of lung cancer often mistaken for large-cell neuroendocrine carcinoma. *Am J Surg Pathol.* 2025;49(1):83-93. doi:10.1097/PAS.0000000000002318. PMID: 39450943.
109. Park SK, Cho LY, Yang JJ, et al. Lung cancer risk and cigarette smoking, lung tuberculosis according to histologic type and gender in a population based case-control study. *Lung Cancer.* 2010;68(1):20-26.
110. Hammerman PS, Lawrence MS, Voet D, et al. Comprehensive genomic characterization of squamous cell lung cancers. *Nature.* 2012;489(7417):519-525.
111. Gupta A, Harris K, Dhillon SS. Role of bronchoscopy in management of central squamous cell lung carcinoma in situ. *Ann Transl Med.* 2019;7(15):354.
112. Au NH, Gown AM, Cheang M, et al. p63 expression in lung carcinoma: a tissue microarray study of 408 cases. *Appl Immunhistochem Mol Morphol.* 2004;12:240-247.
113. Seagliotti GV, Parikh P, von Pawel J, et al. The differential efficacy of pemetrexed according to NSCLC histology: a review of two phase III studies. *Oncologist.* 2009;14:253-263.
114. Cohen MH, Gootemberg J, Keegan P, Pazdur R. FDA drug approval summary: bevacizumab (Avastin) plus carboplatin and paclitaxel as first-line treatment of advanced/metastatic recurrent nonsquamous non-small cell lung cancer. *Oncologist.* 2007;12:713-718.
115. Zhang H, Liu J, Cagle PT, Allen TC, Laga AC, Zander DS. Distinction of pulmonary small cell carcinoma from poorly differentiated squamous cell carcinoma: an immunohistochemical approach. *Mod Pathol.* 2005;18:111-118.
116. Renshaw AA, Voytek TM, Haja J, Wilbur DC; Cytology Committee; College of American Pathologists. Distinguishing small cell carcinoma from non-small cell carcinoma of the lung: correlating cytologic features and performance in the College of American Pathologists Non-Gynecologic Cytology Program. *Arch Pathol Lab Med.* 2005;129:619-623.

117. Xie L, Duven JD, Pambuccian SE. Paranuclear blue bodies in a CT-guided fine-needle aspirate of a poorly differentiated, small-cell variant of squamous-cell carcinoma of the lung. *Diagn Cytopathol.* 2012;40(3):236-238.

118. Moro-Sibilot D, Lantuejoul S, Diab S, et al. Lung carcinomas with a basaloid pattern: a study of 90 cases focusing on their poor prognosis. *Eur Respir J.* 2008;31(4):854-859.

119. Lin L, Lin T, Zeng B. Primary lymphoepithelioma-like carcinoma of the lung: an unusual cancer and clinical outcomes of 14 patients. *Oncol Lett.* 2017;14(3):3110-3116.

120. Yeh YC, Kao HL, Lee KL, Wu MH, Ho HL, Chou TY. Epstein-Barr virus-associated pulmonary carcinoma: proposing an alternative term and expanding the histologic spectrum of lymphoepithelioma-like carcinoma of the lung. *Am J Surg Pathol.* 2019;43(2):211-219.

121. Jung M, Kim S, Lee JK, et al. Clinicopathological and preclinical findings of NUT carcinoma: a multicenter study. *Oncologist.* 2019;24(8):e740-e748.

122. Lemelle L, Pierron G, Fréneaux P, et al. NUT carcinoma in children and adults: a multicenter retrospective study. *Pediatr Blood Cancer.* 2017;64(12):e26693.

123. Benito BC, Romero MC, Almadana PV. NUT midline carcinoma of the lung, a rare form of lung cancer [in Spanish]. *Arch Bronconeumol.* 2016;52(12):619-621.

124. Hung YP, Sholl LM. Diagnostic and predictive immunohistochemistry for non-small cell lung carcinomas. *Adv Anat Pathol.* 2018;25(6):374-386.

125. Rao N. Adenosquamous carcinoma. *Semin Diagn Pathol.* 2014;31(4):271-277.

126. Pan F, Cui S, Wang W, Gu A, Jiang L. Survival analysis for lung adenosquamous carcinoma patients with brain metastasis. *J Cancer.* 2018;9(20):3707-3712.

127. Vassella E, Langsch S, Dettmer MS, et al. Molecular profiling of lung adenosquamous carcinoma: hybrid or genuine type? *Oncotarget.* 2015;6(27):23905-23916.

128. Pelosi G, Barbareschi M, Cavazza A, Graziano P, Rossi G, Papotti M. Large cell carcinoma of the lung: a tumor in search of an author. A clinically oriented critical reappraisal. *Lung Cancer.* 2015;87(3):226-231.

129. Cheung AH, Wong KY, Chau SL, et al. SMARCA4 deficiency and mutations are frequent in large cell lung carcinoma and are prognostically significant. *Pathology.* 2024;56(4):504-515. doi:10.1016/j.pathol.2023.12.414. PMID: 38413251.

130. Boucher LD, Yoneda K. The expression of trophoblastic cell markers by lung carcinomas. *Hum Pathol.* 1995;26(11):1201-1206.

131. Liu X, Adams AL. Mucoepidermoid carcinoma of the bronchus: a review. *Arch Pathol Lab Med.* 2007;131(9):1400-1404.

132. Belgod SR, Reddy RHV, Kumar SP. Mucoepidermoid carcinoma of the lung: a rare entity. *Oxf Med Case Rep.* 2015;2015(2):203-205.

133. Moran CA. Primary salivary gland type tumors of the lung. *Semin Diagn Pathol.* 1995;12:106-122.

134. Zhang XP, Hu PZ, Shen SS, Li XY. Clinical characteristics and prognostic analyses of 87 patients with pulmonary mucoepidermoid carcinoma [in Chinese]. *Zhonghua Zhong Liu Za Zhi.* 2018;40(6):452-455.

135. Fink DD, Lomas AM, Roden AC, Shah PC, Zreik RT. Primary mucoepidermoid carcinoma of the lung with prominent clear cells. *Proc (Baylor Univ Med Cent).* 2017;30(3):322-324.

136. Bell D, El-Naggar AK. Molecular heterogeneity in mucoepidermoid carcinoma: conceptual and practical implications. *Head Neck Pathol.* 2013;7(1):23-27.

137. Shen W, Yang T, Fan Y, et al. Pulmonary mucoepidermoid carcinoma: a clinicopathological study of 45 patients. *Thorac Cancer.* 2022;13(16):2385-2389.

138. Moran CA, Suster S, Koss MN. Primary adenoid cystic carcinoma of the lung: a clinicopathologic and immunohistochemical study of 16 cases. *Cancer.* 1994;73:1390-1397.

139. Ben Salha I, Bhide S, Mourtzoukou D, Fisher C, Thway K. Solid variant of adenoid cystic carcinoma: difficulties in diagnostic recognition. *Int J Surg Pathol.* 2016;24(5):419-424.
140. Chen Z, Jiang J, Fan Y, Lu H. Pulmonary adenoid cystic carcinoma: molecular characteristics and literature review. *Diagn Pathol.* 2023;18(1):65. doi:10.1186/s13000-023-01354-4. PMID: 37198615; PMCID: PMC10190020.
141. Roden AC, Greipp PT, Knutson DL, et al. Histopathologic and cytogenetic features of pulmonary adenoid cystic carcinoma. *J Thorac Oncol.* 2015;10(11):1570-1575. doi:10.1097/JTO.0000000000000656. PMID: 26309189.
142. Moran CA, Suster S, Koss MN. Acinic cell carcinoma of the lung ("Fechner tumor"): a clinicopathologic, immunohistochemical and ultrastructural study of five cases. *Am J Surg Pathol.* 1992;16:1039-1050.
143. Yang MQ, Wang ZQ, Li XF, et al. Primary acinic cell carcinoma of the trachea: a case report and literature review. *Medicine (Baltimore).* 2023;102(6):e32871. doi:10.1097/MD.0000000000032871. PMID: 36820581; PMCID: PMC9907908.
144. Nibid L, Frasca L, Sabarese G, et al. DOG-1 positive primary acinic cell carcinoma of the lung and investigation of molecular status. *Pathologica.* 2022;114(5):385-390. doi:10.32074/1591-951X-786. PMID: 36305026; PMCID: PMC9614299.
145. Moran CA, Suster S, Askin FB, Koss MN. Benign and malignant salivary gland type tumors of the lung: clinicopathologic and immunohistochemical study of 8 cases. *Cancer.* 1994;73:2481-2490.
146. Chen L, Zhang W, Li X. Analysis of clinical features of 7 cases of primary pleomorphic adenoma of lower respiratory tract and review of literature. *Medicine (Baltimore).* 2023;102(49):e36258. doi:10.1097/MD.0000000000036258. PMID: 38065895; PMCID: PMC10713184.
147. Asahina M, Hayashi T, Takamochi K, et al. Identification of CTNNB1-PLAG1 gene rearrangement in a patient with pulmonary pleomorphic adenoma. *Virchows Arch.* 2020;477(5):739-742. doi:10.1007/s00428-020-02810-y. PMID: 32307573.
148. Nguyen CV, Suster S, Moran CA. Pulmonary epithelial–myoepithelial carcinoma: a clinicopathologic and immunohistochemical study of 5 cases. *Hum Pathol.* 2009;40:366-374.
149. Morgado S, Santos AF, Nogueira F. Primary pulmonary epithelial-myoepithelial carcinoma: a case report and comprehensive literature review of a rare lung neoplasm. *Cureus.* 2025;17(3):e80188. doi:10.7759/cureus.80188. PMID: 40061844; PMCID: PMC11886455.
150. Deb PQ, Suster DI. Outcome of primary lung salivary gland-type carcinoma: a population-based study. *Int J Surg Pathol.* 2025;33(1):49-58. doi:10.1177/10668969241256107 PMID:38839261.
151. Jian CH, Luo S, Wang JJ. Primary pulmonary hyalinizing clear cell carcinoma with *EWSR1* gene translocation: a case report. *Front Oncol.* 2024;14:1509132. doi:10.3389/fonc.2024.1509132
152. Su YJ, Wu YS, How CH, Hsieh MS. Hyalinizing clear cell carcinoma of the lung: a case report and literature review. *Diagn Pathol.* 2024;19(1):154. doi:10.1186/s13000-024-01579-x
153. Ishikawa A, Fujisawa H, Yasumura N, et al. Histopathology and cytology of pulmonary myoepithelial neoplasms: 2 cases. *Case Rep Oncol* 2022;15(2):599-605. doi:10.1159/000524769
154. Sharma S, Tayal A, Khatri S, Mohapatra SG, Mohanty SK. Primary pulmonary epithelial-myoepithelial carcinoma: report of a rare and under-diagnosed low-grade malignancy. *J Cancer Res Ther.* 2022;18(3):795-800. doi:10.4103/jcrt.JCRT_559_20
155. Berho M, Moran CA, Suster S. Mixed malignant epithelial/mesenchymal lung neoplasms. *Semin Diagn Pathol.* 1995;12:123-139.

156. Kilic D, Yilmaz C, Tepeoglu M, Vural C, Caner H. Biphasic pulmonary blastoma associated with cerebral metastasis. *Turk Neurosurg.* 2016;26(1):169-172.

157. Liman ST, Altinok T, Topcu S, et al. Survival of biphasic pulmonary blastoma. *Respir Med.* 2006;100(7):1174-1179.

158. Takahashi K, Kohno T, Matsumoto S, et al. Clonality and heterogeneity of pulmonary blastoma from the viewpoint of genetic alterations: a case report. *Lung Cancer.* 2007;57(1):103-108.

159. Alirezaie N, Chong AL, Kommoss FKF, et al. Exomic and epigenomic analysis of pulmonary blastoma. *Lung Cancer.* 2024;195:107916. doi:10.1016/j.lungcan.2024.107916 PMID:39121796.

160. Yao H, Jiang X, Zeng Y, Wang X, Tang X. Classic biphasic pulmonary blastoma: a case report and review of the literature from 2000 to 2022. *Clin Respir J.* 2023;17(11):1103-1116. doi:10.1111/crj.13701. PMID: 37772674; PMCID: PMC10632085.

161. Mekheal E, Kapoor A, Roman S, et al. Pulmonary carcinosarcoma: a rare disease with challenging diagnosis and treatment. *Cureus.* 2022;14(7):e26901. doi:10.7759/cureus.26901. PMID: 35983399; PMCID: PMC9376117.

162. Ohtaki Y, Kawabata-Iwakawa R, Nobusawa S, et al. Molecular and expressional characterization of tumor heterogeneity in pulmonary carcinosarcoma. *Mol Carcinog.* 2022;61(10):924-932. doi:10.1002/mc.23448. PMID: 35848137.

163. Zhang MY, Tang LS, Qin ZJ, Hao YT, Cheng K, Zheng A. Clinical features and prognostic factors of pulmonary carcinosarcoma: a nomogram development and validation based on surveillance epidemiology and end results database. *Front Med (Lausanne).* 2022;9:988830. doi:10.3389/fmed.2022.988830. PMID: 36330063; PMCID: PMC9622765.

13

NEUROENDOCRINE LUNG NEOPLASMS

Neuroendocrine lung tumors are relatively rare neoplasms that have undergone a number of revisions in their nomenclature and diagnostic approach during the past several years. In particular, the terminology applied to these tumors has been a topic of much debate and controversy in the literature.[1] Most authors today seem to accept the concept that neuroendocrine tumors form part of a family of neoplasms that can show a wide spectrum of differentiation and morphologic appearances. In previous years, the term "carcinoid tumor" was applied to tumors belonging to the more benign end of the spectrum, and the majority of poorly differentiated tumors were designated as "small cell carcinoma." Eventually, the realization that intermediate forms also exist led to the creation of the category of "atypical carcinoid." This was followed by the creation of "large cell neuroendocrine carcinoma (LCNEC)" to describe tumors with high-grade features but that demonstrated large cell morphology. The situation is complicated by the fact that the tumors often refuse to adhere to these artificially created categories. Low- and intermediate-grade tumors can present with highly proliferative areas that preclude them from being classified according to the established mitotic count cutoffs. Intermediate-grade tumors ("atypical carcinoids") can show significant morphologic overlap and proliferative indexes with LCNECs. High-grade neuroendocrine carcinomas can present as combined tumors with adenocarcinoma or squamous cell carcinoma, including as a secondary treatment resistance mechanism. Some small cell carcinomas are recognized to have low neuroendocrine marker expression and may be difficult to identify with immunohistochemistry. Some tumors can present with combined features of both small cell neuroendocrine carcinoma and LCNEC leading to difficulty in classification. Conventional adenocarcinoma and squamous cell carcinoma may show aberrant expression of neuroendocrine-associated immunohistochemical markers or neuroendocrinelike morphology that may be confused for true neuroendocrine differentiation. It goes to follow that the diagnosis of these unusual variants may be difficult or impossible on small biopsy material, and even larger resection specimens may still pose a problem for diagnosis and classification. However, for the purposes of this chapter, we will focus on conventional neuroendocrine tumor types as they comprise the majority of tumors encountered in clinical practice and form the basis for developing an approach to diagnosis of these tumors.

The general trend in most organ systems is to subdivide neuroendocrine tumors according to their morphologic features and potential behavior into well-differentiated, moderately differentiated, and poorly differentiated tumors or by grade into low-, intermediate-, and high-grade tumors.[2-4] It is unfortunate that the current World Health Organization (WHO) classification of tumors of the lung continues to retain the terms "carcinoid tumor" and "atypical carcinoid" for designating these lesions, as such terms are generally acknowledged to be outdated and may be misleading with regard to their malignant potential. Though we expect some of this terminology may change in the upcoming edition of the WHO.[5] In any case, the lack of uniformity in terminology has created ambiguity and the potential for confusion among clinicians, patients, and pathologists.[6] The terminology we use divides these tumors into a three-tiered system: low, intermediate, and high grades, using the term "neuroendocrine carcinoma" for all tumor types. The system is as follows: (1) **low-grade neuroendocrine carcinoma**, considered equivalent to a "grade 1 neuroendocrine tumor," "typical carcinoid tumor," or "well-differentiated neuroendocrine tumor" as used in other classification systems, (2) **intermediate-grade neuroendocrine carcinoma**, considered equivalent to a "grade 2 neuroendocrine tumor" or "grade 3 neuroendocrine tumor," "atypical carcinoid," or "moderately differentiated neuroendocrine tumor," and (3) **high-grade neuroendocrine carcinoma**, considered equivalent to "small cell carcinoma," "large cell neuroendocrine carcinoma," or "poorly differentiated neuroendocrine carcinoma." We designate the high-grade neuroendocrine carcinomas as either "small cell type" or "large cell type." This classification system is roughly equivalent to some currently proposed grading systems for pulmonary neuroendocrine neoplasms (Table 13.1).[7] Though we acknowledge that the tumors at the low-grade end of the spectrum (mostly typical carcinoid tumor) often behave in an exceedingly indolent fashion, these tumors still have some degree of malignant potential, and thus, we prefer the more precise term of "carcinoma" over the term "tumor." The same rationale applies to intermediate-grade lesions that show significantly more aggressive biologic behavior with up to a 50% mortality at 5 years.

As mentioned above, the diagnosis of neuroendocrine neoplasms of the lung continues to be a problem area for pathologists. Although there have been many attempts over the years at refining our criteria for their diagnosis, reproducibility remains poor, even among expert pulmonary pathologists. In a study by Travis et al,[8] a unanimous agreement among five experienced pulmonary pathologists could only be achieved in 58% of cases for carcinoid tumors, 50% for atypical carcinoids, and 40% for LCNECs. Since then additional studies have been undertaken that confirm

TABLE 13.1 Neuroendocrine Neoplasms of the Lung

Tumor	Older Nomenclature	Features
Low-grade neuroendocrine carcinoma (aka Grade 1 NET)	Carcinoid tumor Bronchial adenoma Kulchitsky cell tumor Typical carcinoid Well-differentiated neuroendocrine carcinoma Well-differentiated neuroendocrine tumor	Prominent "neuroendocrine" (organoid) growth pattern No cytologic atypia Stippled chromatin ("salt and pepper") Low mitotic activity ($<2 \times 2$ mm^2) Absence of tumor cell necrosis Strong expression of neuroendocrine markers by immunohistochemistry
Intermediate-grade neuroendocrine carcinoma (aka grade 2 and/or grade 3 NET)	Atypical carcinoid Moderately differentiated neuroendocrine carcinoma	Preservation of neuroendocrine growth pattern Increased cytologic atypia Prominent nucleoli Moderately increased mitotic activity (2-10 $\times$ 2 mm^2) Frequent areas of comedonecrosis Retained expression of neuroendocrine immunohistochemical markers
High-grade neuroendocrine carcinoma, small cell or large cell type	Small cell carcinoma Oat cell carcinoma Kulchitsky cell carcinoma Large cell neuroendocrine carcinoma Undifferentiated small cell carcinoma Poorly differentiated neuroendocrine carcinoma	Poorly developed, or only focal, neuroendocrine growth pattern Marked cytologic atypia Small cell or large cell morphology High mitotic activity ($>10 \times 2$ mm^2) Extensive areas of necrosis Reduced expression of neuroendocrine immunohistochemical markers

NET, neuroendocrine tumor; aka, also known as.

the high degree of interobserver variability of the WHO criteria.[9,10] Studies have also pointed out that prognosis based on the assessment of histology of neuroendocrine neoplasms can vary, especially with regard to intermediate-grade neuroendocrine carcinomas (atypical carcinoids).[11] Morphometric studies carried out on surgically resected tissues in patients with poorly differentiated lung cancers have underscored the difficulties inherent in separating these tumors based on morphology by demonstrating considerable overlap in nuclear size between “small cells” and “large cells” in examples of small cell neuroendocrine carcinoma and LCNECs.[12] Thus, it follows that making a specific diagnosis based on cell size and cytologic features can be extremely problematic and sometimes unreliable when applied to these lesions, especially in small biopsy samples. Another factor, in addition to the difficulties involved in evaluating cell size, has been the emphasis placed by many experts on mitotic activity as a means for distinguishing among the various categories. Mitotic activity, although consistently high in the high-grade lesions and consistently low in the low-grade lesions, can show significant variability within intermediate-grade neuroendocrine carcinomas, making strict separation based on this criterion alone very difficult and sometimes arbitrary. Moreover, the requirement for assessing mitotic counts has been based on review of resection specimens and may not be applicable to small biopsy samples, thus further limiting the use of this feature for the evaluation of small lung biopsies.

An additional aspect that has been either neglected or underemphasized in most of the current classification schemes is the architecture and growth pattern. Low-grade and intermediate-grade neuroendocrine neoplasms are generally characterized by a well-developed “endocrine” or “organoid” pattern of growth (nests, ribbons, trabeculae, peripheral palisading of tumor cells, etc.), whereas high-grade neuroendocrine neoplasms are characterized by loss of organotypic architecture, usually with complete absence of any well-defined architectural growth pattern (ie, showing only sheets of tumor cells without any particular organization). Tumors that show a combination of well-preserved features of an endocrine growth pattern in combination with high histologic grade are likely to be located along the middle of the spectrum (ie, intermediate-grade neuroendocrine carcinoma/atypical carcinoid), rather than at the extremes. Lack of inclusion of the assessment of growth pattern for the classification, thus, detracts from our ability to properly evaluate their degree of differentiation and biologic potential.

An additional difficulty that is commonly encountered in clinical practice is how to distinguish between intermediate-grade neuroendocrine carcinomas (atypical carcinoid) and LCNEC (currently regarded as belonging in the high-grade, poorly differentiated end of the spectrum). In fact, critical reading of the proposed criteria for the diagnosis of these tumor types shows significant overlap. The main diagnostic feature that permits separation of LCNEC from other types of nonneuroendocrine large cell carcinomas is precisely the well-developed “neuroendocrine” growth pattern (ie, organoid architecture) in the former.[13] This organotypic growth also suggests that some LCNECs may lie closer on the spectrum of neuroendocrine tumors to intermediate-grade neuroendocrine carcinomas than to high-grade neuroendocrine carcinomas, although this has not been entirely borne out in survival studies of LCNEC, which have shown poor overall survival.[14] Clearly, a better understanding of this family of tumors is still required. In the setting of an endoscopic biopsy, in particular, it may be nearly impossible to separate these two categories with absolute certainty, regardless of the results of special stains, molecular testing, or morphologic features.

LOW-GRADE NEUROENDOCRINE CARCINOMA (CARCINOID TUMOR, GRADE 1 NEUROENDOCRINE TUMOR)

Low-grade neuroendocrine carcinoma (or "carcinoid tumor" of the older literature) has traditionally been regarded as the prototype neuroendocrine tumor of the lung. Because up to 15% of conventional "carcinoids" of the lung can metastasize to regional lymph nodes, these tumors are now generally regarded as low-grade malignant neoplasms with some degree of metastatic potential though overall as a group they tend to behave in a very indolent fashion.[14] By current definitions, these tumors must be at least greater than 5 mm or they are instead termed "pulmonary tumorlet." Tumorlets are a frequent incidental finding in resections done for alternative reasons and are generally clinically silent.[15,16] The majority of these lesions are sporadic; however, they may rarely arise in association with multiple neuroendocrine neoplasia (MEN) Type I or in association with diffuse idiopathic pulmonary neuroendocrine cell hyperplasia, a condition in which patients develop multiple low-grade tumorlets or low-grade neuroendocrine carcinomas (carcinoids) that involve the lungs bilaterally in a diffuse fashion.[17-20] This putative precursor condition cannot be diagnosed on small biopsy material or even on larger wedge resections in most cases and requires sampling of multiple lobes of the lungs for confirmation; alternatively, it may be suggested in the appropriate radiologic context.[21] Low-grade neuroendocrine carcinomas occur predominantly in adults and are more often centrally located within the lung, although some tumors can also be present in peripheral locations away from cartilage-bearing airways.[22] The tumors may be rarely be associated with paraneoplastic syndromes (such as Cushing syndrome) owing to aberrant synthesis of peptide hormones, and they can give rise to the carcinoid syndrome when they metastasize to the liver.[23] The majority of the tumors are characterized by endobronchial growth into the bronchial lumen and are thus readily amenable to sampling by endoscopic biopsies. They usually present as tan, polypoid, and smooth endobronchial lesions that cause obstruction and hemoptysis. Bleeding is a common complication of the endoscopic biopsy procedure.[24] The influence of nodal metastases in low-grade neuroendocrine carcinomas on overall survival appears to be an important prognostic factor; however, some studies have been unable to demonstrate a significant correlation. Patients generally have a very good prognosis, with overall survival rates greater than 90% following surgical resection of the primary lesions.[25-29] Sporadic low-grade neuroendocrine carcinomas of the lung show frequent somatic *MEN1* mutations as well as mutations in other chromatin remodeling genes in the SWI/SNF complex including *PSIP1* and *ARID1A*.[5,30,31] Rare cases have been shown to have a hypermutated phenotype with damaging *POLQ* mutations. Although the WHO reports the rate of *RB1* alterations to be below 5% in "carcinoid" tumors, at least one study has shown the rate to be as high as 25%. Interestingly enough the rate of *RB1* alterations in "atypical carcinoids" in that study was approximately 10%, significantly lower than that reported by the WHO.[32] The rate of *TP53* alterations in low-grade neuroendocrine carcinomas is low as compared to high-grade tumors.[32] The known molecular alterations of neuroendocrine neoplasms of the lung are listed in Table 13.2.

The histologic diagnosis of low-grade neuroendocrine carcinomas on endoscopic biopsy is generally straightforward (eFigs. 13.1-13.3). The tumors are characterized by their striking neuroendocrine ("organoid") growth pattern, comprising nests of monotonous tumor cells separated by thin fibrovascular septa (Zellballen), serpiginous trabeculae, or ribbons of tumor cells, and epithelial pseudorosettes (Fig. 13.1A and B). The tumor cells are round to oval, with round, centrally located nuclei showing a characteristically stippled ("salt and pepper") chromatin pattern and

TABLE 13.2 Molecular Alterations in Neuroendocrine Neoplasms of the Lung

Tumor	Primary Molecular Alterations
Low-grade neuroendocrine carcinoma (carcinoid)	Somatic mutations in *MEN1* and alterations of chromatin remodeling genes
Intermediate-grade neuroendocrine carcinoma (atypical carcinoid)	Somatic mutations in *MEN1* and alterations of chromatin remodeling and DNA repair genes
High-grade neuroendocrine carcinoma–small cell type (small cell carcinoma)	Concurrent loss-of-function mutations in *RB1* and *TP53*, *MYC* amplification
High-grade neuroendocrine carcinoma–large cell type (large cell neuroendocrine carcinoma [LCNEC])	1. SCLC-like LCNEC–Concurrent mutations in *RB1* and *TP53*, *MYC* amplification 2. NSCLC-like LCNEC–Mutually exclusive mutations in *RB1* and *TP53* combined with NSCLC-associated mutations (*KEAP1*, *STK11*, *KRAS*) and loss of *CDKN2A* 3. "Carcinoidlike" LCNEC–*MEN1* mutations

NSCLC, non–small cell lung carcinoma; SCLC, small cell lung cancer.

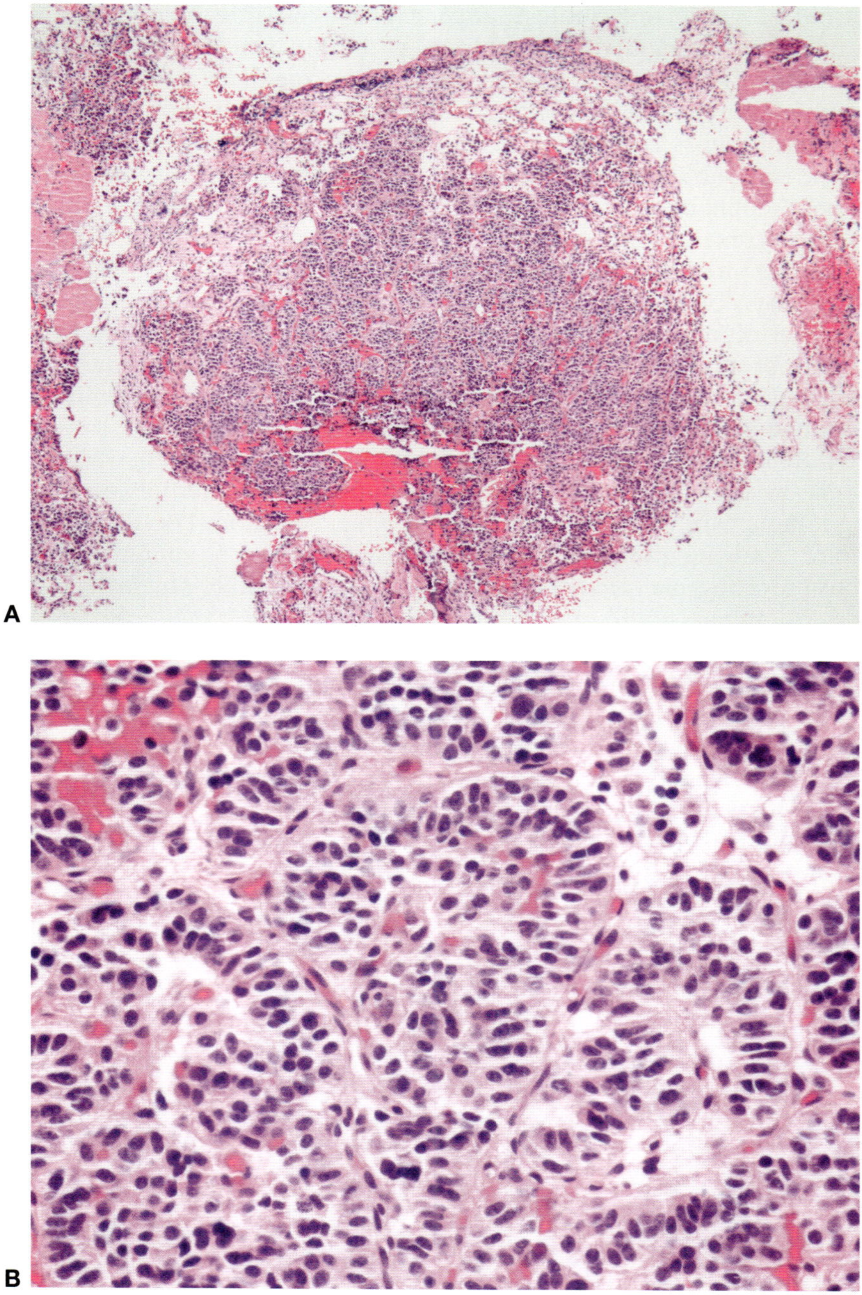

FIGURE 13.1 **A.** Bronchial biopsy showing uniform nests of tumor cells beneath a denuded bronchial mucosa showing the typical "Zellballen" appearance of low-grade neuroendocrine carcinoma of the lung (bronchial carcinoid). **B.** Higher magnification showing a monotonous population of tumor cells with stippled chromatin pattern and rim of eosinophilic cytoplasm.

devoid of significant cytologic atypia. The nuclei are surrounded by an ample rim of eosinophilic cytoplasm, with a normal nuclear to cytoplasmic ratio. The cells can also be spindled, pigmented (owing to melanin granules), or contain abundant granular eosinophilic cytoplasm (oncocytic variant). Tumors comprising spindle cells show a tendency to present as peripheral, subpleural lesions and for that reason are seldom encountered in endoscopic biopsies (Fig. 13.2). Rare mitoses can be observed, but they should normally not exceed 2 mitoses per 2 mm^2. An accurate mitotic count can often be difficult to establish in small endoscopic biopsies where there may not be 2 mm^2 available for a proper assessment, making this criterion difficult to apply in endoscopic biopsy material. However, the finding of more than one mitosis in a small endoscopic biopsy, coupled with mild or moderate cytologic atypia, should raise the possibility of an intermediate-grade neuroendocrine carcinoma.

Some unusual morphologic variants of low-grade neuroendocrine carcinomas have been observed that may pose difficulties for interpretation, including tumors with metaplastic cartilage or bone formation (Fig. 13.3A and B), tumors containing abundant mucinous stroma that may be confused for mucinous bronchogenic carcinomas or a metastasis from other organs (Fig. 13.4A and B), tumors with prominent angiectatic features that may resemble vascular neoplasms, tumors with prominent cystic changes, tumors with a glandular arrangement resembling adenocarcinoma (Fig. 13.5A and B), and

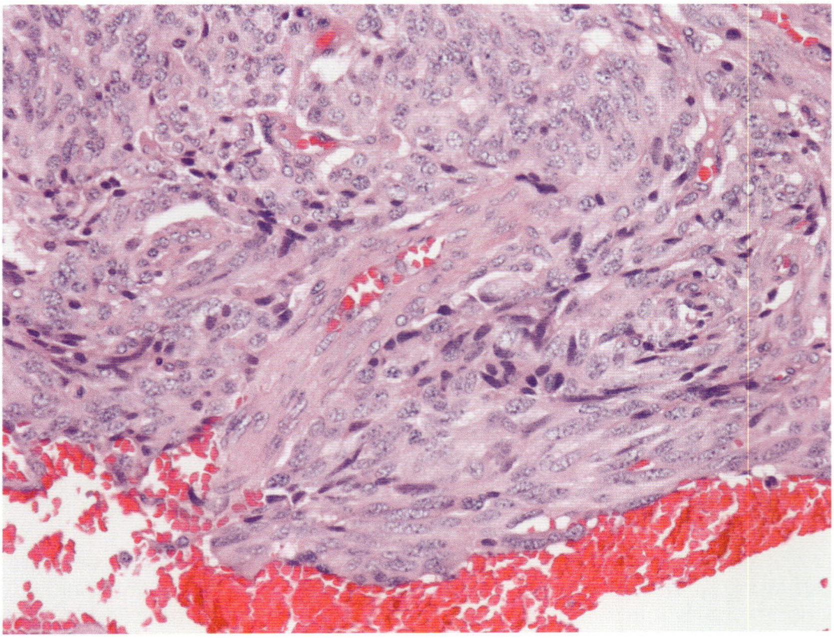

FIGURE 13.2 Low-grade neuroendocrine carcinoma of the lung showing spindling of the tumor cells (*lower right*).

A

B

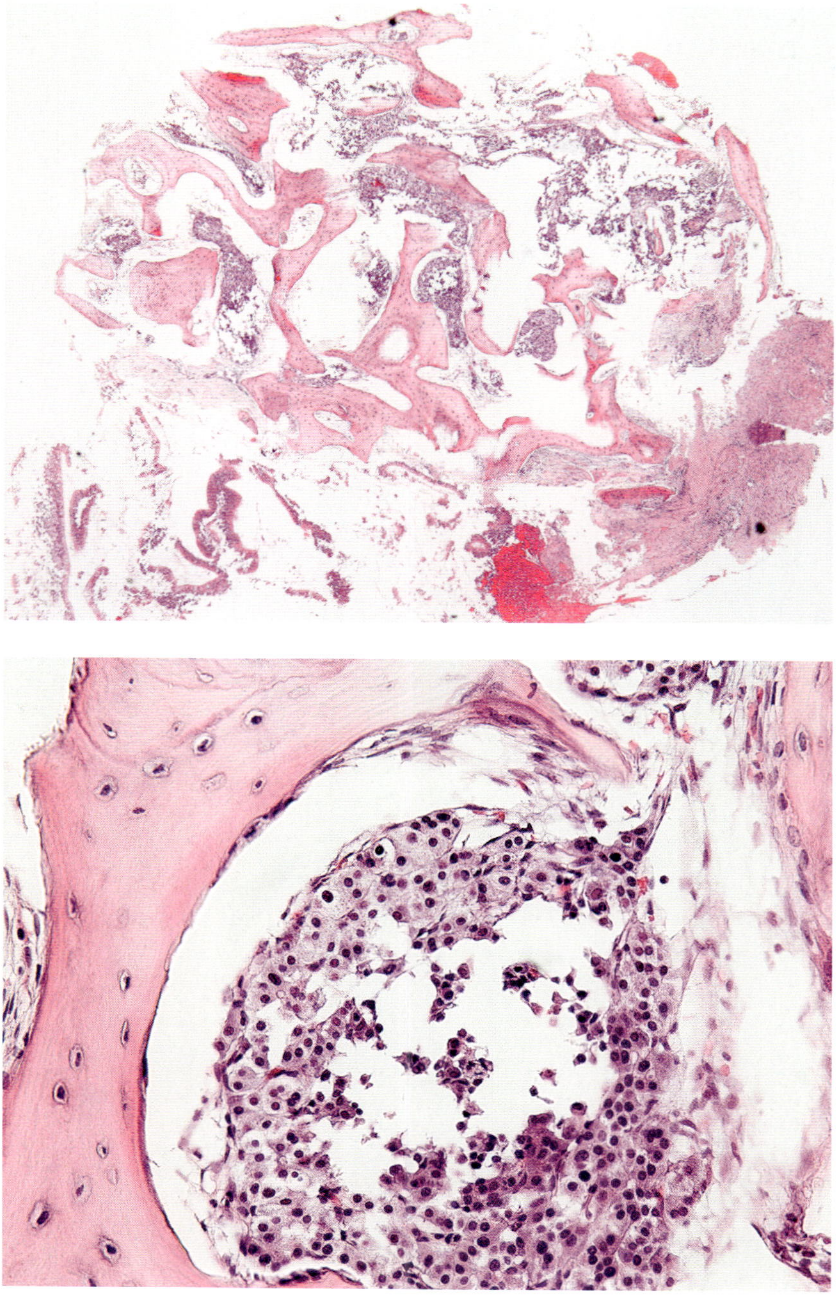

FIGURE 13.3 **A.** Bronchial biopsy showing extensive bony deposition circumscribing small cellular islands of tumor cells. **B.** Higher magnification showing a monotonous population of bland-appearing tumor cells surrounded by bone in low-grade neuroendocrine carcinoma of the lung with extensive osseous metaplasia.

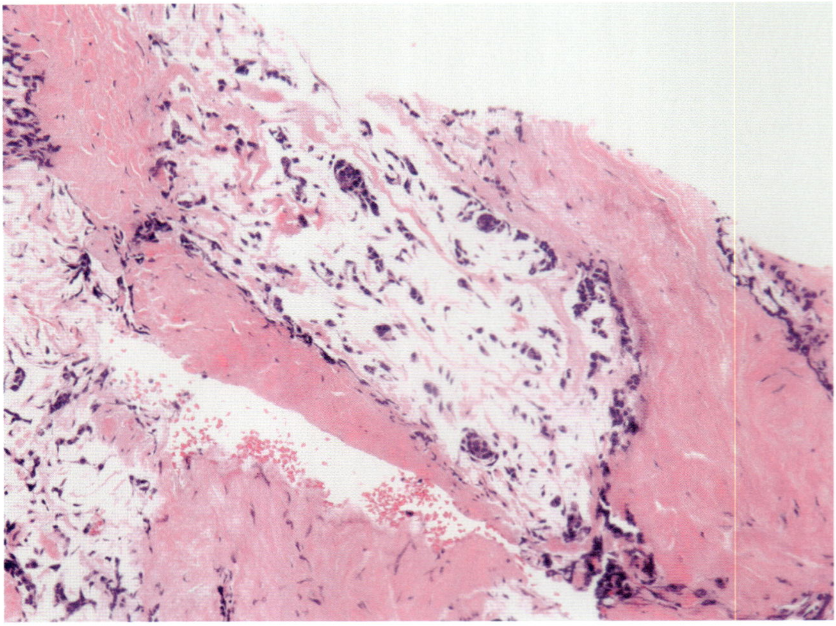

A

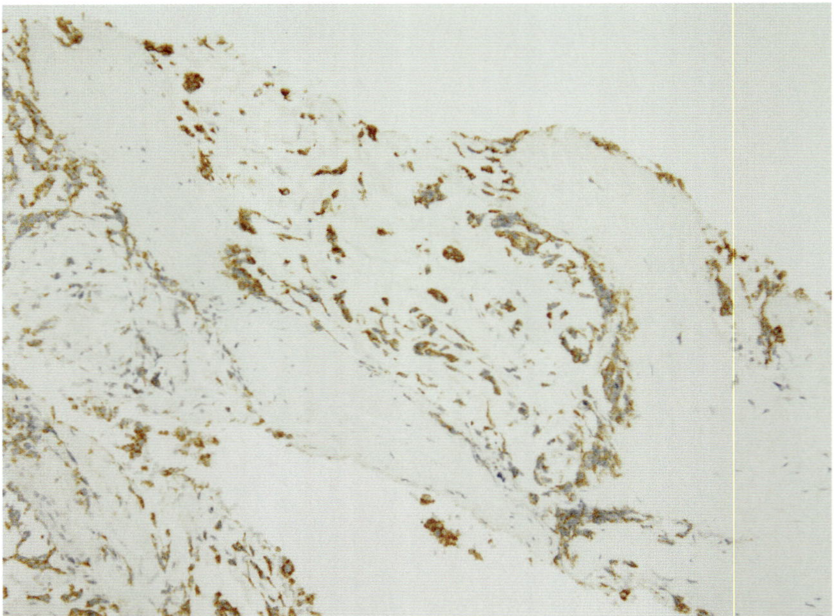

B

FIGURE 13.4 **A.** Core biopsy of low-grade neuroendocrine carcinoma of the lung shows small clusters and cords of small, monotonous tumor cells embedded in a mucinous stroma simulating metastatic mucin-secreting (colloid) carcinoma. **B.** Immunohistochemical staining for synaptophysin demonstrates cytoplasmic positivity of the tumor cells, indicating a diagnosis of low-grade neuroendocrine carcinoma with abundant mucinous stroma. Such tumors must be distinguished from metastases from breast and gastrointestinal tract carcinomas.

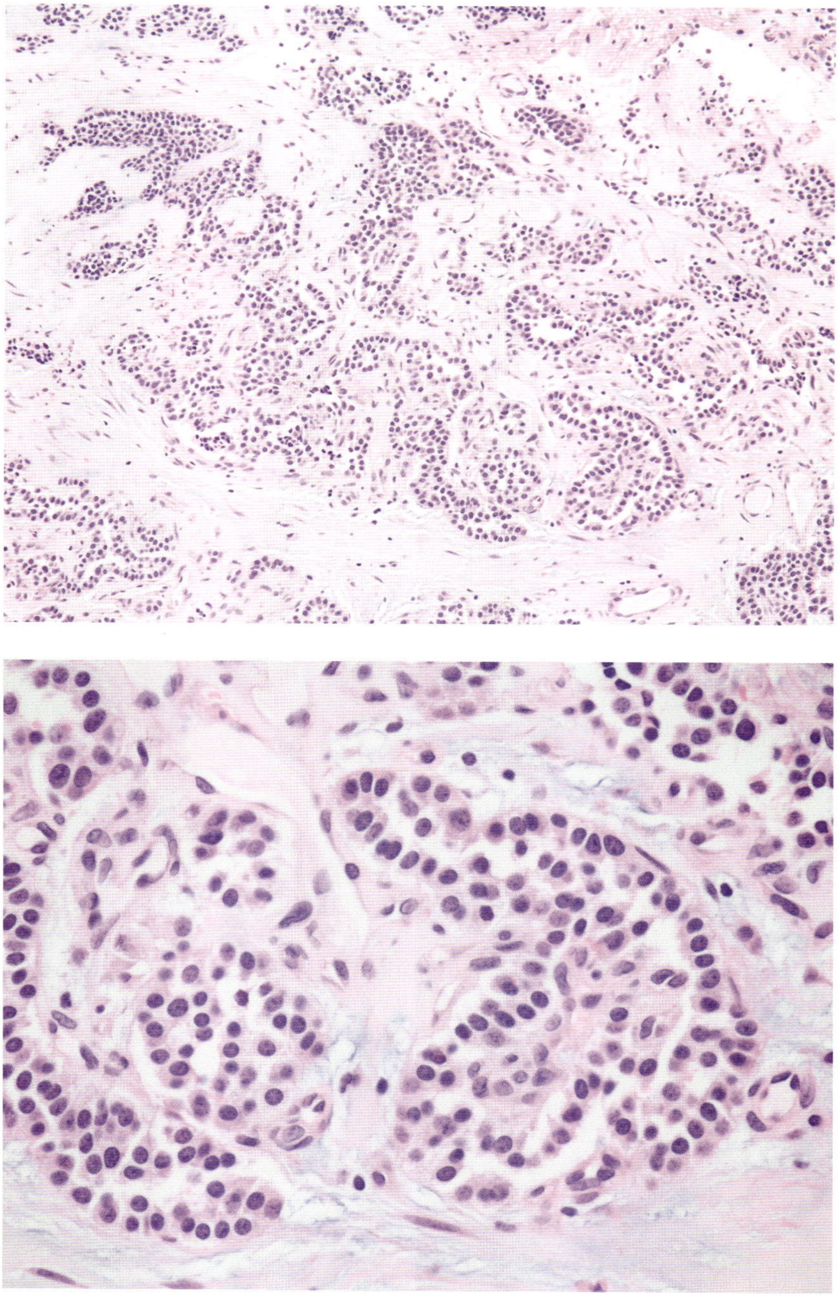

A

B

FIGURE 13.5 **A.** Endoscopic biopsy of low-grade neuroendocrine carcinoma with pseudoglandular pattern simulating low-grade adenocarcinoma. **B.** Higher magnification showing a monotonous population of small tumor cells lining the pseudoglandular structures; these cells reacted strongly with chromogranin and synaptophysin.

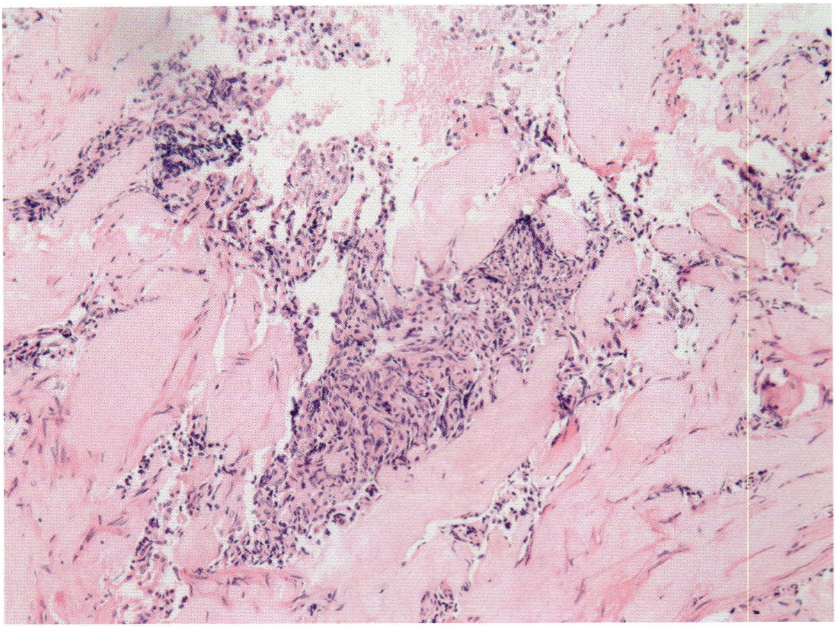

FIGURE 13.6 **Low-grade neuroendocrine carcinoma of the lung with abundant stromal sclerosis; notice bland-appearing population of tumor cells with focal crushing artifact.** These tumors need to be distinguished from metastases or desmoplastic carcinomas.

tumors with amyloidlike or sclerotic stroma (Fig. 13.6).[33-37] In small biopsies, the tumors may often display a solid, sheetlike pattern of growth with bland-appearing, monotonous small tumor cells without any particular architectural organization that can resemble a lymphoma or be suggestive of a higher-grade neoplasm (Fig. 13.7A and B). Attention to the bland nuclear morphology, ample rim of eosinophilic cytoplasm, and absence of mitotic activity should prompt investigation with neuroendocrine markers to confirm the diagnosis. Another potential pitfall for diagnosis is artifactual distortion of the tumor cells in small biopsy samples leading to spindling or crushing of the tumor cells, making recognition of the underlying process very difficult (Fig. 13.8A and B). Use of immunohistochemical stains in such instances can facilitate the diagnosis (Fig. 13.8C).

An important distinction to make for low-grade neuroendocrine carcinomas is with the so-called pulmonary tumorlet. As mentioned previously, the latter is generally an incidental finding usually seen away from cartilage-bearing airways in lung resection specimens and, therefore, generally not amenable to sampling by endoscopic techniques. The pulmonary tumorlet is histologically indistinguishable from low-grade neuroendocrine tumors and is separated from it by an arbitrary size criterion (<0.5 cm). The diagnosis of pulmonary tumorlet should not be made on endoscopic

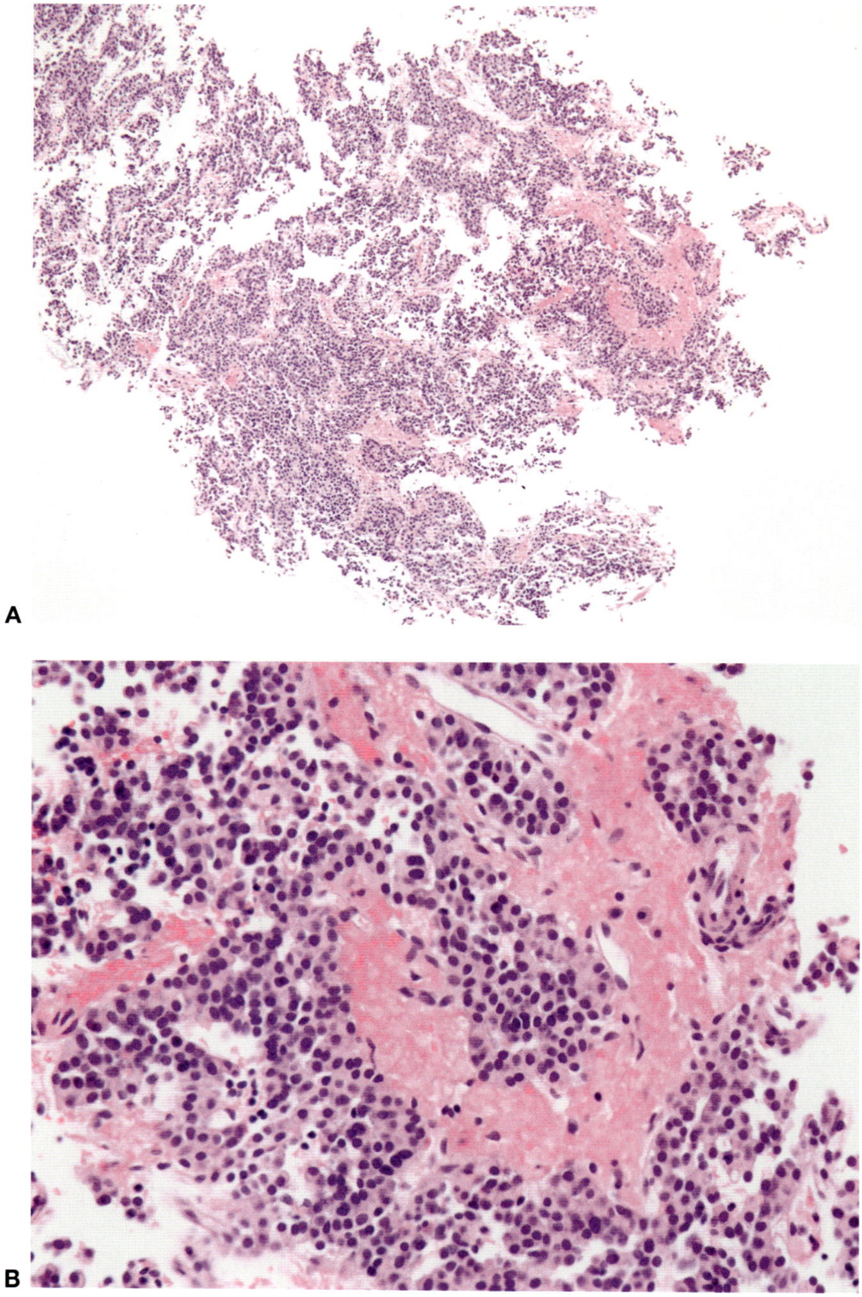

FIGURE 13.7 **A.** Bronchial biopsy of low-grade neuroendocrine carcinoma of the lung shows a solid proliferation of uniform small cells without any particular organization or distinctive growth pattern. This is a frequently encountered presentation for these tumors in small endoscopic biopsies. **B.** Higher magnification shows a monotonous tumor cell population with no evidence of cytologic atypia or mitotic activity. This finding should prompt ordering of stains for neuroendocrine markers to confirm the diagnosis.

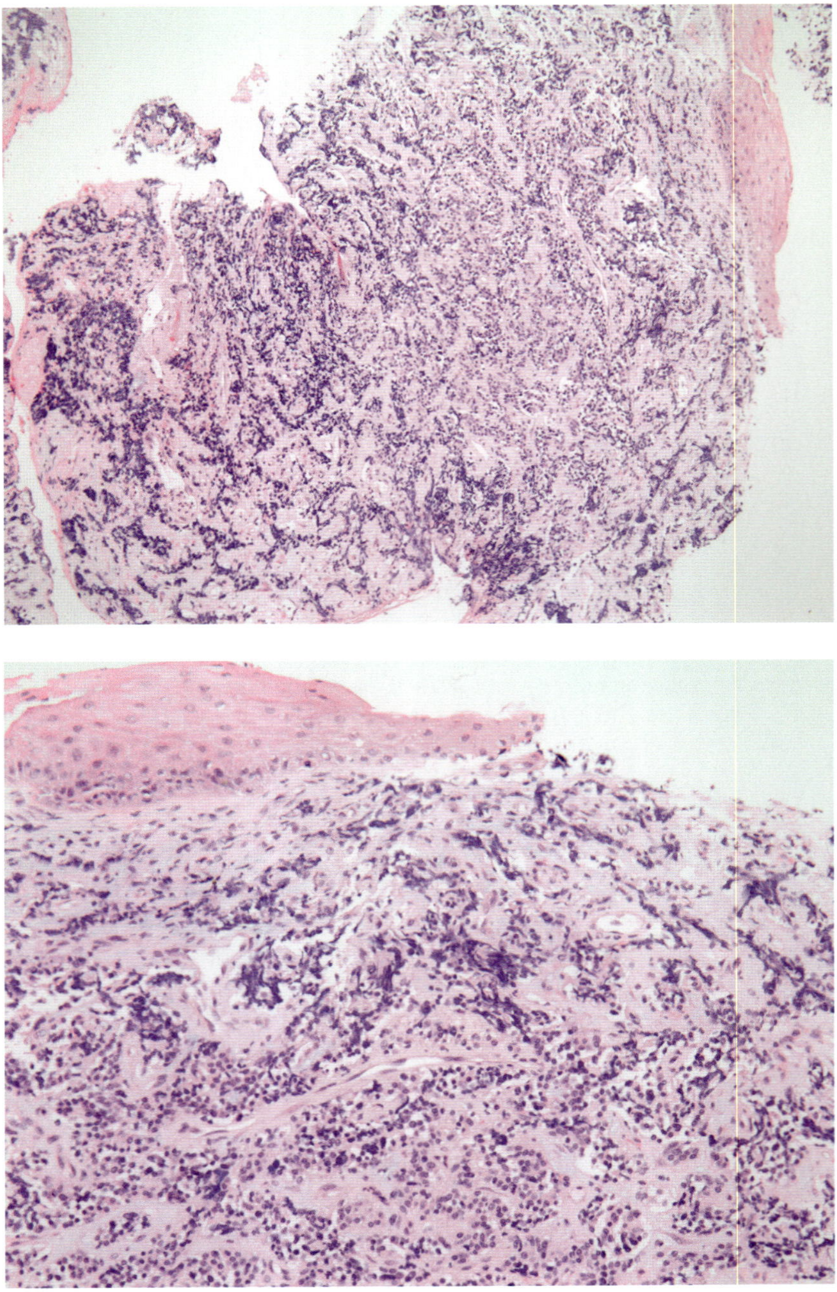

A

B

FIGURE 13.8 **A.** Bronchial biopsy of low-grade neuroendocrine carcinoma showing a monotonous population of tumor cells lying beneath the squamous bronchial epithelium and showing focal crush artifact. **B.** Higher magnification shows clusters of cells with prominent crush artifact underlying the squamous mucosa with more well-preserved round, uniform tumor cells lying underneath.

C
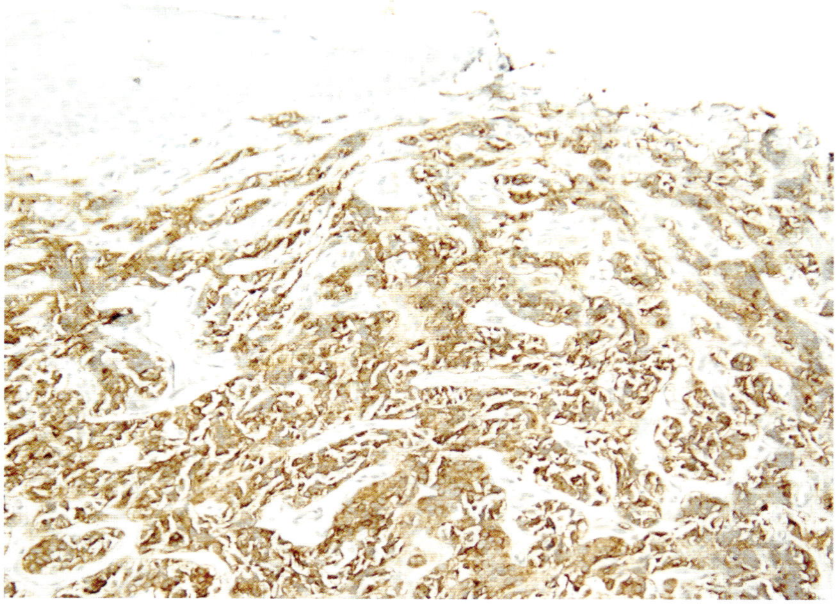

FIGURE 13.8 (*continued*) **C.** Immunohistochemical stain for synaptophysin shows strong cytoplasmic positivity in both the crushed and viable tumor cells.

biopsy specimens and should be reserved only for the incidental finding of this lesion in resected lung specimens or larger wedge biopsies taken for other reasons.

Immunohistochemistry plays an important role in the diagnosis of neuroendocrine neoplasms of the lung. Low-grade neuroendocrine carcinomas are characterized by the strong expression of neuroendocrine-associated markers, including chromogranin A, synaptophysin, neuron-specific enolase, and CD56. The staining pattern is cytoplasmic and diffuse (Fig. 13.9). A transcription factor, INSM1, will also stain neuroendocrine lesions and offers the advantage of being a nuclear stain. These tumors are also strongly positive for cytokeratins, in particular CK7 and low molecular weight cytokeratins.[38] The tumors can also express specific peptide hormones, including gastrin, somatostatin, and bombesin. A subpopulation of S100 protein–positive sustentacular cells can sometimes be identified in some of these tumors. Of interest, thyroid transcription factor-1 (TTF-1), an intranuclear transcription factor frequently expressed in high-grade neuroendocrine carcinomas of the lung, is only weakly expressed or absent in low-grade neuroendocrine carcinomas.[39] Demonstration of numerous dense-core, membrane-bound neurosecretory granules by electron microscopy is another way to establish the diagnosis in equivocal cases, but this methodology has largely fallen in disuse owing to the broad availability of immunohistochemical markers in routine practice. Use of

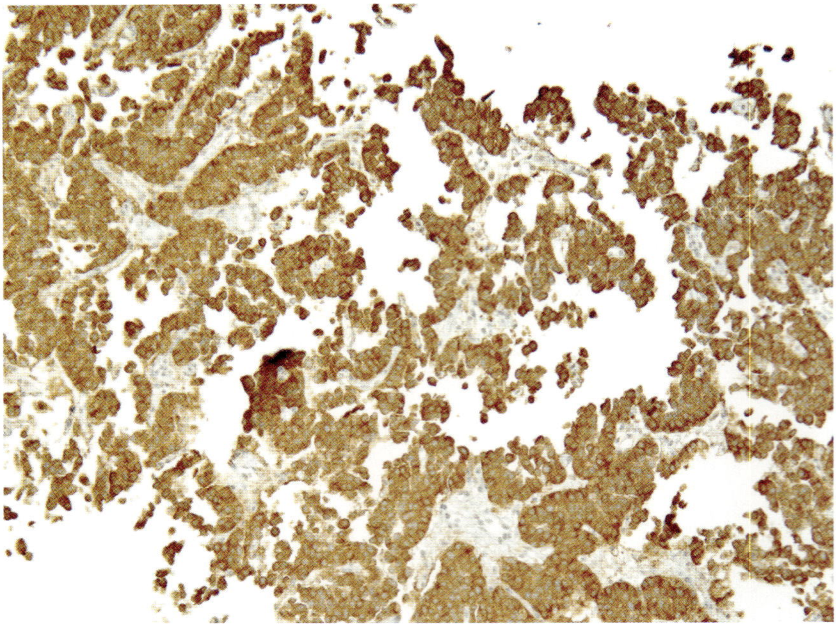

FIGURE 13.9 Immunohistochemical stain for chromogranin in low-grade neuroendocrine carcinoma of the lung shows strong cytoplasmic positivity in the majority of the tumor cells.

proliferation markers such as Ki-67 can be of help in equivocal cases for distinguishing low-grade neuroendocrine carcinomas from intermediate-grade and high-grade neuroendocrine carcinomas; low-grade neuroendocrine carcinomas are characterized by low expression of this marker (<5% nuclear positivity), although a subset with bland cytologic features and well-differentiated neuroendocrine growth pattern have been reported to display a Ki-67 labeling index of greater than 20%.[40] An unusual pitfall that can be posed by these tumors and in which the use of proliferation markers may be useful is the occasional absence of the distinctive speckled chromatin pattern of the nuclei in the tumor cells, with the nuclei showing dense and evenly dispersed nuclear chromatin resembling a small cell carcinoma (Fig. 13.10A and B). This feature may lead to misinterpreting the lesion as a small cell neuroendocrine carcinoma on small biopsy material. Special stains for neuroendocrine markers may not be helpful in this setting given that both can be expected to be positive for the same tumor markers; however, immunostaining for a Ki-67 proliferation marker will be helpful for separating the two, as small cell neuroendocrine carcinoma should be expected to show a very high proliferative index, unlike low-grade neuroendocrine carcinomas that characteristically have a low proliferation fraction (Fig. 13.10C).

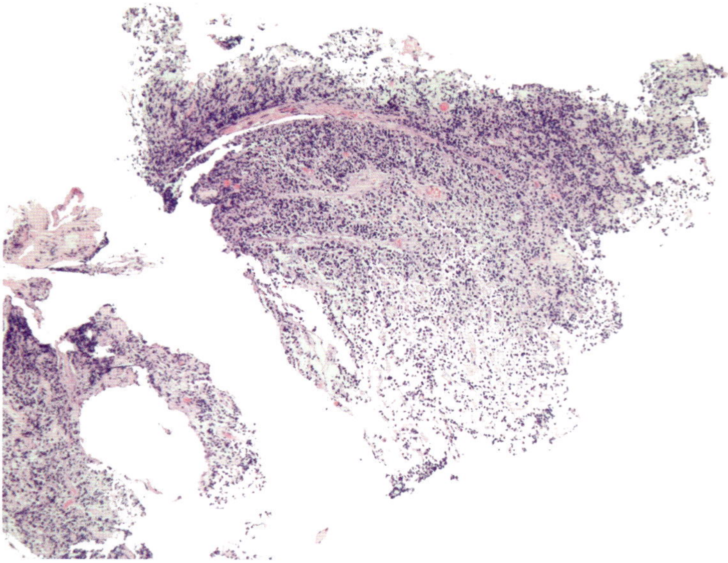

A

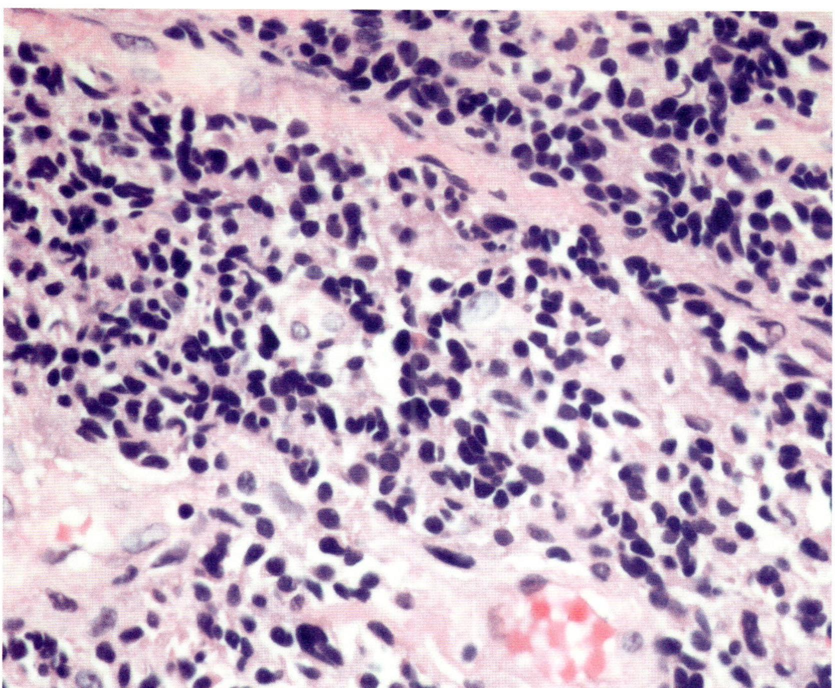

B

FIGURE 13.10 **A.** Endoscopic biopsy of low-grade neuroendocrine lung carcinoma showing islands of monotonous small, round to oval cells with hyperchromatic nuclei. **B.** Higher magnification of the same tumor showing small round to oval nuclei with dense chromatin pattern simulating those of small cell neuroendocrine carcinoma. The tumor cells were strongly positive for chromogranin and synaptophysin.

C
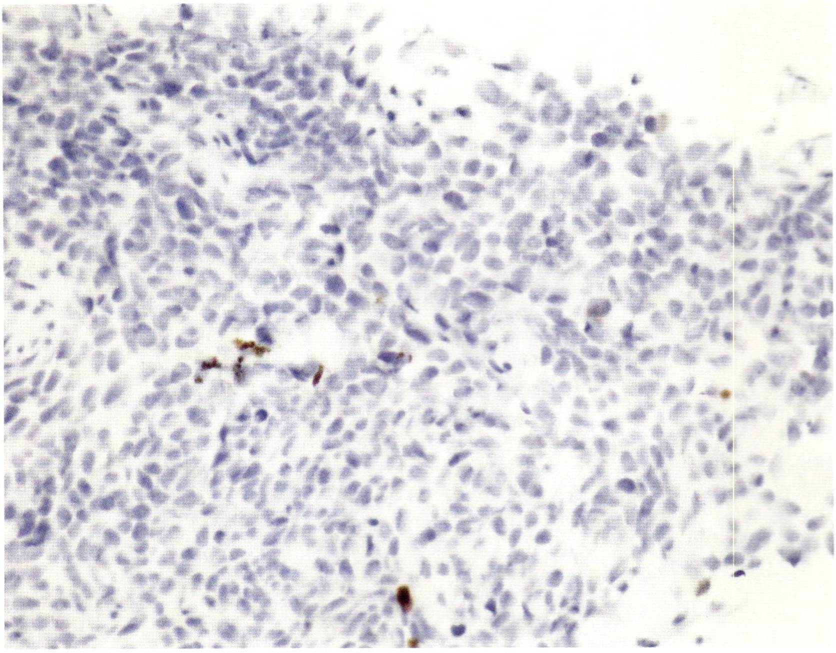

FIGURE 13.10 (*continued*) **C.** Almost complete absence of nuclear staining for Ki-67 proliferation marker in the same case, essentially eliminating a diagnosis of high-grade neuroendocrine carcinoma, small cell type.

INTERMEDIATE-GRADE NEUROENDOCRINE CARCINOMA (ATYPICAL CARCINOID, GRADE 2, AND/OR GRADE 3 NEUROENDOCRINE TUMOR)

The first recognition of this intermediate category of tumors was in a study by Arrigoni et al[41] who introduced the term "atypical carcinoid" for tumors that closely resembled histologically carcinoid tumors but showed increased nuclear pleomorphism and cytologic atypia, with increased mitotic activity and foci of necrosis. Unlike conventional "carcinoid" tumors, intermediate-grade neuroendocrine carcinomas are associated with cigarette smoking and are more often peripheral in location. They are usually unassociated with a bronchus and present as a well-circumscribed intraparenchymal lung mass. Because these tumors occupy a middle position in the spectrum of neuroendocrine lung neoplasms, their biologic behavior may vary depending on whether they are closer in the spectrum to low-grade or to high-grade lesions. In general, the majority of published studies have demonstrated that intermediate-grade neuroendocrine carcinomas follow a more aggressive behavior with a higher incidence of distant metastases and tumor-associated deaths in up to 50% of patients.[5] As compared to low-grade neuroendocrine carcinomas, they have a lower overall 5-year survival (~60%).[5,42] As with most other forms of lung cancer, clinical stage will also play a significant role in the outcome of these patients. Genetically, intermediate-grade neuroendocrine carcinomas appear to share many of the somatic mutational profile described for the low-grade lesions; however, additional aberrations in DNA repair genes including *E2F1*, *p14ARF*, and *cyclin E* have been reported to occur at a higher rate.[43-45] Copy number alterations of *RB1* have been reported to be between 10% and 20% in intermediate-grade neuroendocrine tumors. Rates of *TP53* alterations are low as compared to high-grade neuroendocrine carcinomas.[5,32]

The criteria for the histologic diagnosis of "atypical carcinoid" remain controversial and have varied widely depending on the investigator.[14,46] In general terms, we reserve the designation of intermediate-grade neuroendocrine carcinoma for tumors that still retain a recognizable neuroendocrine architectural growth pattern (ie, show evidence of organoid architectural differentiation), but in which the tumor cells show increased cytologic atypia, including enlargement of nuclei and hyperchromasia, prominent nucleoli, decreased nuclear to cytoplasmic ratio, and increased mitotic activity (Fig. 13.11A and B; eFigs. 13.4-13.6).[3] A stippled chromatin pattern can be retained by these tumors, similar to that seen in low-grade neuroendocrine carcinomas. Another important discriminating feature for these tumors is the presence of tumor cell necrosis. This is characteristically seen as pinpoint or central, comedolike areas of necrosis within large islands of tumor cells (Fig. 13.12A and B). The cells in intermediate-grade neuroendocrine carcinomas can be round or polygonal, but they also often adopt an oval or spindle configuration. Peripheral palisading of tumor cells within large tumor cell islands is also seen in many cases. The main criterion adopted by the WHO for the definition of atypical carcinoid is mitotic activity; tumors containing from 2 to 10 mitoses per 2 mm^2 are considered to fall within this category. In practice, this criterion may be very difficult to apply, as mitotic activity in these tumors can vary widely, and some tumors may have low mitotic activity in the presence of necrosis and nuclear atypia, whereas others may have high mitotic counts (>10 per 2 mm^2) despite being well circumscribed and displaying a perfectly well-developed organoid architecture. Review of the literature reveals that mitotic activity in "atypical carcinoid" has ranged from 2 to 80 per 10 high power field (HPF) (many of these studies were performed before the introduction of mm^2 nomenclature), depending on the study quoted.[41,47-50] The current WHO classifies these tumors as "atypical carcinoid tumors with elevated mitotic activity."[5] Mitotic counts can thus be a poor discriminating factor for making this diagnosis. This is particularly true in small endoscopic biopsies where an adequate mitotic count may not be possible owing to the limited amount of tissue present in the specimen. In our opinion, architectural features and growth pattern play a more important role in the diagnosis of these tumors than mitotic counts as they constitute the most important parameter for assessing the degree of differentiation of the tumor. High-grade neuroendocrine carcinoma, small cell type seldom displays a well-developed "organoid"

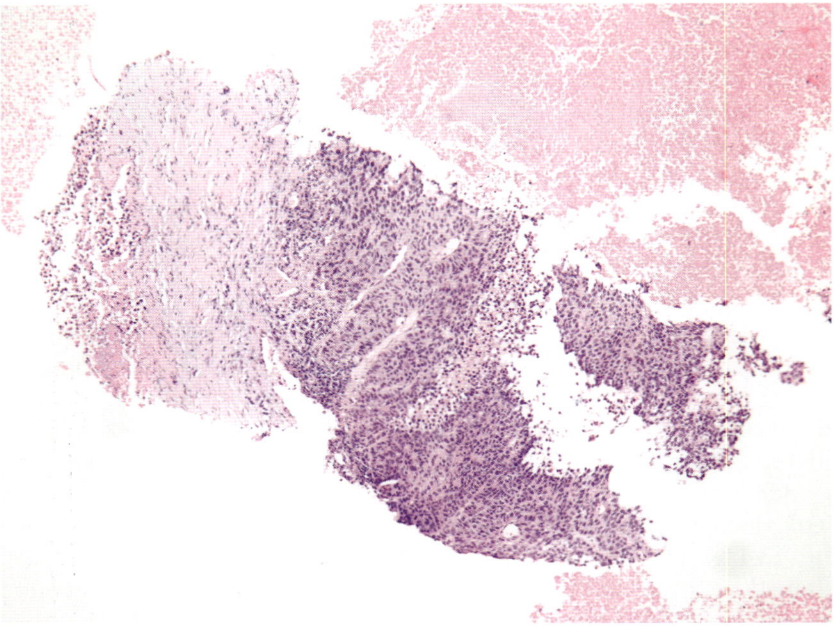

A

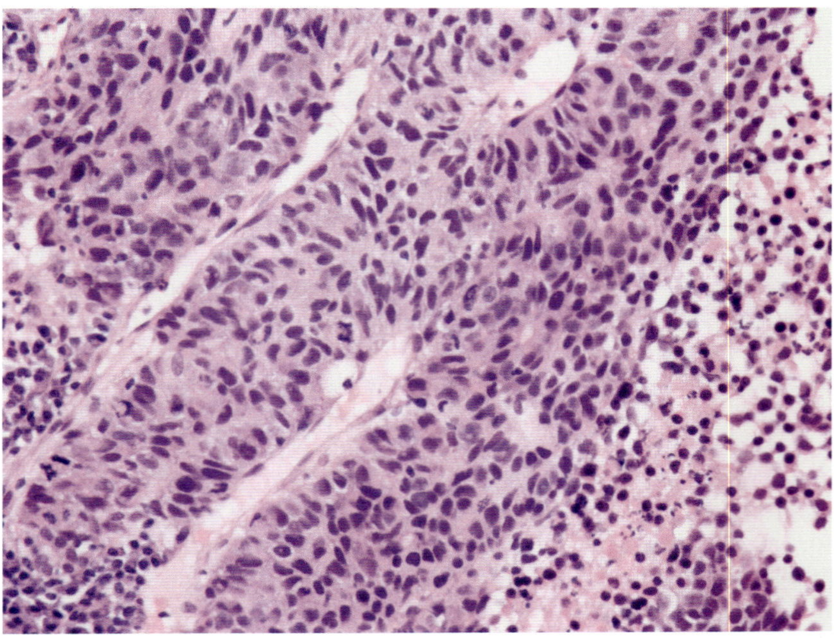

B

FIGURE 13.11 **A.** Core biopsy of intermediate-grade neuroendocrine carcinoma of the lung (atypical carcinoid) shows cords of large tumor cells with focal pinpoint areas of necrosis within the tumor and adjacent necrotic debris. **B.** Higher magnification shows a population of atypical cells with increased nuclear pleomorphism and frequent mitoses.

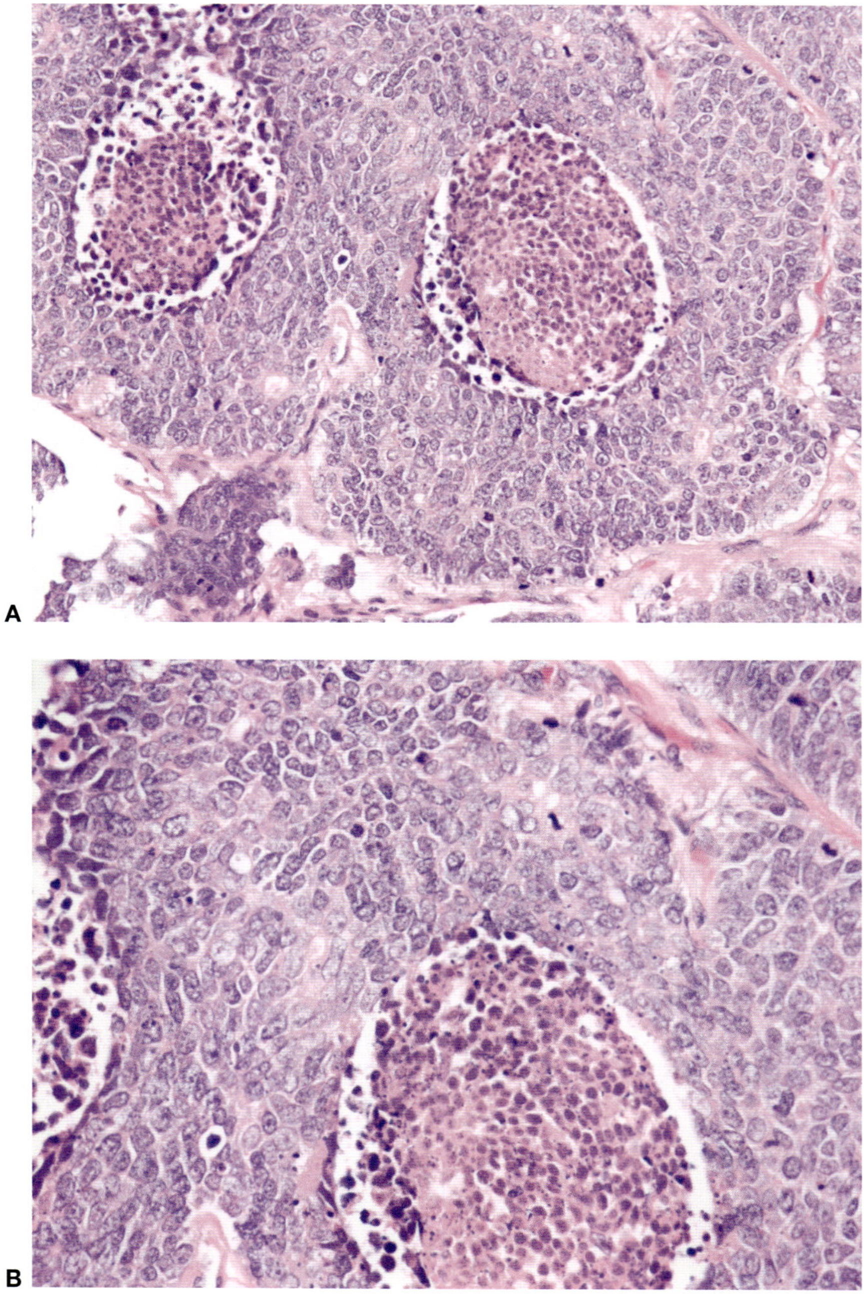

FIGURE 13.12 **A.** Intermediate-grade neuroendocrine carcinoma shows areas with central comedolike foci of necrosis surrounded by an atypical population of cells with large nuclei, visible nucleoli, and ample rim of cytoplasm. **B.** Higher magnification showing cytologic atypia of the tumor cells and abundant mitoses.

growth pattern, although it may be focally present in some cases, usually at the periphery of the tumor. The identification of a recognizable endocrine pattern of growth in a tumor with cytologic atypia and positive neuroendocrine markers should prompt consideration of a diagnosis of intermediate-grade neuroendocrine carcinoma ("atypical carcinoid"); if mitotic activity is highly elevated consideration should be given to a high-grade neuroendocrine carcinoma, large cell type, as these tumors can often demonstrate well-differentiated organoid morphology.

The lack of clearly defined criteria for diagnosis in this group of tumors has also led to considerable confusion and overlap with the group of tumors known as high-grade neuroendocrine carcinoma, large cell type. Making this distinction on endoscopic biopsies can, thus, be highly problematic. A diagnosis of intermediate-grade neuroendocrine carcinoma in small biopsy samples should be considered when the cytologic features of the tumor display marked atypia, with prominent nucleoli, tumor cell necrosis, and more than two mitoses in a tumor that is still showing a well-preserved neuroendocrine architectural growth pattern, features which unfortunately overlap in many cases with high-grade neuroendocrine carcinoma, large cell type. In many instances, it may not be possible to distinguish these two entities on biopsy material. This situation must be acknowledged in the report, and a generic diagnosis of neuroendocrine neoplasm can be rendered with a note indicating the diagnostic possibilities and recommending complete excision and further sampling for a more definitive diagnosis (Fig. 13.13A and B).

The immunohistochemical features of intermediate-grade neuroendocrine carcinomas are similar to those of low-grade neuroendocrine carcinomas, except that the extent of immunoreactivity for neuroendocrine markers may be somewhat diminished and not as intense.[51] TTF-1 will often be positive in these tumors, although the extent and intensity of staining is not as strong as that of high-grade tumors. Proliferation markers will show increased proliferative activity compared with low-grade neuroendocrine carcinoma, but it will also not be as high in high-grade tumors. A general guideline proposed by the WHO and adopted by most pulmonary experts is that a Ki-67 proliferation index in the neighborhood of 6% to 30% is consistent with an intermediate-grade neuroendocrine carcinoma ("atypical carcinoid").[5]

HIGH-GRADE NEUROENDOCRINE CARCINOMA (SMALL CELL AND LARGE CELL TYPE)

This designation refers to primary lung neoplasms located at the more aggressive end of the spectrum of neuroendocrine tumors. These tumors comprise approximately 95% of all lung neuroendocrine neoplasms.[52] The prototype of high-grade neuroendocrine carcinoma over the years has been the small cell type of lung carcinoma, colloquially referred to as "small cell carcinoma." More recently, an additional category of tumor

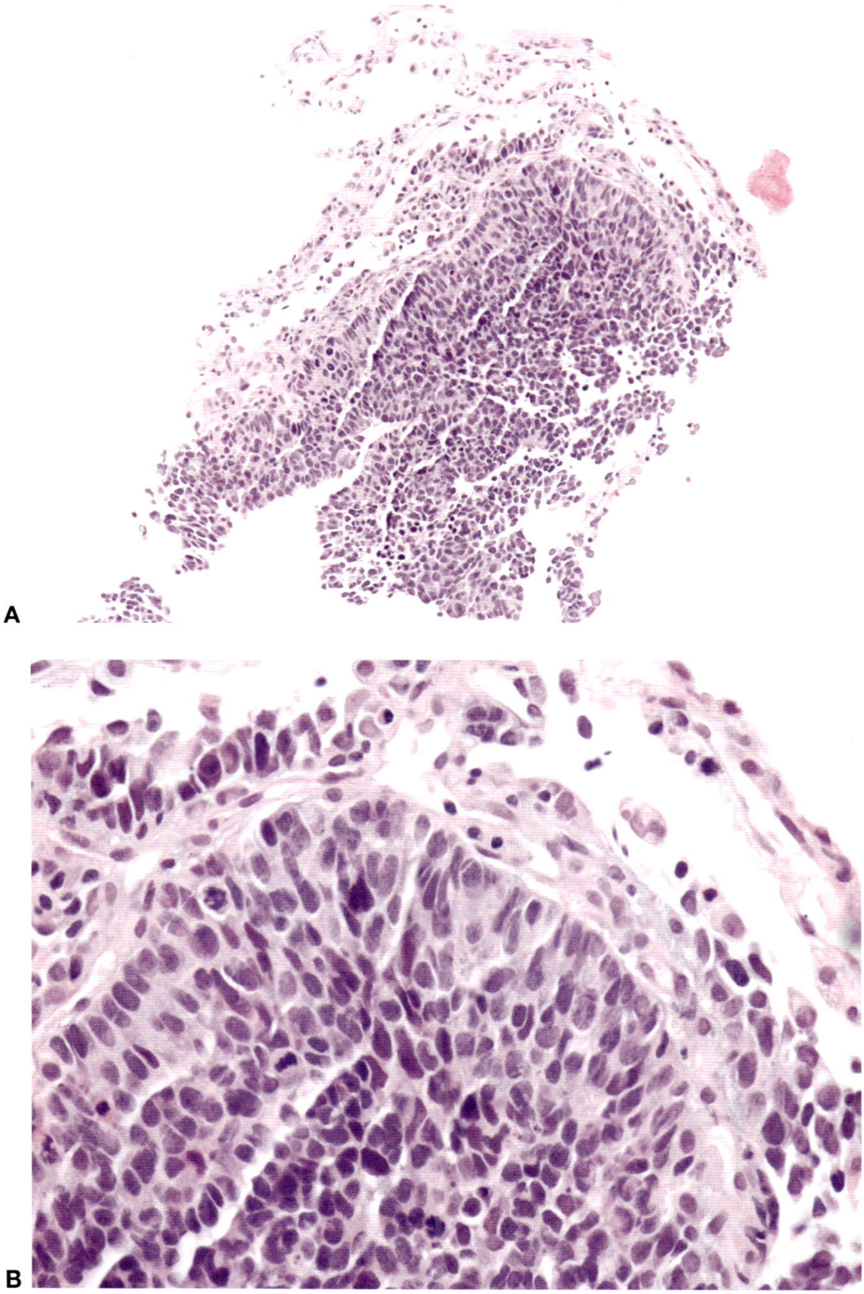

FIGURE 13.13 **A.** Endoscopic biopsy of neuroendocrine carcinoma with borderline features between atypical carcinoid and high-grade neuroendocrine carcinoma, large cell type. The tumor shows sheets of large tumor cells with abundant cytoplasm displaying a vague organoid pattern. **B.** Higher magnification shows large cells with speckled chromatin pattern, a hint of peripheral palisading of nuclei, and frequent mitotic figures. The tumor cells showed positivity for neuroendocrine markers. Tumors like this may be best categorized as "intermediate- to high-grade neuroendocrine carcinoma, not otherwise specified."

termed "large cell neuroendocrine carcinoma" has been added to this group. Some debate remains as to whether tumors showing the features of "atypical carcinoid" but with marked nuclear pleomorphism or high mitotic counts can also be regarded as belonging in the high-grade category owing to their more aggressive biologic behavior. These tumors are currently classified by the WHO as "atypical carcinoids with elevated mitotic activity" and from a conceptual standpoint would likely be classified under "grade 3 neuroendocrine tumors" in the classification systems of neuroendocrine tumors in other organs.[5]

High-grade neuroendocrine carcinomas of the lung (small cell and large cell types) share some similar genetics. The primary genetic alterations driving these tumors are loss-of-function mutations within the *RB1* and *TP53* genes (with loss of function of *RB1* being the defining molecular change in small cell carcinomas).[53] Small cell type carcinomas in addition show a complex genomic signature, with many smoking-related changes as well as a plethora of additional driver mutations including mutations in *CREBBP*, *EP300*, *MLL*, *PTEN*, *SLIT2*, *MYCL*, *E2F2*, and *FGFR1*.[54,55] Numerous other abnormalities have been described including aberrations in numerous cell cycle regulators, chromosomal abnormalities affecting tumor suppressor genes other than *RB1* and *TP53*, and *MYC* gene amplification among others.[43-45,56-58] Recent transcriptomic and immunohistochemical analysis of these tumors has shown four distinct subtypes based on expression levels of ASCL1, NEUROD1, POU2F3, and YAP1 with associated prognostic implications and possible future therapeutic implications.[59-61] The POU2F3 variant is of particular interest since it has been noted that these tumors are a challenging diagnosis due to low or completely absent expression of standard neuroendocrine markers.[62] Molecular analysis of large cell type neuroendocrine carcinomas have demonstrated variable subclasses, though many cases are also characterized by *RB1* and *TP53* mutations similar to the small cell subtype[63-65]; however, additional studies are needed to confirm those findings as many of the tumors examined in these studies have shown genetic alterations commonly found in non–small cell lung carcinoma (NSCLC), raising the possibility that many of these tumors are simply poorly differentiated NSCLC with aberrant neuroendocrine differentiation.

High-grade neuroendocrine carcinoma, small cell type ("small cell carcinoma" or "small cell lung carcinoma") is characterized by a close association with cigarette smoking and highly aggressive behavior; it accounts for approximately 15% to 25% of all lung carcinomas.[66,67] The tumors can be associated with paraneoplastic syndromes, including hypercalcemia, hyponatremia, or Cushing syndrome owing to ectopic production of peptide hormones. Symptoms include cough, hemoptysis, weight loss, hypertrophic osteoarthropathy, and fatigue.[5] The commonest location is central in association with a proximal bronchus, although they can originate in peripheral locations in rare instances, sometimes in association with interstitial lung disease.[68] Peribronchial or mediastinal adenopathy is a prominent finding and can be massive. The lesions can sometimes be cystic. Pleural involvement with pleural effusion is a common complication. Small cell carcinoma is characterized clinically by early dissemination. Chemotherapy combined with immunotherapy (primarily anti-PD1 or anti-PDL1 therapies) is now the mainstay of treatment for advanced disease.[69-72] PD-L1 immunohistochemistry may be requested by treating oncologists on these tumors and may be incorporated into the standard workup of these cases. Additional biomarkers such as DLL3, an inhibitory NOTCH ligand, have also shown some promise and may see an increased role in the management of this disease in the future, though this marker is not yet widely available in most histology laboratories.[73,74]

These tumors are not generally regarded as candidates for surgical excision (with the exception of early, limited disease in peripheral locations).[75] The endoscopic biopsy is therefore the only tissue that will be available for final diagnosis in the majority of patients. A diagnosis of high-grade neuroendocrine carcinoma, small cell type rendered on an endoscopic biopsy usually precludes surgery as a therapeutic option. Unfortunately, the limited size of the sample and frequent artifactual distortion caused by the forceps can sometimes make the diagnosis quite difficult. In general, most authors are in agreement that the diagnosis of high-grade neuroendocrine carcinoma, small cell type is a straightforward morphologic diagnosis, largely based on the histologic features as observed by the examination of hematoxylin and eosin–stained sections. Immunohistochemical stains, however, can be of help in problematic or equivocal cases.

High-grade neuroendocrine carcinoma, small cell type can exhibit a spectrum of microscopic features (eFigs. 13.7-13.10). The most common form is characterized by cells that are two to three times the size of a small lymphocyte. The cell nuclei are large, hyperchromatic, with densely scattered or smudged chromatin and absent or inconspicuous nucleoli imparting the cells with a “primitive” or undifferentiated appearance. The latter feature, that is, absent or inconspicuous nucleoli, is a particularly important feature to remember in the evaluation of small endoscopic biopsies to avoid making a mistaken diagnosis of high-grade neuroendocrine carcinoma of small cell type in tumors comprising sheets of “small” cells that exhibit prominent or easily discernible nucleoli. This feature is of particular importance for the distinction between the small cell or “basaloid” variant of squamous cell carcinoma. In well-preserved samples, the cells of high-grade neuroendocrine carcinoma, small cell type often show a tendency for molding. The nuclei are surrounded by an indistinct and very scant rim of cytoplasm (Fig. 13.14A and B). Ample cytoplasm essentially disqualifies a tumor from this diagnosis. The tumors often contain numerous apoptotic bodies and are characterized by high mitotic activity (>10 mitoses per 2 mm^2). Tumor cell necrosis is a frequent finding, and the necrosis is irregular and “geographic” (with jagged, irregular borders, as opposed to the comedolike areas seen in intermediate-grade neuroendocrine tumors). A well-developed neuroendocrine growth pattern is usually not observed in

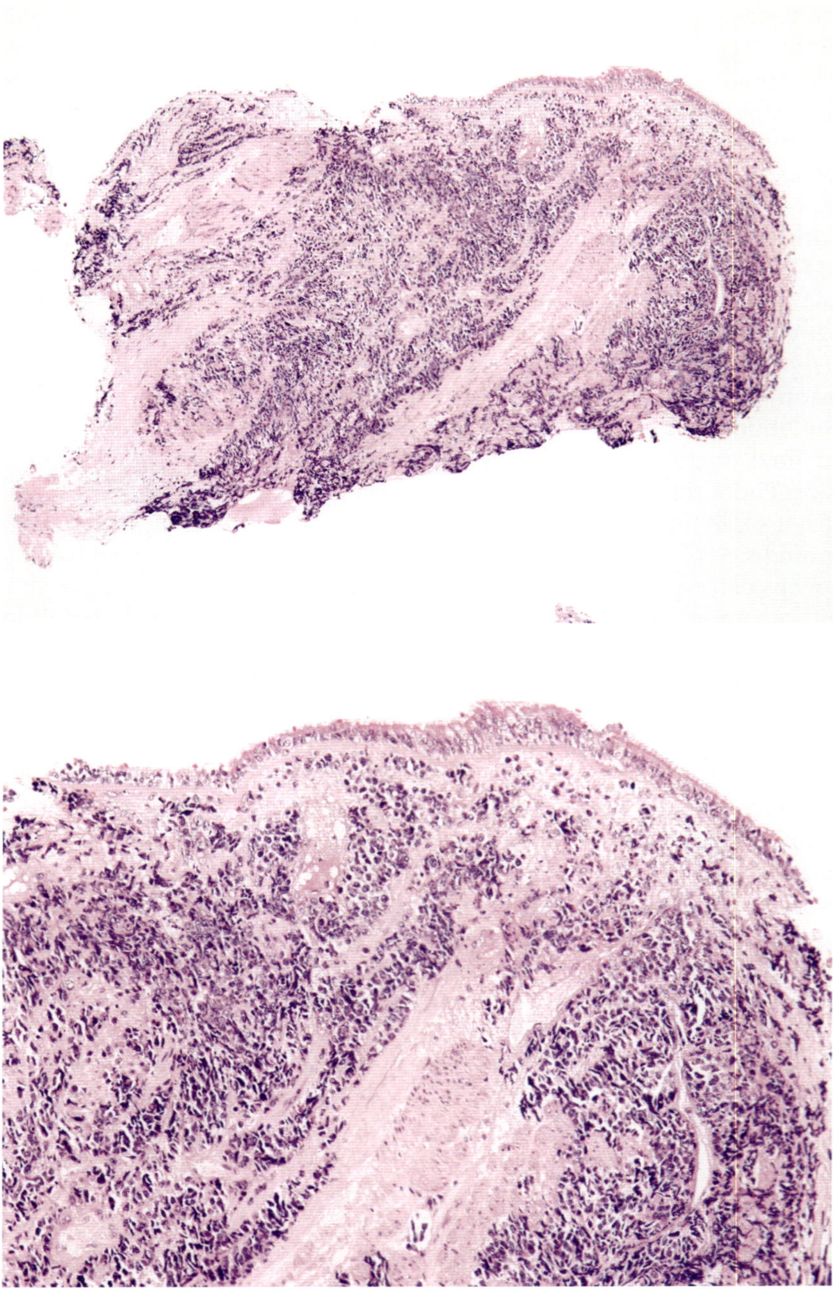

A

B

FIGURE 13.14 **A.** Endoscopic biopsy of small cell lung cancer showing an overlying intact respiratory mucosa with a population of tumor cells infiltrating the connective tissue in the submucosa. **B.** Higher magnification shows preserved small islands and clusters of primitive small tumor cells typical of small cell carcinoma.

small cell lung cancer, although resected specimens can sometimes demonstrate a vague organoid growth pattern focally. Identification of a neuroendocrine growth pattern is even harder in small endoscopic biopsies and is rarely seen under such circumstances. Incrustation of basophilic nucleic acid material around vessel walls (Azzopardi phenomenon) is another frequent occurrence. Crush artifact, with distortion of the nuclei, is a common event that is frequently encountered in small endoscopic biopsies owing to the scant connective tissue stroma of these tumors. The distortion of the tumor cells may be massive and affect virtually the entire sample, making definitive interpretation difficult (Fig. 13.15A and B). Close correlation with the clinical history and radiographic findings is important in such instances before making a final diagnosis.

Endoscopic biopsies can often present challenges for diagnosis not only on account of the extensive crush artifact but also owing to the paucity of well-preserved tumor cells, making reliable interpretation of nuclear features difficult. The cells in high-grade neuroendocrine carcinoma, small cell type can sometimes be very small and round and closely resemble lymphocytes, thus simulating a lymphoma (Fig. 13.16A-D). Attention to the nuclear detail will be of importance for correct diagnosis between the two; immunohistochemical stains can also be of help in separating the two conditions. Another morphologic variant of high-grade neuroendocrine carcinoma, small cell type is one characterized by prominent spindling of the tumor cells. Such cases can be confused for a sarcomatous lesion in small biopsy samples; immunohistochemical stains may also be of help in separating them from its mimics (Fig. 13.17A-C). Another unusual morphologic variant is tumors with mixed small cell and large cell cytology. In previous classification schemes, a *polygonal cell type* or *intermediate cell type* of high-grade neuroendocrine carcinoma, small cell type was also recognized. These categories have been merged in the current WHO schema with the conventional small cell type and are no longer regarded as clinically significant histologic variants of these tumors. The cells in the latter type were described as being larger, oval to polygonal in shape, with sharp cell membranes, prominent nucleoli, and abundant rim of cytoplasm. The description of this cell type thus significantly overlaps with that of intermediate neuroendocrine tumors ("atypical carcinoid") and high-grade neuroendocrine carcinoma, large cell type. Many of the cases diagnosed as polygonal or intermediate cell type in the past, thus, most likely, corresponded to intermediate grade neuroendocrine tumors or high-grade neuroendocrine carcinoma, large cell type.[12] It follows that distinction of these three types of tumors can be a veritable challenge in small endoscopic biopsies.

The role of ancillary techniques in the diagnosis of high-grade neuroendocrine carcinomas varies depending on the specific type of tumor examined. The small cell type consistently labels with keratin antibodies but may show variable and inconsistent expression of neuroendocrine markers. An immunohistochemical study of these tumors showed reactivity for chromogranin in transbronchial biopsy specimens in only 47% of

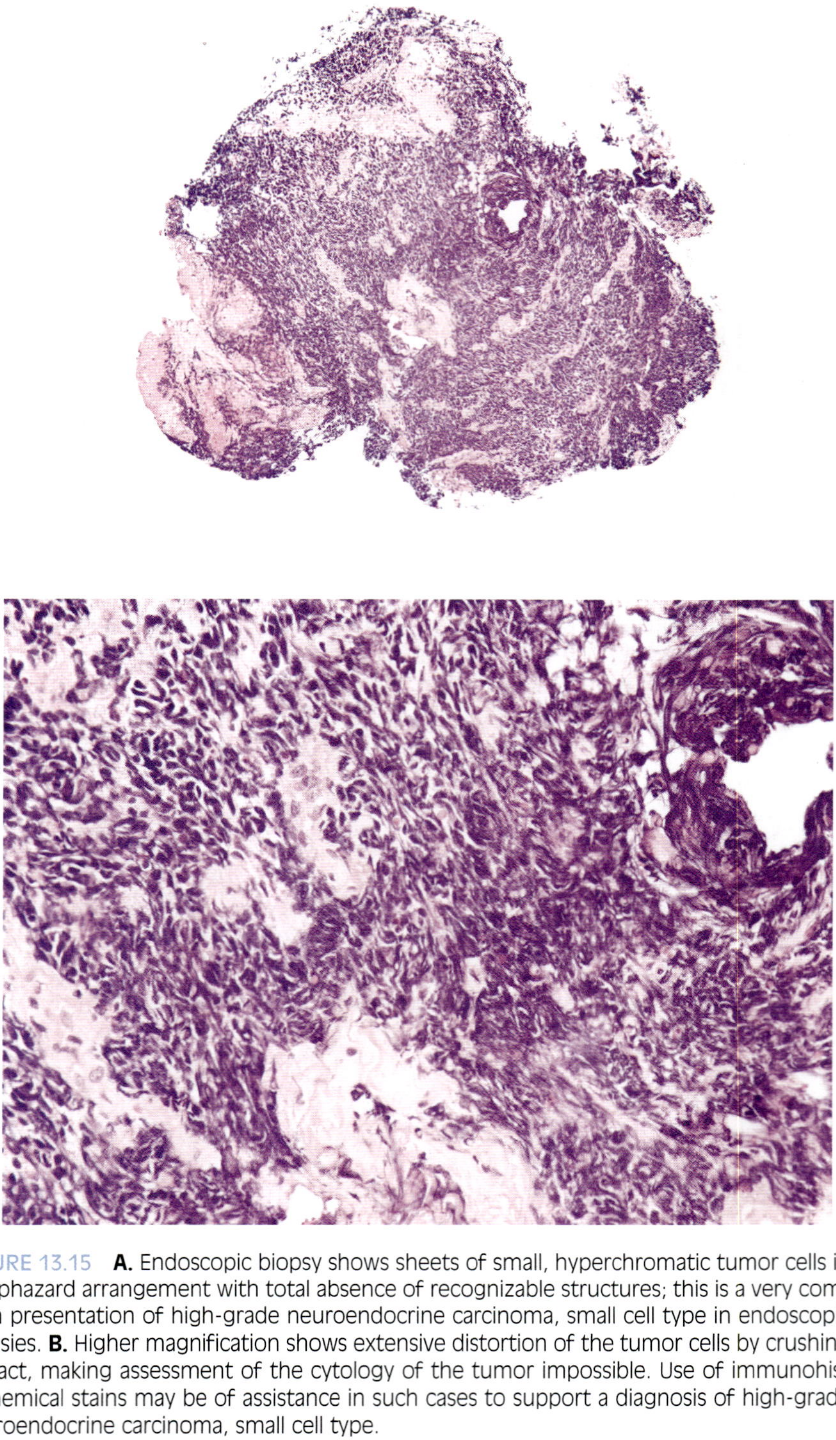

A

B

FIGURE 13.15 **A.** Endoscopic biopsy shows sheets of small, hyperchromatic tumor cells in a haphazard arrangement with total absence of recognizable structures; this is a very common presentation of high-grade neuroendocrine carcinoma, small cell type in endoscopic biopsies. **B.** Higher magnification shows extensive distortion of the tumor cells by crushing artifact, making assessment of the cytology of the tumor impossible. Use of immunohistochemical stains may be of assistance in such cases to support a diagnosis of high-grade neuroendocrine carcinoma, small cell type.

A

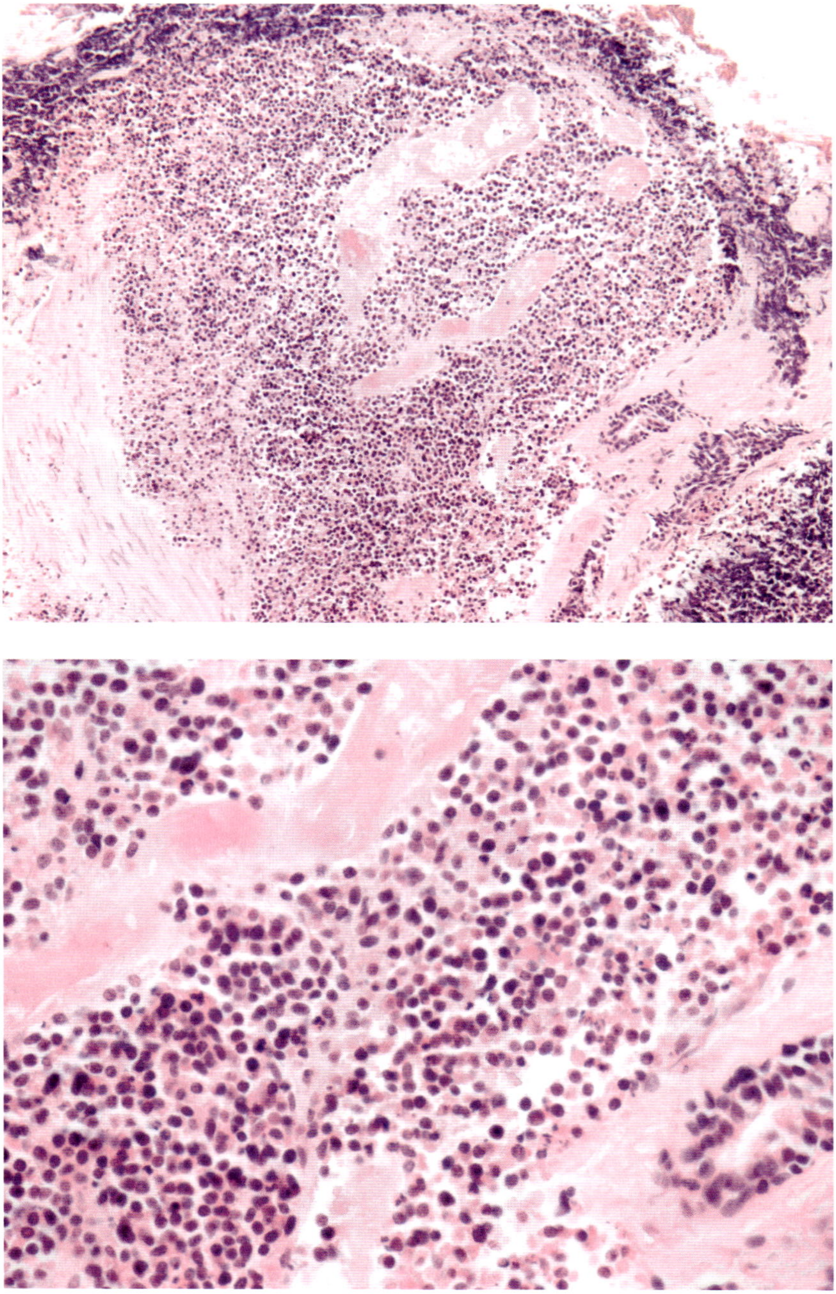

B

FIGURE 13.16 **A.** Bronchial biopsy of high-grade neuroendocrine carcinoma, small cell type ("small cell carcinoma") with lymphocytelike features shows a monotonous population of small round cells with peripheral areas of necrosis; tumors like this may be mistaken for lymphomas. **B.** Higher magnification shows a monotonous round blue cell population with no nuclear detail and scant mitotic activity.

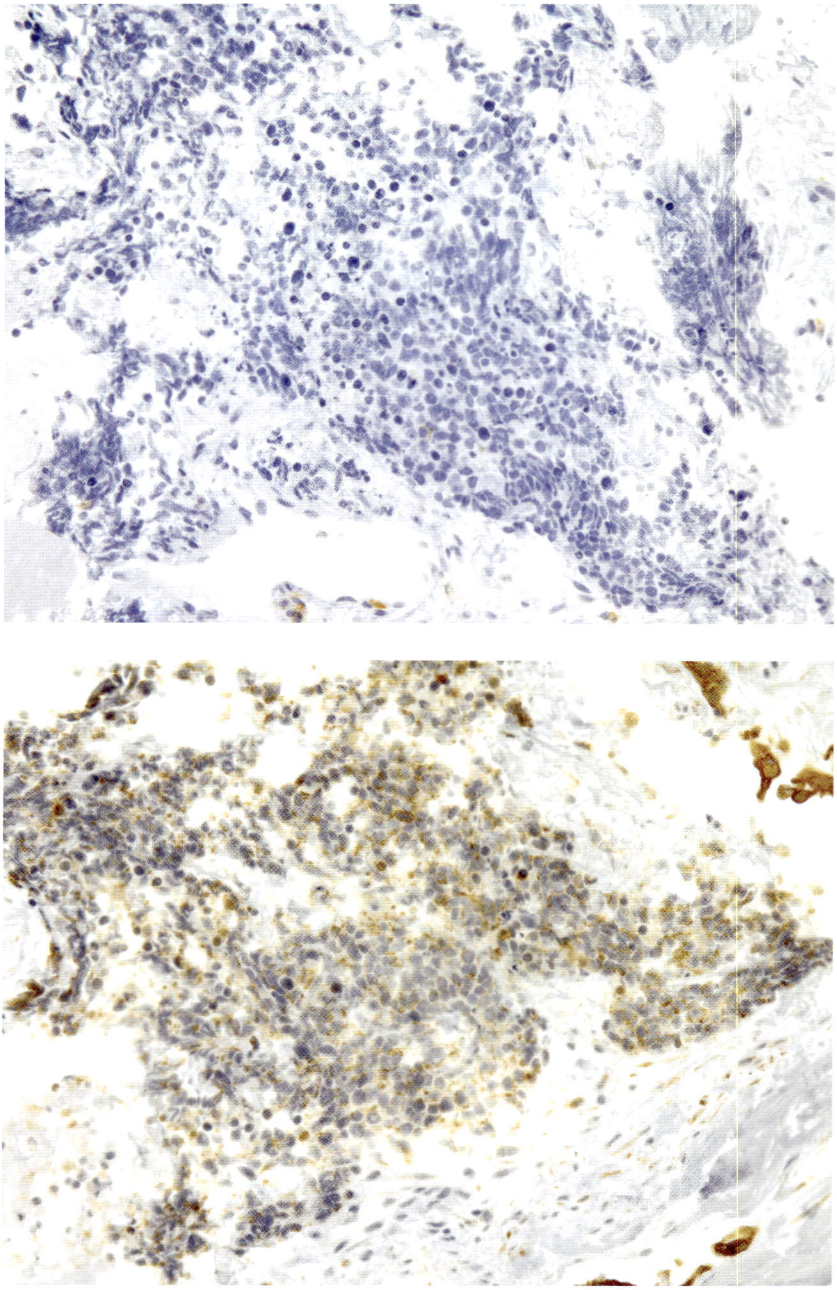

C

D

FIGURE 13.16 (*continued*) **C.** Immunohistochemical stain for leukocyte common antigen (ie, CD45) shows negative reaction in the tumor cells. **D.** Immunohistochemical stain for CK7 shows dotlike, paranuclear positivity in the tumor cells supporting the diagnosis of high-grade neuroendocrine carcinoma (small cell lung cancer).

A

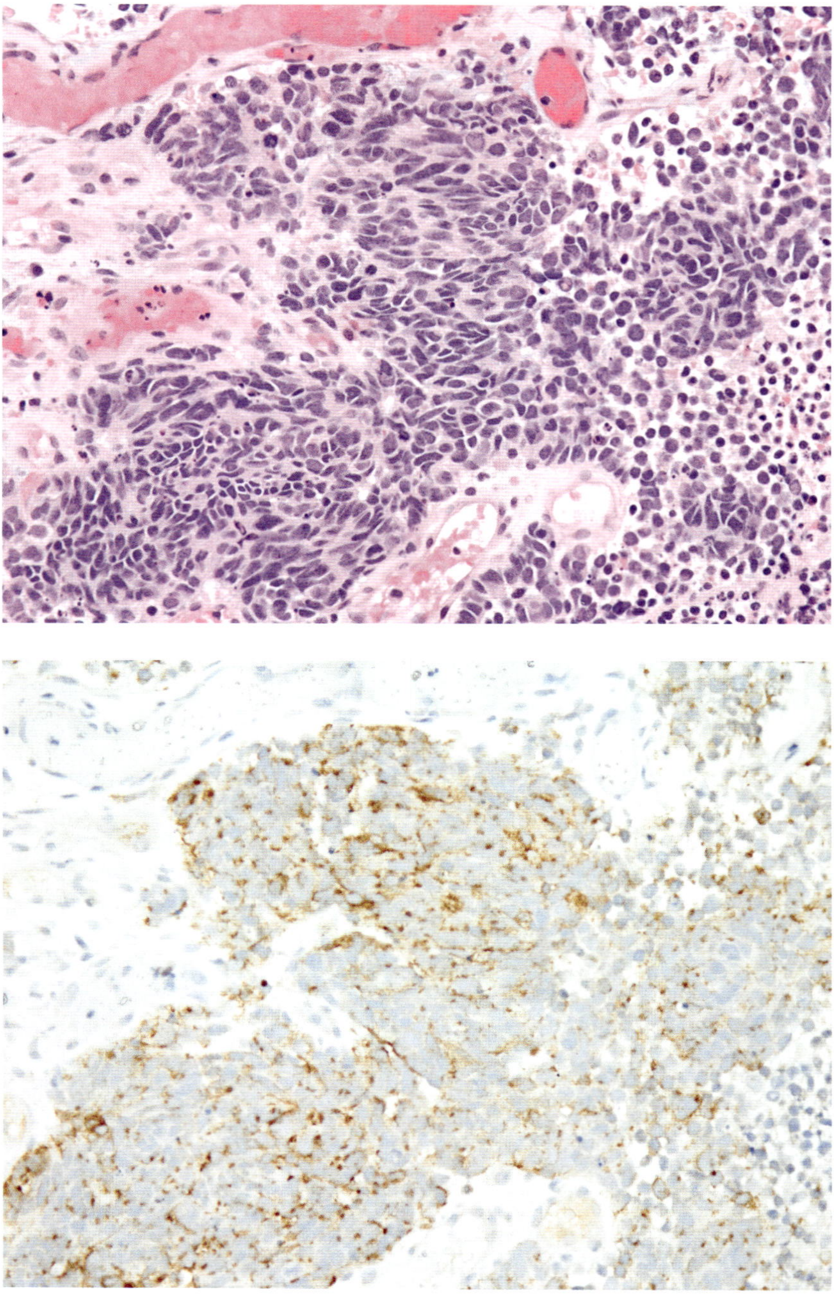

B

FIGURE 13.17 **A.** High-grade neuroendocrine carcinoma, small cell type showing admixture of small round cells with a prominent spindle cell component containing elongated nuclei with scant cytoplasm and distinct molding. **B.** Immunohistochemical stain for chromogranin shows cytoplasmic staining in many of the tumor cells.

C 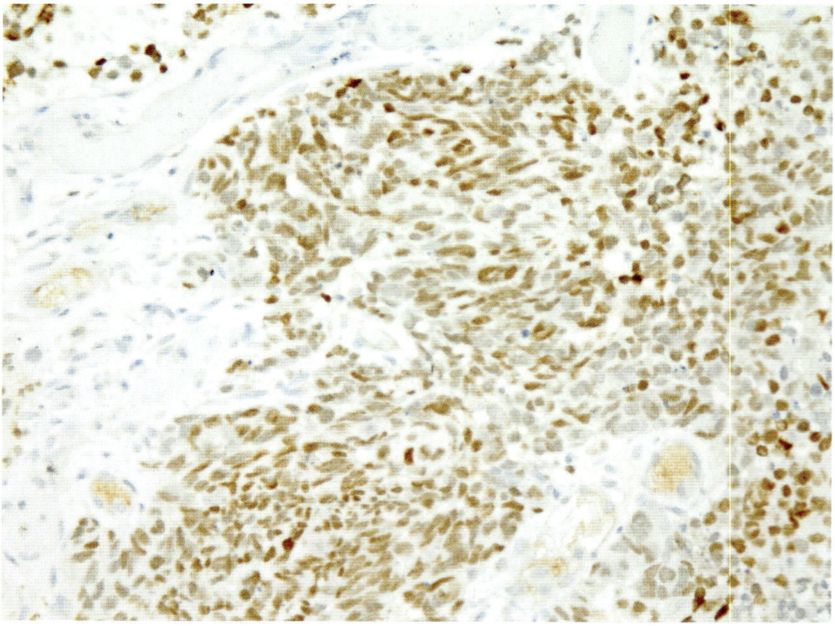

FIGURE 13.17 (*continued*) **C.** Immunohistochemical stain for thyroid transcription factor-1 shows strong nuclear positivity of the tumor cells.

cases and for synaptophysin in only 19%.[76] Pan-cytokeratin antibodies and low molecular weight cytokeratins are particularly useful for the diagnosis, and in many instances, when the cells are well preserved, they will show a characteristic dotlike paranuclear staining pattern. Another marker that has been found to be of utility, particularly for the evaluation of metastases to the skin, is CK7 (Fig. 13.18A), which is strongly expressed in lung tumors as opposed to primary small cell carcinoma of the skin (Merkel cell carcinoma), which preferentially expresses CK20 and is usually negative for CK7. Neuroendocrine markers may show variable degrees of positivity and can be a source of confusion in small biopsy samples when they are negative. Stains such as chromogranin A, synaptophysin, neuron-specific enolase, and CD56 can all be positive in small cell carcinoma (Fig. 13.18B), but in tumors with extensive crush artifact or poorly preserved samples, the results of these stains may be quite difficult to evaluate. Absence of reactivity for any particular neuroendocrine marker should, therefore, not be regarded as an indication that the tumor is not a high-grade neuroendocrine carcinoma of small cell type; in fact, negative staining for neuroendocrine markers should not be used as a criterion for eliminating this diagnosis. The final interpretation should rely heavily on the hematoxylin and eosin and can be supported by strong cytokeratin positivity. Another marker that is quite helpful for making the diagnosis is TTF-1, a nuclear transcription factor, that is strongly expressed in the majority of high-grade

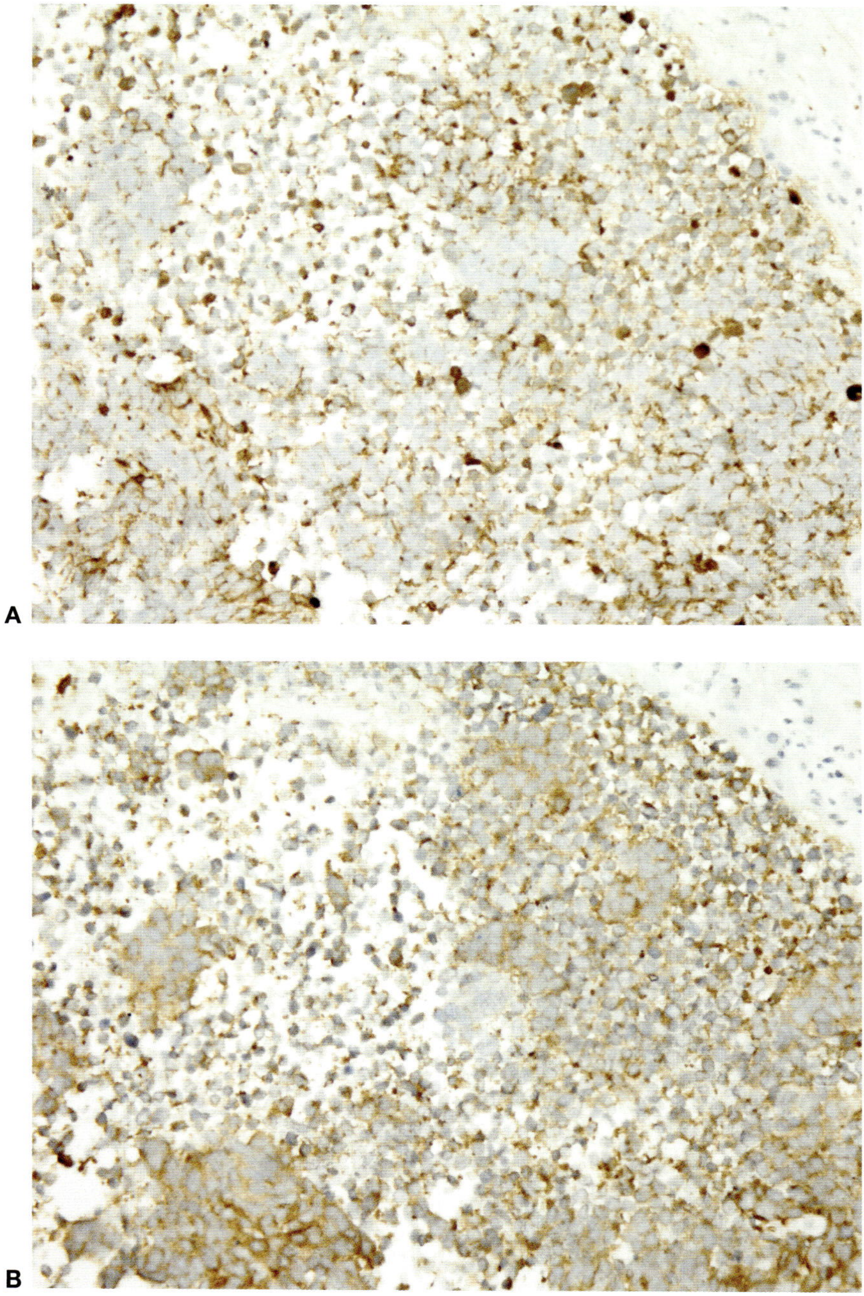

FIGURE 13.18 **Immunohistochemical reactions in small cell lung cancer of the lung. A.** Immunohistochemical stain for CK7 shows faint cytoplasmic positivity in this high-grade neuroendocrine carcinoma, small cell type, with dotlike paranuclear accentuation in many of the cells. **B.** Immunostaining for chromogranin also shows faint cytoplasmic positivity in the tumor cells.

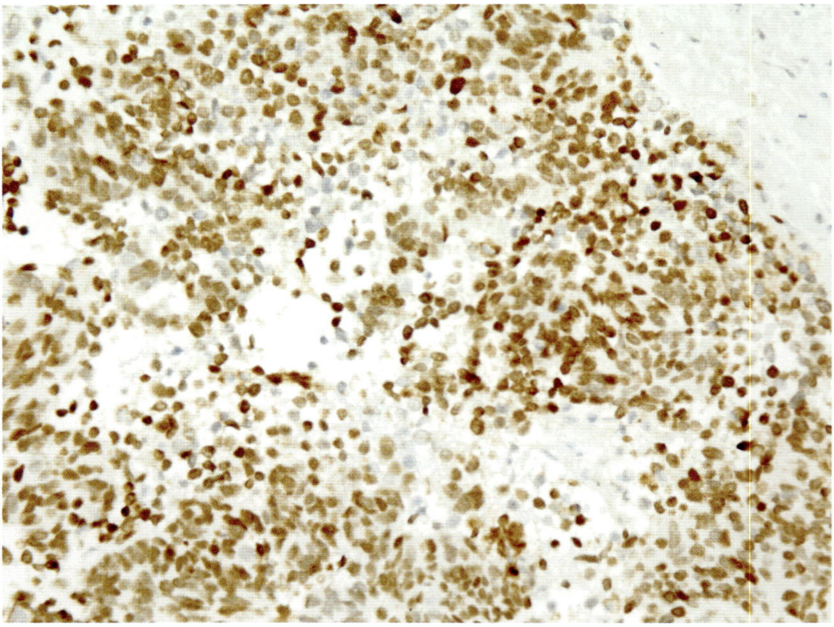

C

FIGURE 13.18 (*continued*) **C.** A thyroid transcription factor-1 stain shows strong nuclear positivity in the majority of the tumor cells.

neuroendocrine carcinomas (Fig. 13.18C). Because TTF-1 is a nuclear protein, it may be very helpful in instances where the biopsy is poorly preserved or shows extensive crush artifact with loss of cytoplasmic contents. INSM1, a recently introduced neuroendocrine marker, may also be of help in these situations as it also shows a nuclear staining pattern and has been shown to be very sensitive and relatively specific for neuroendocrine differentiation in the lung (Figs. 13.19-13.21), although it should be noted that recent literature has identified that this immunostain can demonstrate strong positivity in poorly differentiated squamous cell carcinomas of the thorax (as well as other organs) and thus should not be used in isolation.[77-80] In cases showing a lymphocytelike morphology (comprising small round cells that resemble a lymphoma), addition of a stain for leukocyte common antigen (LCA/CD45) or other lymphoid marker (such as CD3 or CD20) may be of help to separate small cell type tumors from lymphoma or other lymphoid infiltrates. In small biopsies with extensive crush artifact, it is a good practice to add an LCA/CD45 stain to the panel to ensure that the crushed cells are not lymphocytes, which may also be subject to the same type of artifact. Unfortunately, strong extracellular reactivity for either LCA or keratin can be observed in extensively crushed biopsies, so care must be taken when examining these stains. Another useful marker for the diagnosis of small cell type tumors on small biopsy samples in equivocal cases is p16. This marker was shown to display nuclear positivity

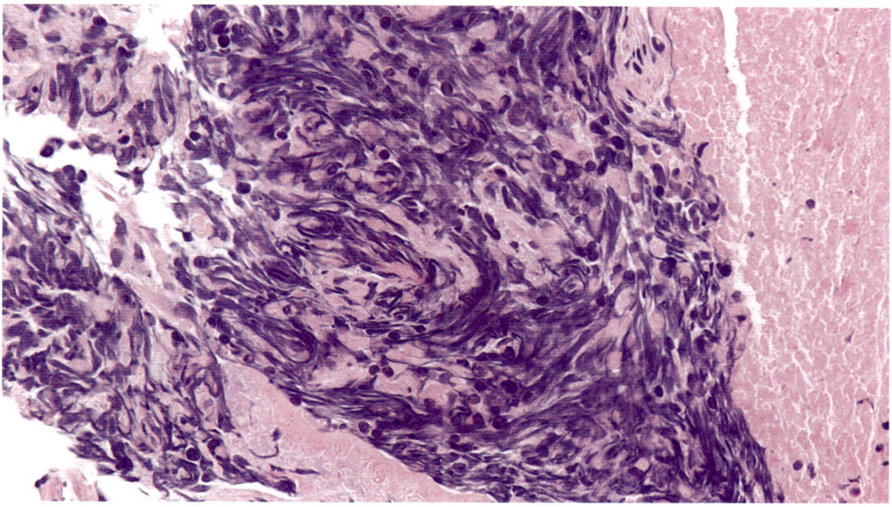

FIGURE 13.19 **Core needle biopsy of a high-grade neuroendocrine carcinoma, small cell type shows extensive crush artifact characteristic of this tumor type.**

in 95/101 cases tested with a diagnostic sensitivity of 94%, particularly when combined with CD56 and synaptophysin.[81] Electron microscopy can also be utilized to demonstrate cytoplasmic membrane–bound dense-core granules; however, this technique has been abandoned in recent years and is often feasible only in resection specimens and will be of very limited utility in endoscopic biopsy samples.

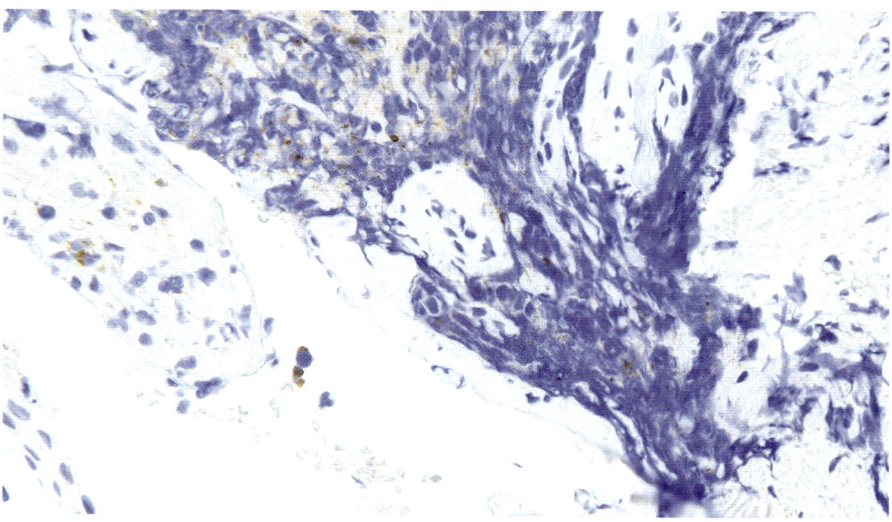

FIGURE 13.20 **Chromogranin immunohistochemistry in the previous tumor shows some very focal cytoplasmic positivity.** The other neuroendocrine markers were negative in this case leading to difficulty with the diagnosis.

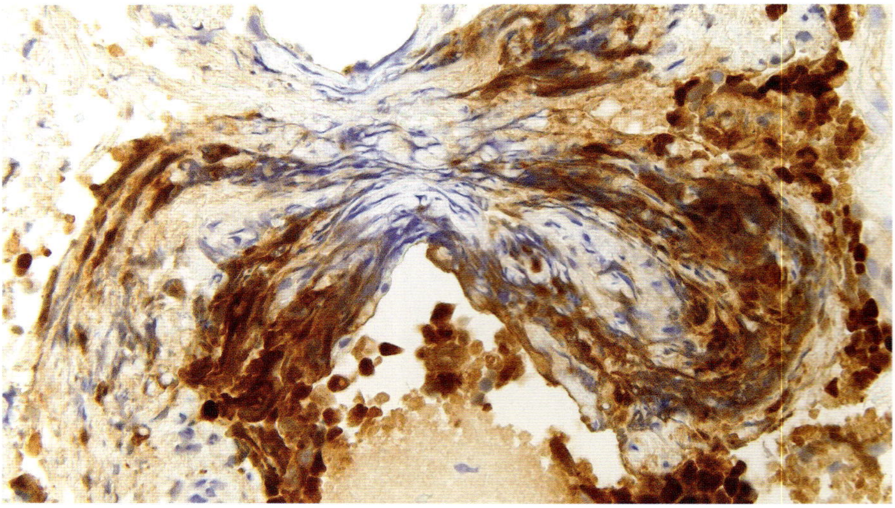

FIGURE 13.21 **INSM1 immunohistochemistry performed on the same biopsy showed relatively strong staining with convincing nuclear positivity even within many of the crushed cells confirming the focal chromogranin positivity.**

High-grade neuroendocrine carcinoma, large cell type (also referred to as "large cell neuroendocrine carcinoma" or "LCNEC") is a subtype of high-grade neuroendocrine carcinoma that has also been the subject of much confusion and debate.[13] It has been noted across most organ systems that aberrant neuroendocrine differentiation is a common occurrence in poorly differentiated neoplasms arising in epithelial organs. The lines that separate large cell carcinoma of the lung with aberrant neuroendocrine differentiation from high-grade neuroendocrine carcinoma, large cell type have not yet been clearly defined. Current recommendations by the International Association for the Study of Lung Cancer/American Thoracic Society/European Respiratory Society classification for small biopsy samples are that tumors showing morphologic features that are consistent with the large cell type of neuroendocrine carcinoma be reported as (1) "nonsmall cell carcinoma with neuroendocrine morphology and positive neuroendocrine markers, possible LCNEC" or (2) "nonsmall cell carcinoma with neuroendocrine morphology and negative neuroendocrine markers, LCNEC suspected," thus betraying a bias to force consideration of this diagnosis in such instances.[82] Unfortunately, the situation is not that simple, and currently, at least three categories of tumors that may share similar features have been recognized: (1) high-grade neuroendocrine carcinoma, large cell type, for tumors characterized by a neuroendocrine histologic growth pattern plus obvious positivity for neuroendocrine markers; (2) large cell carcinoma with neuroendocrine morphology, for tumors characterized by a neuroendocrine histologic growth pattern but without positive neuroendocrine immunohistochemical markers; and (3) large cell carcinoma with neuroendocrine differentiation, which refers to tumors with large cell morphology but without histologic neuroendocrine growth pattern that display positivity for neuroendocrine markers.[33,83-86]

Clinically, high-grade neuroendocrine carcinoma, large cell type presents with similar signs and symptoms as other conventional lung cancers and is closely associated with cigarette smoking.[87-89] The tumors may occur in a central location but are more often located at the periphery or in subpleural portions of the lung. They are therefore more often sampled by core needle biopsy or open lung biopsy than through the endoscope. The biologic behavior of these tumors has varied depending on the study cited, but most studies are in agreement that the tumors behave aggressively.[90] Therapeutic guidelines for these tumors have not been entirely standardized though they are often treated with similar regimens to small cell type neuroendocrine carcinomas.[91-94]

The current definition of high-grade neuroendocrine carcinoma, large cell type is that of a lung neoplasm comprising large, atypical cells (five times larger than a small lymphocyte) displaying a "neuroendocrine" light microscopic growth pattern and demonstrating evidence of neuroendocrine differentiation at the immunohistochemical or ultrastructural level (Fig. 13.22A-C). Per the current WHO definition, tumors should

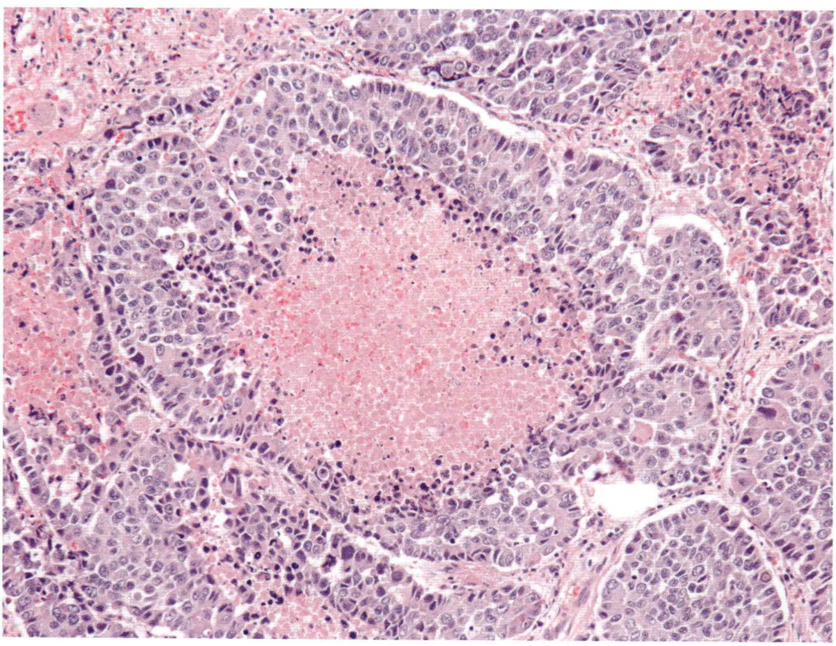

A

FIGURE 13.22 **A.** High-grade neuroendocrine carcinoma, large cell type ("large cell neuroendocrine carcinoma [LCNEC]") of the lung shows islands of large tumor cells with central comedonecrosis and peripheral palisading of nuclei; notice close similarity with intermediate-grade neuroendocrine carcinoma of the lung (atypical carcinoid).

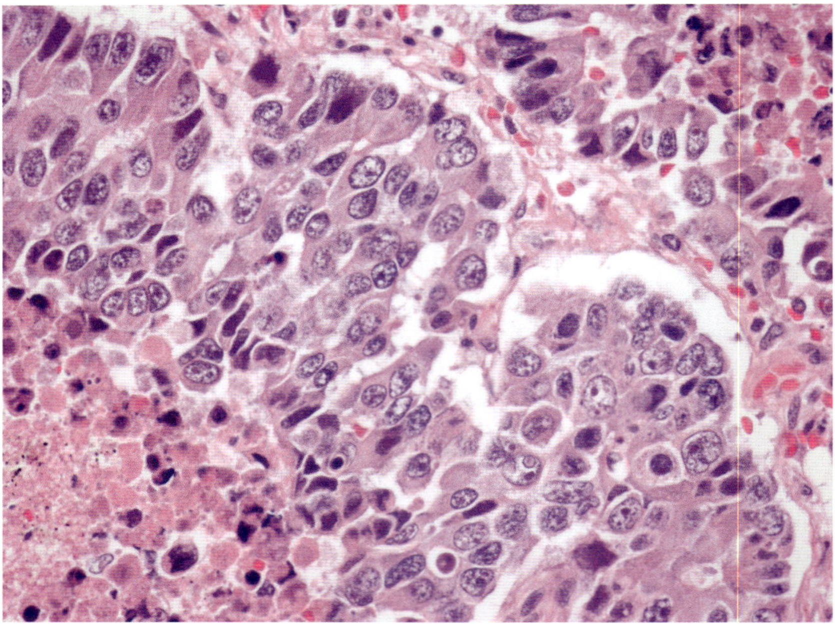

B

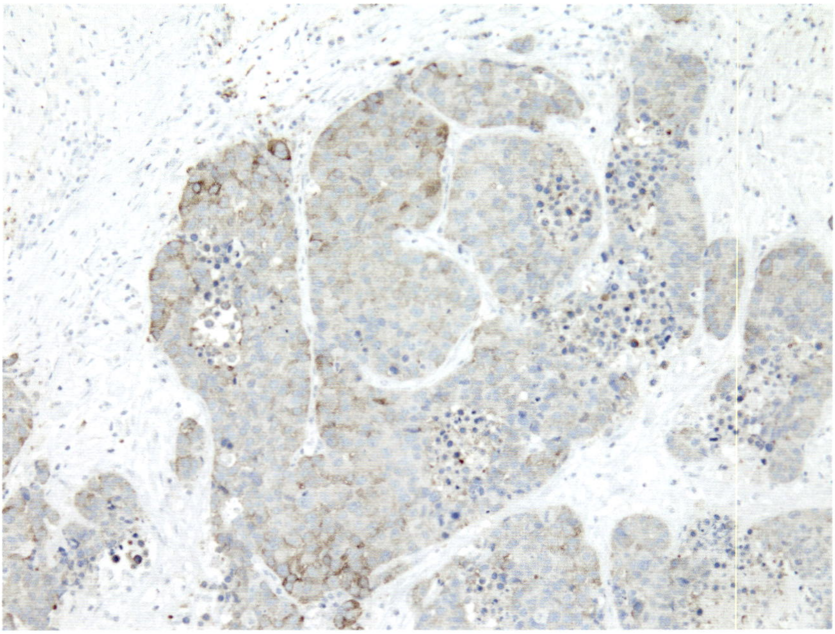

C

FIGURE 13.22 (*continued*) **B.** Higher magnification of high-grade neuroendocrine carcinoma, large cell type shows cells with enlarged nuclei and prominent nucleoli. **C.** Immunohistochemical staining for chromogranin in high-grade neuroendocrine carcinoma, large cell type shows cytoplasmic positivity of the tumor cells. Positive staining for neuroendocrine markers is an indispensable requirement for making this diagnosis.

demonstrate greater than 10 mitoses per 2 mm^2. Tumors should generally demonstrate relatively high Ki-67 proliferation indexes; usually from 50% to 85%, though not quite as high as the small cell type of high-grade neuroendocrine carcinoma. The "organoid" or neuroendocrine growth pattern has been described as comprising islands or cords of tumor cells with central areas of comedonecrosis and with peripheral palisading of nuclei. Such features are said to be best appreciated in resection specimens and may be often difficult to discern in small endoscopic biopsies. Moreover, these features are not distinctive or specific for neuroendocrine tumors and may be observed in several other lung neoplasms that do not have immunohistochemical or ultrastructural evidence of neuroendocrine differentiation. The only reliable criterion for neuroendocrine differentiation in these tumors is, therefore, the demonstration of neuroendocrine features by immunohistochemistry, electron microscopy, or molecular testing. As noted earlier, it may be very difficult, sometimes bordering on arbitrary, to determine whether the aforesaid features are the result of aberrant expression of neuroendocrine markers in an otherwise poorly differentiated carcinoma or whether they truly represent evidence of neuroendocrine differentiation. In addition, as previously mentioned, mitotic activity may vary in these tumors and also overlap with intermediate-grade neuroendocrine carcinomas. The diagnosis of high-grade neuroendocrine carcinoma, large cell type should, thus, always be made with caution in small endoscopic biopsies. It may be preferable to make a generic diagnosis of "Neuroendocrine carcinoma with large cell morphology" with a comment that the differential diagnosis includes a high-grade neuroendocrine carcinoma, large cell type and to wait for the examination of the resected specimen before a final diagnosis is rendered in equivocal cases.

The role of immunohistochemical markers is more critical in the diagnosis of high-grade neuroendocrine carcinoma, large cell type than in the small cell type. The demonstration of unequivocal evidence of neuroendocrine differentiation is part of the requirements for the current definition of this entity and, therefore, must be applied in every case. All cases of high-grade neuroendocrine carcinoma, large cell type should demonstrate cytokeratin positivity and at least one neuroendocrine associated marker. Chromogranin A is the most consistently detected specific neuroendocrine marker; synaptophysin and CD56 are less frequently observed.[95] The extent or intensity of labeling that is necessary to separate high-grade neuroendocrine carcinoma, large cell type from large cell carcinoma with aberrant neuroendocrine differentiation has not been determined. Electron microscopy has also been claimed to demonstrate dense-core neurosecretory granules in the cytoplasm of the tumor cells in all cases and can be used as alternative evidence of neuroendocrine differentiation in cases where adequately fixed material is available. For the time being, high-grade neuroendocrine carcinoma, large cell type remains a controversial diagnosis because of the difficulties in separating this condition from large cell carcinoma with aberrant (or spurious) neuroendocrine differentiation, large cell carcinoma with an architectural growth pattern that may be suggestive of neuroendocrine differentiation, intermediate-grade neuroendocrine carcinomas (atypical carcinoid) and large-cell basaloid adenocarcinoma (see Chapter 12 for discussion on this new entity), for which precise criteria for distinction do not exist.

OTHER NEUROENDOCRINE LUNG TUMORS

Neuroendocrine tumors of the lung of nonepithelial origin are quite rare and include primary intrapulmonary paraganglioma and primary primitive neuroectodermal tumors (PNETs) of the lung.

Pulmonary Paraganglioma

The existence of this tumor has been controversial for many years, with some authors claiming that primary tumors of this type do not exist in the lung and represent either metastases or misdiagnosed carcinoid tumors and others who support their existence. There are reports of a few rare examples of primary lung tumors that exhibited all the features of paraganglioma in whom an extrapulmonary source of the tumor could not be detected on thorough clinical and radiographic examination.[33,96] The majority of patients reported in the literature have been middle-aged adults with a slight male predominance. Rare reports exist of the gangliocytic subtype of paraganglioma similar to those that occur within the duodenum; it is unclear whether these represent primary tumors or metastasis from occult lesions.[97] Some tumors in these patients have been associated with the MEN-II syndrome. Many of the tumors described in the literature were clinically characterized by the active production of neuropeptides leading to clinical manifestations of Cushing syndrome, Verner-Morrison syndrome, or episodes of sustained hypertension. Nonfunctional tumors usually come to the attention of the physician owing to symptoms caused by the growing intrapulmonary mass lesion. The tumors can be central and close to major airways, or they can be peripheral; the latter is most commonly found incidentally on chest X-rays. Histologically, the tumors are characterized by their prominent nested neuroendocrine growth pattern (Zellballen) separated by thin fibrovascular septa.[98] Unlike low-grade neuroendocrine carcinomas ("carcinoid" tumors), ribbons, trabeculae, festoons, and rosettes are not a feature of paragangliomas. The tumor cells are usually large, round to oval with centrally placed nuclei and often show nucleomegaly with bizarre nuclear forms, large hyperchromatic nuclei, and intranuclear pseudoinclusions owing to cytoplasmic invaginations. Despite the marked nuclear pleomorphism and atypia, however, mitotic activity and tumor cell necrosis are minimal or absent. Some tumors may not display atypical nuclear features at all. The presence of mitotic activity is not a very reliable indicator of malignancy as it may be seen in both benign and malignant forms. By immunohistochemistry, paragangliomas uniformly react with neuroendocrine markers, particularly chromogranin A and synaptophysin. A distinctive feature of paragangliomas that is very useful for separating them from other epithelial neuroendocrine neoplasms is the absence of reactivity for cytokeratins. Because of the positivity for neuroendocrine markers and the frequent presence of focal cytologic atypia, the lesions must also be distinguished from LCNEC. This is best accomplished by the demonstration of the absence of cytokeratin reactivity and by noting the lack of brisk mitotic activity in paraganglioma. The most important differential diagnosis of paraganglioma is with low-grade lesions ("carcinoid tumor"), particularly in small biopsy samples or when the characteristic nucleomegaly is not evident. Absence of cytokeratin reactivity will also be critical for making this distinction, as carcinoids are almost universally positive for cytokeratin. In previous years, the presence of a rich network of S100 protein–positive sustentacular cells surrounding the tumor cell islands was regarded as a valuable criterion for establishing the above distinction, but more recent studies have demonstrated that these sustentacular cells can also be seen in carcinoid tumors, thus severely limiting their value for making this diagnosis.

Pulmonary Primitive Neuroectodermal Tumor

PNETs (also known as extraskeletal Ewing's sarcoma) are rare neoplasms of the lung. Few cases have been reported so far in the literature.[99-105] The tumors essentially show features of small blue cell tumors at other locations with strong membrane positivity for CD99 and also harbor a t(11;22) chromosomal translocation typical of this family of tumors. The differential diagnosis involves other small round cell tumors of the lung, including lymphoma/leukemia and small cell carcinoma, metastases to the lung from extrapulmonary PNET, melanoma metastases, and metastases from other round cell sarcomas. Molecular testing for *EWSR1* will generally be of help for distinguishing them from other round blue cell tumors.

REFERENCES

1. Moran CA, Suster S, Coppola D, Wick MR. Neuroendocrine carcinomas of the lung: a critical analysis. *Am J Clin Pathol.* 2009;131:206-221.
2. Suster S, Moran CA. Tumors of the lung and pleura. In: Fletcher CDM, ed. *Diagnostic Histopathology of Tumors*. 4th ed. Saunders; 2013:207-245.
3. Suster S, Moran CA. The lung. In: Weidner N, Cote R, Suster S, et al., eds. *Modern Surgical Pathology*. 2nd ed. Saunders; 2009:363-433.
4. Wick MR, Ritter JH. Neuroendocrine neoplasia of the lung. *Ann Thorac Surg.* 2000;69:307-308.
5. Travis WD, Brambilla E, Allan B, et al; World Health Organization Classification of Tumors. *Pathology & Genetics, Tumors of the Lung, Pleura, Mediastinum and Heart.* IARC Press; 2015.
6. McMullan DM, Wood DE. Pulmonary carcinoid tumors. *Semin Thorac Cardiovasc Surg.* 2003;15(3):289-300.

7. Pelosi G, Pattini L, Morana G, et al. Grading lung neuroendocrine tumors: controversies in search of a solution. *Histol Histopathol.* 2017;32(3):223-241.
8. Travis WD, Gal AA, Colby TV, Klimstra DS, Falk R, Koss MN. Reproducibility of neuroendocrine lung tumor classification. *Hum Pathol.* 1998;29:272-279.
9. Volante M, Gatti G, Papotti M. Classification of lung neuroendocrine tumors: lights and shadows. *Endocrine.* 2015;50(2):315-319.
10. Den Bakker MA, Willemsen S, Grünberg K, et al. Small cell carcinoma of the lung and large cell neuroendocrine carcinoma interobserver variability. *Histopathology.* 2010;56(3):356-363.
11. Swarts DRA, van Suylen RJ, den Bakker MA, et al. Interobserver variability for the WHO classification of pulmonary carcinoids. *Am J Surg Pathol.* 2014;38(10):1429-1436.
12. Marchevsky AM, Gal AA, Shah S, Koss MN. Morphometry confirms the presence of considerable nuclear size overlap between "small cells" and "large cells" in high-grade pulmonary neuroendocrine neoplasms. *Am J Clin Pathol.* 2001;116:466-472.
13. Travis WD, Linnoila RI, Tsokos MG, et al. Neuroendocrine tumors of the lung with proposed criteria for large-cell neuroendocrine carcinoma: an ultrastructural, immunohistochemical, and flow cytometric study of 35 cases. *Am J Surg Pathol.* 1991;15:529-553.
14. Travis WD, Rush W, Flieder DB, et al. Survival analysis of 200 pulmonary neuroendocrine tumors with clarification of criteria for atypical carcinoid and its separation from typical carcinoid. *Am J Surg Pathol.* 1998;22:934-944.
15. Wang J, Ren S, Liu Y, et al. Carcinoid tumorlets co-existing with chronic pulmonary inflammatory processes: imaging findings and histological appearances. *Med Sci Monit.* 2020;26:e926014.
16. La Rosa S, Volante M, Uccella S, et al. ACTH-producing tumorlets and carcinoids of the lung: clinico-pathologic study of 63 cases and review of the literature. *Virchows Arch.* 2019;475:587-597.
17. Oliveira AM, Tazelaar HD, Wentzlaff KA, et al. Familial pulmonary carcinoid tumors. *Cancer.* 2001;91(11):2104-2109.
18. Samhouri BF, Halfdanarson TR, Koo CW, et al. DIPNECH: pragmatic approach, uncertainties, notable associations, and a proposal for an improved definition. *Endocr Relat Cancer.* 2023;30:e230051.
19. Almquist DR, Ernani V, Sonbol MB. Diffuse idiopathic pulmonary neuroendocrine cell hyperplasia: DIPNECH. *Curr Opin Pulm Med.* 2021;27:255-261.
20. Ramirez RA, Cass AS, Das S, et al. A multidisciplinary approach to the work up and management of pulmonary carcinoid tumors and DIPNECH: a narrative review. *Transl Lung Cancer Res.* 2022;11:2567-2587.
21. Silva Torres PPTE, Ximenes Salustiano L, Marchiori E. DIPNECH: when computed tomography may suggest the diagnosis. *Arch Bronconeumol.* 2021;57:544.
22. Papaxoinis G, Lamarca A, Quinn AM, Mansoor W, Nonaka D. Clinical and pathologic characteristics of pulmonary carcinoid tumors in central and peripheral locations. *Endocr Pathol.* 2018;29(3):259-268.
23. Fink G, Krelbaum T, Yellin A, et al. Pulmonary carcinoid: presentation, diagnosis, and outcome in 142 cases in Israel and review of 640 cases from the literature. *Chest.* 2001;119:1647-1651.
24. Dixon RK, Britt EJ, Netzer GA, et al. Ten-year single center experience of pulmonary carcinoid tumors and diagnostic yield of bronchoscopic biopsy. *Lung.* 2016;194(6):905-910.
25. Okereke IC, Taber AM, Griffith RC, Ng TT. Outcomes after surgical resection of pulmonary carcinoid tumors. *J Cardiothorac Surg.* 2016;11:35.
26. Herde RF, Kokeny KE, Reddy CB, et al. Primary pulmonary carcinoid tumor: a long-term single institution experience. *Am J Clin Oncol.* 2018;41(1):24-29.

27. Brown LM, Cooke DT, Jett JR, David EA. Extent of resection and lymph node assessment for clinical stage T1aN0M0 typical carcinoid tumors. *Ann Thorac Surg.* 2018;105(1):207-213.
28. Johnson R, Trocha S, McLawhorn M, et al. Histology, not lymph node involvement, predicts long-term survival in bronchopulmonary carcinoids. *Am Surg.* 2011;77(12):1669-1674.
29. Filosso PL, Oliaro A, Ruffini E, et al. Outcome and prognostic factors in bronchial carcinoids: a single-center experience. *J Thorac Oncol.* 2013;8(10):1282-1288.
30. Rossi G, Bertero L, Marchiò C, Papotti M. Molecular alterations of neuroendocrine tumours of the lung. *Histopathology.* 2018;72(1):142-152.
31. Asiedu MK, Thomas CF, Tomaszek SC, et al. Generation and sequencing of pulmonary carcinoid tumor cell lines. *J Thorac Oncol.* 2014;9(12):1763-1771.
32. Simbolo M, Mafficini A, Sikora KO, et al. Lung neuroendocrine tumours: deep sequencing of the four World Health Organization histotypes reveals chromatin-remodeling genes as major players and a prognostic role for TERT, RB1, MEN1 and KMT2D. *J Pathol.* 2017;241(4):488-500.
33. Moran CA, Suster S. *Tumors and Tumor-Like Conditions of the Lung and Pleura.* WB Saunders; 2010:137-164.
34. Kalhor N, Suster S, Moran CA. Primary sclerosing neuroendocrine carcinomas of the lung: a clinicopathologic and immunohistochemical study of 10 cases. *Am J Clin Pathol.* 2010;133:618-622.
35. Moran CA, Suster S. Cystic well-differentiated neuroendocrine carcinoma (carcinoid tumor): a clinicopathologic and immunohistochemical study of two cases. *Am J Clin Pathol.* 2006;126:377-380.
36. Sklar JL, Churg A, Bensch KG. Oncocytic carcinoid tumor of the lung. *Am J Surg Pathol.* 1980;4:287-292.
37. Gal AA, Koss MN, Hochholzer L, DeRose PB, Cohen C. Pigmented pulmonary carcinoid tumor. *Arch Pathol Lab Med.* 1993;117:832-836.
38. Cai YC, Banner B, Glickman J, Odze RD. Cytokeratin 7 and 20 and thyroid transcription factor 1 can help distinguish pulmonary from gastrointestinal carcinoid and pancreatic endocrine tumors. *Hum Pathol.* 2001;32:1087-1093.
39. Sturm N, Rossi G, Lantuejoul S, et al. Expression of thyroid transcription factor-1 in the spectrum of neuroendocrine cell lung proliferations with special interest in carcinoids. *Hum Pathol.* 2002;33:175-182.
40. Kasajima A, Konukiewitz B, Oka N, et al. Clinicopathological profiling of lung carcinoids with a Ki-67 index > 20. *Neuroendocrinology.* 2019;108:109-120.
41. Arrigoni MG, Woolner LB, Bernatz PE. Atypical carcinoid tumors of the lung. *J Thorac Cardiovasc Surg.* 1972;64:413-421.
42. Marciello F, Mercier O, Ferolla P, et al. Natural history of localized and locally advanced atypical lung carcinoids after complete resection: a joined French-Italian retrospective multicenter study. *Neuroendocrinology.* 2018;106(3):264-273.
43. Eymin B, Gazzeri S, Brambilla C, Brambilla E. Distinct pattern of E2F1 expression in human lung tumours: E2F1 is upregulated in small cell lung carcinoma. *Oncogene.* 2001;20(14):1678-1687.
44. Gazzeri S, Della Valle V, Chaussade L, Brambilla C, Larsen CJ, Brambilla E. The human p19ARF protein encoded by the beta transcript of the p16INK4a gene is frequently lost in small cell lung cancer. *Cancer Res.* 1998;58(17):3926-3931.
45. Salon C, Merdzhanova G, Brambilla C, Brambilla E, Gazzeri S, Eymin B. E2F-1, Skp2 and cyclin E oncoproteins are upregulated and directly correlated in high-grade neuroendocrine lung tumors. *Oncogene.* 2007;26(48):6927-6936.

46. Soga J, Yakuwa Y. Bronchopulmonary carcinoids: an analysis of 1875 reported cases with special reference to a comparison between typical carcinoids and atypical varieties. *Ann Thorac Cardiovasc Surg.* 1999;5:211-219.
47. Gould VE, Linnoila RI, Memoli VA, Warren WH. Neuroendocrine cells and neuroendocrine neoplasms of the lung. *Pathol Annu.* 1983;18:287-330.
48. Paladugu RR, Benfield JR, Pak HY, Ross RK, Teplitz RL. Bronchopulmonary Kulchitsky cell carcinoma: a new classification scheme for typical and atypical carcinoids. *Cancer.* 1985;55:1303-1311.
49. Valli M, Fabris GA, Dewar A, Hornall D, Sheppard MN. Atypical carcinoid tumors of the lung: a study of 33 cases with prognostic features. *Histopathology.* 1994;24:363-369.
50. Mills SE, Cooper PH, Walker AN, Kron IL. Atypical carcinoid tumor of the lung: a clinicopathologic study of 17 cases. *Am J Surg Pathol.* 1982;6:643-654.
51. Wick MR. Immunohistology of neuroendocrine and neuroectodermal tumors. *Semin Diagn Pathol.* 2000;17:194-203.
52. Siegel RL, Miller KD, Jemal A. Cancer statistics, 2020. *CA Cancer J Clin.* 2020;70:7-30.
53. Peifer M, Fernández-Cuesta L, Sos ML, et al. Integrative genome analyses identify key somatic driver mutations of small-cell lung cancer. *Nat Genet.* 2012;44(10):1104-1110.
54. Pleasance ED, Stephens PJ, O'Meara S, et al. A small-cell lung cancer genome with complex signatures of tobacco exposure. *Nature.* 2010;463(7278):184-190.
55. Brambilla E, Travis WD, Brennan P, et al. Lung cancer. In: Steward BW, Wild CP, eds. *World Cancer Report.* IARC; 2014:350-362.
56. D'Angelo SP, Pietanza MC. The molecular pathogenesis of small cell lung cancer. *Cancer Biol Ther.* 2010;10(1):1-10.
57. Staaf J, Isaksson S, Karlsson A, et al. Landscape of somatic allelic imbalances and copy number alterations in human lung carcinoma. *Int J Cancer.* 2013;132(9):2020-2031.
58. Kim YH, Girard L, Giacomini CP, et al. Combined microarray analysis of small cell lung cancer reveals altered apoptotic balance and distinct expression signatures of MYC family gene amplification. *Oncogene.* 2006;25(1):130-138.
59. Baine MK, Hsieh MS, Lai WV, et al. SCLC subtypes defined by ASCL1, NEUROD1, POU2F3, and YAP1: a comprehensive immunohistochemical and histopathologic characterization. *J Thorac Oncol.* 2020;15:1823-1835.
60. Megyesfalvi Z, Barany N, Lantos A, et al. Expression patterns and prognostic relevance of subtype-specific transcription factors in surgically resected small-cell lung cancer: an international multicenter study. *J Pathol.* 2022;257:674-686.
61. Qu S, Fetsch P, Thomas A, et al. Molecular subtypes of primary SCLC tumors and their associations with neuroendocrine and therapeutic markers. *J Thorac Oncol.* 2022;17:141-153.
62. Baine MK, Febres-Aldana CA, Chang JC, et al. POU2F3 in SCLC: clinicopathologic and genomic analysis with a focus on its diagnostic utility in neuroendocrine-low SCLC. *J Thorac Oncol.* 2022;17:1109-1121.
63. Hiroshima K, Mino-Kenudson M. Update on large cell neuroendocrine carcinoma. *Transl Lung Cancer Res.* 2017;6(5):530-539.
64. Rekhtman N, Pietanza MC, Hellmann MD, et al. Next-generation sequencing of pulmonary large cell neuroendocrine carcinoma reveals small cell carcinoma-like and non-small cell carcinoma-like subsets. *Clin Cancer Res.* 2016;22(14):3618-3629.
65. Miyoshi T, Umemura S, Matsumura Y, et al. Genomic profiling of large-cell neuroendocrine carcinoma of the lung. *Clin Cancer Res.* 2017;23(3):757-765.
66. Leslie KO, Colby TV. Pathology of lung cancer. *Curr Opin Pulm Med.* 1997;3:252-256.
67. Byers LA, Rudin CM. Small cell lung cancer: where do we go from here? *Cancer.* 2015;121(5):664-672.

68. Kanaji N, Sakai K, Ueda Y, et al. Peripheral-type small cell lung cancer is associated with better survival and higher frequency of interstitial lung disease. *Lung Cancer.* 2017;108:126-133.

69. Reck M, Heigener D, Reinmuth N. Immunotherapy for small-cell lung cancer: emerging evidence. *Future Oncol.* 2016;12(7):931-943.

70. Lehman JM, Gwin ME, Massion PP. Immunotherapy and targeted therapy for small cell lung cancer: there is hope. *Curr Oncol Rep.* 2017;19(7):49.

71. Horn L, Mansfield AS, Szczesna A, et al. First-line atezolizumab plus chemotherapy in extensive-stage small-cell lung cancer. *N Engl J Med.* 2018;379:2220-2229.

72. Liu SV, Reck M, Mansfield AS, et al. Updated overall survival and PD-L1 subgroup analysis of patients with extensive-stage small-cell lung cancer treated with atezolizumab, carboplatin, and etoposide (IMpower133). *J Clin Oncol.* 2021;39:619-630.

73. Giffin MJ, Cooke K, Lobenhofer EK, et al. AMG 757, a half-life extended, DLL3-targeted bispecific T-cell engager, shows high potency and sensitivity in preclinical models of small-cell lung cancer. *Clin Cancer Res.* 2021;27:1526-1537.

74. Owonikoko TK, Champiat S, Johnson ML, et al. Updated results from a phase 1 study of AMG 757, a half-life extended bispecific T-cell engager (BiTE) immuno-oncology therapy against delta-like ligand 3 (DLL3), in small cell lung cancer (SCLC). *J Clin Oncol.* 2021;39(15_Suppl):8510.

75. Johnson DH. Management of small cell lung cancer: current state of the art. *Chest.* 1999;116(6 suppl):525S-530S.

76. Guinee DG Jr, Fishback NF, Koss MN, Abbondanzo SL, Travis WD. The spectrum of immunohistochemical staining of small-cell lung carcinoma in specimens from transbronchial and open-lung biopsies. *Am J Clin Pathol.* 1994;102:406-414.

77. Sakakibara R, Kobayashi M, Takahashi N, et al. Insulinoma-associated protein 1 (INSM1) is a better marker for the diagnosis and prognosis estimation of small cell lung carcinoma than neuroendocrine phenotype markers such as chromogranin A, synaptophysin, and CD56. *Am J Surg Pathol.* 2020;44:757-764.

78. Staaf J, Tran L, Söderlund L, et al. Diagnostic value of insulinoma-associated protein 1 (INSM1) and comparison with established neuroendocrine markers in pulmonary cancers. *Arch Pathol Lab Med.* 2020;144:1075-1085.

79. Suster DI, Mackinnon AC, Suster S. Insulinoma-associated protein-1 expression in lymphoepithelial carcinoma of the thymus: a potential pitfall for diagnosis with neuroendocrine carcinomas of the thymus. *Arch Pathol Lab Med.* 2025;149: e31-e35.

80. Wang M, Abi-Raad R, Baldassarri R, Adeniran AJ, Cai G. Expression of insulinoma-associated protein 1 in non-small cell lung cancers: a diagnostic pitfall for neuroendocrine tumors. *Hum Pathol.* 2021;115:104-111.

81. Svajdler M, Mezencev R, Ondic O, Šašková B, Mukenšnábl P, Michal M. P16 is a useful supplemental diagnostic marker of pulmonary small cell carcinoma in small biopsies and cytology specimens. *Ann Diagn Pathol.* 2018;33:23-29.

82. Travis WD, Brambilla E, Noguchi M, et al. International Association for the Study of Lung Cancer/American Thoracic Society/European Respiratory Society international multidisciplinary classification of lung adenocarcinoma. *J Thorac Oncol.* 2011;6:244-285.

83. Iyoda A, Hiroshima K, Baba M, Saitoh Y, Ohwada H, Fujisawa T. Pulmonary large cell carcinomas with neuroendocrine features are high-grade neuroendocrine tumors. *Ann Thorac Surg.* 2002;73:1049-1054.

84. Howe MC, Chapman A, Kerr K, Dougal M, Anderson H, Hasleton PS. Neuroendocrine differentiation in non-small cell lung cancer and its relation to prognosis and therapy. *Histopathology.* 2004;46:195-201.

85. Ionescu DN, Treaba D, Gilks CB, et al. Nonsmall cell lung carcinoma with neuroendocrine differentiation: an entity of no clinical or prognostic significance. *Am J Surg Pathol.* 2007;31:26-32.
86. Iyoda A, Hiroshima K, Toyozaki T, Haga Y, Fujisawa T, Ohwada H. Clinical characterization of pulmonary large cell neuroendocrine carcinoma and large cell carcinoma with neuroendocrine morphology. *Cancer.* 2001;91:1992-2000.
87. Dresler CM, Ritter JH, Patterson GA, Ross E, Bailey MS, Wick MR. Clinical–pathologic analysis of 40 patients with large cell neuroendocrine carcinoma of the lung. *Ann Thorac Surg.* 1997;63:180-185.
88. Takei H, Asamura H, Maeshima A, et al. Large cell neuroendocrine carcinoma of the lung: a clinicopathologic study of eighty-seven cases. *J Thorac Cardiovasc Surg.* 2002;124:285-292.
89. Paci M, Cavazza A, Annessi V, et al. Large cell neuroendocrine carcinoma of the lung: a 10-year clinicopathologic retrospective study. *Ann Thorac Surg.* 2004;77:1163-1167.
90. Battafarano RJ, Fernandez FG, Ritter J, et al. Large cell neuroendocrine carcinoma: an aggressive form of non-small cell lung cancer. *J Thorac Cardiovasc Surg.* 2005;130(1):166-172.
91. Rossi G, Cavazza A, Marchioni A, et al. Role of chemotherapy and the receptor tyrosine kinases KIT, PDGFRalpha, PDGFRbeta, and Met in large-cell neuroendocrine carcinoma of the lung. *J Clin Oncol.* 2005;23(34):8774-8785.
92. Yang L, Fan Y, Lu H. Pulmonary large cell neuroendocrine carcinoma. *Pathol Oncol Res.* 2022;28:1610730.
93. Buium C, Negru S, Ionescu DN, Dediu M. The unmet diagnostic and treatment needs in large cell neuroendocrine carcinoma of the lung. *Curr Oncol.* 2023;30:7218-7228.
94. Lo Russo G, Pusceddu S, Proto C, et al. Treatment of lung large cell neuroendocrine carcinoma. *Tumour Biol.* 2016;37:7047-7057.
95. Jiang SX, Kameya T, Shoji M, Dobashi Y, Shinada J, Yoshimura H. Large cell neuroendocrine carcinoma of the lung: a histologic and immunohistochemical study of 22 cases. *Am J Surg Pathol.* 1998;22:526-537.
96. Huang X, Liang QL, Jiang L, et al. Primary pulmonary paraganglioma: a case report and review of literature. *Medicine (Baltimore).* 2015;94(31):e1271.
97. Lin D, Hu Y, Xing X, et al. Pulmonary gangliocytic paraganglioma: a case report and review of the literature. *Int J Clin Exp Pathol.* 2014;7(1):432-437.
98. Aubertine CL, Flieder DB. Primary paraganglioma of the lung. *Ann Diagn Pathol.* 2004;8:237-241.
99. Imamura F, Funakoshi T, Nakamura S, Mano M, Kodama K, Horai T. Primary primitive neuroectodermal tumor of the lung: report of two cases. *Lung Cancer.* 2000;27:55-60.
100. Mikami Y, Nakajima M, Hashimoto H, et al. Primary pulmonary primitive neuroectodermal tumor (PNET): a case report. *Pathol Res Pract.* 2001;197:113-119.
101. Shet N, Stanescu L, Deutsch G. Primary extraosseous Ewing sarcoma of the lung: case report and literature review. *Radiol Case Rep.* 2013;8(2):832.
102. Takahashi D, Nagayama J, Nagatoshi Y, et al. Primary Ewing's sarcoma family tumors of the lung a case report and review of the literature. *Jpn J Clin Oncol.* 2007;37(11):874-877.
103. Deokar KK, Kunjir NG, Ghorpade S. Primary Ewings sarcoma of the lung. *J Clin Diagn Res.* 2015;9(1):XD01-XD03.
104. Hwang SK, Kim DK, Park SI, Kim Y-H, Kim HR. Primary Ewing's sarcoma of the lung. *Korean J Thorac Cardiovasc Surg.* 2014;47(1):47-50.
105. Hirano H, Maeda H, Takeuchi Y, et al. Primary pulmonary Ewing sarcoma. *Pathol Int.* 2016;66(4):239-241.

14

UNUSUAL LUNG TUMORS, MESENCHYMAL TUMORS, AND TUMORLIKE CONDITIONS

A series of unusual lung tumors and tumorlike conditions can be occasionally encountered in lung biopsies. These include primary and metastatic sarcomas, lung tumors derived from presumed ectopic tissues, various lung tumors of uncertain histogenesis, and a few rare benign tumors and tumorlike conditions.

MESENCHYMAL NEOPLASMS

Varied mesenchymal neoplasms can arise in the lung; however, the presence of a sarcoma in the lung is most often the result of a metastasis from a distant soft tissue site.[1] Clinicopathologic correlation and a thorough clinical history are, therefore, essential for a correct interpretation.

Benign Mesenchymal Neoplasms

Benign mesenchymal neoplasms that can originate in the lung include cartilaginous hamartoma, pulmonary adenofibroma, endobronchial lipoma, leiomyoma, schwannoma, neurofibroma, and other less common mesenchymal entities that have been rarely reported in the literature.

Cartilaginous hamartoma is probably the most common benign mesenchymal neoplasm of the lung. The term "hamartoma" was coined because of the presence of an admixture of mature cartilage with mature adipose tissue, myxoid stroma, or a fibroblastic spindle cell component. Studies have demonstrated a high frequency of mutations in these tumors, as well as the presence of microsatellite instability and alterations in mitochondrial DNA copy number, suggestive of a neoplastic process.[2,3] The majority of these lesions present as a solitary "coin lesion" within lung parenchyma, but they may also present as endobronchial tumors causing bronchial obstruction. Histologically, they are characterized by lobules comprising mature hyaline cartilage surrounded by other mesenchymal elements such as fat, bone, smooth muscle, and occasional myxoid matrix with sparse fibroblastic spindle cells (Fig. 14.1). A characteristic feature is the entrapment of benign

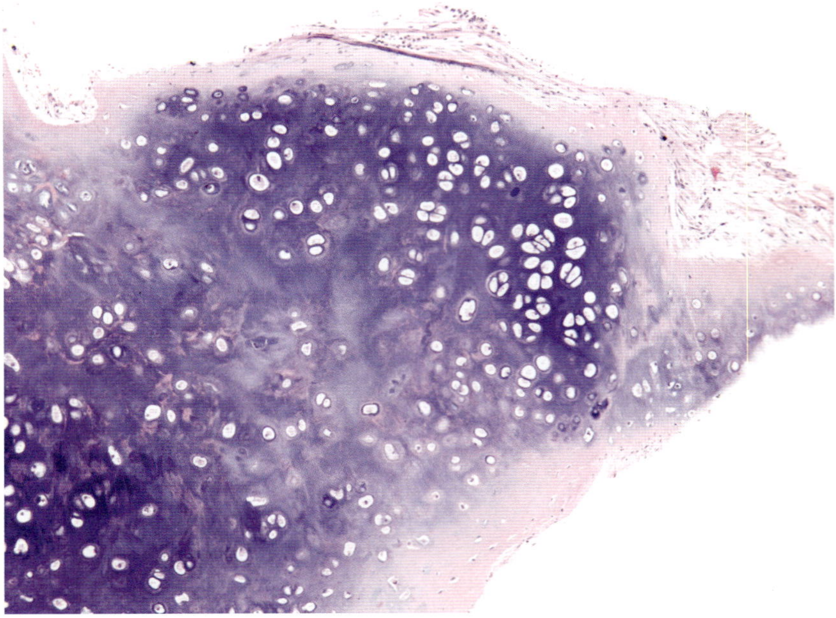

FIGURE 14.1 Endoscopic biopsy of cartilaginous hamartoma shows mature hyaline cartilage surrounded by fibroconnective tissue.

respiratory epithelium from the surrounding lung parenchyma inside the cartilaginous lesion (eFig. 14.1). The latter feature serves to separate them from bronchopulmonary chondromas, which tend to be multiple when seen as part of Carney triad. *Pulmonary adenofibroma* is a rare lesion of disputed histogenesis that is characterized by clublike papillae lined by cuboidal or columnar cells that contain a bland fibroblastic spindle cell proliferation in the cores of the papillae.[4] The histologic appearance of the lesion is reminiscent of müllerian adenofibromas of the female genital tract and ovary. The lesions are usually small (1-2 cm) and intraparenchymatous, with no relationship to the bronchial tree. The spindle cells stain only with vimentin and are negative for all other specific markers such as smooth muscle actin (SMA), desmin, S-100 protein, and CD34. Similar tumors that show expression of smooth muscle–associated markers, such as SMA, h-caldesmon, and desmin, have been designated as adenomyomas. It has been postulated that they may represent hamartomatous lesions, similar to cartilaginous hamartoma but lacking the cartilaginous component. However, recent studies have shown recurrent *NAB2::STAT6* translocations in some pulmonary adenofibromas, suggesting that these lesions may represent a histologic variant of solitary fibrous tumor that shares the same translocation.[5] *Endobronchial lipomas* affect adult patients in their fifth or sixth decade of life and present with clinical signs and symptoms of bronchial obstruction.[6] The tumors can range in size from 1 to 5 cm in greatest diameter and are soft, yellow, and well circumscribed (Fig. 14.2).

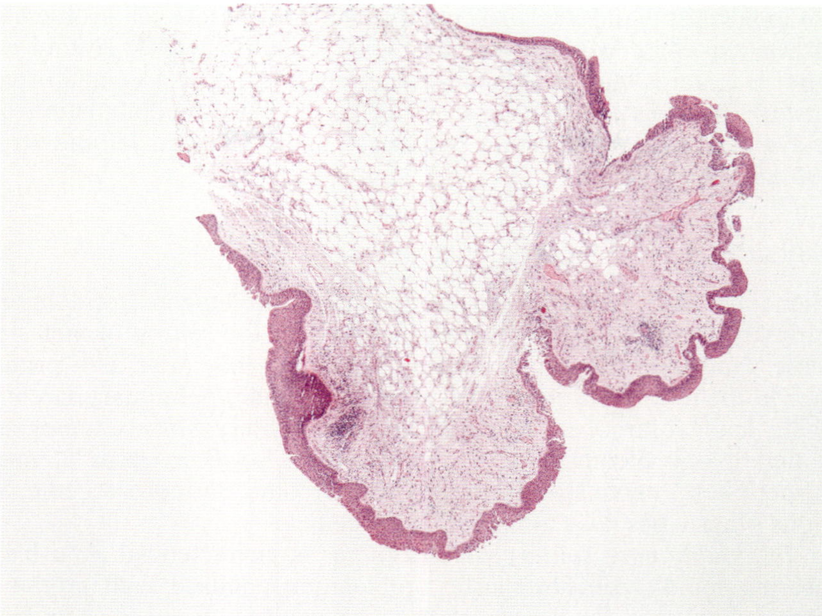

FIGURE 14.2 Endoscopic biopsy of endobronchial lipoma shows an intact overlying squamous mucosa overlying a well-circumscribed proliferation of mature adipose tissue.

They are histologically characterized by mature adipose tissue without any evidence of cytologic atypia. Tumors characterized by a prominent vascular component associated with a perivascular epithelioid smooth muscle proliferation, in addition to adipose tissue, are diagnostic of *angiomyolipoma*.[7] Such tumors are most often seen in the background of tuberous sclerosis complex and are characterized by coexpression of melanocytic (HMB45, Melan-A) and smooth muscle markers (SMA) in the epithelioid perivascular cells. *Pulmonary leiomyoma* is a rare tumor that has been the subject only of case reports. Care must be taken not to confuse them with *benign metastasizing leiomyoma*, a condition that occurs mainly in young women with a history of prior hysterectomy for uterine leiomyomas and presents as multifocal lesions (see Chapter 15). Intrapulmonary leiomyomas are usually single and can present as endobronchial masses, making them amenable to diagnosis through endoscopic biopsies.[8] The tumor is characterized by a bland-appearing population of spindle cells with large nuclei showing blunted ends and surrounded by a rim of finely fibrillary cytoplasm. The tumor cells are devoid of cytologic atypia or mitotic activity and strongly stain with muscle markers such as SMA, smooth muscle myosin, desmin, calponin, and h-caldesmon. *Intrapulmonary schwannomas* are rare tumors that can occur in any age group and usually present as polypoid endobronchial masses or as an intraparenchymal peripheral nodule.[9] They are usually well circumscribed and unencapsulated and measure from 1 to

5 cm in greatest diameter. They comprise a bland spindle cell proliferation with wavy nuclei devoid of nuclear atypia or mitotic activity. Antoni A or Antoni B features may be difficult to identify in small endoscopic or core biopsies. The diagnosis can be made by observing the combination of a bland spindle cell proliferation with wavy or fusiform nuclei and strong S-100 protein reactivity.

Malignant Mesenchymal Neoplasms

Malignant mesenchymal neoplasms are rare in the lung and seldom arise as primary tumors; they are most often seen in the setting of metastatic disease. However, virtually any type of sarcoma may arise as a primary tumor in the lung.[1] The commonest types of primary pulmonary sarcomas include leiomyosarcoma, synovial sarcoma, solitary fibrous tumor, and undifferentiated pleomorphic sarcoma (UPS); however, cases of malignant peripheral nerve sheath tumor, osteosarcoma, chondrosarcoma, and various other types have also been described.

Intrapulmonary solitary fibrous tumor is characterized by a bland-appearing spindle cell fibroblastic proliferation admixed with prominent sclerotic changes in the stroma, with a particular tendency to show linear deposition of hyalinized collagen alongside the spindle cells (ie, "ropelike" collagen) (Fig. 14.3A; eFigs. 14.2 and 14.3).[10] The tumors can be difficult to

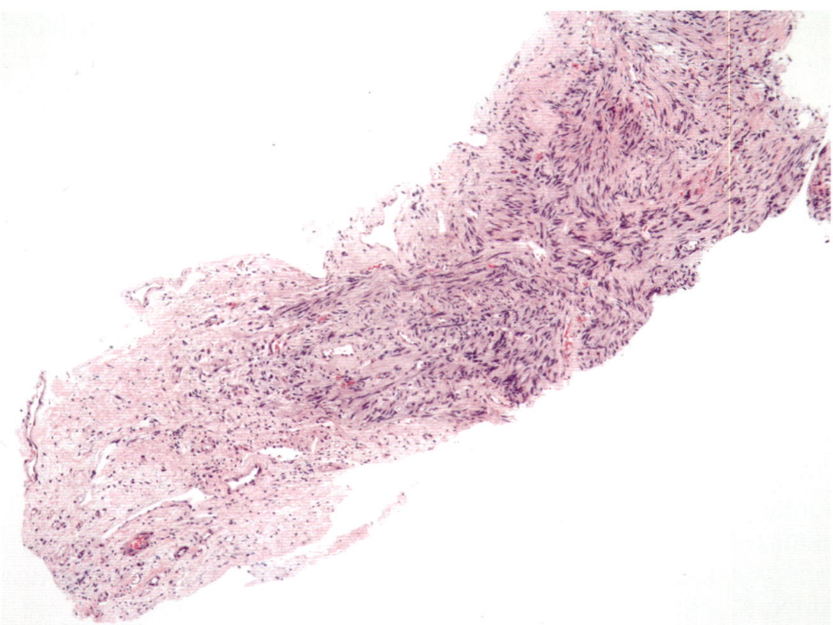

A

FIGURE 14.3 **A.** Core biopsy of peripherally located intrapulmonary solitary fibrous tumor showing a bland-appearing spindle cell proliferation with abundant collagenous stroma.

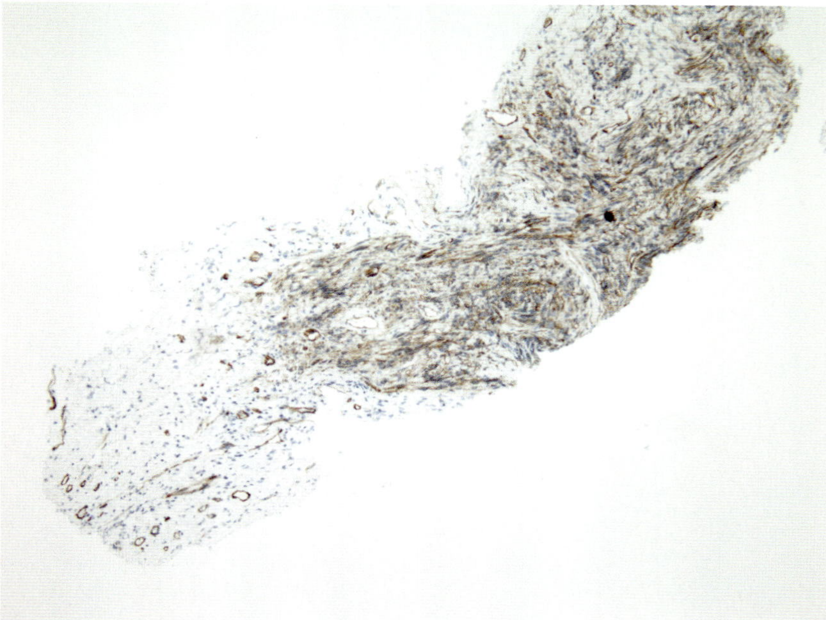

B

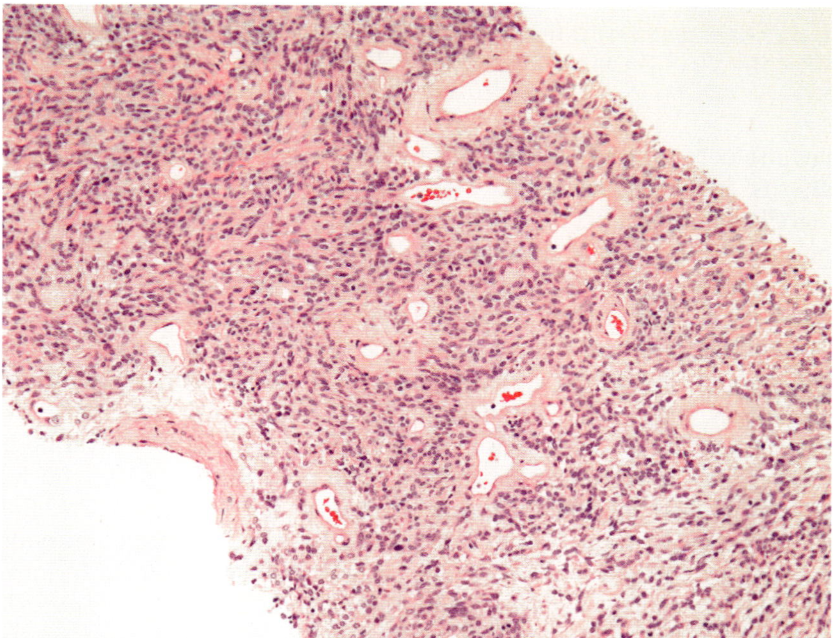

C

FIGURE 14.3 (*continued*) **B.** Immunohistochemical staining for CD34 shows strong cytoplasmic positivity in the tumor cells. **C.** Core biopsy of intrapulmonary solitary fibrous tumor showing the bland spindle cell proliferation with numerous irregularly shaped "hemangiopericytic" vessels.

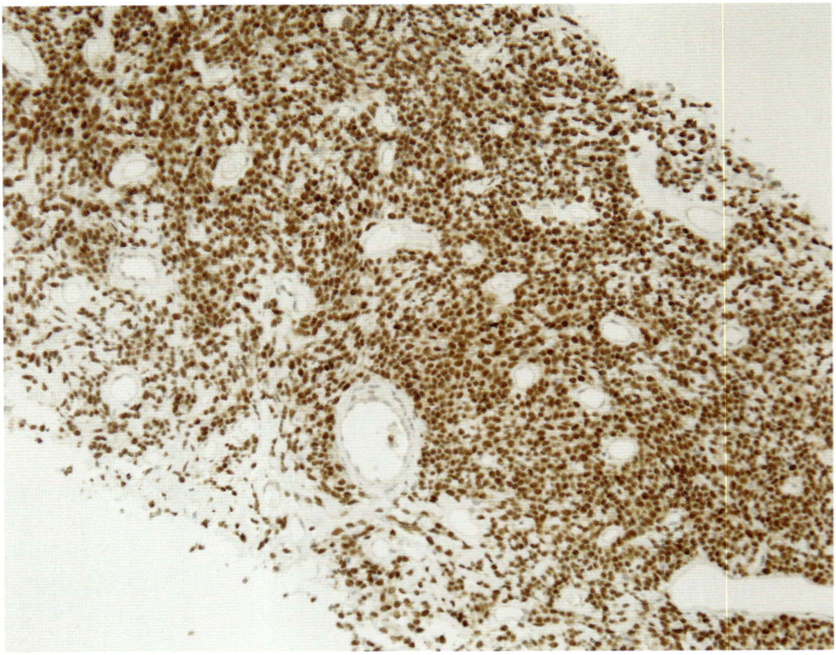

D

FIGURE 14.3 (*continued*) **D.** Immunohistochemical staining for STAT6 shows diffuse strong nuclear staining of the tumor cells in intrapulmonary solitary fibrous tumor.

diagnose because of their tendency to show a great heterogeneity of growth patterns, including fascicular, storiform, herringbone, hemangiopericytic, angiofibromatous, and neural-like with wavy nuclei.[11] In years past, these tumors were frequently misdiagnosed as pulmonary hemangiopericytoma. It is currently acknowledged that tumors reported under the latter designation most likely correspond to intrapulmonary solitary fibrous tumors. Immunohistochemical stains can play a helpful role in diagnosis; the tumors usually react with CD34 and are negative for other specific markers of differentiation, such as keratin, desmin, actin, and S-100 protein (Fig. 14.3B; eFig. 14.4). Patchy CD99 positivity and positivity for bcl-2 may be seen, though these markers are recognized to be nonspecific and are no longer commonly used for the diagnosis of solitary fibrous tumor. The tumors are molecularly characterized by a distinctive translocation involving an inversion of chromosome 12 leading to a *NAB2::STAT6* gene fusion. The translocation can be assessed by immunohistochemistry utilizing a STAT6 antibody, which has been shown to successfully identify these tumors in up to 98% of cases[12] (Fig. 14.3C and D). The overwhelming majority of solitary fibrous tumors behave in an indolent fashion and show a very bland morphologic appearance; however, all solitary fibrous tumors harbor some degree of malignant potential and should be treated as sarcomas. So-called malignant forms are characterized by increased cellularity, nuclear atypia with prominent nucleoli, nuclear pleomorphism, bizarre and multinucleated tumor cells, increased mitotic activity (>3 mitoses per 10 high-power fields), and areas of necrosis. Occasionally, cases presenting with bland histologic appearances can also behave aggressively and metastasize.[13] Given that all solitary fibrous tumors are considered to have some degree of malignant potential, in current practice, these tumors are usually risk stratified with regard to metastatic potential rather than being diagnosed as "benign" or "malignant." Risk stratification is most commonly performed using a system based on the age of the patient, presence of necrosis, mitotic count, and size of the tumor.[14] Caution should be observed in the wording of the report when interpreting small biopsy samples, and a note should always be added to indicate that even if the cytology of the lesion appears benign, the biologic behavior of the tumor cannot be predicted with certainty, and complete excision is recommended.

Pulmonary leiomyosarcoma usually presents as a well-circumscribed tumor mass that can be either endobronchial or peripheral and can vary in size from 1 to 10 cm in greatest diameter.[15] These tumors can occur in any age group without gender predilection. The tumors are characterized by a fascicular spindle cell proliferation that often shows nuclei with blunted ends and variable mitotic activity. Well-differentiated tumors tend to retain the normal low-power architecture of smooth muscle, with fascicles that are cut at 90° angles (Fig. 14.4); poorly differentiated tumors will display marked

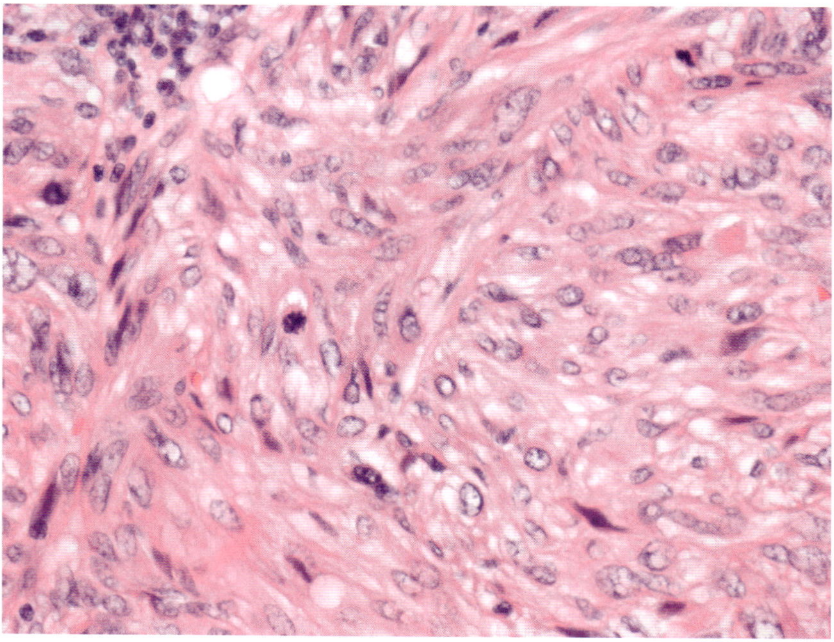

FIGURE 14.4 Low-grade pulmonary leiomyosarcoma shows fascicles of atypical spindle cells that intersect at 90° angles and show scattered mitoses.

nuclear pleomorphism with bizarre mitotic figures, closely resembling an UPS; in fact, it may be impossible to make any distinction other than by the application of immunohistochemical stains. Leiomyosarcoma should stain strongly positive for muscle-associated markers, such as desmin, SMA, smooth muscle myosin, h-caldesmon, and calponin. The lung is a common site of metastases for uterine leiomyosarcomas; a diagnosis of primary leiomyosarcoma of the lung should be made with caution in women with a history of hysterectomy or in whom recent pelvic examination has not been done. These tumors in addition need to be separated from intimal sarcomas that are a group of sarcomas that will commonly display smooth muscle histology; these tumors tend to arise from the great vessels and may secondarily involve the lungs.[16] Intimal sarcomas molecularly are characterized by amplification of *MDM2*, *CDK4*, and *CDK6*, which may be helpful in making the distinction from leiomyosarcomas, though in practice this distinction may be extremely difficult.[17]

Intrapulmonary synovial sarcoma has become increasingly recognized in recent years as one of the most common primary spindle cell sarcomas in this organ.[18] The tumors can occur in patients of any age but are more common in young to middle-aged adults (mean age 38 years), with a slight female predilection. The lesions are usually well circumscribed but unencapsulated and are most often peripheral but may also present as endobronchial masses that are amenable to examination by endoscopy. The majority of cases (>80%) show a characteristic X;18(p11.2;q11.2) translocation that fuses the *SS18* gene to either the *SSX1* or *SSX2* genes (or less commonly other *SSX* genes or non-*SSX* partner genes). Some studies have shown a genotype-phenotype correlation, indicating that *SS18::SSX1* fusion synovial sarcomas are more likely to show epithelial differentiation. These genetic alterations can be detected on formalin-fixed, paraffin-embedded tissues by fluorescence in situ hybridization (FISH), polymerase chain reaction (PCR) techniques, or by next-generation sequencing (NGS) fusion assays.[19-21] The majority of synovial sarcomas of the lung are of the monophasic spindle cell type: they are characterized by a monotonous population of atypical spindle cells with scant stroma and variable mitotic activity (1 to 10 mitoses per 2 mm^2). The tumors can show varied growth patterns, including herringbone, storiform, hemangiopericytic, and palisading (resembling a neural neoplasm) that can sometimes obscure the diagnosis (Fig. 14.5A-C; eFigs. 14.5 and 14.6). Tumors in central location may show entrapment of residual respiratory structures by the spindle cell proliferation, simulating a biphasic malignancy (Fig. 14.6). Some tumors can show prominent myxoid degeneration of the stroma, particularly following treatment. Another morphologic variant is characterized by round, rather than oval, cells, with an epithelioid appearance; such tumors have been termed "poorly differentiated" synovial sarcoma. Immunohistochemical stains will usually show focal positivity in small clusters of spindle cells for cytokeratin stains or epithelial membrane antigen (EMA), and strong cytoplasmic positivity in the majority of the tumor cells for vimentin and bcl-2, though these markers are recognized as nonspecific and are rarely used for the diagnosis of

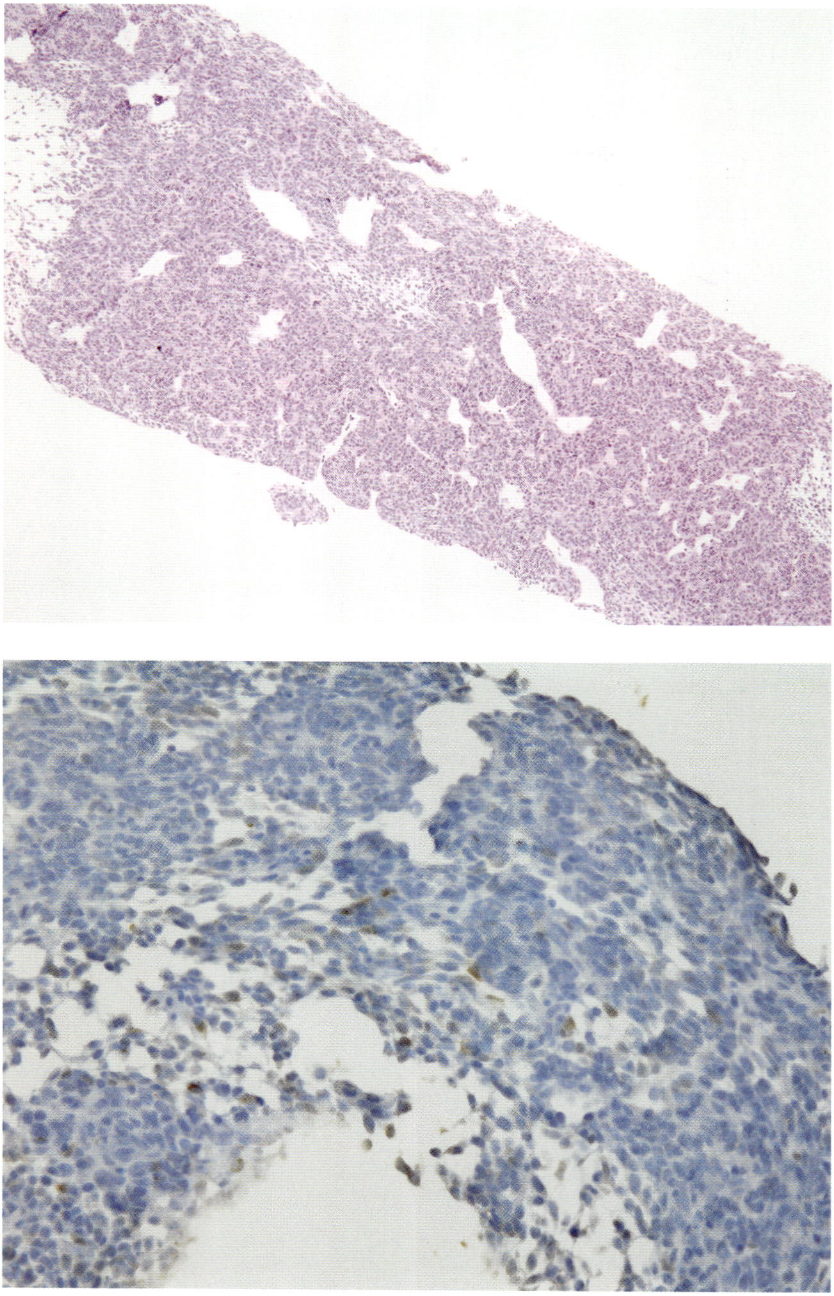

A

B

FIGURE 14.5 **A.** Core biopsy of pulmonary synovial sarcoma showing monotonous small spindle cells with a hemangiopericytic vascular pattern. **B.** Immunohistochemical staining of the tumor cells in synovial sarcoma for cytokeratin AE1/AE3; notice the patchy, focal staining in only a few scattered cells.

C
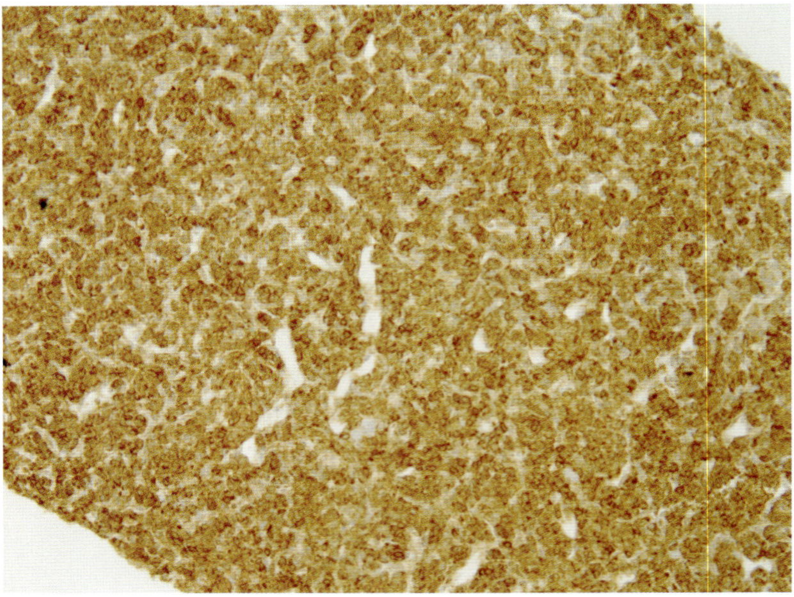

FIGURE 14.5 (*continued*) **C.** Immunohistochemical staining of pulmonary synovial sarcoma for bcl-2; notice strong, diffuse cytoplasmic staining in the majority of the tumor cells, a pattern that is quite characteristic for this tumor.

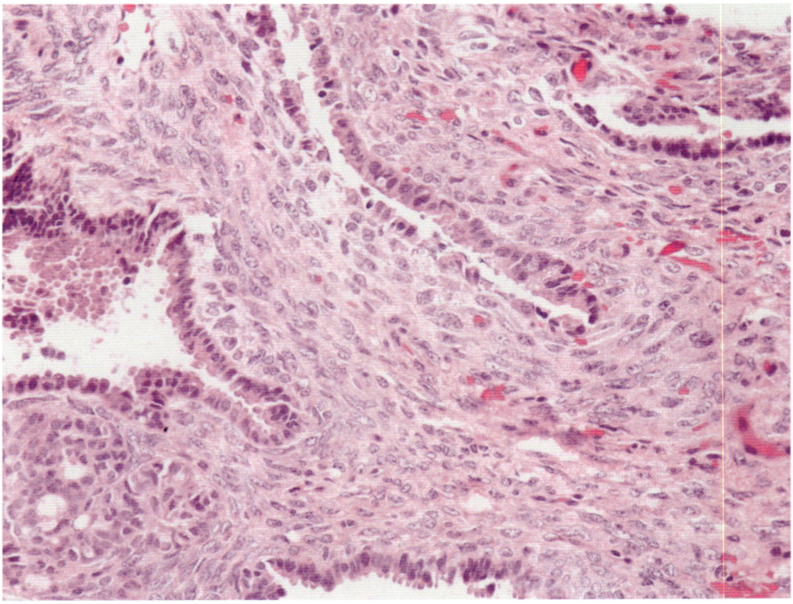

FIGURE 14.6 **Endoscopic biopsy of pulmonary synovial sarcoma showing entrapment of respiratory structures by the monotonous spindle cell proliferation, resembling a biphasic neoplasm.** The bland morphology of the lining of the glands and thyroid transcription factor-1 positivity serve to identify them as entrapped benign elements.

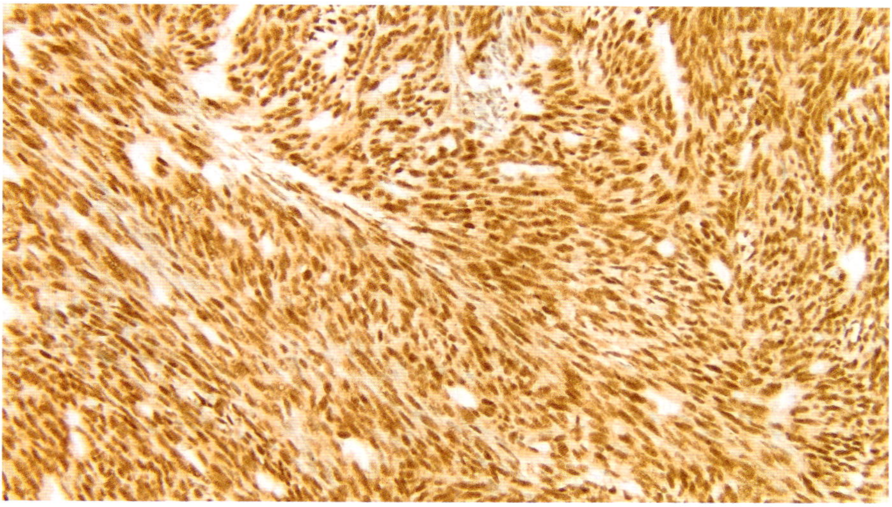

FIGURE 14.7 Immunohistochemical staining for SS18-SSX in monophasic synovial sarcoma shows strong nuclear positivity.

synovial sarcoma in modern practice (eFigs. 14.7 and 14.8).[22] Other markers that have been demonstrated to be positive in synovial sarcoma include calponin, TLE-1, calretinin, S-100 protein, HBME-1, and CD117. More recently, monoclonal antibodies directed against the *SS18::SSX* fusion protein and the C terminus of *SSX* have been introduced for the diagnosis of synovial sarcoma and serve as specific markers (Figs. 14.7 and 14.8).[23,24] The demonstration of the *SS18::SSX* fusion product in these tumors is an extremely helpful adjunct

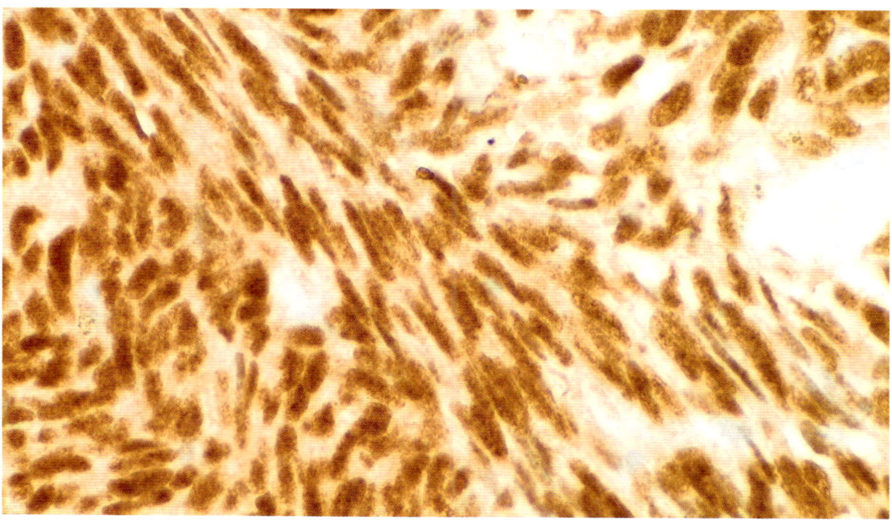

FIGURE 14.8 Immunohistochemical staining for SSX-C terminus in monophasic synovial sarcoma shows strong nuclear positivity.

for diagnosis in equivocal cases and may be very useful for separating these tumors from sarcomatoid carcinoma or from the spindle cell component of a biphasic pulmonary blastoma, which it may closely resemble. Because the lung is the second most common site of metastasis for synovial sarcoma of soft tissues, ruling out a primary source outside of the lungs is necessary before a diagnosis of primary pulmonary synovial sarcoma can be rendered.

Primary pulmonary myxoid sarcoma (PPMS) and *pulmonary angiomatoid fibrous histiocytoma* are exceedingly rare entities characterized by variable histology ranging from a bland spindled to ovoid cell population embedded within a myxoid stroma to a more inflammatory, cellular, spindle cell neoplasm with a vague histiocytoid appearance that resembles inflammatory myofibroblastic tumor (IMT).[25] PPMS is classified as a low- to intermediate-grade sarcoma of uncertain histogenesis, although it has been postulated to originate from primitive peribronchial mesenchymal cells undergoing myofibroblastic differentiation.[26] This tumor, however, has a controversial relationship with angiomatoid fibrous histiocytoma with which it shares a similar *EWSR1* translocation. Recent cases have been described in which tumors showing overlapping features of both harbored *EWRS1::CREB1* and *EWRS1::ATF1* fusions.[27,28] It has been suggested that PPMS and the myxoid variant of angiomatoid fibrosus histiocytoma may represent a continuum with overlapping histologic, immunohistochemical, and genetic features. PPMS commonly present as endobronchial masses and occur more often in females than in males (Figs. 14.9 and 14.10).[29] They usually occur in younger patients but have been reported in patients as old as 80 years. Although the recurrent *EWSR1* fusion is characteristic and appears to define these tumors, a single case of an *EWSR1* fusion negative,

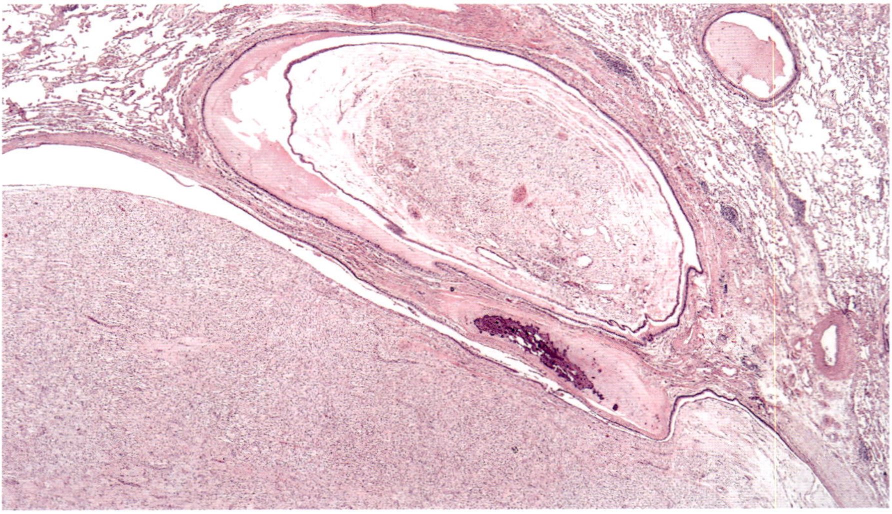

FIGURE 14.9 Low-power magnification of primary pulmonary myxoid sarcoma shows a myxoid neoplasm growing in an endobronchial location.

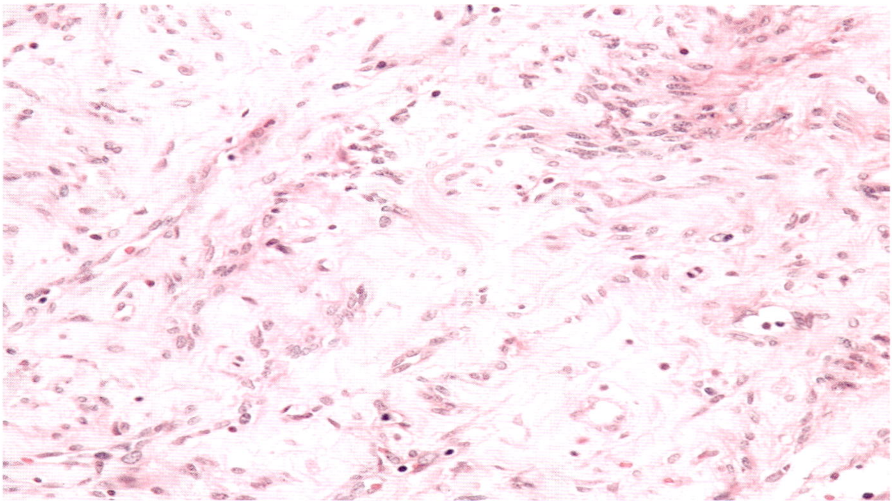

FIGURE 14.10 **Higher-power magnification highlights small spindled to ovoid cells embedded in a myxoid stroma.** Notice in some areas the cells almost begin to adopt a single file conformation.

SMARCB1 lost, PPMS has been reported, suggesting that there may be possible alternative driver events.[25,26,29-31] The tumors appear to behave in an indolent fashion, although some patients have developed metastasis and succumbed to their disease.[25] Pulmonary angiomatoid fibrous histiocytoma usually presents as multinodular islands of spindle to epithelioid cells with bland, ovoid vesicular nuclei and abundant cytoplasm devoid of cytologic atypia or nuclear pleomorphism lying within a loose stroma that can be often myxoid and accompanied by a lymphocytic inflammatory infiltrate, particularly at the periphery (Figs. 14.11 and 14.12).[32,33] The differential diagnosis for both tumors is primarily with metastases from extraskeletal myxoid chondrosarcoma and myoepithelioma/myoepithelial carcinoma as well as other myxoid tumors of the lung.[25] Immunohistochemistry is noncontributory because they tend to have a nonspecific immunophenotype; they are usually positive for vimentin and have also shown focal positivity for EMA. They are negative for keratins and other markers of myoepithelial differentiation. The diagnosis of these rare lesions requires awareness of the entity, correlation with clinicopathologic features, and demonstration of the characteristic fusion.

Pulmonary artery sarcoma (intimal sarcoma) is an extremely rare tumor characterized by a varied histomorphology and aggressive behavior.[34] Patients present with dyspnea, chest pain, back pain, cough, and hemoptysis, which may mimic thromboembolism.[35-37] Surgery is the treatment of choice, and patients generally have a poor prognosis.[38] The histologic features are quite variable in pulmonary artery sarcoma, and the lesions may present as low-grade myofibroblastic lesions, high-grade undifferentiated

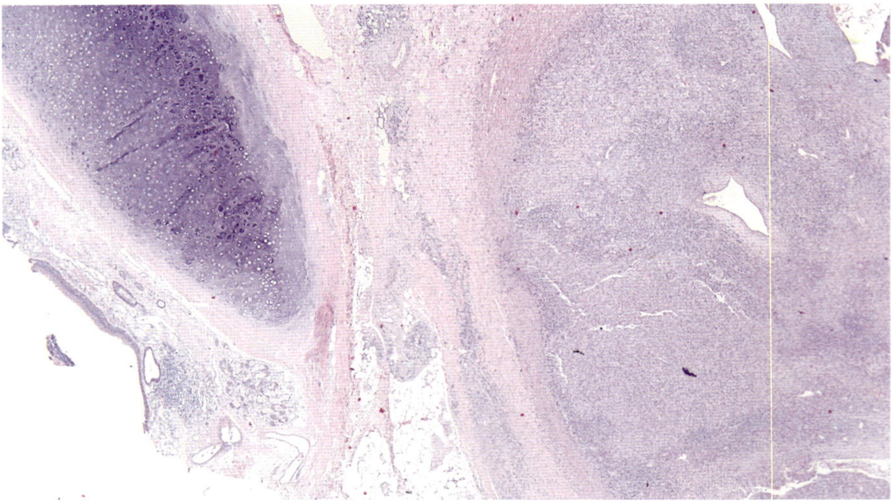

FIGURE 14.11 Low-power magnification of angiomatoid fibrous histiocytoma of the lung demonstrates a relatively well-circumscribed, nodular lesion with a peripheral rim of inflammation located in a parabronchial location.

sarcomas, or with many types of heterologous differentiation such as bone or cartilage.[39] Genetically, the lesions are characterized by amplifications of *MDM2*, *CDK4*, *CDK6*, and *PDGFRA*.[40,41] Owing to its variegated appearance, the diagnosis of pulmonary artery sarcoma requires strict correlation with clinical and radiologic features, and caution should be employed when interpreting biopsy specimens.

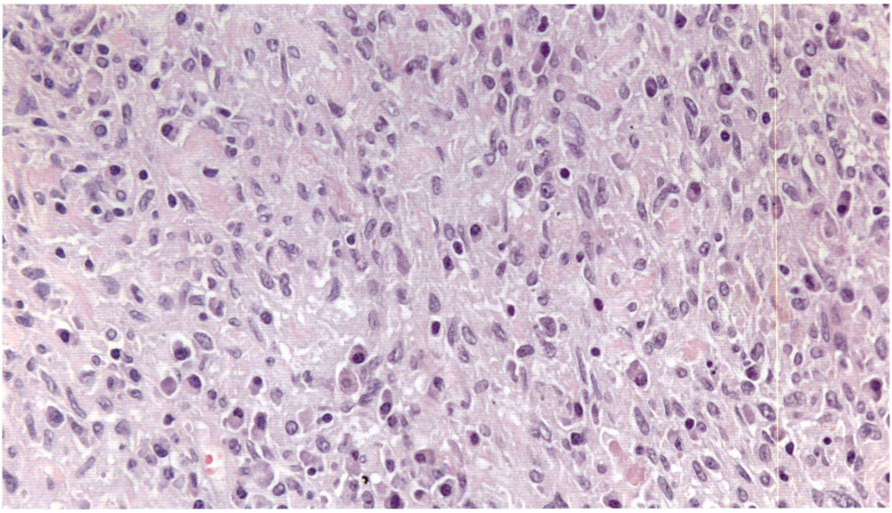

FIGURE 14.12 Higher-power magnification of angiomatoid fibrous histiocytoma of the lung shows a bland spindle cell population with admixed inflammatory cells; notice the vague myxoid change to the background sharing some overlap with primary pulmonary myxoid sarcoma.

Undifferentiated pleomorphic sarcoma arising in the lung has been the subject only of case reports in the literature. The tumors are, by definition, high-grade and are characterized by high cellularity, marked nuclear pleomorphism with bizarre multinucleated tumor cells, and frequent abnormal mitotic figures.[42,43] The tumors can show a prominent storiform pattern or grow as sheets of atypical tumor cells with a haphazard arrangement. Some tumors may display prominent myxoid stromal changes; hemorrhage and necrosis are also a common finding. There are no specific markers associated with UPS; the tumors generally type only for vimentin, although some may show aberrant expression of desmin, keratin, S-100, or other immunohistochemical stains in isolated tumor cells; they, thus, represent a "wastebasket" category for poorly differentiated sarcomas. The diagnosis of UPS must be made with caution, particularly in small biopsy material, because of the difficulties for separating them from other pleomorphic poorly differentiated tumors of the lung, in particular, large cell carcinoma and pleomorphic carcinomas, including SMARCA4-deficient undifferentiated thoracic tumors. Immunohistochemical stains for cytokeratins should be routinely ordered to rule out the possibility of an undifferentiated carcinoma of the lung.

In general terms, a definitive diagnosis of primary sarcoma of the lung may be impossible to render on a small biopsy sample because of the difficulties on limited biopsy material for determining whether other epithelial components may be present, such as in carcinosarcoma and pulmonary blastoma. Moreover, metastases from soft tissue sarcomas to the lung greatly outnumber primary lung sarcomas. Clinicopathologic correlation, thorough radiographic studies, and a very detailed clinical history are, therefore, necessary to establish whether the tumor is primary or metastatic. This applies even when dealing with a solitary lesion. As mentioned above, the most important consideration when dealing with biopsies of sarcoma-like tumors in the lung is the need to rule out the possibility of a sarcomatoid carcinoma. The latter are generally positive for epithelial markers, such as cytokeratin, p40/p63, or EMA. Some types of sarcoma may also express cytokeratin, either aberrantly or as part of the inherent makeup of the lesion (ie, epithelioid sarcoma, synovial sarcoma, and angiosarcoma), but the reactivity in such cases may be spotty and weak, and the tumors will also express other markers that are not normally expressed in carcinomas, such as CD99, bcl-2, ERG, and CD34. Unless very specific features associated with a given tumor are identified or the results of special studies such as immunohistochemistry and molecular pathology yield convincing evidence in favor of a specific diagnosis, it is preferable to diagnose the lesion descriptively and generically as a "low-grade or high-grade sarcoma," with a note detailing the diagnostic possibilities.

Vascular Endothelial Neoplasms

Different types of neoplasms of vascular endothelium may arise in the lung, including hemangiomas, epithelioid hemangioendothelioma (EHE), Kaposi sarcoma, and angiosarcoma. Of these, EHE is the one most frequently encountered as a primary vascular tumor of the lung. Another condition that can be encountered in endoscopic biopsy samples and that needs to be distinguished from a malignant vascular neoplasm is capillary hemangiomatosis which, although not a neoplastic process, will be included in the discussion here because of its potential for confusion with a vascular tumorlike process.

Epithelioid hemangioendothelioma is a malignant vascular neoplasm characterized by a proliferation of large, epithelioid cells with abundant eosinophilic cytoplasm and large, vesicular nuclei with prominent nucleoli. The tumors are most common in young adults but can occur at any age with a female predilection.[44] The tumor is usually multifocal and bilateral and presents as multiple pulmonary nodules within lung parenchyma that measure from a few millimeters to a few centimeters in greatest diameter. Some lesions have been known to regress spontaneously.[45] EHE harbors a consistent and characteristic translocation in chromosomes 1 and 3 that result in the fusion of the *WWTR1* and *CAMTA1* genes.[46] A smaller subset of cases have been identified that harbor a *YAP1*::*TFE3* fusion.[47,48] Molecular testing by FISH and NGS can thus be utilized as an adjunct modality for diagnosis in these tumors in equivocal cases. The lesions have a tendency to fill up the lumen of alveolar spaces in a polypoid fashion, resembling glomerular structures (Fig. 14.13A). The epithelioid cells are usually embedded in abundant chondromyxoid matrix and are characterized

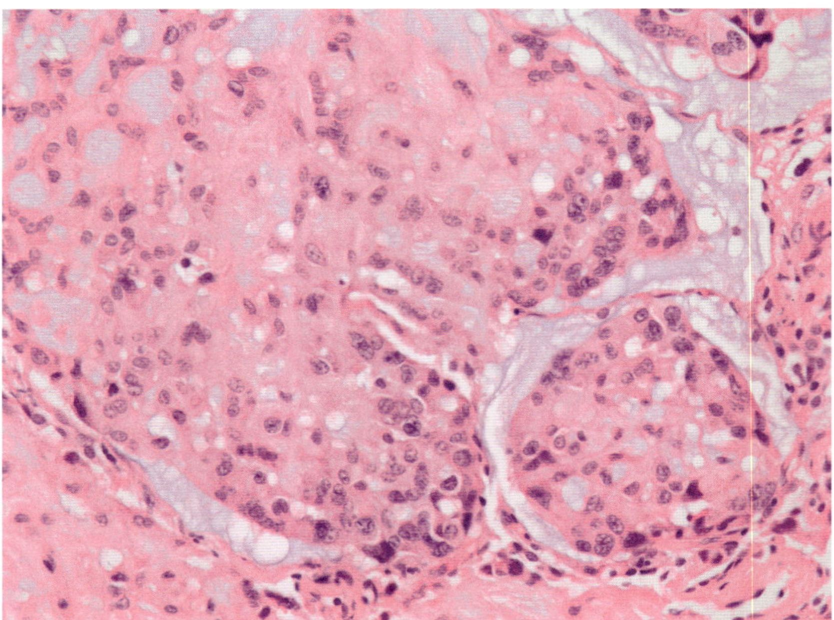

A

FIGURE 14.13 **A**. Epithelioid hemangioendothelioma (EHE) of lung shows polypoid cellular structures filling the alveoli comprising large epithelioid cells with prominent myxoid stroma and numerous cytoplasmic empty vacuoles.

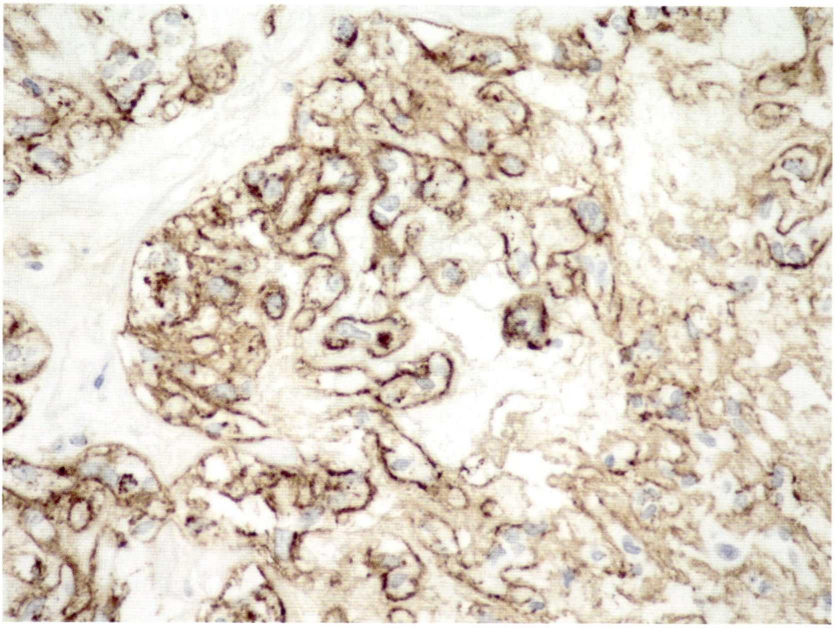

B

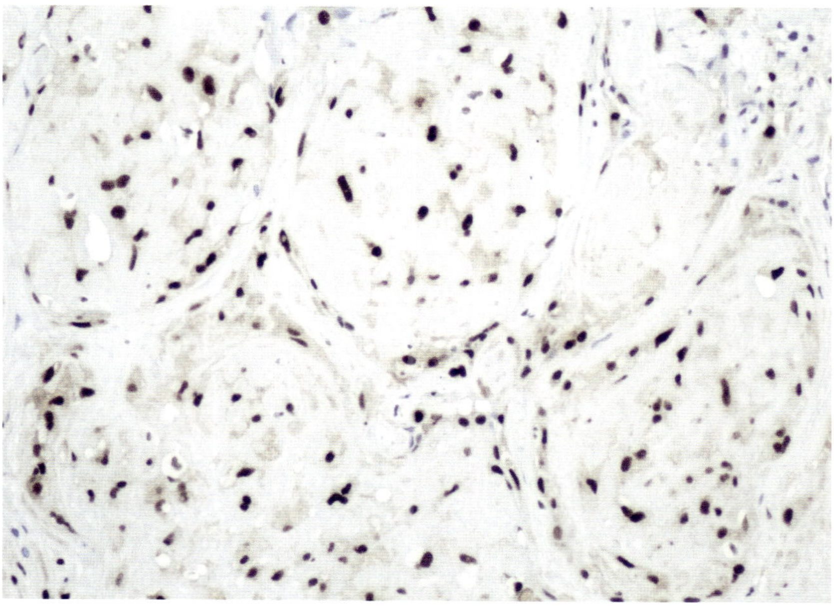

C

FIGURE 14.13 (*continued*) **B.** Immunohistochemical staining of EHE with factor VIII–related antigen highlights the positive epithelioid cells embedded in the myxoid stroma. **C.** Immunohistochemical staining of EHE with ERG shows strong nuclear staining and highlights the vascular nature of the epithelioid cells embedded in the myxoid stroma.

by prominent cytoplasmic vacuoles. Stromal sclerosis is a common finding, and some cases may show foci of calcification or develop a cartilagelike matrix. The tumor cells are positive for vascular endothelium–associated markers, including CD31, CD34, ERG, and FVIII-RA (Fig. 14.13B and C). The use of an antibody for CAMTA1, if available, is recommended because it is relatively sensitive for EHE, whereas TFE3 immunohistochemistry has thus far proved unreliable.[49,50] Of note, the tumor cells can also be positive for cytokeratins, and another potential diagnostic pitfall is the expression of CD10 in these tumors.[51] The lesions need to be distinguished mainly from metastases of chondrosarcoma, chordoma, or metastatic carcinoma.

Kaposi sarcoma is a low-grade vascular malignancy that is associated with human herpes virus 8.[52,53] When it involves the lung, the condition is associated with a poor prognosis. It presents clinically as bilateral interstitial pulmonary infiltrates with ill-defined nodularity, most commonly occurring in a patient with a history of human immunodeficiency virus infection and acquired immunodeficiency syndrome but may be seen in any patient under immunosuppression such as transplant patients or intravenous drug abusers. Histologically, it is characterized by a fascicular spindle cell proliferation that follows intrapulmonary fibrous septa and lymphatics with a perivascular and peribronchial distribution.[54] The cells show mild to moderate atypia with scattered mitoses, and they are admixed with extravasated red blood cells and inflammatory cells (Fig. 14.14A). Dense, eosinophilic hyaline globules can also be seen scattered in the interstitium. The spindle cells are positive for CD31, ERG, and, to a lesser extent, CD34, and they also show strong nuclear staining for human herpes virus 8 (Fig. 14.14B). The diagnosis should be suspected in endoscopic biopsies of patients with a history of immunodeficiency presenting with multiple nodules containing a dense spindle cell proliferation surrounding vessels or lymphatics; appropriate stains should always be ordered to support the diagnosis.

Angiosarcoma of the lung is a rare condition that most often represents a metastasis to the lung rather than a primary tumor.[55] It can present either as a single nodule or as multiple hemorrhagic nodules.[56-58] Occasionally, it may present as diffuse pulmonary hemorrhage.[59] The tumor can exhibit the whole spectrum of features commonly associated with angiosarcoma in their more common locations, from anastomosing vascular spaces lined by atypical endothelial cells, to an atypical spindle cell proliferation with abortive vasoformative structures, to a highly anaplastic malignant neoplasm with epithelioid or pleomorphic features and prominent stromal hemorrhage (Fig. 14.15). The tumor cells are usually positive for vascular markers (CD31, CD34, ERG) but may show patchy or inconsistent staining with FVIII-RA.

Pulmonary capillary hemangiomatosis is a rare cause of pulmonary hypertension and is characterized by uncontrollable capillary proliferation in the pulmonary interstitium and the alveolar walls secondary to postcapillary obstruction.[60] The condition has a peak incidence in the second or third

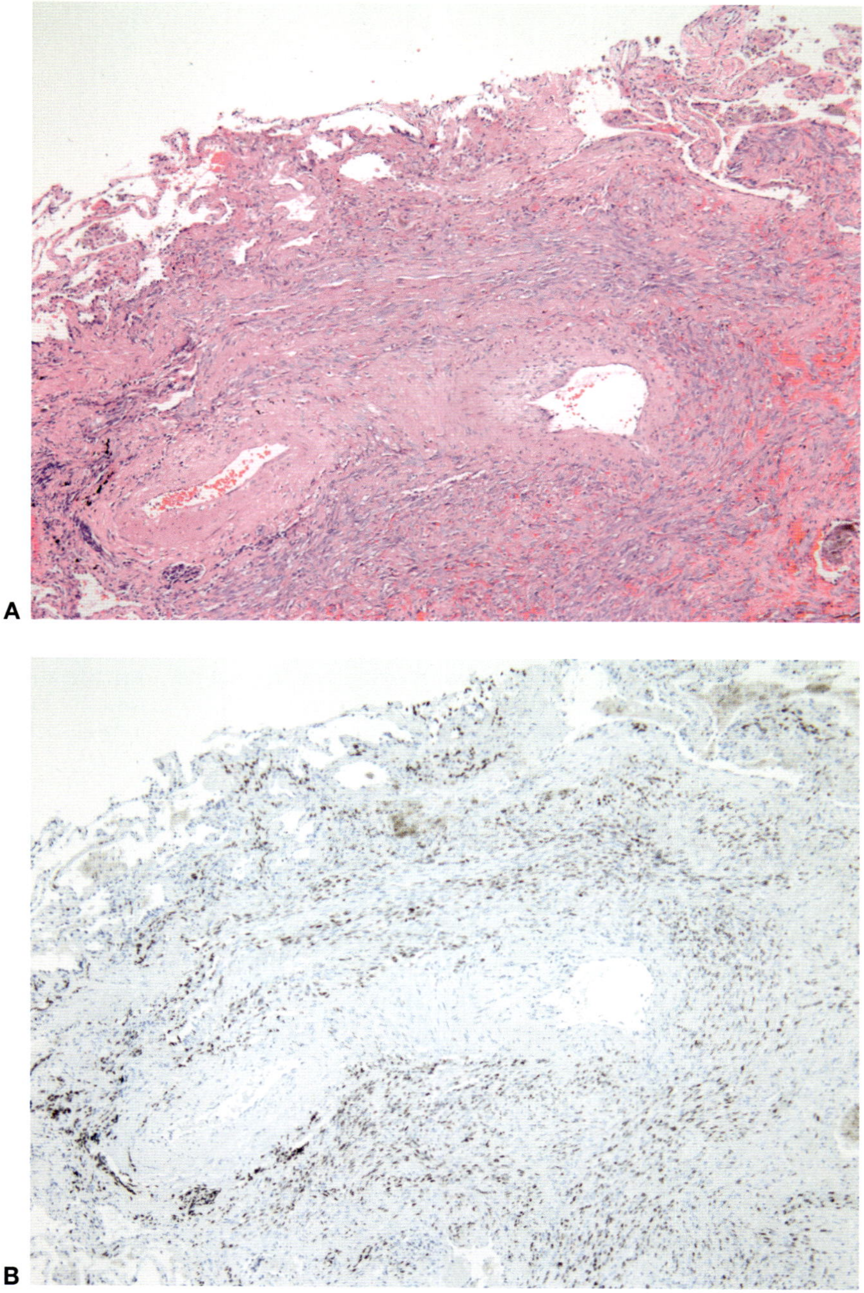

FIGURE 14.14 **A.** Endobronchial biopsy of pulmonary lesion in Kaposi sarcoma shows a dense spindle cell proliferation in a perivascular location admixed with extravasated red blood cells. **B.** Immunohistochemical staining for human herpes virus 8 in Kaposi sarcoma shows strong nuclear staining in the spindle cells.

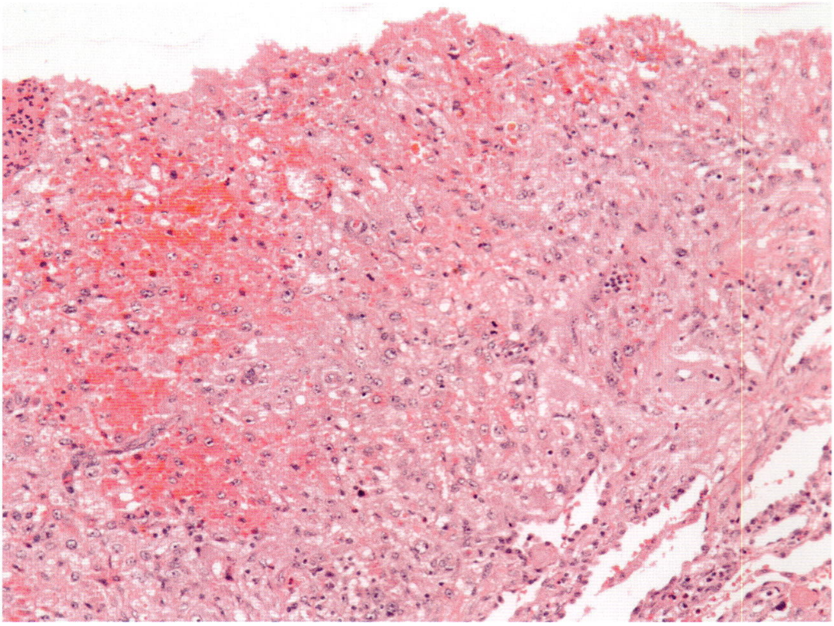

FIGURE 14.15 Endoscopic biopsy in a patient with angiosarcoma of the lung shows an atypical, primitive cell population with extensive stromal hemorrhage and no distinctive growth pattern; such tumors can be diagnosed properly only by the application of immunohistochemical stains for vascular endothelium–associated markers.

decade of life without any gender predilection and presents clinically with worsening dyspnea on exertion in patients with signs of primary pulmonary hypertension. Imaging studies can show multiple, diffuse, centrilobular ground-glass nodules.[61] The process is benign and commonly regarded as nonneoplastic and reactive in nature. Histologically, it is characterized by a striking capillary proliferation infiltrating vascular, bronchial, and interstitial pulmonary structures (Fig. 14.16A and B). Similar findings can be seen in patients with pulmonary veno-occlusive disease, but unlike the latter, pulmonary capillary hemangiomatosis is not accompanied by venulitis or infarction, and there is no identifiable cause of the venous obliteration. Some authors, however, have suggested that these two conditions may be closely related and may represent opposite ends of the same spectrum.[62]

TUMORS DERIVED FROM ECTOPIC TISSUES

Tumors with melanocytic, meningothelial, or thymic phenotype; glomus tumors; and teratomas can occasionally arise in the lung and can display features or evidence of certain lines of differentiation that are not normally present in the lung. Such tumors are presumed to arise from ectopic or embryologically displaced elements.

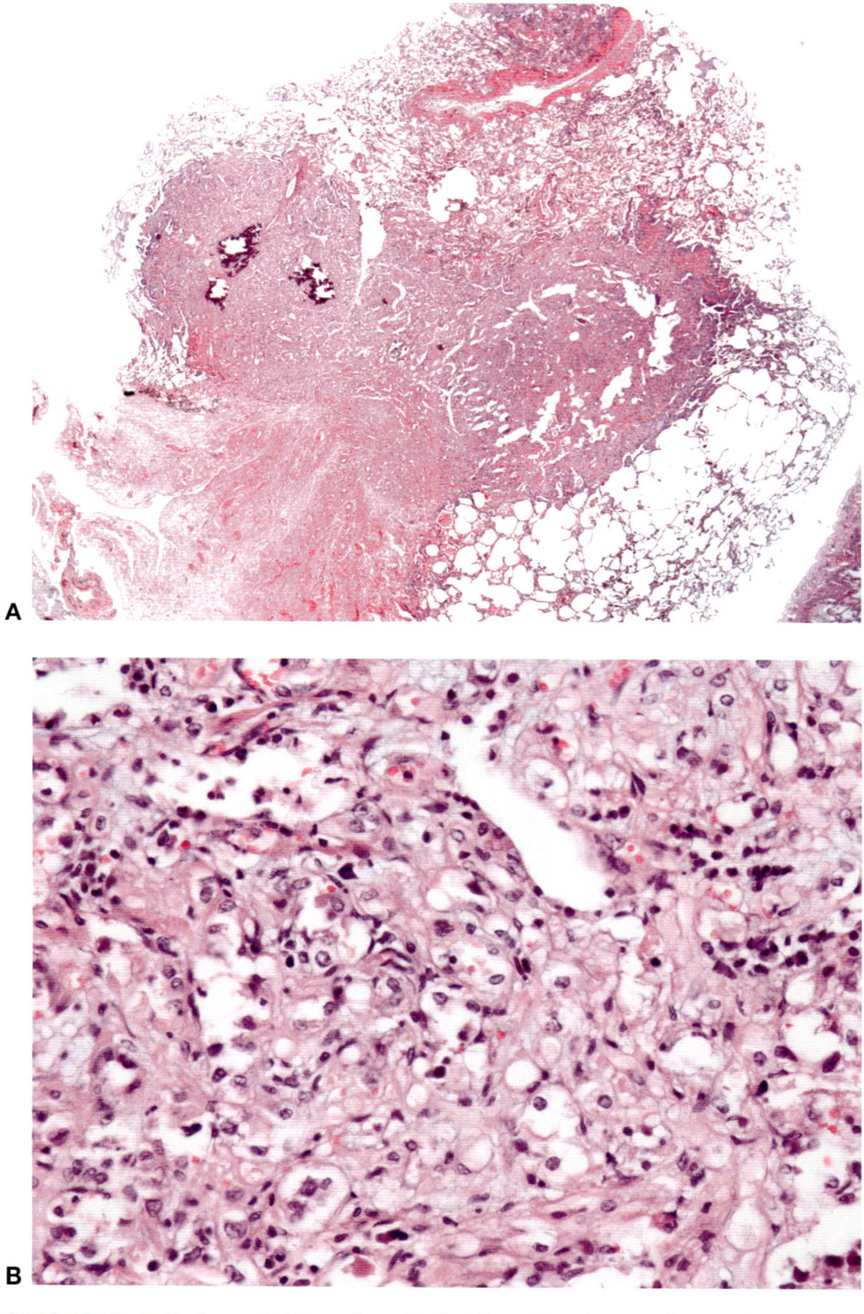

FIGURE 14.16 **A.** Endoscopic biopsy in patient with capillary hemangiomatosis shows focal replacement of lung parenchyma by a dense cellular proliferation, causing consolidation of air spaces. **B.** Higher magnification shows a compact proliferation of minute capillary vessels replacing the normal underlying architecture.

Pulmonary Melanoma

Primary melanoma of the lung is a rare and controversial entity.[63] Because the lung is a common site of metastases from cutaneous melanoma, care must be taken to obtain a very thorough clinical history before a diagnosis of primary melanoma of the bronchus is rendered.[64] Recent studies have suggested that at least some primary pulmonary melanomas actually represent metastatic disease from occult or regressed cutaneous primaries, based off the presence of UV-related signatures and constellation of cutaneous melanoma–associated mutations identified in these tumors.[65] The tumors can present as polypoid, endobronchial lesions that obstruct the bronchial lumen, or they may grow as an intraparenchymatous mass.[66] Histologically, the tumors may show an in situ component in the bronchial mucosa that can be confused for squamous carcinoma in small endoscopic biopsies. The lesions, however, extensively infiltrate the bronchial wall and grow as sheets or nests of epithelioid to spindle cells with marked cytologic atypia, prominent nucleoli, and frequent mitotic figures. Melanin pigment may or may not be seen. Identification of the characteristic nested growth pattern is a helpful clue for diagnosis. Immunohistochemical stains will show strong positivity of the tumor cells for melanoma-associated markers, including S-100 protein, HMB45, SOX10, Melan-A, and tyrosinase. Melanoma may also be positive for epithelial markers, in particular, carcinoembryonic antigen (CEA); caution must be exercised in interpreting such results, and adding melanocytic markers in the panel to avoid a misdiagnosis should always be considered.

Pulmonary Meningioma and Pulmonary Minute Meningothelial Nodules

Cellular proliferations arising from presumed ectopic or misplaced meningothelial elements in the lung are rare but may be the source of confusion on small biopsy samples. *Primary meningioma* of the lung has been described in the absence of any past history or synchronous evidence of intracranial lesions.[67] The possibility of a late metastasis from an intracranial tumor needs to always be ruled out by means of a thorough clinical history; metastases to the lung from intracranial meningioma have been reported up to 19 years after the initial diagnosis.[68] Primary meningioma usually occurs in adults between 30 and 72 years of age and are usually discovered incidentally on routine chest X-rays. They present as well-circumscribed, subpleural lesions that measure on average 3 to 4 cm in greatest dimension. Histologically, they resemble their intracranial counterpart and are characterized by a proliferation of spindle to oval cells with bland cytologic appearance and occasional intranuclear cytoplasmic inclusions that tend to display focally a marked whorling pattern. Psammoma bodies may be seen scattered throughout the tumor. Mitoses are rare or absent. Immunohistochemical stains show positivity of the tumor cells for EMA and vimentin, and some tumors may stain focally for S-100 protein, cytokeratin, and CD34. Many tumors will also show strong nuclear positivity for progesterone receptors. The tumors are almost always benign and adequately treated by surgical excision. *Pulmonary minute meningothelial nodules* usually represent an incidental finding at autopsy or in resected lung specimens removed for other conditions. They are characterized by minute (1-5 mm) cellular aggregates that show all of the histologic and immunophenotypic attributes of meningothelial cells and are located in the pulmonary interstitium, in the vicinity of small- and medium-sized vessels (Fig. 14.17A and B).[69,70] Some early clonality studies showed that these lesions represented a reactive process;[71] however, more recent studies have demonstrated that they share genetic abnormalities with meningiomas of the central nervous system, including deletion of the *NF2* gene and chromosomal gains in 22q, suggesting that they have a common histogenesis and may represent precursor lesions to meningioma.[72] Because the lesions are microscopic and asymptomatic, they are often missed when other dominant pathology is present. A rare presentation of this condition has also been described, which has been designated as *diffuse pulmonary meningotheliomatosis.*[73] Such lesions are usually multiple and bilateral and can present with symptoms of progressive shortness of breath and bilateral interstitial reticulonodular lung infiltrates on imaging studies. Endoscopic or open lung biopsies performed in such patients

A

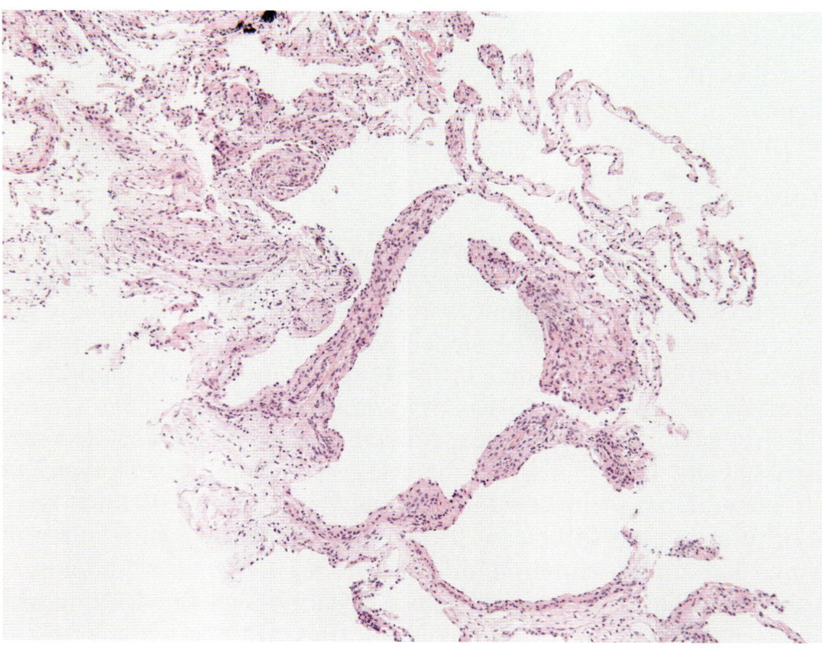

FIGURE 14.17 **A.** Transbronchial lung biopsy in a symptomatic patient with diffuse reticulonodular disease shows focally very subtle thickening of alveolar septae by a spindle cell proliferation.

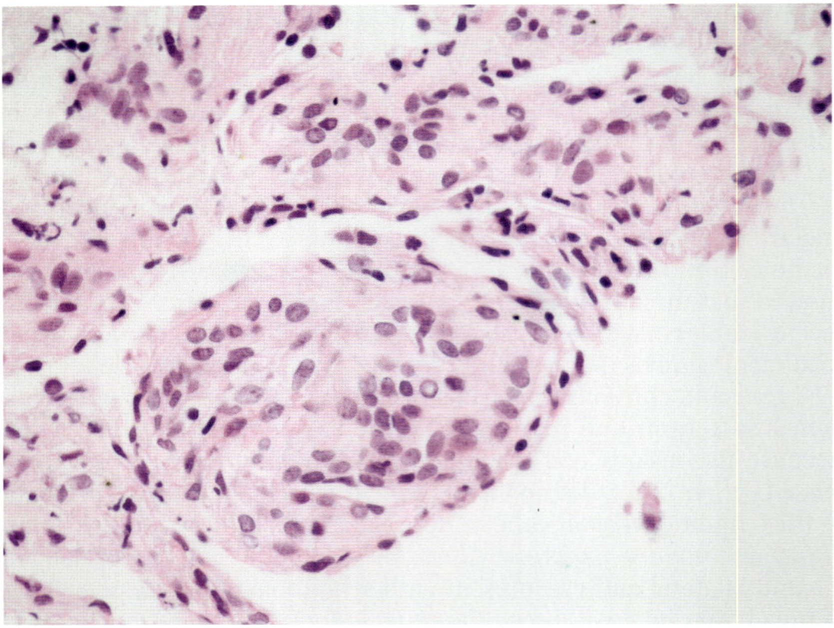

B

FIGURE 14.17 (*continued*) **B.** Higher magnification reveals minute meningothelial-like nodules in the walls of the alveoli composed of plump oval to spindle cells adopting a whorled appearance.

will show the meningothelial nodules to be the sole pathology. Correct diagnosis in such instances will be of importance in explaining the symptoms and the results of imaging studies.

Intrapulmonary Thymoma

Intrapulmonary thymoma represents a rare form of presentation for these tumors, which are normally located in the anterior mediastinum. When arising as primary tumors in the lung, they can essentially display the entire spectrum of histologic features of mediastinal thymomas.[74] The tumors can be located either in the lung hilum or in the periphery and can range in size from 1 to 10 cm in greatest diameter. They are usually well circumscribed and unencapsulated and have a rubbery cut surface. Histologically, they can show the features of spindle cell, lymphocyte-rich, mixed lymphoepithelial, or epithelial-rich (atypical) thymoma. The majority of tumors will retain some of the organotypical features of the thymus, including lobulation, dilated perivascular spaces, and admixture of the epithelial cells with immature T lymphocytes in varying proportions (Fig. 14.18A and B). The lymphocyte-rich tumors can be confused for lymphoma, particularly in small biopsies in which the lobulation or perivascular spaces are not easily identified. Immunohistochemical stains for cytokeratin or p63 will be indicated to identify the scattered

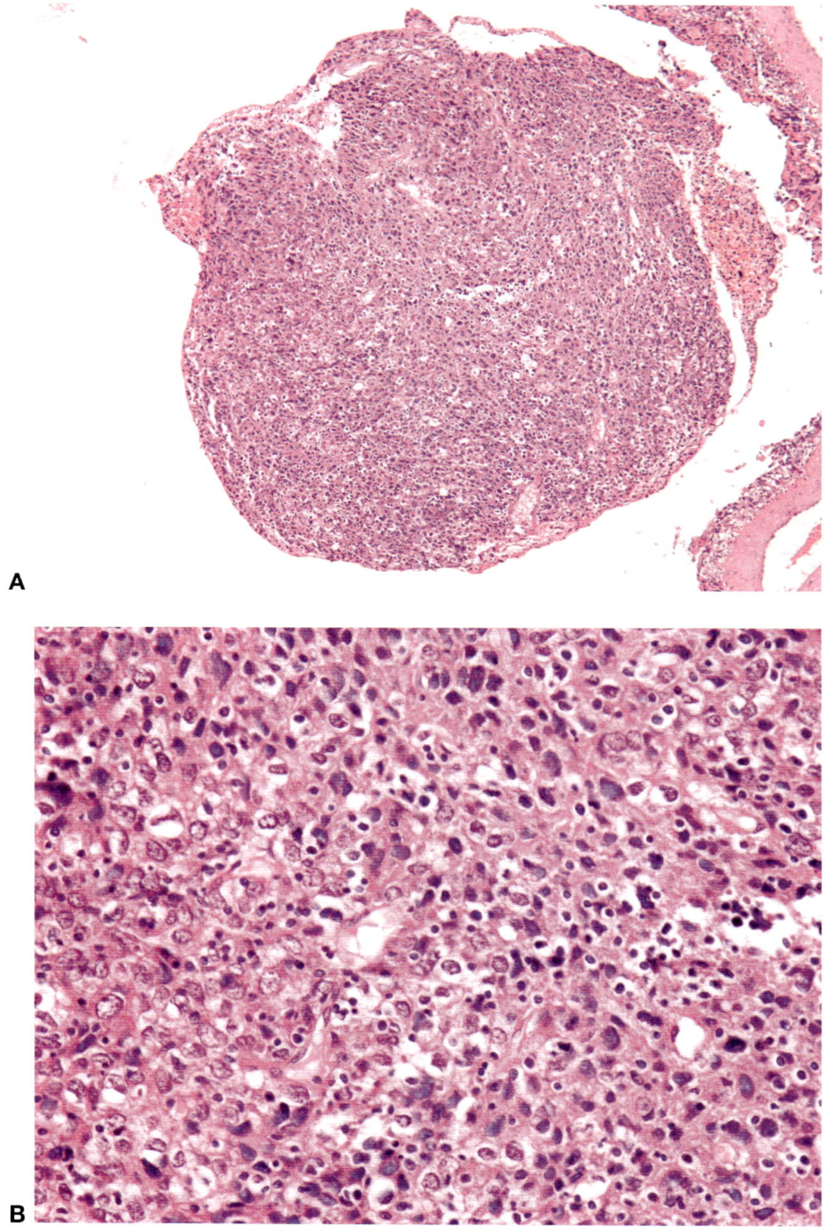

FIGURE 14.18 **A.** Endoscopic biopsy of intrapulmonary thymoma (atypical thymoma) shows a cluster of cells showing sheets of small lymphocytes admixed with larger epithelioid cells. **B.** Higher magnification showing admixtures of small lymphocytes with larger cells with vesicular nuclei and indistinct rim of amphophilic cytoplasm. Immunohistochemical stains are necessary to make the correct diagnosis; the large cells with vesicular nuclei should be strongly positive for cytokeratin and p63, and the surrounding lymphocytes should type as immature T lymphocytes (CD1a+, CD3+, TdT+, CD99+).

proliferating epithelial cells admixed with the lymphocytes. In addition, the lymphocytes will stain strongly with CD1a, TdT, and CD99, indicating their immature lymphoblastic phenotype.[75] Epithelial-rich tumors may be confused with well-differentiated squamous cell carcinomas; the lack of small, infiltrative islands of tumor cells and of marked cytologic atypia will be a helpful clue to separate them from the latter. Use of immunohistochemical markers is recommended when evaluating a bland-appearing spindle or epithelioid cell population of the lung showing an intimate admixture of epithelial cells with scattered small T lymphocytes.

Benign and Malignant Glomus Tumors

Tumors bearing the morphologic and immunohistochemical features of both benign and malignant glomus tumors have been reported in the lung. Because glomus tumors can sometimes metastasize late in the course of the disease, care must be taken to rule out the possibility of a late metastasis in patients with such lesions. Glomus tumors can encompass a range of morphologic features and biologic behavior that ranges from benign glomangioma to malignant glomus tumor, or glomangiosarcoma.[76-78] Glomus tumors can present either as a central or as a peripheral solitary lesion located within lung parenchyma. They range in size from 1 to 6 cm in greatest dimension and can occur across a broad age range (20-65 years).[79-81] Histologically, pulmonary glomus tumors resemble their soft tissue counterpart and are characterized by a monotonous population of round to polygonal cells containing dark, round nuclei and ample eosinophilic or clear cytoplasm. The tumor cells show a tendency to surround vascular spaces, which can often display striking perivascular hyalinization. The malignant variant, glomangiosarcoma, is characterized by more pronounced cytologic atypia with mitotic activity and focal areas of tumor necrosis. The tumor cells are positive for vimentin and muscle-specific actin and do not stain for other differentiation markers such as cytokeratins, EMA, CEA, S-100 protein, HMB45, CD31, CD34, and FVIII-RA. Of note, one study has described *BRAF* V600E mutations in a small subset of glomus tumors that acted in a malignant fashion; however, additional studies are required to determine the sensitivity and specificity of this finding.[82]

Teratoma

Teratoma is defined as a germ cell tumor that contains elements derived from all three germ layers. Such tumors are exceedingly rare in the lung and may be present either in endobronchial location or as a solitary intraparenchymatous nodule. In some instances, the diagnosis may become quite evident when hair is found on endoscopic examination.[83] Well-formed teeth can also be sometimes observed on imaging studies. The majority of the tumors are identified as cystic structures on chest X-rays that may vary from a few centimeters to 10 cm in size. The clue to the diagnosis lies in identifying the various normal cellular elements of diverse histogenesis present in the lesion, including glandular and epithelial structures of skin, sebaceous adnexa, enteric or other origin admixed with mature cartilage, neural tissue, bone, and other mesodermal elements. Such lesions will only rarely be sampled endoscopically, and the diagnosis is most often established on completely resected specimens following a high index of suspicion on the imaging studies. Testicular malignant teratomas can also occasionally metastasize to the lung as mature teratomas; care must be employed to obtain a careful clinical history before a diagnosis of primary lung teratoma is rendered.[84]

LUNG TUMORS OF UNCERTAIN HISTOGENESIS

Several lung tumors of uncertain histogenesis can infrequently be encountered in biopsy material. The majority represent benign conditions in which the histogenesis is either disputed or unknown, but they have sufficiently distinctive morphologic and/or immunophenotypic features that will permit accurate diagnosis in the majority of instances.

Sclerosing Pneumocytoma (Sclerosing Hemangioma)

Sclerosing pneumocytoma (sclerosing hemangioma) is a tumor of unknown histogenesis that tends to occur more frequently in women in their fourth or fifth decade of life. They are usually found incidentally on routine chest X-rays as a solitary coin lesion. The tumors are most often found in a peripheral subpleural location with a predilection for the lower lobes and are usually well circumscribed, measuring from 1 to 6 cm in greatest dimension.[85] Rare cases have been found in endobronchial locations.[86] The tumors are characterized by varying histologic appearances; four major growth patterns that can be present in varying proportions are identified: solid, papillary, sclerosing, and angiomatous. The solid pattern is characterized by sheets of monotonous round to polygonal tumor cells with small, round, bland-appearing nuclei surrounded by abundant, lightly eosinophilic cytoplasm (Fig. 14.19A; eFigs. 14.9 and 14.10). The tumor cells in these areas are strongly positive for EMA, vimentin, and thyroid transcription factor-1 (TTF-1) and are negative for cytokeratins, vascular endothelium–associated markers, and surfactant apoprotein.[87] The papillary pattern is characterized by papillary structures lined by round to cuboidal cells with a hobnail appearance that contain large, hyperchromatic nuclei with scant cytoplasm. These cells are positive for CK7, TTF-1, napsin A, and p40/p63 and also react with surfactant apoprotein and Clara cell markers, indicating a close kinship with normal alveolar lining epithelial cells and suggesting that it may arise from pneumocytic epithelial elements.[88] The cuboidal cells lining the papillae have also been recently demonstrated to show membranous staining for E-cadherin and β-catenin, two cell adhesion molecules that can be expressed in hyperplastic type II pneumocytes.[89] Although the two cell types have traditionally

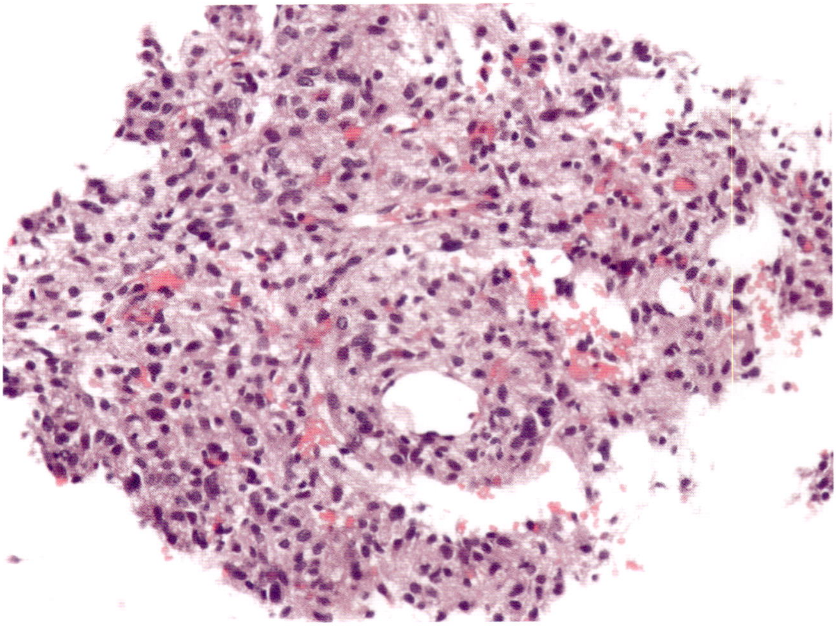

A

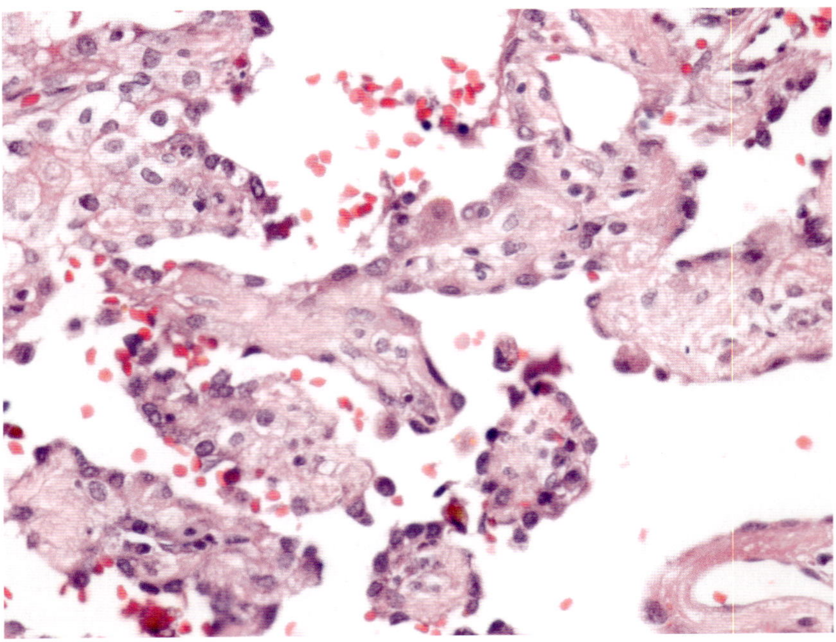

B

FIGURE 14.19 **A.** Endobronchial biopsy of sclerosing pneumocytoma shows a small fragment containing solid population of monotonous, bland-appearing, round to polygonal tumor cells devoid of cytologic atypia; tumor cells in these areas label with epithelial membrane antigen and thyroid transcription factor-1. **B.** Papillary areas in sclerosing pneumocytoma show characteristic hyperchromatic hobnail cells lining the papilla; notice, however, the distinctive round cells with clear cytoplasm located within the cores of the papillae.

been regarded as being neoplastic in nature, the latter finding raises the interesting possibility that the cuboidal cells lining the papillae may actually represent reactive type II pneumocytes entrapped within the growing tumor and that the only neoplastic component is the round polygonal cells present in the more solid portions of the tumor. This is further supported by transcriptomic analysis using RNA sequencing, which demonstrated that the cuboidal cells exhibit characteristics of type II alveolar epithelial cells.[90] The cores of the papillae may also contain monotonous round or polygonal cells identical to those seen in the solid areas (Fig. 14.19B). The sclerosing pattern is characterized by confluent areas of stromal hyalinization, particularly around vessels, admixed with the solid monotonous round cell population. The angiomatous pattern is characterized by clusters of dilated vascular spaces filled with pools of blood, showing a superficial resemblance on scanning magnification to cavernous hemangioma; the stroma surrounding the dilated vascular spaces is occupied by the same type of cells as in the solid pattern. On small biopsy samples, making a diagnosis of sclerosing pneumocytoma can be quite challenging because it will not be feasible to appreciate the admixture of the various patterns, which is one of the hallmarks of this lesion. A high level of suspicion needs to be observed to make the correct diagnosis. In general, the diagnosis should be suspected when dealing with a bland-appearing cell population comprising monotonous round or polygonal tumor cells with clear cytoplasm and absence of nuclear pleomorphism or mitotic activity. The presence of papillary structures lined by hobnail cells should prompt a search for the characteristic monotonous round cells with clear cytoplasm in the stroma, with application of an appropriate panel of immunohistochemical stains. A tentative diagnosis can be rendered under such circumstances with the recommendation that the tumor be completely excised for further histologic examination and definitive characterization.

Pulmonary PEComa (Clear Cell "Sugar" Tumor)

Pulmonary PEComa, originally described as clear cell "sugar" tumor, is a rare type of tumor that usually presents as a solitary, well-circumscribed intraparenchymatous pulmonary nodule discovered incidentally on routine chest X-rays. The term "sugar" tumor derives from the fact that its cytoplasm is rich in glycogen. Although for many years thought to be of unknown histogenesis, this tumor has more recently been demonstrated to show expression of SMA as well as HMB45, Melan-A, and S-100 protein—markers of myogenic and melanocytic differentiation. This tumor is now acknowledged to be part of the family of tumors comprised of perivascular epithelioid cells (PECs) currently designated as PEComas or myomelanocytic tumors.[91,92] Histologically, the tumors are characterized by a solid, sheetlike proliferation of large round, oval, or polygonal cells with abundant clear to lightly eosinophilic cytoplasm. The tumor cells usually have distinct cytoplasmic borders and contain small, dark nuclei with inconspicuous nucleoli (Fig. 14.20). The tumors often display a prominent

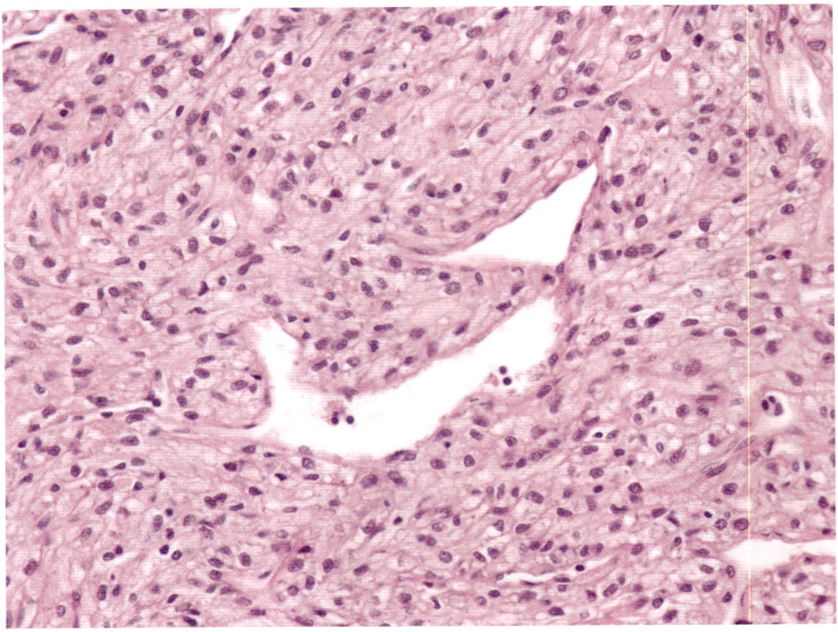

FIGURE 14.20 **Clear cell "sugar" tumor of lung shows sheets of round to oval cells with small nuclei and abundant clear to lightly eosinophilic cytoplasm.** Branching vessels with open lumens are a constant feature of these tumors.

stromal vascular component characterized by large, dilated vessels with branching lumens, resulting in a hemangiopericytic growth pattern. The tumors are negative for all epithelial markers (keratin, EMA, CEA, etc.), distinguishing them from metastatic clear cell carcinomas, as well as for other specific differentiation markers. HMB45 is a marker consistently expressed in these tumors; some cases may also show positivity for CD34, synaptophysin, neuron-specific enolase, CD68, and cathepsin-K.[93] More recently, genetic abnormalities with rearrangement of the *TFE3* gene have also been demonstrated in a subset of cases.[94] The presence of cytoplasmic glycogen in these tumors can be generally demonstrated with a periodic acid-Schiff (PAS) stain with diastase.

Clear Cell Stromal Tumor of the Lung

Clear cell stromal tumor of the lung was originally described by Falconieri et al[95] as "hemangioblastoma-like clear cell stromal tumor" due to its close resemblance with central nervous system hemangioblastoma. The tumors affect principally middle-aged patients and present as solitary nodules ranging from 1 to 9 cm in diameter, although multifocal cases have also been described.[96] The majority of tumors reported so far have behaved in a benign fashion, with only two cases showing distant metastases.[97,98] The tumors are histologically characterized by sheets of round to oval cells with clear to lightly eosinophilic cytoplasm, round monomorphic nuclei with inconspicuous nucleoli, and absence of cytologic atypia (Figs. 14.21 and 14.22). Rare cells with enlarged nuclei and degenerative atypia can also be seen in some cases. Dilated, thin-walled staghorn-shaped vessels are easily identified; small lymphocytes can also be seen scattered among the tumor cells or forming discrete small aggregates. Mitotic activity is either absent or very low, and the tumors are not associated with necrosis. The histologic features are closely reminiscent of clear cell sugar tumor (pulmonary PEComa); unlike PEComas, however, the tumor cells do not express myomelanocytic markers such as SMA, HMB45, S-100, and Melan-A. Recent studies have demonstrated recurrent *YAP1::TFE3* gene fusions in these tumors.[97,98] The *TFE3* rearrangement can be demonstrated by FISH or sequencing studies, or by using YAP1 and TFE3 antibodies by immunoperoxidase techniques.[99] The morphologic similarities and the shared translocation with PEComa has led to the proposal that both tumors may be closely related and represent parts of a spectrum of the same disease.[100] Because many of the reported cases were found in endobronchial location, these tumors are amenable to endoscopic biopsy. The main differential diagnosis is with metastatic clear cell tumors to the lung; appropriate use of immunohistochemical stains and clinical history are required. If metastatic disease is successfully ruled out, the differential diagnosis is with a pulmonary PEComa. Positive diagnosis, however, must

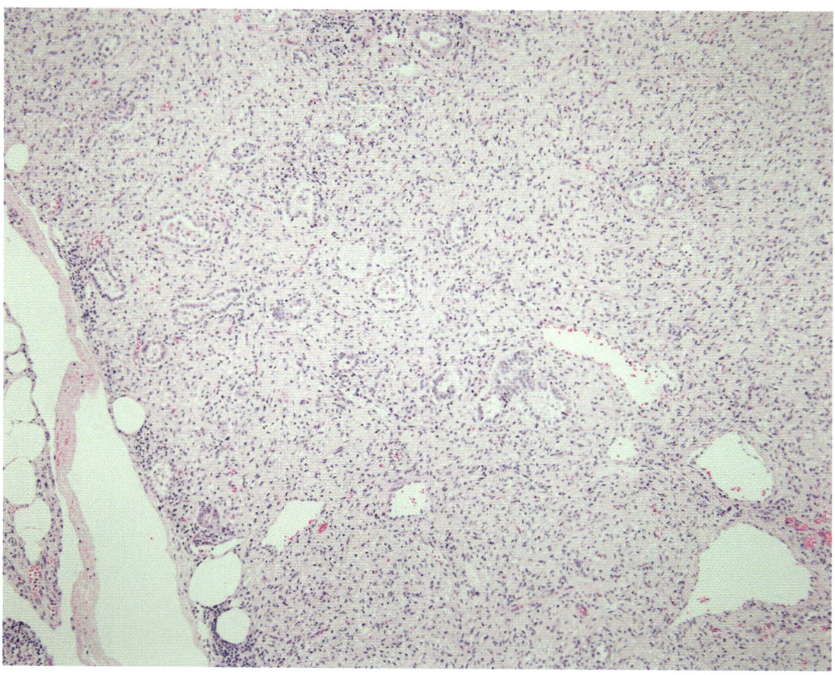

FIGURE 14.21 A Low-power magnification of clear cell stromal tumor of the lung shows a tumor composed of bland spindled cells with admixed irregular blood vessels and entrapped residual pulmonary structures at the periphery of the tumor.

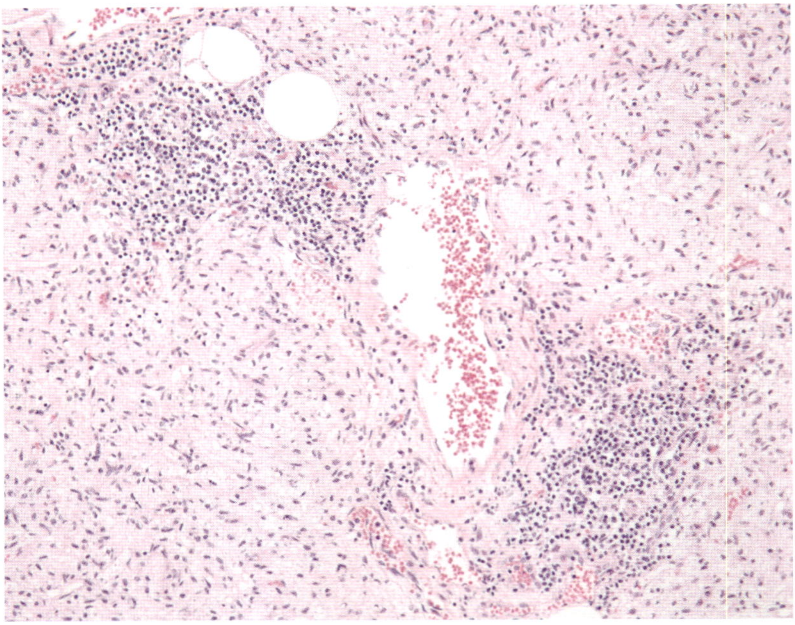

FIGURE 14.22 Higher magnification highlights lightly eosinophilic cytoplasm with clear cell changes.

be based on a combination of negative immunohistochemical stains for myomelanocytic markers and positive staining for TFE3 or molecular demonstration of the translocation.

Granular Cell Tumor

Granular cell tumors occur in middle-aged adults (but can also occur in children) and characteristically present as an endobronchial centrally located mass.[101] They can measure from 1 to 5 cm in diameter and present as polypoid tumors obstructing the airway. Because of the proximal endobronchial location, they are amenable to diagnosis on endoscopic biopsies.[102] These tumors are regarded as being of unknown histogenesis; however, many modern authors consider this to represent the granular cell variant of schwannoma. Histologically, the tumor shows sheets of large, round to polygonal cells with abundant eosinophilic granular cytoplasm and small, centrally placed nuclei devoid of atypia (Fig. 14.23A-C). The tumors are unencapsulated and may show infiltrative borders, with a tendency to entrap normal bronchial structures in its path as well as small nerve trunks. The overlying bronchial epithelium may show squamous metaplasia and can ulcerate. Similar to their soft tissue counterparts, these tumors rarely can display marked cytologic atypia, mitotic activity, and necrosis, heralding a process of transformation to malignancy.[103] The tumor cells consistently express S-100 protein in their nuclei and cytoplasm, and the cytoplasmic granules react positively with PAS stain. The tumor cells also show cytoplasmic positivity for inhibin. The tumors do not react

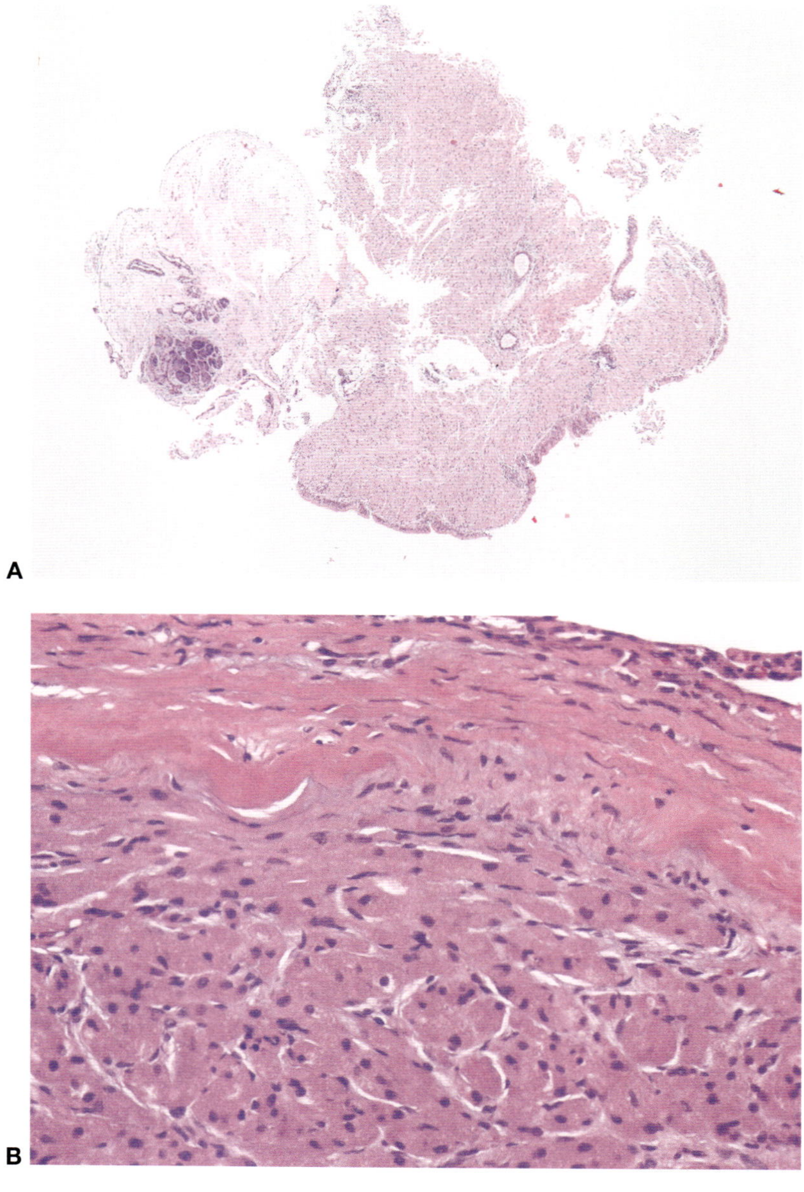

FIGURE 14.23 **A.** Endoscopic biopsy of granular cell tumor of the bronchus shows replacement of the submucosa by sheets of large cells with abundant eosinophilic cytoplasm. **B.** The cells in granular cell tumor sometimes display a vague nested appearance.

with epithelial, muscle, neuroendocrine, or melanocyte-specific markers such as HMB45 or Melan-A. The diagnosis is usually straightforward on endoscopic biopsies. The only significant differential diagnosis is with an oncocytic carcinoid tumor of the bronchus (low-grade neuroendocrine carcinoma), which will be characterized, in addition to the abundant granular cytoplasm, by larger nuclei showing a "salt and pepper" chromatin pattern.

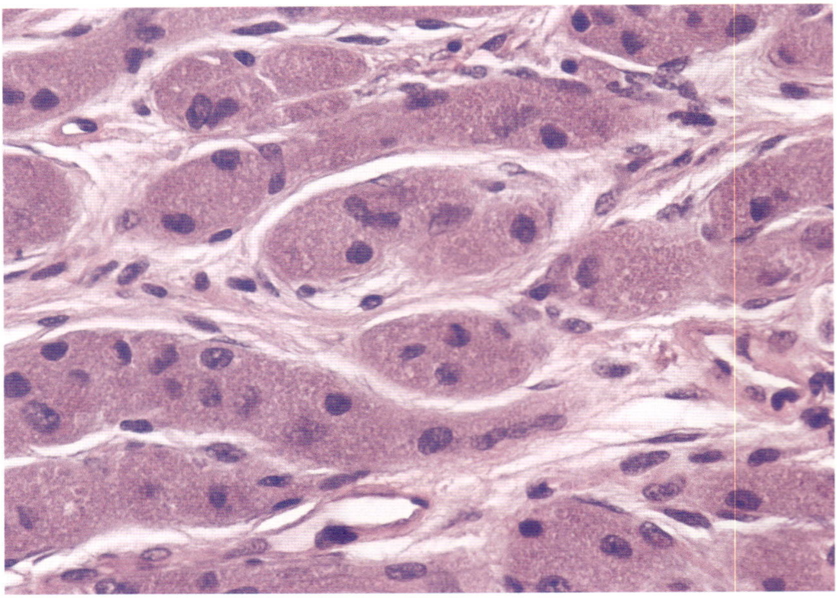
C

FIGURE 14.23 (*continued*) **C.** Higher magnification shows large cells with small, centrally placed nuclei containing abundant granular eosinophilic cytoplasm.

Inflammatory Myofibroblastic Tumor

Inflammatory myofibroblastic tumor (IMT), historically known as inflammatory pseudotumor and plasma cell granuloma, is a process of unknown etiology that has been felt to possibly represent an inflammatory response to previous injury but that has in some cases the attributes of a neoplastic process with the capability for infiltration and destruction of lung parenchyma and invasion of adjacent structures. The fact that some of these lesions can recur and progress to a fully malignant tumor has also been cited as evidence of their neoplastic nature. Cytogenetic and molecular features have been more recently identified that also strongly support a neoplastic process.[104,105] The tumors are rare and have a predilection for children and young adults and may have either a central or a peripheral location. Tumors in peripheral locations can often extend into the pleura and involve extrapulmonary structures. Tumors in central locations show a tendency to grow in a polypoid fashion into the bronchial lumen, causing symptoms of obstruction. Two patterns can be observed histologically: a fibrohistiocytic spindle cell type and a plasma cell type. The fibrohistiocytic type is characterized by fascicles of spindle cells with focal storiform pattern admixed with inflammatory cells (Fig. 14.24A). The spindle cells show elongated nuclei with inconspicuous nucleoli surrounded by a rim of amphophilic to eosinophilic cytoplasm and are generally devoid of cytologic atypia or mitotic activity. Foamy macrophages can be frequently seen admixed with the spindle cells. The plasma cell type is characterized by a predominance of mature plasma cells in the stroma admixed with a

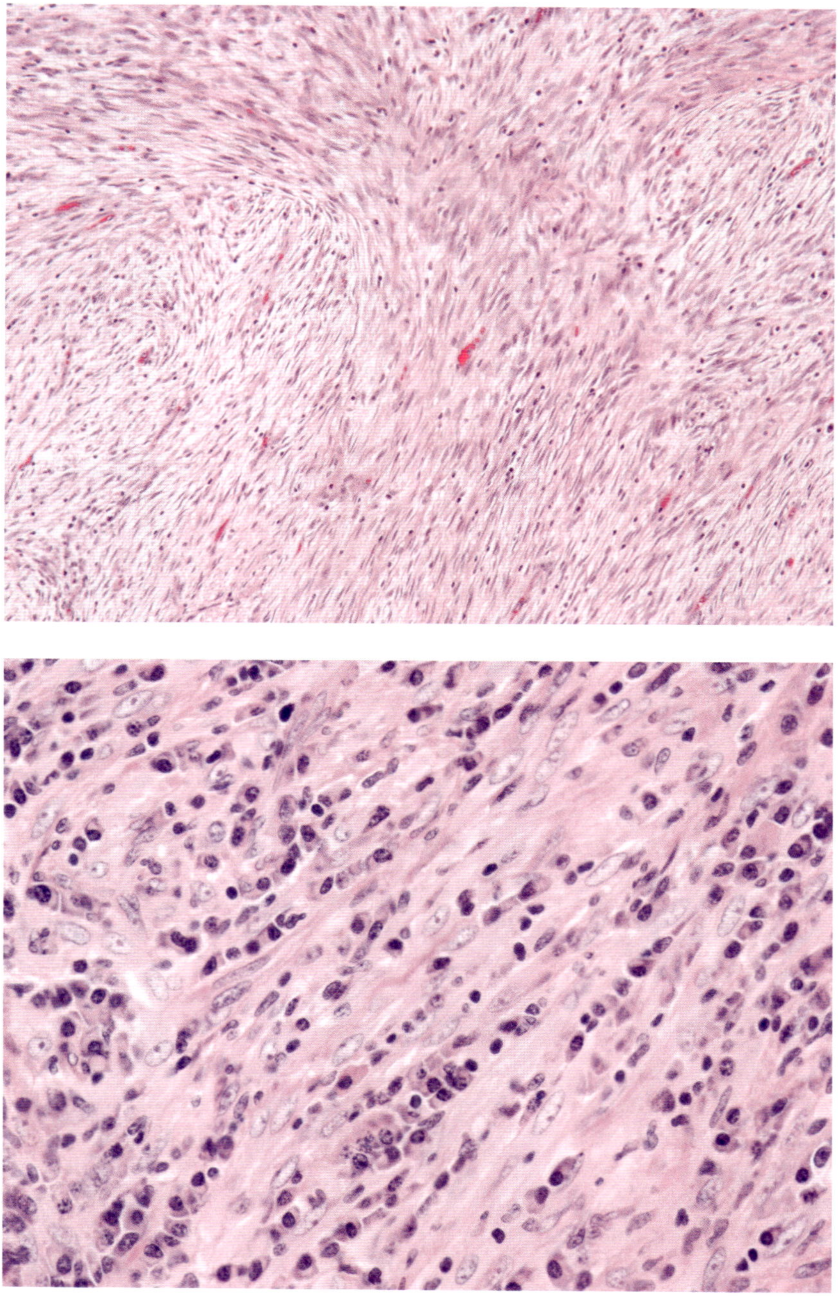

A

B

FIGURE 14.24 **A.** Inflammatory myofibroblastic tumor of the lung, fibrohistiocytic type, shows a bland-appearing fascicular spindle cell proliferation with minor inflammatory component. **B.** Inflammatory myofibroblastic tumor, plasma cell type, shows a fibroblastic spindle cell proliferation accompanied by numerous mature plasma cells.

lesser component of fibroblastic spindle cells (Fig. 14.24B). The plasma cell population will type as polyclonal by immunoperoxidase or other techniques. The spindle cells will show positivity for SMA and vimentin. About one-half of cases have been shown to harbor an anaplastic lymphoma kinase (*ALK*) rearrangement, which can be detected by FISH or NGS or by immunohistochemistry using the ALK antibody-1 (ALK-1).[105] ALK-1 positivity, however, has been observed mostly in children, and absence of this stain does not rule out the diagnosis. A subset of these tumors have also been shown to harbor non-*ALK* fusion events, including rearrangements of *ROS1*, *PDGFR*, and an *ETV6::NTRK3* translocation, an abnormality that is shared with infantile fibrosarcoma.[106,107] Although the behavior of these tumors is generally that of an indolent process, it may be difficult to adequately predict the biologic behavior of these lesions.[108] It may also be difficult in some cases to draw the line between an IMT and a spindle cell sarcoma. The presence of marked cytologic atypia, nuclear pleomorphism, mitotic activity, and tumor cell necrosis favors a diagnosis of sarcoma over that of IMT. The other important differential diagnosis to consider is with *IgG4-related disease (IgG4-RD)*, which may also present as a focal fibroinflammatory lesion with increased numbers of plasma cells; clinical correlation with serum immunoglobulin levels and immunohistochemistry can help differentiate these two lesions. The diagnosis of IMT should be made with caution in endoscopic or core biopsies in the absence of ALK-1 positivity. A descriptive diagnosis and recommendation for complete excision of the lesion is appropriate under such circumstances.

OTHER BENIGN TUMORS AND TUMORLIKE CONDITIONS

A number of other benign tumors and tumorlike conditions can occur in the lung that may be amenable to sampling through endoscopy or by core biopsies.

Immunoglobulin G4–Related Disease

IgG4-related disease (IgG4-RD), or IgG4 sclerosing disease, is a rare systemic fibroinflammatory condition associated with typical histologic features and elevated serum levels of circulating IgG4.[109] The condition was originally described in the pancreas (as autoimmune pancreatitis) but is now acknowledged to involve numerous and diverse organ systems, including organs within the head and neck, thorax, retroperitoneum, and genitourinary system as well as lymph nodes and hepatic and pancreaticobiliary structures.[110] Clinically, IgG4-RD often presents in older individuals aged 50 to 80 years when a tumorlike mass (or masses) or organ enlargement is detected. Other presenting signs and symptoms include weight loss, weakness, cough, chest pain, and exertional dyspnea.[111,112] In some cases, pulmonary involvement may be the first manifestation of the disease.[113] The lesions will often present as a solid nodule within the lung but may also present as organizing pneumonia, multiple masses, airway disease, and pleural disease.[114,115] Elevated serum IgG4 levels are commonly associated with the disease; however, recent studies have shown that a high percentage of patients with IgG4-RD can have normal IgG4 serum levels, while some patients may have elevated serum IgG4 levels unrelated to IgG4-RD.[116] Intrathoracic disease, however, appears to have a slightly higher rate of elevated serum IgG4 compared to extrathoracic disease, so circulating levels may be more helpful in establishing a diagnosis when lung disease is involved.[115] Histologically, the process presents with three primary features: (1) a lymphoplasmacytic infiltrate, (2) fibrosis with at least a focal "storiform" appearance, and (3) obliterative phlebitis (Fig. 14.25A and B).[109] IgG4-RD may also display areas in which the fibrosis appears as small fascicles of bland spindle cells with admixed plasma cells closely resembling IMT (Fig. 14.25C). It is important to note that these features can present in varying proportions, and lesions can have a heterogeneous distribution, making interpretation on biopsy specimens difficult when some features are missing or only seen focally. Immunohistochemical examination of plasma cells with IgG and IgG4 is essential to the diagnosis of IgG4-RD. With respect to lung biopsies, consensus guidelines have established that both the overall number of IgG4+ cells (>20 IgG4+ plasma cells per 10 high-powered fields) and the ratio of IgG4+:IgG+ plasma cells (IgG4+:IgG+ plasma cell ratio >40%) are required for the diagnosis (Fig. 14.25D).[110] These immunohistochemical

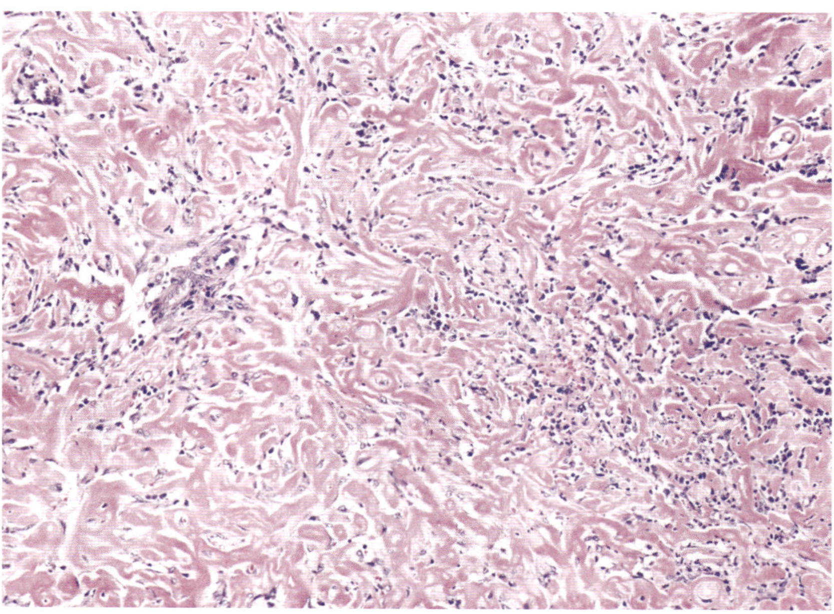

A

FIGURE 14.25 **A.** IgG4-related disease of the lung showing dense fibrosis with focal areas of a storiform pattern and entrapped lymphocytes and plasma cells.

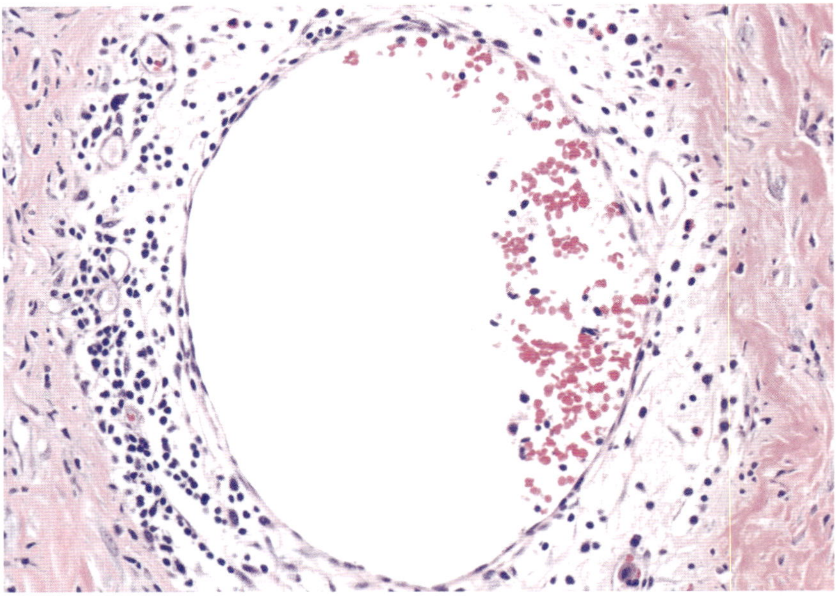

B

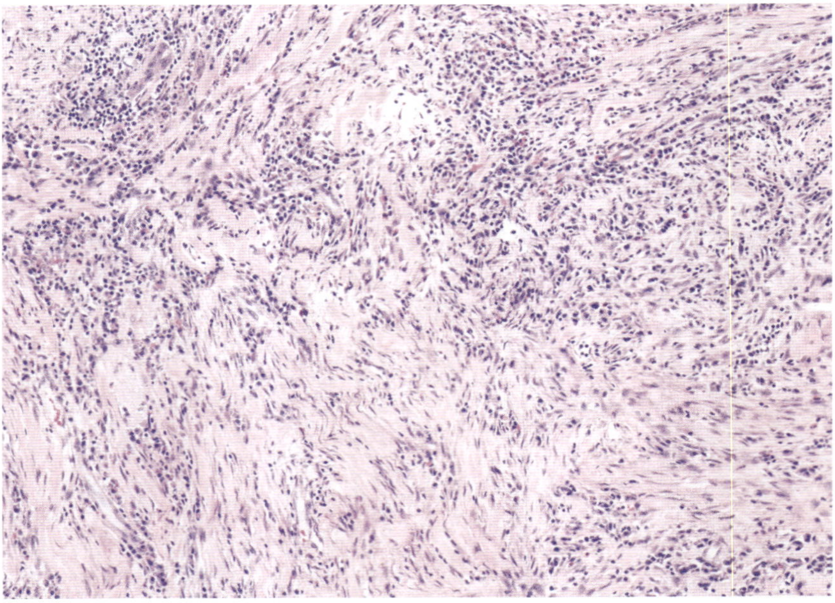

C

FIGURE 14.25 (*continued*) **B.** Focal area of phlebitis with infiltration of a thin-walled vessel by lymphoplasmacytic inflammation. **C.** Portion of a lesion showing increased lymphoplasmacytic inflammation and small wavy fascicles of bland-appearing spindle cells that may be confused with inflammatory myofibroblastic tumor.

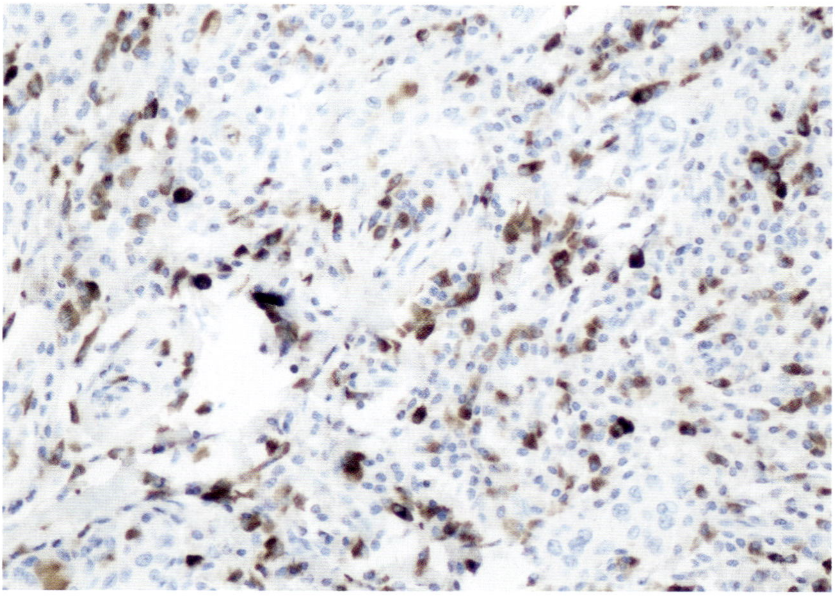

D

FIGURE 14.25 (*continued*) **D.** Immunohistochemistry for IgG4 shows increased numbers of IgG4+ plasma cells.

features must be used in conjunction with the typical histologic features as well as clinical features to establish a definitive diagnosis. On small biopsy material, this may be difficult because some histologic features may be absent or a plasma cell poor area may have been sampled. As the diagnostic features of IgG4-RD can be easily missed on an endoscopic biopsy owing to sampling error, an open biopsy is preferable for definitive diagnosis. When dealing with a biopsy of a fibroinflammatory lesion, care must be taken to rule out other potential causes of lymphoplasmacytic lesions, including underlying infection (cultures and special stains for microorganisms), lymphoma (clonality assessment), and IMT (*ALK/ROS* rearrangements).

Alveolar Adenoma

Alveolar adenoma is a rare benign tumor that usually presents as a small coin lesion within the pulmonary parenchyma and is characterized by multiple large cystic spaces filled with eosinophilic proteinaceous material that superficially resembles dilated lymphatics. The cystic spaces are lined by cuboidal cells with a hobnail appearance, resembling alveolar type II pneumocytes (Fig. 14.26A and B). The interstitium separating the cystic spaces shows collagenous stroma containing scattered bland-appearing spindle cells. The epithelial cells lining the dilated cystic spaces are type II alveolar pneumocytes and stain for keratin, CEA, surfactant apoprotein, and TTF-1. The stromal spindle cells stain for SMA and vimentin.[117]

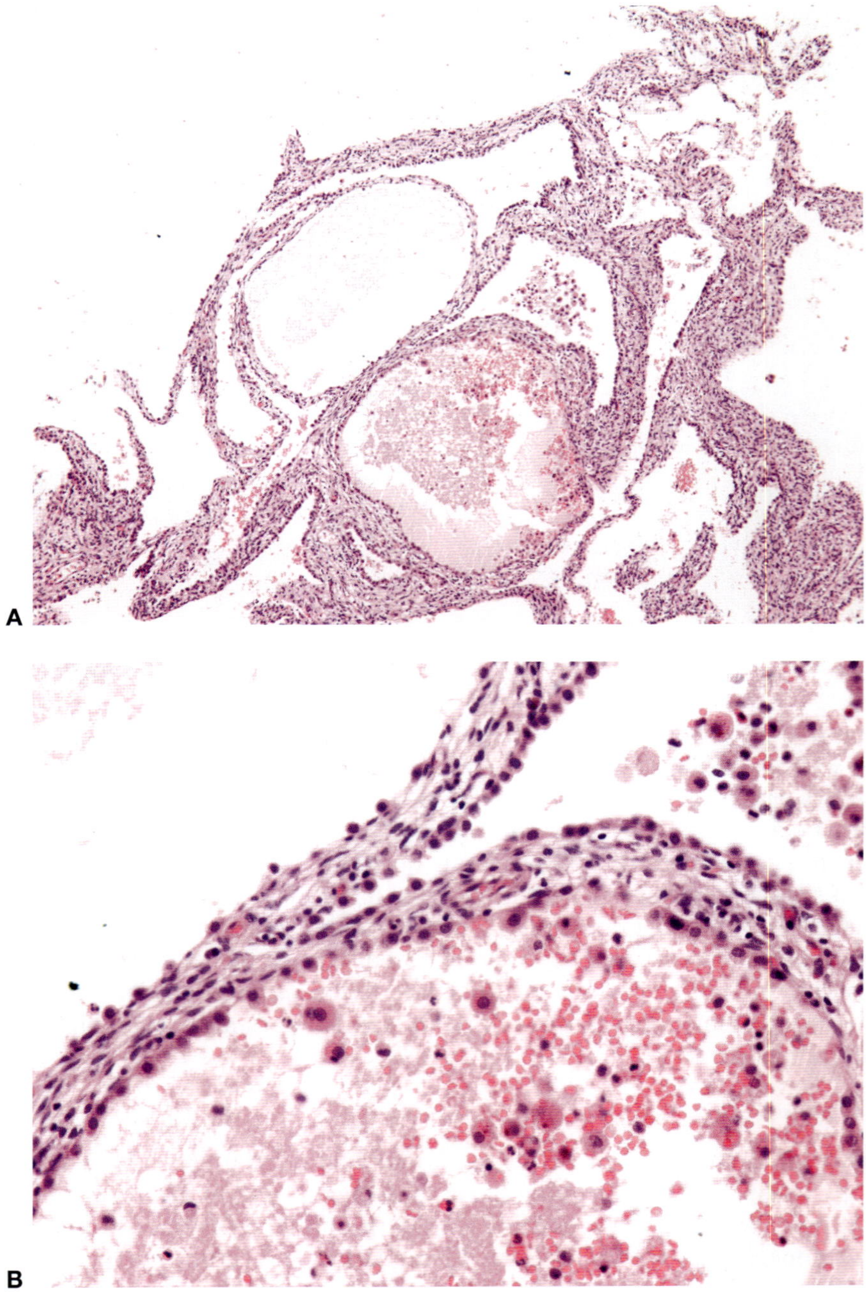

FIGURE 14.26 **A.** Endobronchial biopsy of alveolar adenoma shows dilated spaces filled with proteinaceous fluid simulating distended lymphatics. **B.** Higher magnification shows lining of the cystic spaces by hobnailed type II pneumocytes. Notice the primitive fibroblastic spindle cell proliferation in the septal stroma.

The lesion thus appears to represent a mixed proliferation of alveolar pneumocytes and septal mesenchyme. Very rare cases with few or single cysts have been described.[118] Cytogenetic studies have supported a neoplastic genotype. The main differential diagnosis is with lymphangioma and sclerosing hemangioma. The presence of hobnail cells lining the cystic spaces and cytokeratin/TTF-1 positivity will help distinguish the lesion from lymphangioma. The absence of sheets of monotonous TTF-1+ clear cells in the interstitium surrounding the cystic spaces and the absence of pools of blood in the lumen of the cystic spaces will serve to distinguish it from sclerosing hemangioma.

Mucous Gland Adenoma

Mucous gland adenoma is a rare benign tumor that originates from submucosal seromucinous glands of the proximal airways, leading to bronchial obstruction, mostly in adult patients. They usually appear on endoscopic examination as polypoid endobronchial tumors obstructing the lumen. Small studies have suggested that these tumors represent neoplastic counterparts of mucinous bronchial glands and show upregulation of genes associated with salivary gland tissue.[119] The tumors are usually well circumscribed, with a mucoid consistency and multicystic appearance. Histologically, the tumors are characterized by a proliferation of dilated seromucinous glands as well as nondilated glands and tubules in the submucosa. A distinctive feature of these tumors is the fact that the process is restricted to the submucosa up to the cartilaginous plate and never extends beyond the cartilaginous plate.[120] On higher magnification, the dilated glandular structures are lined mainly by mucinous epithelium, although bland columnar, cuboidal, or flattened mucus-secreting cells as well as foci of squamous metaplasia may also be present. Papillary structures can also be occasionally seen protruding into the lumens. The stroma separating the dilated glands contains a dense inflammatory reaction. The dilated glands may be empty or filled with mucinous material admixed with inflammatory cells. The main differential diagnosis is with a mucoepidermoid carcinoma, and the distinction can be challenging, especially on a small endoscopic biopsy. The complete absence of cytologic atypia, absence of "intermediate" cells or squamoid foci admixed with scattered mucocytes, and the normal appearance of the dilated glands should raise the possibility of a benign process. Mucous gland adenoma is a hematoxylin and eosin diagnosis; immunohistochemical stains play a very limited role in the evaluation of this condition.

Bronchiolar Adenoma/Ciliated Muconodular Papillary Tumor

Bronchiolar adenoma and ciliated muconodular papillary tumor comprise a spectrum of lesions composed of benign bilayered bronchiolar-type epithelium with an associated basal cell layer. The tumors often display a ciliated lining of the epithelium.[121,122] Ciliated muconodular papillary tumors were previously stratified into classic and nonclassic type based on the presence of papillary architecture and ciliated/mucinous cells, though it has been proposed that these tumors now be reclassified under the umbrella term of bronchiolar adenoma.[123] The diagnosis of these tumors is facilitated by identifying the continuous layer of basal cells that are often strongly p40 and CK5/6 positive.[123] The tumors are often misclassified as mucinous adenocarcinoma at time of intraoperative consultation and can be difficult to identify owing to their rare nature. Various molecular alterations, most commonly *BRAF* V600E, have been described supporting a neoplastic origin to these tumors.[123] The tumors appear to almost always behave in a benign fashion, although very rare cases of malignant transformation have been reported.[124]

Pulmonary Alveolar Proteinosis

Pulmonary alveolar proteinosis is a diffuse process that has been observed in association with immunosuppression, autoimmune conditions, fume and dust inhalation, drugs, and hematologic malignancies.[125,126] The process is characterized by alveolar macrophage dysfunction in which the inability to properly catabolize surfactant leads to its accumulation within the alveolar spaces. There appears to be a genetic component in some cases, primarily mutations in surfactant proteins or granulocyte-macrophage colony-stimulating factor.[126,127] The condition affects patients of all ages and may manifest with cough, dyspnea, and diffuse reticulonodular infiltrates in both lung fields. Coalescence of nodules can lead to areas of consolidation. The treatment of the condition is primarily through whole-lung lavages to remove the accumulated infiltrates.[128] The histologic hallmark of the process is filling of the alveoli by acellular proteinaceous eosinophilic material that characteristically stains brightly with PAS (Fig. 14.27). The eosinophilic material tends to show prominent granularity, reminiscent of the frothy exudates seen in *Pneumocystis jirovecii* pneumonia. Electron microscopy has demonstrated lamellar osmiophilic bodies, annular inclusions, and dense granules in the exudate. The underlying pulmonary architecture is preserved, with the absence of fibrosis or other significant alteration in the interstitium. The differential diagnosis is with *P jirovecii* pneumonia; simple histochemical stains can be of assistance for separating the two. PAS stain is positive in alveolar proteinosis but will not stain the frothy infiltrates in *P jirovecii* pneumonia; conversely, Gomori methenamine silver stain will highlight the organisms in *P jirovecii* pneumonia and will be negative in alveolar proteinosis.

Placental Transmogrification

Placental transmogrification refers to a rare condition characterized by extensive replacement of lung parenchyma by structures resembling edematous placental villi.[129,130] The lesions have been described mainly in young adults in association with congenital giant bullous emphysema

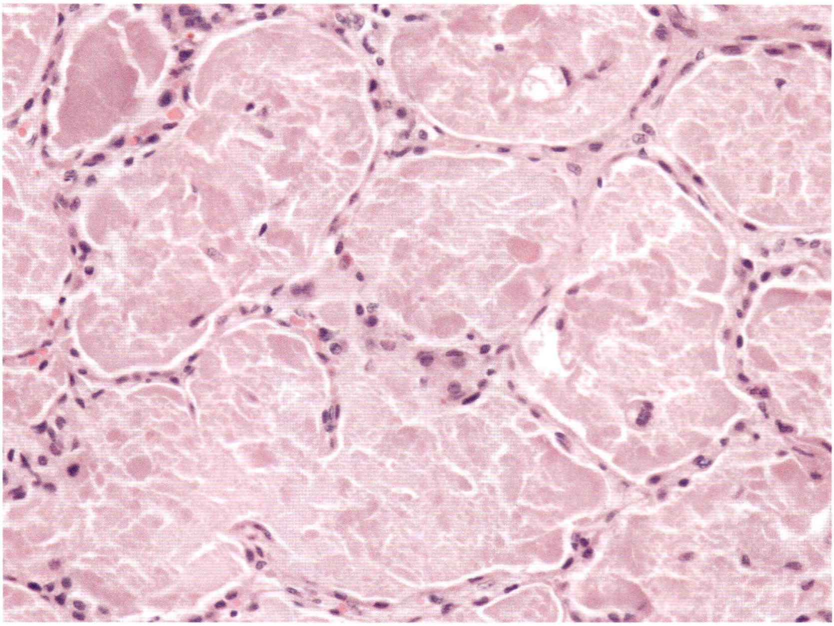

FIGURE 14.27 **Alveolar proteinosis is characterized by distention of alveolar spaces with proteinaceous granular eosinophilic material.** Notice the absence of inflammation or fibrosis in the alveolar walls, a clue to its noninfectious etiology.

and in older adults with severe emphysema related to smoking.[131-133] The alveoli in this condition develop a peculiar villous configuration, resulting from edema and fibrosis of residual strands of alveolar tissue in lungs affected by severe emphysema, leading to the development of grapelike structures and softening of lung parenchyma. The villous-like structures are usually lined on their outer surface by a single layer of cuboidal epithelium (Fig. 14.28). The cores of the papillary-like structures are filled with edema fluid or may show myxoid stroma with scattered small vessels. Some cases may display mature adipose tissue or focal smooth muscle proliferation in the cores. Cases with prominent mature adipose tissue have been interpreted as examples of pulmonary lipomatosis. The striking resemblance to edematous chorionic villi is quite distinctive and greatly facilitates the diagnosis.

Lymphangioleiomyomatosis

Lymphangioleiomyomatosis is a rare multisystem process that occurs predominantly in premenopausal women and is associated in some cases with tuberous sclerosis, with which it shares an alteration in the tumor suppressor gene *TSC2* at chromosomal locus 16p13. Patients present clinically with recurrent bouts of pneumothorax and show the characteristic imaging findings of multiple bilateral nodular and cystic changes

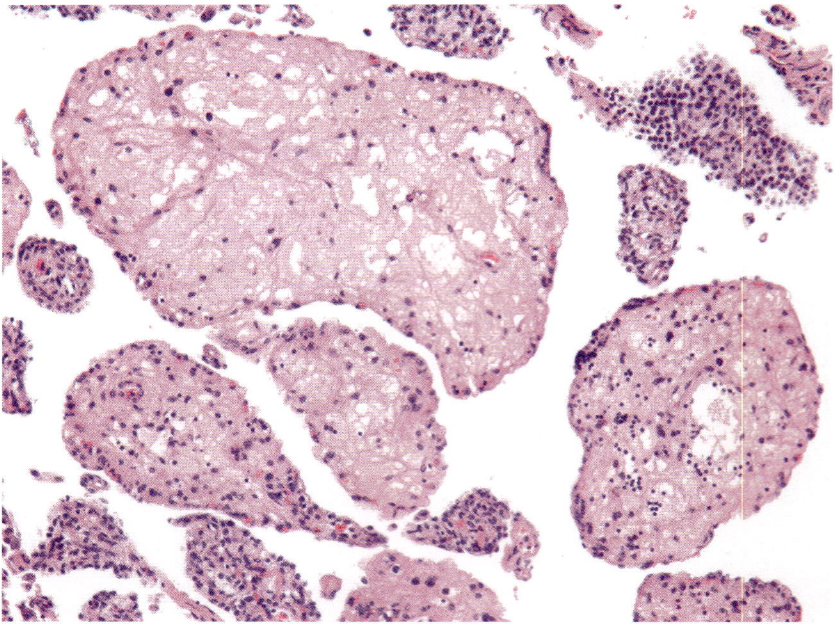

FIGURE 14.28 **Transbronchial biopsy in placental transmogrification of the lung shows distended villous-like structures lined by a single layer of small cuboidal cells on the surface and containing small vessels admixed with myxoid material in their cores.** The structures resemble chorionic villi.

of lung parenchyma with a honeycomb appearance on computerized tomography scans.[134] Although open lung biopsies are the preferred method for establishing a tissue diagnosis, transbronchial biopsies have also been utilized, with good results.[135,136] Histologic examination shows cystic dilatation of air spaces, some of which are at least partially lined by a discrete spindle cell proliferation attached to the walls of the cysts (Fig. 14.29A and B). The spindle cells in these areas resemble smooth muscle and contain elongated nuclei surrounded by lightly eosinophilic to amphophilic fibrillary cytoplasm. The spindle cells may adopt a more epithelioid appearance focally and display abundant clear cytoplasm (Fig. 14.29C). The spindle cell proliferation is not associated with cytologic atypia or mitotic activity and can be extremely subtle and easily missed on initial examination. Attention to the presence of cystically dilated spaces with focal areas of thickening of the walls should prompt closer examination to identify the smooth muscle proliferation. The spindle cells in lymphangioleiomyomatosis have a dual phenotype and coexpress SMA and HMB45; they thus also belong in the family of myomelanocytic proliferations, also known as PEComas. The spindle cells can also stain positive for estrogen and progesterone receptors as well as S-100 protein. The lesions can hardly be confused with any other condition; the differential diagnosis is thus quite limited. The most important consideration is

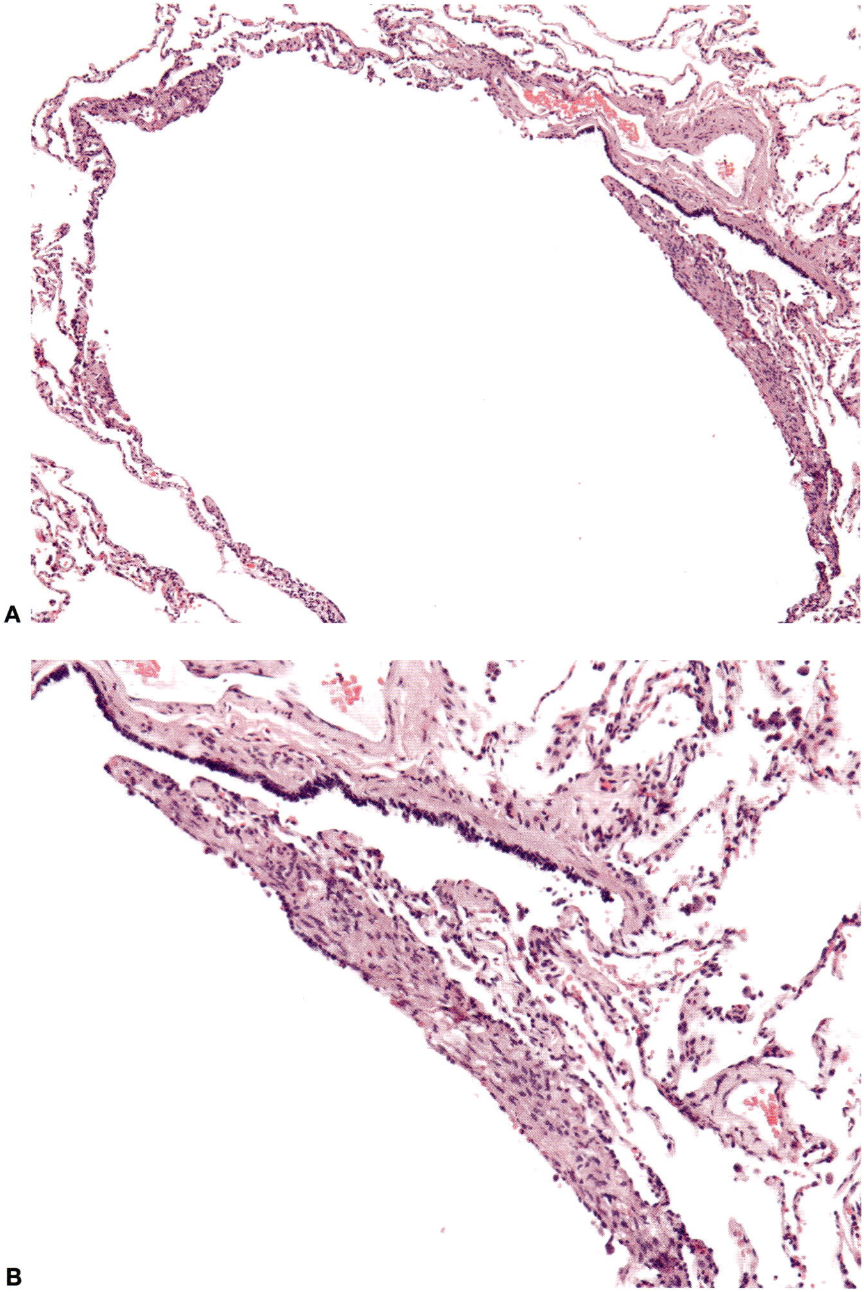

FIGURE 14.29 **Changes seen in endoscopic lung biopsies in lymphangioleiomyomatosis (LAM). A.** Cystic dilatation of air space shows very subtle and focal thickening of the wall. **B.** Higher magnification from same field shows a subtle proliferation of spindle cells beneath the lining mucosa; such a case may be very difficult to diagnose in the absence of clinical information suggestive of LAM.

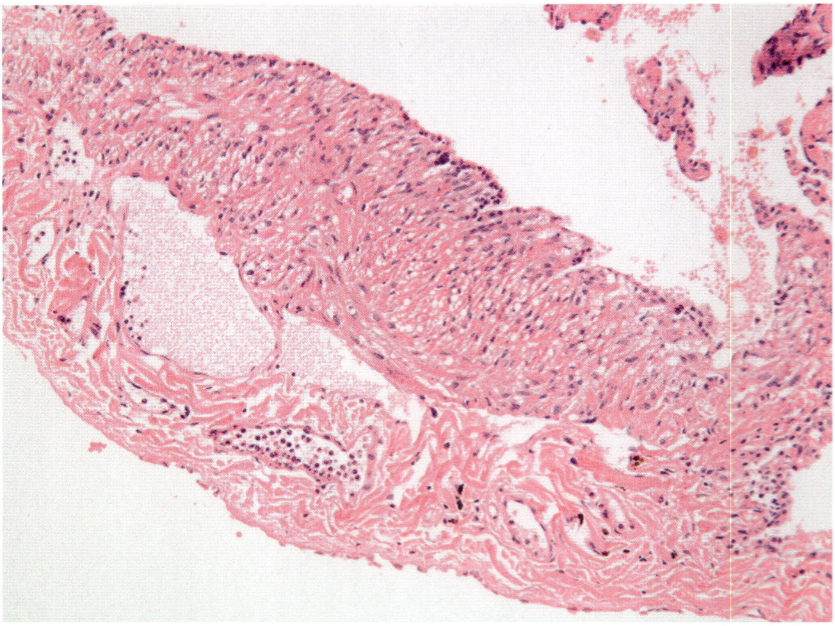

C

FIGURE 14.29 (*continued*) **C.** Another area showing more characteristic spindle cell proliferation with clearing of the cytoplasm. The cells in these areas were positive for actin and HMB45.

simply not missing the lesion, something that can occur quite often when a proper clinical history has not been provided or attention is not paid to the subtle thickening of the cystic spaces and the focal spindle cell proliferation. Use of immunohistochemical stains, in particular, SMA and HMB45, is helpful in highlighting such foci in suspicious cases or in cases with a positive history and typical radiographic findings.

REFERENCES

1. Suster S. Primary sarcomas of the lung. *Semin Diagn Pathol.* 1995;12:140-157.
2. Xiao S, Lux ML, Reeves R, Hudson TJ, Fletcher JA. HMGI(Y) activation by chromosome 6p21 rearrangements in multilineage mesenchymal cells from pulmonary hamartoma. *Am J Pathol.* 1997;150:901-910.
3. Lee DH, Lee JH, Keum DY, Kim DK. Variable alterations of mitochondrial microsatellite instability and DNA copy number in pulmonary hamartomas. *Cancer Biomark.* 2016;17(4):473-478.
4. Suster S, Moran CA. Pulmonary adenofibroma: report of two cases of an unusual type of hamartomatous lesion of the lung. *Histopathology.* 1993;23:547-551.
5. Fusco N, Guerini-Rocco E, Augello C, et al. Recurrent NAB2-STAT6 gene fusions and oestrogen receptor-α expression in pulmonary adenofibromas. *Histopathology.* 2017;70(6):906-917.
6. Moran CA, Suster S, Koss MN. Endobronchial lipomas: a clinicopathologic study of four cases. *Mod Pathol.* 1994;7:212-214.

7. Marcheix B, Brouchet L, Lamarche Y, et al. Pulmonary angiomyolipoma. *Ann Thorac Surg*. 2006;82:1504-1506.
8. Yellin A, Rosenman Y, Lieberman Y. Review of smooth muscle tumors of the lower respiratory tract. *Br J Dis Chest*. 1984;78:337-351.
9. Bosch X, Ramirez J, Font J, et al. Primary intrapulmonary benign schwannoma. A case with ultrastructural and immunohistochemical confirmation. *Eur Respir J*. 1990;3:234-237.
10. Yousem SA, Flynn SD. Intrapulmonary localized fibrous tumor: intraparenchymal so-called localized fibrous mesothelioma. *Am J Clin Pathol*. 1988;89:365-369.
11. Moran CA, Suster S, Koss MN. The spectrum of histologic growth patterns in benign and malignant fibrous tumors of the pleura. *Semin Diagn Pathol*. 1992;9:169-180.
12. Doyle LA, Vivero M, Fletcher CDM, Mertens F, Hornick JL. Nuclear expression of STAT6 distinguishes solitary fibrous tumor from histologic mimics. *Mod Pathol*. 2014;27:390-395.
13. Rao N, Colby TV, Falconieri G, Cohen H, Moran CA, Suster S. Intrapulmonary solitary fibrous tumors: clinicopathologic and immunohistochemical study of 24 cases. *Mod Pathol*. 2011;24:422A.
14. Demicco EG, Wagner MJ, Maki RG, et al. Risk assessment in solitary fibrous tumors: validation and refinement of a risk stratification model. *Mod Pathol*. 2017;30:1433-1442.
15. Moran CA, Suster S, Abbondanzo SL, Koss MN. Primary leiomyosarcomas of the lung: a clinicopathologic and immunohistochemical study of 18 cases. *Mod Pathol*. 1997;10:121-128.
16. Wang HQ, Sun AQ, Liu P, et al. Clinicopathological features of pulmonary artery and vein intimal sarcomas: case series of rare pulmonary vessel intimal sarcoma. *Transl Cancer Res*. 2021;10:3033-3043.
17. Koelsche C, Benhamida JK, Kommoss FKF, et al. Intimal sarcomas and undifferentiated cardiac sarcomas carry mutually exclusive MDM2, MDM4, and CDK6 amplifications and share a common DNA methylation signature. *Mod Pathol*. 2021;34:2122-2129.
18. Zeren H, Moran CA, Suster S, Fishback NF, Koss MN. Primary pulmonary sarcomas with features of monophasic synovial sarcoma: a clinicopathological, immunohistochemical, and ultrastructural study of 25 cases. *Hum Pathol*. 1995;26:474-480.
19. Vlenterie M, Hillebrandt-Roeffen MHS, Flucke UE, et al. Next generation sequencing in synovial sarcoma reveals novel gene mutations. *Oncotarget*. 2015;6(33):34680-34690.
20. Pei J, Zhao X, Patchefsky AS, et al. Clinical application of RNA sequencing in sarcoma diagnosis: an institutional experience. *Medicine (Baltimore)*. 2019;98(25):e16031.
21. Kaplan MA, Goodman MD, Satish J, Bhagavan BS, Travis WD. Primary pulmonary sarcoma with morphologic features of monophasic synovial sarcoma and chromosome translocation t(X;18). *Am J Clin Pathol*. 1996;105:195-199.
22. Suster S, Fisher C, Moran CA. The spectrum of bcl-2 oncoprotein reactivity in benign and malignant spindle cell tumors of soft tissue, skin, serosal surfaces, and gastrointestinal tract. An immunohistochemical study of 380 cases. *Am J Surg Pathol*. 1998;22:863-872.
23. Baranov E, McBride MJ, Bellizi AM, et al. A novel SS18-SSX fusion-specific antibody for the diagnosis of synovial sarcoma. *Am J Surg Pathol*. 2020;44:922-933.
24. Zaborowski M, Vargas AC, Pulvers J, et al. When used together SS18-SSX fusion-specific and SSX C-terminus immunohistochemistry are highly specific and sensitive for the diagnosis of synovial sarcoma and can replace FISH or molecular testing in most cases. *Histopathology*. 2020;77:588-600.
25. Thway K, Nicholson AG, Lawson K, et al. Primary pulmonary myxoid sarcoma with EWSR1-CREB1 fusion: a new tumor entity. *Am J Surg Pathol*. 2011;35(11):1722-1732.
26. Jeon YK, Moon KC, Park SH, Chung DH. Primary pulmonary myxoid sarcomas with EWSR1-CREB1 translocation might originate from primitive peribronchial mesenchymal cells undergoing (myo)fibroblastic differentiation. *Virchows Arch*. 2014;465(4):453-461.

27. Smith SC, Palanisamy N, Betz BL, et al. At the intersection of primary pulmonary myxoid sarcoma and pulmonary angiomatoid fibrous histiocytoma: observation from three new cases. *Histopathology.* 2014;65:144-146.
28. Gui H, Sussman RT, Jian B, Brooks JSJ, Zhang PJL. Primary pulmonary myxoid sarcoma and myxoid angiomatoid fibrous histiocytoma. A unifying continuum with shared and distinct features. *Am J Surg Pathol.* 2020;44:1535-1540.
29. Prieto-Granada CN, Ganim RB, Zhang L, Antonescu C, Mueller J. Primary pulmonary myxoid sarcoma: a newly described entity-report of a case and review of the literature. *Int J Surg Pathol.* 2017;25(6):518-525.
30. Yanagida R, Balzer BL, Mckenna RJ, Fuller CB. Primary pulmonary myxoid sarcoma, a potential mimic of metastatic extraskeletal myxoid chondrosarcoma. *Pathology.* 2017;49(7):792-794.
31. Agaimy A, Duell T, Morresi-Hauf AT. EWSR1-fusion-negative, SMARCB1-deficient primary pulmonary myxoid sarcoma. *Pol J Pathol.* 2017;68(3):261-267.
32. Ren L, Guo P, Zhou XG, Chan JKC. Angiomatoid fibrous histiocytoma: first report of primary lung origin. *Am J Surg Pathol.* 2009;33:1570-1574.
33. Thway K, Nicholson AG, Wallace WA, Al-Nafussi A, Pilling J, Fisher C. Endobronchial pulmonary angiomatoid fibrous histiocytoma: two cases with *EWSR1-CREB1* and *EWSR1-ATF1* fusions. *Am J Surg Pathol.* 2012;36:883-888.
34. Mussot S, Ghigna M-R, Mercier O, et al. Retrospective institutional study of 31 patients treated for pulmonary artery sarcoma. *Eur J Cardiothorac Surg.* 2013;43(4):787-793.
35. Fernandez R, Edgren D, Bharat A. Pulmonary artery sarcoma. *Am J Respir Crit Care Med.* 2017;195(3):e23-e24.
36. Bandyopadhyay D, Panchabhai TS, Bajaj NS, Patil PD, Bunte MC. Primary pulmonary artery sarcoma: a close associate of pulmonary embolism—20-year observational analysis. *J Thorac Dis.* 2016;8(9):2592-2601.
37. Srivali N, Yi ES, Ryu JH. Pulmonary artery sarcoma mimicking pulmonary embolism: a case series. *QJM.* 2017;110(5):283-286.
38. Yin K, Zhang Z, Luo R, et al. Clinical features and surgical outcomes of pulmonary artery sarcoma. *J Thorac Cardiovasc Surg.* 2018;155(3):1109-1115.e1.
39. Tavora F, Miettinen M, Fanburg-Smith J, Franks TJ, Burke A. Pulmonary artery sarcoma: a histologic and follow-up study with emphasis on a subset of low-grade myofibroblastic sarcomas with a good long-term follow-up. *Am J Surg Pathol.* 2008;32(12):1751-1761.
40. Bode-Lesniewska B, Zhao J, Speel EJ, et al. Gains of 12q13-14 and overexpression of mdm2 are frequent findings in intimal sarcomas of the pulmonary artery. *Virchows Arch.* 2001;438(1):57-65.
41. Dewaele B, Floris G, Finalet-Ferreiro J, et al. Coactivated platelet-derived growth factor receptor {alpha} and epidermal growth factor receptor are potential therapeutic targets in intimal sarcoma. *Cancer Res.* 2010;70(18):7304-7314.
42. Yousem SA, Hochholzer L. Malignant fibrous histiocytoma of the lung. *Cancer.* 1987;60:2532-2541.
43. Pleština S, Librenjak N, Marušić A, Vuletić LB, Janevski Z, Jakopović M. An extremely rare primary sarcoma of the lung with peritoneal and small bowel metastases: a case report. *World J Surg Oncol.* 2019;17(1):147.
44. Weiss SW, Ishak KG, Dail DH, Sweet DE, Enzinger FM. Epithelioid hemangioendothelioma and related lesions. *Semin Diagn Pathol.* 1986;3:259-287.
45. Kitaichi M, Nagai S, Nishimura K, et al. Pulmonary epithelioid hemangioendothelioma in 21 patients, including three with partial spontaneous regression. *Eur Respir J.* 1998;12:89-96.
46. Errani C, Zhang L, Sung YS, et al. A novel WWTR1-CAMTA1 gene fusion is a consistent abnormality in epithelioid hemangioendothelioma of different anatomic sites. *Gene Chromosome Cancer.* 2011;50:644-653.

47. Rosenbaum E, Jadeja B, Xu B, et al. Prognostic stratification of clinical and molecular epithelioid hemangioendothelioma subsets. *Mod Pathol.* 2020;33(4):591-602. doi:10.1038/s41379-019-0368-8
48. Lamar JM, Nehru VM, Weinberg G. Epithelioid hemangioendothelioma as a model of YAP/TAZ-driven cancer: insights from a rare fusion sarcoma. *Cancers (Basel).* 2018;10(7):229.
49. Doyle LA, Fletcher CDM, Hornick JL. Nuclear expression of CAMTA1 distinguishes epithelioid hemangioendothelioma from histologic mimics. *Am J Surg Pathol.* 2016;40(1):94-102.
50. Flucke U, Vogels RJC, Somerhausen NDSA, et al. Epithelioid hemangioendothelioma: clinicopathologic, immunohistochemical, and molecular genetic analysis of 39 cases. *Diagn Pathol.* 2014;9:131.
51. Weinreb I, Cunningham KS, Perez-Ordonez B, Hwang DM. CD10 is expressed in most epithelioid hemangioendotheliomas: a potential diagnostic pitfall. *Arch Pathol Lab med.* 2009;133:1965-1968.
52. Meduri GU, Stover DE, Lee M, Myskowski PL, Caravelli JF, Zaman MB. Pulmonary Kaposi's sarcoma in the acquired immune deficiency syndrome. Clinical, radiographic and pathologic manifestations. *Am J Med.* 1986;81:11-18.
53. Howard M, Brink N, Miller R, Tedder R. Association of human herpes virus with pulmonary Kaposi's sarcoma. *Lancet.* 1995;346:712.
54. Nash G, Fligiel S. Kaposi's sarcoma presenting as pulmonary disease in the acquired immunodeficiency syndrome: diagnosis by lung biopsy. *Hum Pathol.* 1984;15:999-1001.
55. Wang H, Shi J, Liu H, et al. Clinical and diagnostic features of angiosarcoma with pulmonary metastases: a retrospective observational study. *Medicine (Baltimore).* 2017;96(36):e8033.
56. Yousem SA. Angiosarcoma presenting in the lung. *Arch Pathol Lab Med.* 1986;110:112-115.
57. Spragg RG, Wolf PL, Haghighi P, Abraham JL, Astarita RW. Angiosarcoma of the lung with fatal pulmonary hemorrhage. *Am J Med.* 1983;74:1072-1076.
58. Grafino M, Alves P, de Almeida MM, et al. Angiosarcoma of the lung. *J Bras Pneumol.* 2016;42(1):68-70.
59. Lin Y, Yu H, Wang C, Zhang D. Primary pulmonary angiosarcoma mimicking diffuse pulmonary hemorrhage: a case report. *Oncol Lett.* 2023;25:211.
60. Wagenvoort CA, Beetstra A, Spijker J. Capillary hemangiomatosis of the lungs. *Histopathology.* 1989;14:212-214.
61. Poletti V, Femia D, Petrarulo S, Marinelli A, Ravaglia C, Piciucchi S. Pulmonary capillary hemangiomatosis/veno-occlusive disease diagnosed by transbronchial cryobiopsy. *Pulmonology*. 2024;30:310-312.
62. Lantuejoul S, Sheppard MN, Corrin B, Burke MM, Nicholson AG. Pulmonary veno-occlusive disease and pulmonary capillary hemangiomatosis: a clinicopathologic study of 35 cases. *Am J Surg Pathol.* 2006;30:850-857.
63. Wilson RW, Moran CA. Primary melanoma of the lung: a clinicopathologic and immunohistochemical study of eight cases. *Am J Surg Pathol.* 1997;21:1196-1202.
64. Littman CD. Metastatic melanoma mimicking primary bronchial melanoma. *Histopathology.* 1991;18:561-563.
65. Yang C, Sanchez-Vega F, Chang JC, et al. Lung-only melanoma: UV mutational signature supports origin from occult cutaneous primaries and argues against the concept of primary pulmonary melanoma. *Mod Pathol.* 2020;33:2244-2255.
66. Barisione E, Boutros A, Mora M, et al. Primary endobronchial melanoma: a case report and clinical management indications. *BMC Pulm Med.* 2024;24:97.
67. Moran CA, Hochholzer L, Rush W, Koss MN. Primary intrapulmonary meningiomas: a clinicopathologic and immunohistochemical study of ten cases. *Cancer.* 1996;78:2328-2333.

68. Kodama K, Doi O, Higashiyama M, Horai T, Nakagawa H. Primary and metastatic meningioma. *Cancer.* 1991;67:1412-1417.
69. Gaffey MJ, Mills SE, Askin FB. Minute pulmonary meningothelial-like nodules: a clinicopathologic study of so-called minute pulmonary chemodectoma. *Am J Surg Pathol.* 1988;12:167-175.
70. Mizutani E, Tsuta K, Maeshima AM, Asamura H, Matsuno Y. Minute pulmonary meningothelial-like nodules: clinicopathologic analysis of 121 patients. *Hum Pathol.* 2009;40(5):678-682.
71. Niho S, Yokose T, Nishiwaki Y, Mukai K. Immunohistochemical and clonal analysis of minute pulmonary meningothelial-like nodules. *Hum Pathol.* 1999;30(4):425-429.
72. Weissferdt A, Tang X, Suster S, Wistuba II, Moran CA. Pleuropulmonary meningothelial proliferations: evidence for a common histogenesis. *Am J Surg Pathol.* 2015;39:1673-1678.
73. Suster S, Moran CA. Diffuse pulmonary meningotheliomatosis. *Am J Surg Pathol.* 2007;31:624-631.
74. Moran CA, Suster S, Fishback NF, Koss MN. Primary intrapulmonary thymoma: a clinicopathologic and immunohistochemical study of eight cases. *Am J Surg Pathol.* 1995;19:304-312.
75. Suster S, Moran CA. Histologic classification of thymoma: the World Health Organization and beyond. *Hematol Oncol Clin North Am.* 2008;22:381-392.
76. Folpe AL, Fanburg-Smith JC, Miettinen M, Weiss SW. Atypical and malignant glomus tumors: analysis of 52 cases, with a proposal for the reclassification of glomus tumors. *Am J Surg Pathol.* 2001;25:1-12.
77. Oide T, Yasufuku K, Shibuya K, Yoshino I, Nakatani Y, Hiroshima K. Primary pulmonary glomus tumor of uncertain malignant potential: a case report with literature review focusing on current concepts of malignancy grade estimation. *Respir Med Case Rep.* 2016;19:143-149.
78. Cunningham JD, Plodkowski AJ, Giri DD, Hwang S. Case report of malignant pulmonary parenchymal glomus tumor: imaging features and review of the literature. *Clin Imaging.* 2016;40(1):144-147.
79. Tang CK, Toker C, Foris NP, Trump BF. Glomangioma of the lung. *Am J Surg Pathol.* 1978;2:103-109.
80. Koss MN, Hochholzer L, Moran CA. Primary pulmonary glomus tumor: a clinicopathologic and immunohistochemical study of two cases. *Mod Pathol.* 1998;11:253-258.
81. Weissferdt A, Kalhor N, Moran CA. Intrathoracic glomus tumors and glomangiosarcomas: a clinicopathological and immunohistochemical study of 14 cases with emphasis on anatomic distribution. *Virchows Arch.* 2016;469:541-546.
82. Dashti NK, Bahrami A, Lee SJ, et al. BRAF V600E mutations occur in a subset of glomus tumors, and are associated with malignant histologic characteristics. *Am J Surg Pathol.* 2017;41(11):1532-1541.
83. Cai C, Zeng Y, Chen H, Gu Y, Zeng Q, Zhong N. Fibrobronchoscopic evidence of endobronchial hairs in intrapulmonary teratoma with hemoptysis but without trichoptysis. *Am J Med Sci.* 2008;336:441-444.
84. Moran CA, Travis WD, Carter D, Koss MN. Metastatic mature teratomas in lung following testicular embryonal carcinoma and teratocarcinoma. *Arch Pathol Lab Med.* 1993;117:641-644.
85. Katzenstein AL, Gmelich JT, Carrington CB. Sclerosing hemangioma of the lung: a clinicopathologic study of 51 cases. *Am J Surg Pathol.* 1980;4:343-356.
86. Devouassoux-Shiosheboran M, de la Fouchardiere A, Thivolet-Bejui F, Sourisseau-Millan ML, Guerin JC, Travis WD. Endobronchial variant of sclerosing hemangioma of the lung: histologic and cytological features of endobronchial material. *Mod Pathol.* 2004;17:252-257.

87. Devouassoux-Shisheboran M, Hayashi T, Linnoila RI, Koss MN, Travis WD. A clinicopathologic study of 100 cases of pulmonary sclerosing hemangioma with immunohistochemical studies: TTF-1 is expressed in both round and surface cells, suggesting an origin from primitive respiratory epithelium. *Am J Surg Pathol.* 2000;24:906-916.

88. Satoh Y, Tsuchiya E, Weng SY, et al. Pulmonary sclerosing hemangioma of the lung. A type II pneumocytoma by immunohistochemical and immunoelectron microscopic studies. *Cancer.* 1989;64:1310-1317.

89. Shun-Dong D, Xiu-Wei Z, Feng-Jie Q, Xu HT, Wang EH. Expression of E-cadherin, beta-catenin and p120^{ctn} in the pulmonary sclerosing hemangioma. *Lung Cancer.* 2007;57:54-59.

90. Shang Z, Xiang C, Ding B, Zhu Q, Yu M, Han Y. Single cell transcriptome analysis reveals 2 subtypes of tumor cells of sclerosing pneumocytoma with distinct molecular features and clinical implications. *Mod Pathol.* 2024;37:100560.

91. Gaffey MJ, Mills SE, Zarbo RJ, Weiss LM, Gown AM. Clear cell tumor of the lung. Immunohistochemical and ultrastructural evidence of melanogenesis. *Am J Surg Pathol.* 1991;15:644-653.

92. Fetsch PA, Fetsch JF, Marincola FM, Travis W, Batts KP, Abati A. Comparison of melanoma antigen recognized by T-cells (MART-1) to HMB-45: additional evidence to support a common lineage for angiomyolipoma, lymphangiomyomatosis, and clear cell sugar tumor. *Mod Pathol.* 1998;11:699-703.

93. Calio A, Mengoli MC, Cavazza A, et al. Cathepsin K expression in clear cell "sugar" tumor (PEComa) of the lung. *Virchows Arch.* 2018;473:55-59.

94. Maloney N, Giannikou K, Lefferts J, Bridge JA, Linos K. Expanding the histomorphologic spectrum of *TFE3*-rearranged perivascular epithelioid cell tumors. *Hum Pathol.* 2018;82:125-130.

95. Falconieri G, Mirra M, Michal M, Suster S. Hemangioblastoma-like clear cell stromal tumor of the lung. *Adv Anat Pathol.* 2013;20:130-135.

96. Weissferdt A, Moran CA. Clear cell stromal tumor of the lung: report of 3 cases with emphasis on multifocal tumors. *Pathol Res Pract.* 2024;264:155722.

97. Agaimy A, Stoehr R, Michal M, et al. Recurrent YAP1-TFE3 gene fusions in clear cell stromal tumor of the lung. *Am J Surg Pathol.* 2021;45:1541-1549.

98. Dehner C, Sadegh D, Boulos F, et al. Clear cell stromal tumor of the lung with YAP1::TFE3 fusion: four cases including a case with highly aggressive clinical course. *Histopathology.* 2022;81:239-245.

99. Odintsov I, Isaacson A, Fritchie KJ, et al. Clear cell stromal tumor of the lung: Clinicopathologic, immunohistochemical, and molecular characterization of eight cases. *Mod Pathol.* 2025;38:100632.

100. Kojima N, Nishino S, Sasahara Y, et al. Inflammatory spindle cell PEComa of the lung with YAP1::TFE3 fusion: a report of two cases and a potential relationship with clear cell stromal tumor. *Histopathology.* 2025;86:365-372.

101. Deavers M, Guinee D, Koss MN, Travis WD. Granular cell tumors of the lung: clinicopathologic study of 20 cases. *Am J Surg Pathol.* 1995;19:627-635.

102. Van der Maten J, Blaauwgeers JL, Sutedja TG, Kwa HB, Postmus PE, Wagenaar SS. Granular cell tumors of the tracheobronchial tree. *J Thorac Cardiovasc Surg.* 2003;126:740-743.

103. Stemm M, Suster D, Wakely PE Jr, Suster S. Typical and atypical granular cell tumors of soft tissue: a clinicopathologic study of 50 patients. *Am J Clin Pathol.* 2017;148(2):161-166.

104. Su LD, Atayde-Perez A, Sheldon S, Fletcher JA, Weiss SW. Inflammatory myofibroblastic tumor: cytogenetic evidence supporting clonal origin. *Mod Pathol.* 1998;11:364-368.

105. Antonescu CR, Suurmeijer AJ, Zhang L, et al. Molecular characterization of inflammatory myofibroblastic tumors with frequent ALK and ROS1 fusions and rare novel RET gene rearrangement. *Am J Surg Pathol.* 2015;39(7):957-967.

106. Alassiri AH, Ali RH, Shen Y, et al. ETV6-NTRK3 is expressed in a subset of ALK-negative inflammatory myofibroblastic tumors. *Am J Surg Pathol.* 2016;40:1051-1061.
107. Lovly CM, Gupta A, Lipson D, et al. Inflammatory myofibroblastic tumors harbor multiple potentially actionable kinase fusions. *Cancer Discov.* 2014;4(8):889-895.
108. Sagar AES, Jimenez CA, Shannon VR. Clinical and histopathologic correlates and management strategies for inflammatory myofibroblastic tumor of the lung. A case series and review of the literature. *Med Oncol.* 2018;35(7):102.
109. Deshpande V, Zen Y, Chan JK, et al. Consensus statement on the pathology of IgG4-related disease. *Mod Pathol.* 2012;25(9):1181-1192.
110. Zen Y, Nakanuma Y. IgG4-related disease: a cross-sectional study of 114 cases. *Am J Surg Pathol.* 2010;34(12):1812-1819.
111. Umehara H, Okazaki K, Nakamura T, et al. Current approach to the diagnosis of IgG4-related disease: combination of comprehensive diagnostic and organ-specific criteria. *Mod Rheumatol.* 2017;27(3):381-391.
112. Bledsoe JR, Della-Torre E, Rovati L, Deshpande V. IgG4-related disease: review of the histopathologic features, differential diagnosis, and therapeutic approach. *APMIS.* 2018;126(6):459-476.
113. Grewal K, Cohen P, Kwon JS, Kaufman DA. IgG4-related disease presenting as a lung mass and weight loss: case report and review of the literature. *Respir Med Case Rep.* 2016;17:27-29.
114. Taniguchi T, Ko M, Seko S, et al. Interstitial pneumonia associated with autoimmune pancreatitis. *Gut.* 2004;53(5):770-771.
115. Ryu JH, Sekiguchi H, Yi ES. Pulmonary manifestations of immunoglobulin G4-related sclerosing disease. *Eur Respir J.* 2012;39(1):180-186.
116. Wallace ZS, Deshpande V, Mattoo H, et al. IgG4-related disease: clinical and laboratory features in one hundred twenty-five patients. *Arthritis Rheumatol.* 2015;67(9):2466-2475.
117. Burke LM, Rush WI, Khoor A, et al. Alveolar adenoma: a histochemical, immunohistochemical, and ultrastructural analysis of 17 cases. *Hum Pathol.* 1999;30:156-167.
118. Matsui H, Utsumi T, Maru N, et al. Alveolar adenoma with a single cyst: A case report. *Med Int (Lond).* 2024;4(2):16.
119. Sasaki E, Masago K, Kogure Y, et al. Mucous gland adenoma of the lung: a neoplastic counterpart of mucinous bronchial glands. *Mod Pathol.* 2023;36:100182.
120. England DM, Hochholzer L. Truly benign "bronchial adenoma": report of 10 cases of mucous gland adenoma with immunohistochemical and ultrastructural findings. *Am J Surg Pathol.* 1995;19:887-899.
121. Zheng Q, Luo R, Jin Y, et al. So-called "non-classic" ciliated muconodular papillary tumors: a comprehensive comparison of the clinicopathological and molecular features with classic ciliated muconodular papillary tumors. *Hum Pathol.* 2018;82:193-201.
122. Takeda-Miyata N, Miyagawa-Hayashino A, Hamada S, et al. A clinicopathologic and molecular analysis of five cases of bronchiolar adenoma with rare mutations. *Pathol Int.* 2022;72:5273-5282.
123. Chang JC, Montecalvo J, Borsu L, et al. Bronchiolar adenoma: expansion of the concept of ciliated muconodular papillary tumors with proposal for revised terminology based on morphologic, immunophenotypic, and genomic analysis of 25 cases. *Am J Surg Pathol.* 2018;42(8):1010-1026.
124. Yang YH, Yin K, Xu JQ, et al. Proximal bronchiolar adenoma with malignant transformation to invasive mucinous adenocarcinoma with 4 years follow-up: a case report and literature review. *Front Oncol.* 2025;15:1491339.
125. Bedrossian CW, Luna MA, Conklin RH, Miller WC. Alveolar proteinosis as a consequence of immunosuppression. A hypothesis based on clinical and pathologic observations. *Hum Pathol.* 1980;11:527-535.

126. Papiris SA, Tsirigotis P, Kolilekas L, et al. Pulmonary alveolar proteinosis: time to shift? *Expert Rev Respir Med.* 2015;9(3):337-349.

127. Borie R, Danel C, Debray MP, et al. Pulmonary alveolar proteinosis. *Eur Respir Rev.* 2011;20(120):98-107.

128. Griese M. Pulmonary alveolar proteinosis: a comprehensive clinical perspective. *Pediatrics.* 2017;140(2):e20170610.

129. Ortiz S, Tortosa F. Pulmonary placental transmogrification: the last 16 years in a reference centre. *Rev Port Pneumol (2006).* 2017;23(3):164-166.

130. Ma DJ, Liu HS, Li SQ, et al. Placental transmogrification of the lung: case report and systematic review of the literature. *Medicine (Baltimore).* 2017;96(35):e7733.

131. Ventura L, Gnetti L, Silini EM, et al. Placental transmogrification of the lung presenting as a giant bulla associated with a pulmonary hamartoma. *Ann Thorac Surg.* 2016;102(1):e61.

132. Lowenthal BM, Saenz NC, Lin GY, Newbury RO. Giant bullous emphysema with placental transmogrification: a case report of a 14-year-old with right middle-and lower-lobe involvement. *Int J Surg Pathol.* 2017;25(8):716-720.

133. Brüstle K, Lema S, Komminoth P, Weder W, Vrugt B, Jungraithmayr W. Placental transmogrification of the lung presenting as progressive symptomatic bullous emphysema. *Thorax.* 2017;72(3):284-285.

134. Gupta N, Vassallo R, Wikenheiser-Brokamp KA, McCormack FX. Diffuse cystic lung disease. Part I. *Am J Respir Crit Care Med.* 2015;191(12):1354-1366.

135. Bonetti F, Chiodera PL, Pea M, et al. Transbronchial biopsy in lymphangioleiomyomatosis of the lung. HMB45 for diagnosis. *Am J Surg Pathol.* 1993;17:1092-1102.

136. Guinee DG Jr, Feuerstein I, Koss MN, Travis WD. Pulmonary lymphangioleiomyomatosis. Diagnosis based on results of transbronchial biopsy and immunohistochemical studies and correlation with high-resolution computed tomography findings. *Arch Pathol Lab Med.* 1994;118:846-849.

15

METASTATIC TUMORS TO THE LUNG

The lung is one of the most frequent visceral sites of metastases for malignancies arising from internal organs. Metastases can reach the lungs through lymphatic or hematogenous routes. The classical presentation of metastatic tumors to the lungs is in the form of multiple bilateral subpleural nodules.[1] Isolated metastases (ie, "coin" lesion) have also been observed in up to 9% of cases.[2,3] Presurgical lung biopsies or intraoperative biopsies are often used for diagnosis of solitary lesions.[4] Distinguishing a primary from metastatic lesion in a lung biopsy may be quite difficult in the absence of a proper clinical history because the morphology of many of the tumors that are capable of metastasizing to the lung can show significant overlap with different primary lung tumors. A multidisciplinary approach that includes clinical and pathologic correlation, results of imaging studies, and comparison of the lesion with previous pathologic material will be critical for accurate diagnosis. Several other factors may also play a role in obscuring the proper identification of metastases in the lungs, including late metastases from low-grade tumors that take place many years after the initial recognition of the primary lesion, changes in morphologic appearance of the metastatic deposits in the lung as compared with the original lesion, unusual mode of spread or distribution of the metastatic deposits in the lung, and unusual or peculiar morphologic appearances of metastatic deposits that may lead to the mistaken assumption of a new or separate, unrelated primary tumor.[5] In addition, a small number of metastases to the lung may correspond to the hematogenous spread of tumors that are deemed by convention to be benign and incapable of metastases; the latter have been categorized as "benign metastasizing" tumors.[1]

METASTASES TO THE LUNGS FROM MALIGNANT EPITHELIAL NEOPLASMS

Because the terminal pulmonary bed is one of the most frequent visceral sites involved in the arrest of circulating tumor cells from internal malignancies, the lung is often one of the first organs, other than the lymph nodes, to be involved by metastatic spread of carcinoma. Metastases of carcinoma to the lungs may occur through hematogenous route, through lymphatics, or by retrograde spread from involved mediastinal or hilar lymph nodes. Most metastases from carcinomas are multiple, sharply circumscribed from the surrounding parenchyma and show rapid growth. The sharp circumscription of the metastatic deposits is a helpful clue on imaging studies to separate them from primary lung cancer that tends to be spiculated on chest X-rays. Solitary metastases from epithelial neoplasms to the lung may be easily mistaken for a primary lung tumor in the absence of a proper clinical history or when the primary tumor remains clinically occult. Clinicopathologic correlation is, thus, indispensable for a correct diagnosis.

Metastases of carcinoma may occasionally adopt a pattern of growth that can closely mimic a primary lung cancer, such as the lepidic growth pattern (Fig. 15.1); this tends to occur particularly with tumors from the colon, breast, pancreas, stomach, and kidney.[5,6] Another unusual presentation for metastases from carcinomas coming from other organs is an endobronchial location; such tumors can present as a polypoid intrabronchial mass, leading to symptoms of obstruction that can closely resemble a primary bronchogenic tumor.[7,8] A common presentation of carcinoma metastases to the lungs is massive lymphangitic spread, particularly from stomach, prostate, breast, or pancreatic cancer, which may lead to the

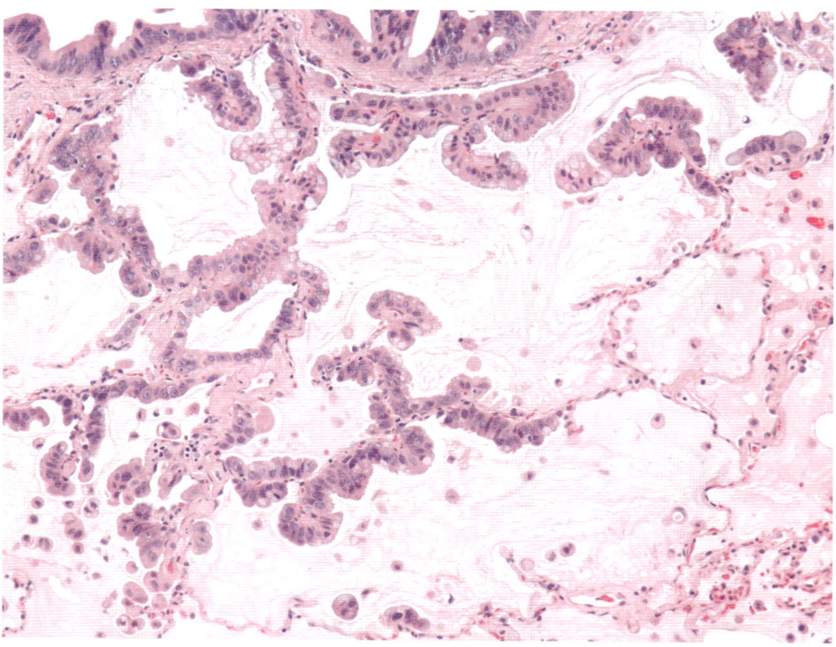

FIGURE 15.1 Metastasis from carcinoma of the pancreas showing lepidic growth along preexisting alveolar septa simulating a mucinous primary lepidic carcinoma of the lung.

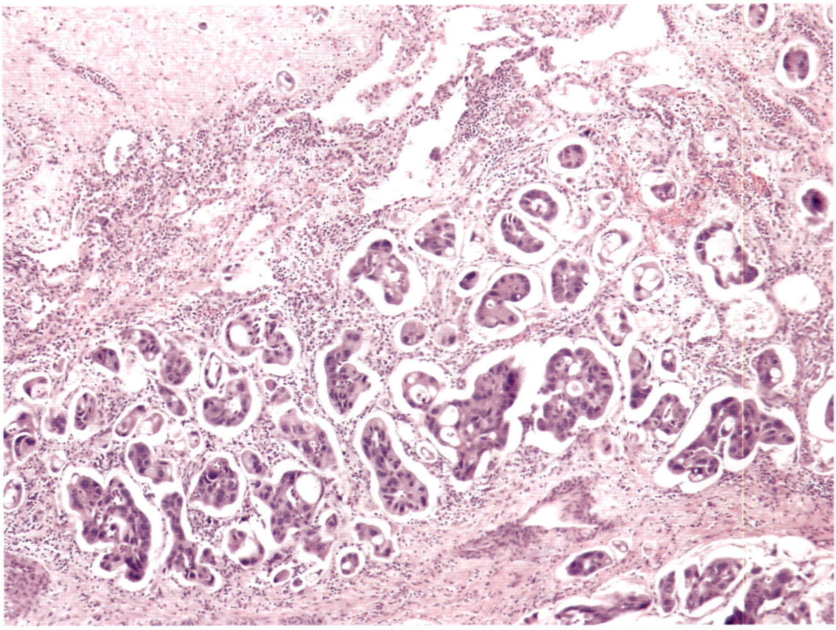

FIGURE 15.2 Metastasis from papillary serous carcinoma of the ovary showing extensive lymphangitic spread throughout septal and bronchial lymphatics ("lymphangitis carcinomatosa").

phenomenon described as "lymphangitis carcinomatosa" characterized by plugging of the peribronchial, septal, and pleural lymphatics by tumor emboli (Fig. 15.2). The diagnosis of metastatic carcinoma to the lung requires communication with the clinician and obtaining a thorough clinical history. Application of immunohistochemical stains or other ancillary techniques may be required in many instances to confirm the lineage of the tumor; review of previous biopsies or resection material will also be necessary to compare with the current lesions, either to confirm the resemblance to the original tumor or to document progression or regression of the malignancy at the metastatic sites.

Metastases From Head and Neck Cancer

Approximately 25% of head and neck cancers metastasize to the lungs.[9] The most common metastatic cancers from the head and neck to the lung originate from the larynx and the oral cavity.[10] The most frequent histologic types are squamous cell carcinoma and basaloid squamous cell carcinoma.[11] The latter can be easily confused for the basaloid/small cell variant of primary squamous cell carcinoma of the lung or for small cell cancer on small endoscopic biopsies (Fig. 15.3). Proper clinical history is, therefore, indispensable for adequate identification of the lesion as a metastasis. Distinction of a metastatic human papillomavirus (HPV)-related head and neck carcinoma

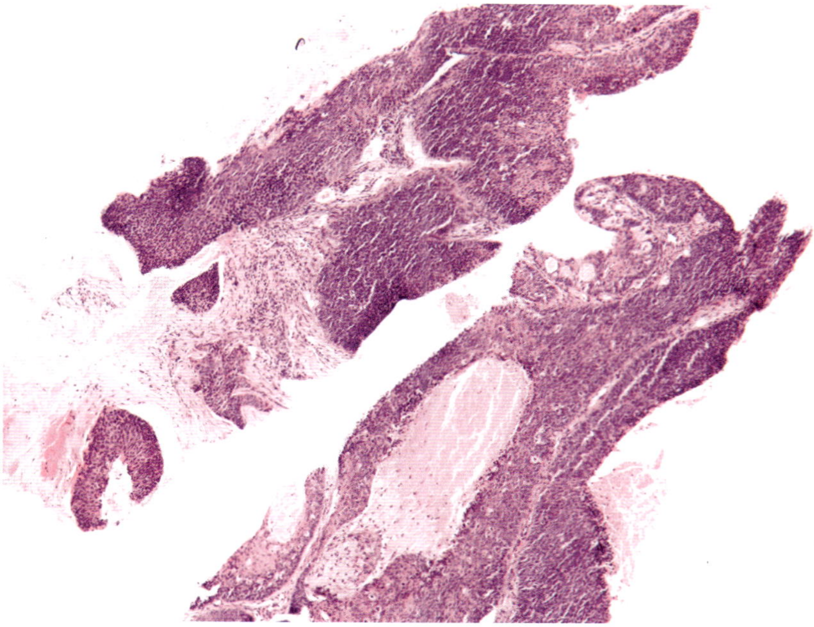

FIGURE 15.3 **Pulmonary metastasis of basaloid squamous carcinoma of the tongue showing islands of tightly packed, uniform small cells with peripheral palisading.** In the absence of a proper history, these tumors can be mistaken for a primary squamous cell carcinoma of the bronchus of the basaloid/small cell variant or neuroendocrine carcinoma of the lung.

from a primary lung squamous cell carcinoma using antibodies to p16 is not reliable because up to 63% of primary squamous cell carcinomas of lung can be positive for this marker.[12] However, polymerase chain reaction–based assays may be of use in identifying the presence of HPV in oropharyngeal metastases by targeting the L1 region and E6/E7 regions of high-risk HPV.[13,14] Salivary gland tumors can also metastasize to the lungs, particularly adenoid cystic carcinoma and acinic cell carcinoma.[15,16] A detailed clinical history is required because salivary gland tumors can often metastasize after a long period of latency and may be easily mistaken for primary salivary gland–type tumors of the lung. Carcinoma of the thyroid, in particular papillary thyroid carcinoma, also metastasizes to the lungs. The clear nuclear features of papillary thyroid carcinoma can sometimes also be observed in some primary lung tumors, such as adenocarcinoma with lepidic growth pattern and in some cribriform-papillary adenocarcinomas.[17-19] Metastases from papillary thyroid carcinomas can also adopt a lepidic pattern of growth that can closely simulate a primary lung adenocarcinoma[5]; use of immunohistochemical stains for thyroglobulin and PAX8 is indicated in such instances to distinguish them from lung primaries because thyroid transcription factor-1 (TTF-1) immunostaining is also positive in thyroid cells (Fig. 15.4A and B). Rarely, Hürthle cell carcinoma from the thyroid can metastasize to the

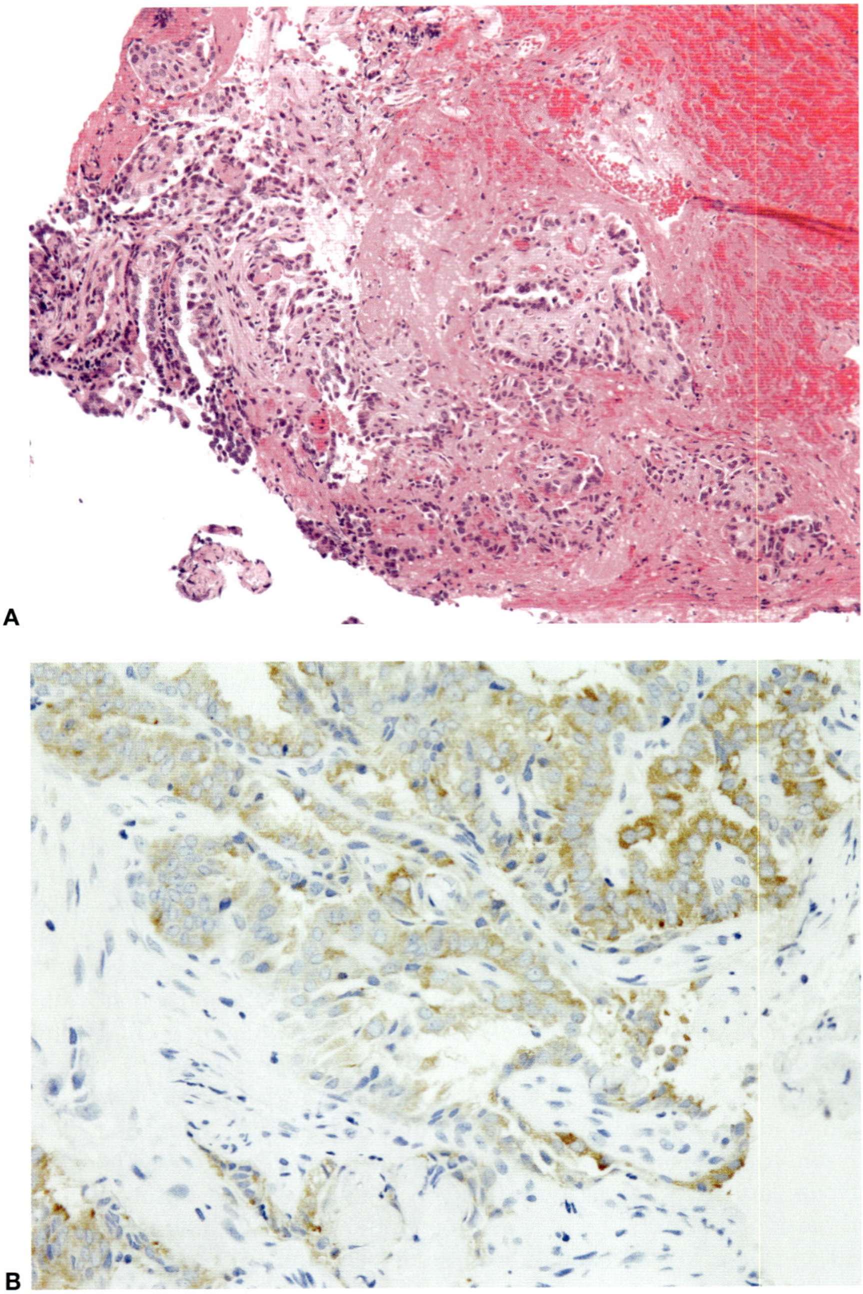

FIGURE 15.4 **A.** Endobronchial biopsy with metastasis of papillary thyroid carcinoma. The tumor can be easily mistaken for a primary papillary carcinoma of the lung on routine microscopy. **B.** Immunohistochemical stain for thyroglobulin showing positivity in the tumor cells supporting thyroid origin.

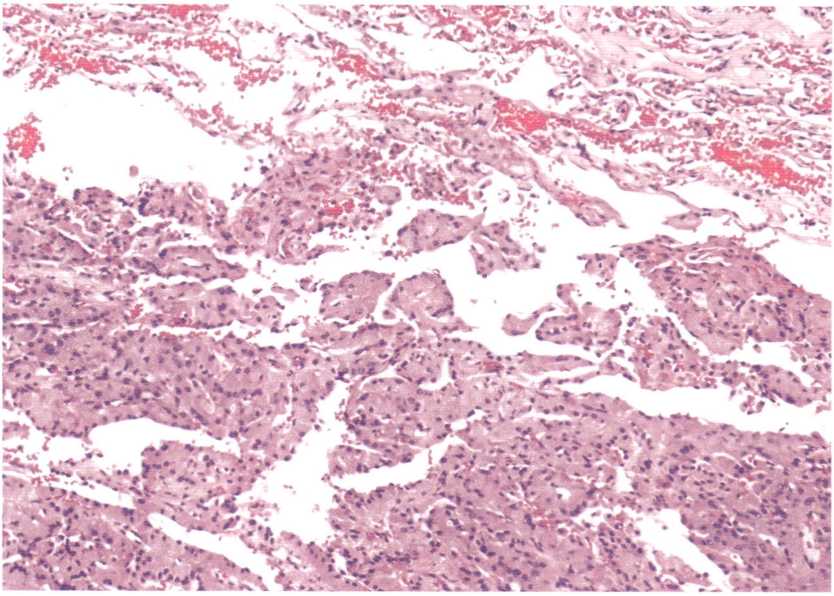

FIGURE 15.5 **Pulmonary metastasis of a Hürthle cell carcinoma of the thyroid.** This tumor must be differentiated from other oncocytic neoplasms such as renal and salivary gland tumors. The patient had a history of a Hürthle cell carcinoma of the thyroid. The lesion stained positive for thyroglobulin.

lung and may be confused for metastases from other oncocytic neoplasms such as renal cell carcinoma or salivary gland tumors (Fig. 15.5).[20] In this scenario, a clinical history and thyroglobulin stains will be important in establishing the thyroid as the primary site; PAX8 may not be of use in this setting because it is also positive in renal cell carcinoma. Parathyroid carcinoma has also been reported to rarely metastasize to the lungs and may resemble a low-grade neuroendocrine neoplasm (Fig. 15.6A and B).[21] As primary lung neuroendocrine tumors and metastasis from the parathyroid may both share neuroendocrine marker positivity and TTF-1 negativity, the use of parathyroid hormone immunohistochemistry along with a detailed clinical history of any prior parathyroid pathology may be helpful in trying to distinguish these entities.[22,23]

Metastases From the Gastrointestinal Tract

Carcinomas arising from the entire length of the gastrointestinal tract can metastasize to the lungs, in particular the colon, stomach, and pancreas. Metastases from the colon have a tendency to display a wreath-like pattern of growth with cribriform structures at the periphery and extensive central areas of necrosis. The cells are usually tall columnar, may be mucin secreting, and may contain interspersed goblet cells (Fig. 15.7A and B). Unlike primary mucinous carcinomas of the lung, colonic metastases usually display

A

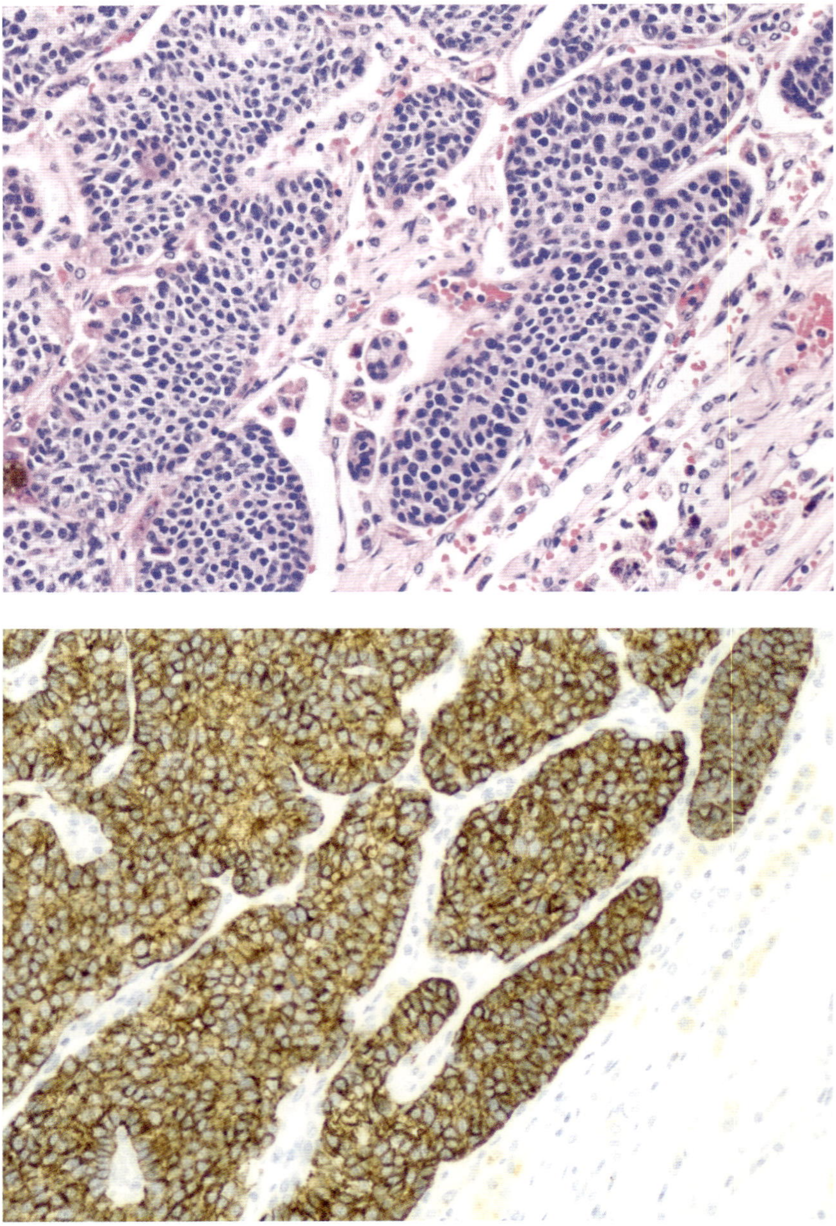

B

FIGURE 15.6 **A.** Metastatic deposit from a parathyroid carcinoma in a patient with a prior history of parathyroid carcinoma. Note the small bland cells growing in nests sharing some resemblance to a neuroendocrine tumor of the lung. **B.** Parathyroid hormone immunohistochemistry showed cytoplasmic staining of the tumor cells consistent with parathyroid origin.

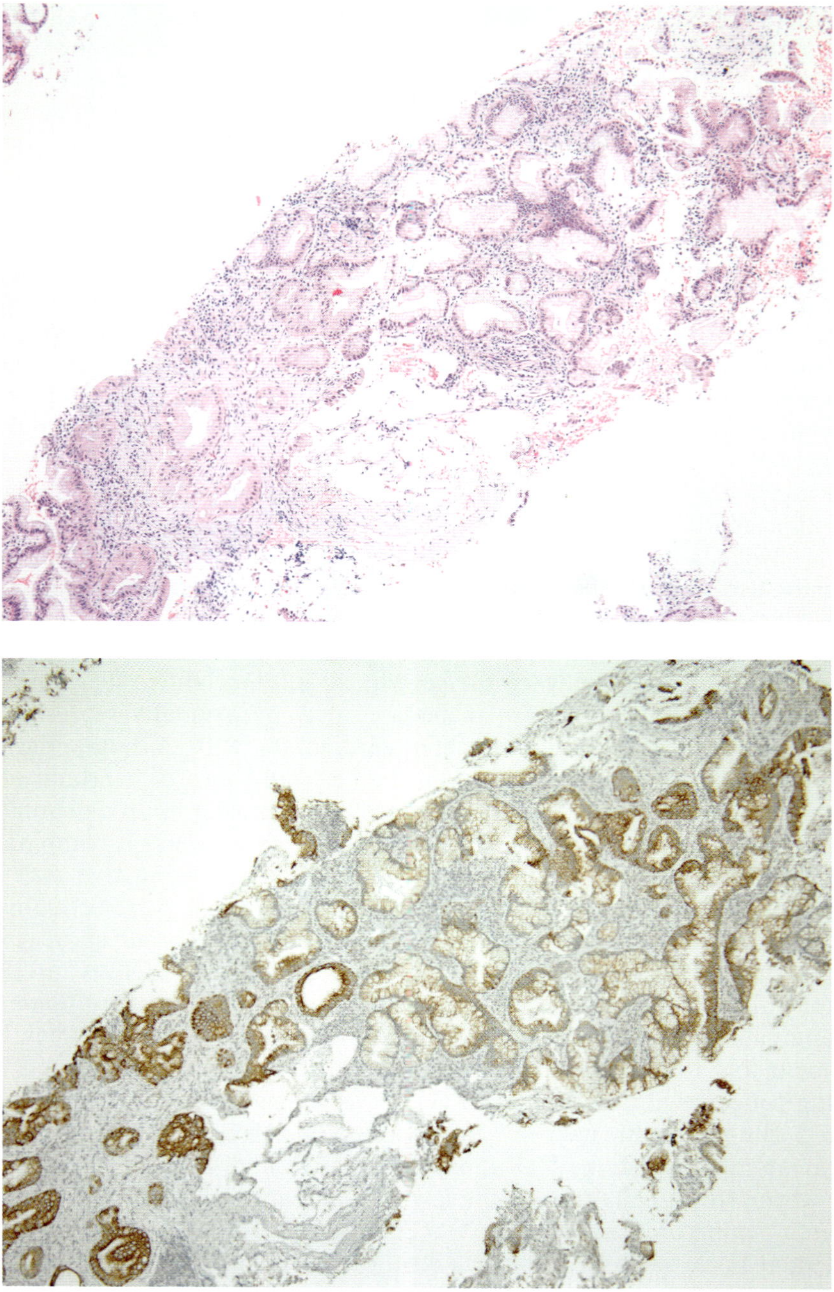

A B

FIGURE 15.7 **A.** Core biopsy of metastatic adenocarcinoma of the colon to the lung showing glands lined by tall columnar cells containing cytoplasmic mucin. **B.** The tumor cells were negative for thyroid transcription factor-1 and CK7 and showed strong positivity for CK20 (shown) and CDX2.

marked cytologic atypia with prominent mitotic activity (eFigs. 15.1-15.3). Immunohistochemical stains may be of limited value in this setting because primary intestinal-type adenocarcinomas of the lung can display an enteric phenotype (CK20+/CDX2+ and CK7−/TTF-1−) or a lung phenotype (CK7+/TTF-1+ and CK20−/CDX2−).[24-26] Strict clinicopathologic correlation and thorough imaging and endoscopic studies may be needed before a definitive diagnosis can be rendered. It is also important to make this distinction because primary lung adenocarcinoma may also adopt a striking cribriform pattern of growth that can be easily confused for a metastasis from the colon or other gastrointestinal organs.[17] Primary mucin-secreting carcinoma of the lung may also adopt certain other unusual morphologic features that can lead to an erroneous diagnosis of metastases when the tumor is, indeed, a primary lung neoplasm, including production of abundant extracellular mucin (the so-called colloid carcinoma) and tumors with signet ring cell features.[27,28] Because such tumors can exhibit either an intestinal or a primary lung immunophenotype, careful clinicopathologic correlation is indicated to establish the correct diagnosis.

Metastases from primary tumors from other parts of the gastrointestinal tract, in particular pancreaticobiliary carcinomas, may pose serious problems for diagnosis. These lesions can sometimes adopt a striking lepidic growth pattern that can closely mimic a primary mucinous carcinoma of the lung with lepidic growth. It is important to keep this fact in mind because pulmonary metastases may occasionally represent the initial manifestation of pancreatic carcinoma, with radiographic and clinical features that are indistinguishable from those of a primary lung cancer (eFigs. 15.4 and 15.5).[29] A careful diagnostic approach must be taken with these specimens. A general guideline is to use a combination of an immunohistochemical panel and molecular testing that will best differentiate a primary lung adenocarcinoma from a pancreaticobiliary metastasis. Given enough diagnostic material, an appropriate strategy is to stain the biopsy material with TTF-1, napsin, CDX2, and CK20 and order molecular testing for *KRAS* mutations. Although both lung carcinoma and pancreaticobiliary carcinoma show *KRAS* mutations, some studies have shown that the *KRAS* G12R variant is more commonly associated with lung cancer, whereas the *KRAS* G12C variant is more commonly associated with pancreatic cancer.[30] As mentioned previously, mucinous lung adenocarcinomas may be TTF-1/napsin negative and CDX2/CK20 positive; however, statistically, this profile favors pancreaticobiliary origin.[30] Adding carcinoembryonic antigen (CEA), CK18, CK19, and SMAD4 may also be of value because positive staining for those markers with loss of SMAD4 is consistent with a pancreaticobiliary origin.[31] It must be kept in mind, however, that all of these markers are nonspecific in this scenario and can be variably positive in both lung cancer and pancreaticobiliary cancer (as well as colorectal-type adenocarcinomas), so they must be evaluated together in the context of clinical, imaging, and molecular findings.[32] Cases such as this should always be discussed with the surgeon and the clinical team.

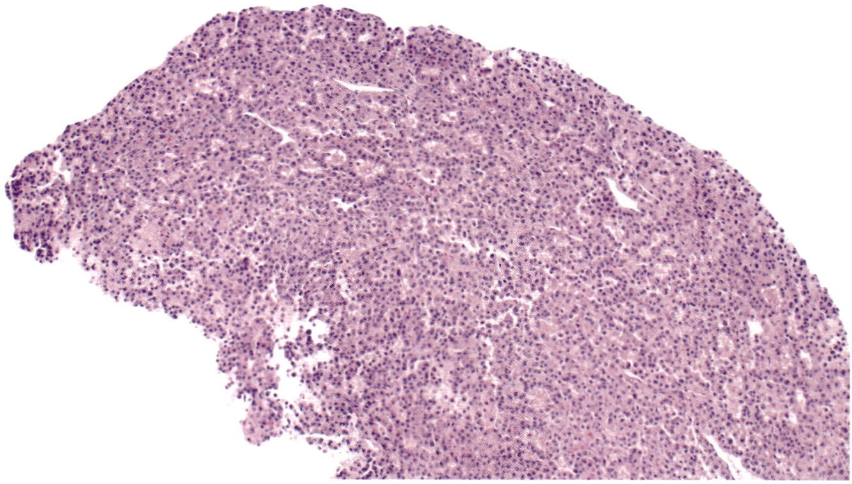

FIGURE 15.8 Biopsy of metastatic hepatocellular carcinoma shows a tumor with large epithelioid cells and abundant eosinophilic cytoplasm; the tumor even demonstrated focal pseudogland formation.

Hepatocellular carcinoma can also metastasize to the lungs in both early and late stages and can present as a solitary nodule (Fig. 15.8). The tumors must be distinguished from different lung primary tumors and other types of metastases comprising cells with abundant eosinophilic cytoplasm (Fig. 15.9A and B). Immunohistochemical staining for HepPar1, arginase-1, and glypican-3 will be helpful if positive, though it should be noted that using HepPar1 by itself may be a pitfall as some primary lung carcinomas can demonstrate strong HepPar1 expression.[33] The demonstration of a canalicular bile duct pattern of staining with CEA can also be of aid in making this distinction.[34]

Metastases From the Genitourinary Tract

The most common metastases to the lung that originate from the genitourinary tract are from renal cell carcinoma (eFigs. 15.6-15.8). Renal cell carcinoma metastases are often multiple but can also present as a solitary lesion; they may precede the clinical detection of the primary tumor or develop several years (>10 years) after detection of the primary tumor in the kidney.[35] Metastatic renal cell carcinoma to the lung can also occur as an endobronchial lesion adopting a polypoid endobronchial configuration, thus clinically simulating a bronchogenic neoplasm.[36] The lung is also the most common site of metastasis for renal cell carcinoma.[37] Proper identification of a renal cell carcinoma metastasis to the lung may be of clinical significance because survival following metastasectomy can be quite significant.[38] The majority of renal cell carcinoma metastases to the lung will show the classical clear cell morphology characteristic of these

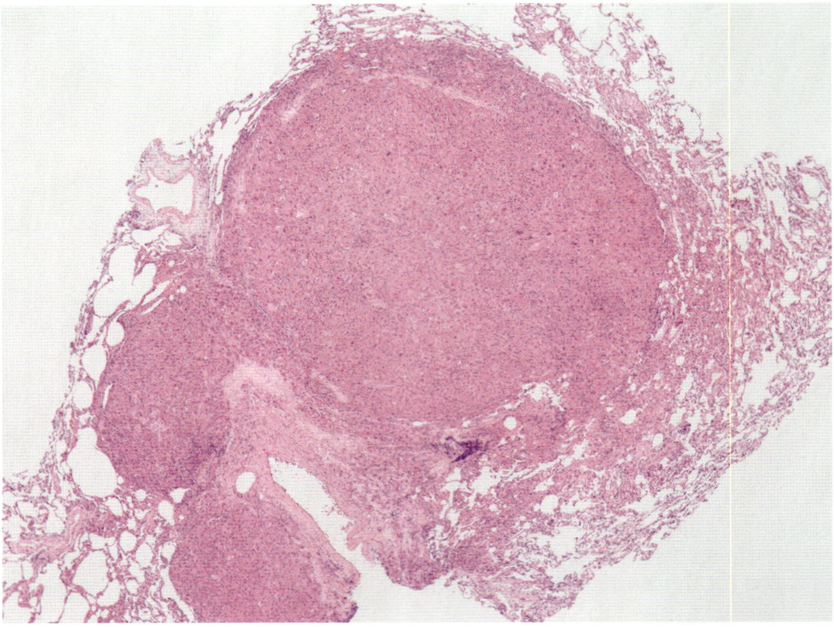

A

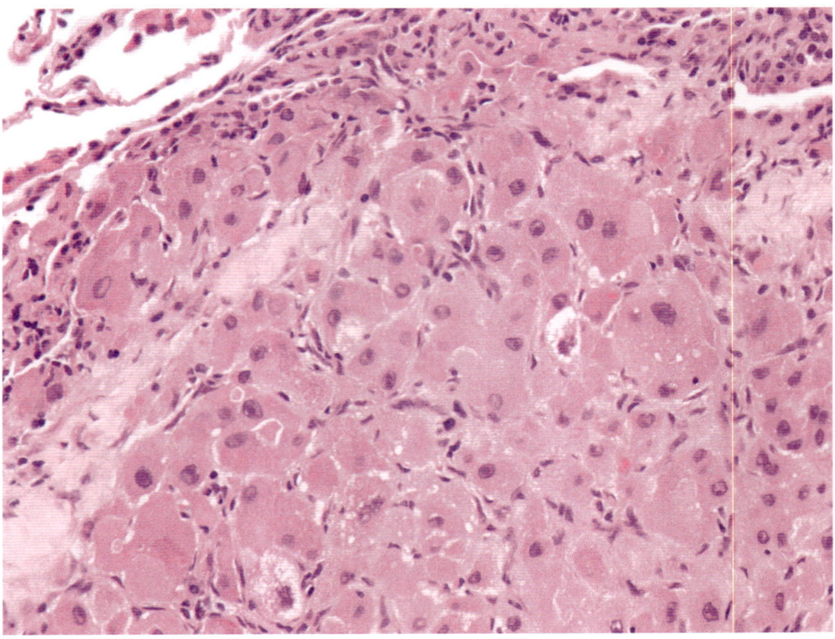

B

FIGURE 15.9 **A.** Metastasis of hepatocellular carcinoma showing a well-circumscribed pulmonary nodule sharply separated from the surrounding parenchyma. **B.** Higher magnification showing large cells with abundant densely eosinophilic cytoplasm and round nuclei with prominent nucleoli.

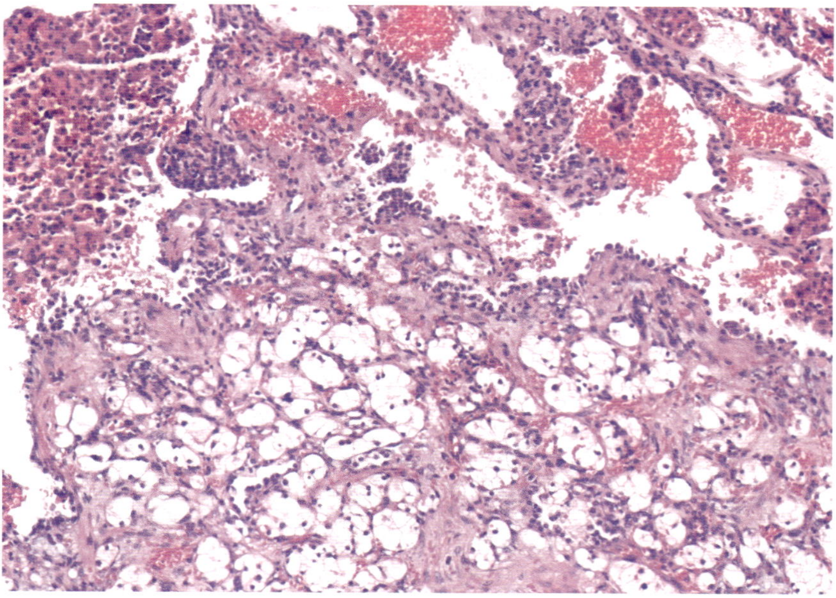

FIGURE 15.10 Metastasis of clear cell renal cell carcinoma in the lung.

tumors (Fig. 15.10); however, unusual variants can also be observed, such as tumors with abundant eosinophilic granular cytoplasm, tumors with a sarcomatoid appearance, tumors with papillary architecture, and tumors with a prominent hemangiopericytic growth pattern (Fig. 15.11A-C).[5] Immunohistochemical stains play an important role in the diagnosis of these tumors. All renal cell carcinoma metastases (including the sarcomatoid variant) are strongly positive for cytokeratin antibodies, in particular low-molecular weight cytokeratins, and they coexpress vimentin intermediate filaments. The tumors are negative for TTF-1, p63, and surfactant apoprotein but can be positive for napsin A. Other helpful markers associated with renal cell carcinoma include CD10, renal cell carcinoma antigen (although the latter is not particularly helpful for metastatic renal cell carcinoma), PAX8, and carbonic anhydrase (CA) IX (Fig. 15.11D). A potential pitfall for diagnosis occurs with metastases from the papillary variant of renal cell carcinoma. Such tumors may display a prominent papillary growth pattern that can be confused for papillary adenocarcinoma of the lung and other metastatic tumors; moreover, they strongly express CK7, thus overlapping with the immunophenotype of primary lung adenocarcinoma. A helpful marker that can serve to distinguish metastases to the lung from papillary renal cell carcinoma is α-methyl-CoA racemase, which is strongly and preferentially expressed in the papillary variant of renal cell carcinoma.[39] Metastases to the lung characterized by clear cell morphology can also occur in patients with adrenal cortical carcinoma; the lesions may be impossible to distinguish from a clear cell renal cell carcinoma by

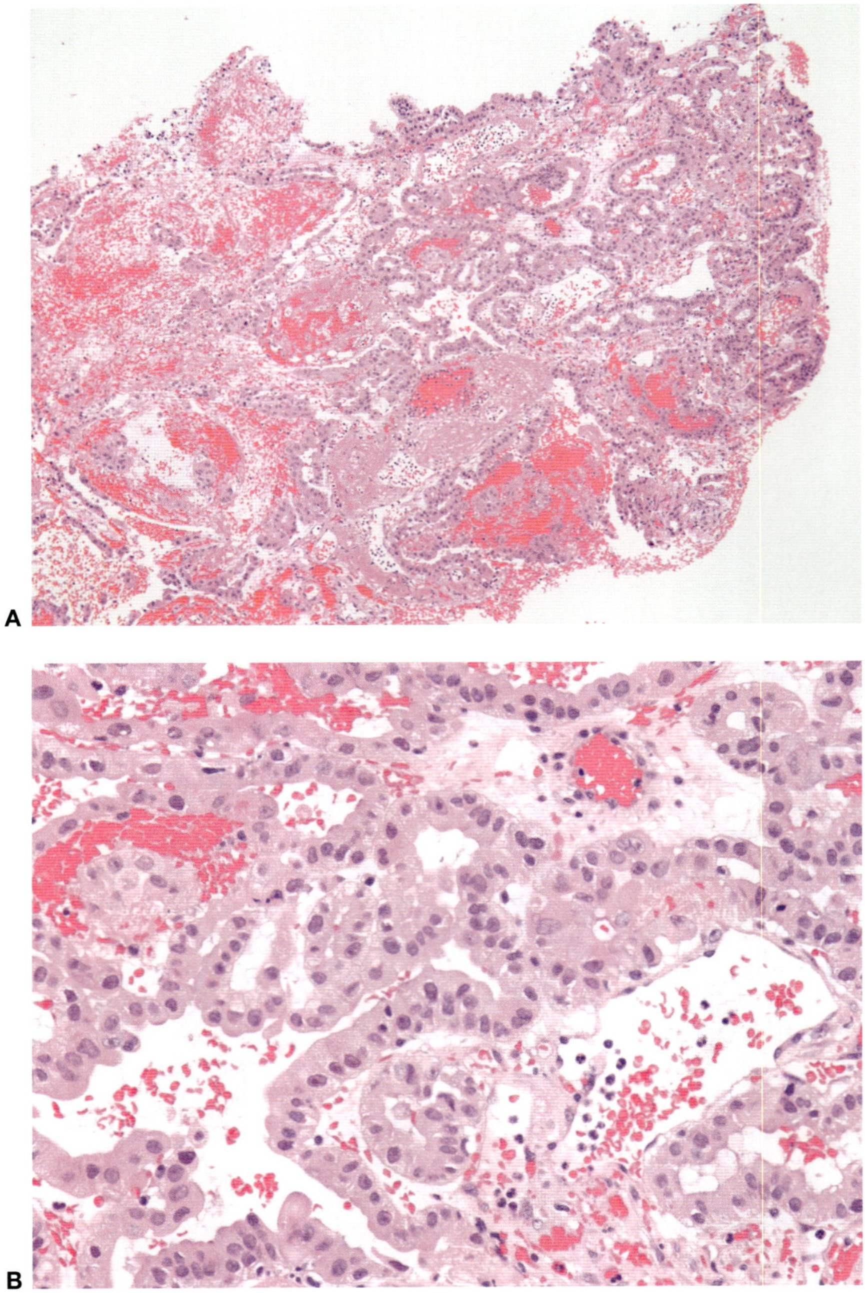

FIGURE 15.11 **A.** Endobronchial biopsy showing metastasis of renal cell carcinoma with abundant oncocytic cytoplasm. The tumor adopts a glandular configuration that can simulate other types of epithelial malignancies. **B.** Higher magnification showing glandular structures lined by large cells with abundant eosinophilic cytoplasm.

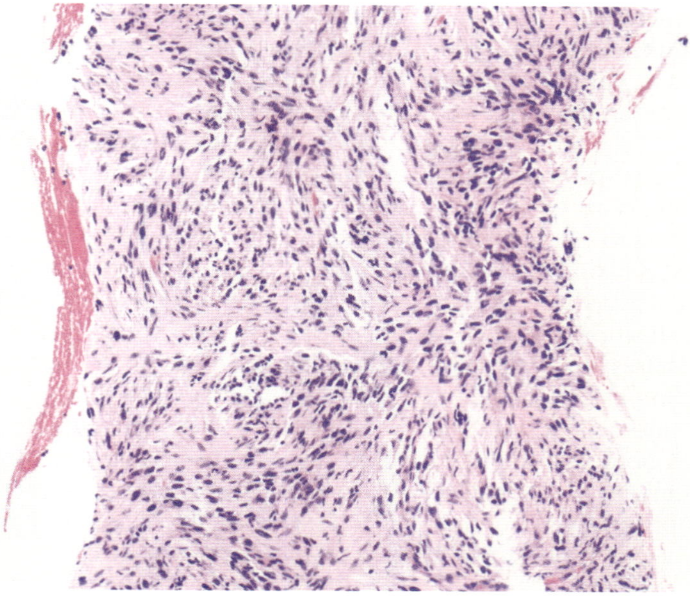

C

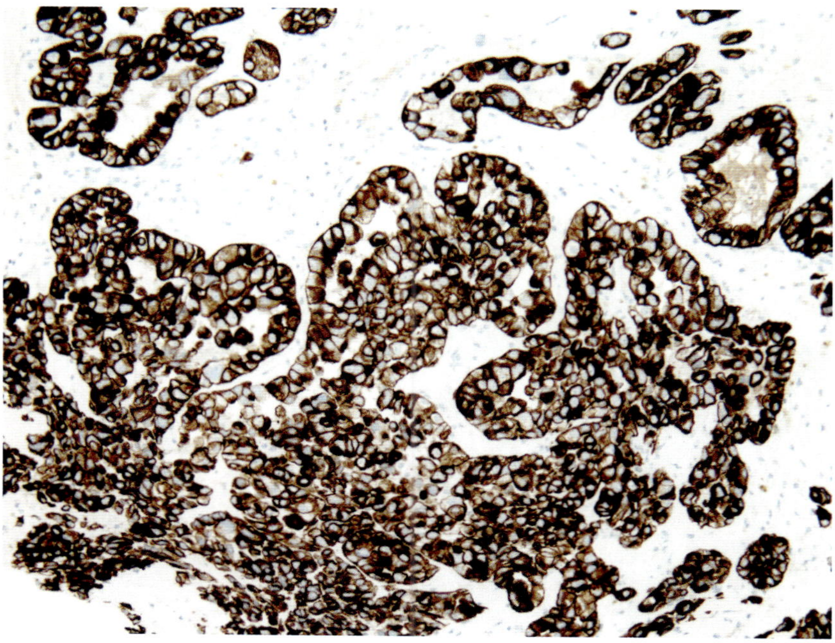

D

FIGURE 15.11 (*continued*) **C.** Core needle biopsy showing a metastatic deposit of sarcomatoid renal cell carcinoma. These tumors must be differentiated from metastatic spindle cell tumors. **D.** Immunohistochemical stain for CD10 showing striking cytoplasmic and membranous positivity of the tumor cells in metastatic renal cell carcinoma.

routine histology. Immunohistochemical stains will be required for proper diagnosis; adrenal cortical carcinoma is most often negative for cytokeratin but will stain strongly with inhibin, Melan-A, and steroidogenic factor 1, whereas renal cell cancer will be negative.[40]

Metastases from urothelial carcinoma of the bladder and renal pelvis and from prostate adenocarcinoma can also occur in the lung, particularly in the more advanced stages of the disease. Metastases of urothelial carcinoma are usually disseminated and multiple and will show the characteristic histology of these tumors (Fig. 15.12). Some high-grade urothelial carcinomas can display marked squamous differentiation that complicates the diagnosis. GATA3 will be a helpful discriminatory marker in equivocal cases and is more sensitive than uroplakin for separating primary squamous cell lung cancer from metastatic poorly differentiated urothelial carcinoma.[41] Carcinoma of the prostate, although usually presenting first with bony and regional lymph node metastases, can rarely also present initially with metastases to the lungs, with no obvious involvement of lymph nodes or bone.[42,43] Metastases to the lung from prostate cancer often resemble conventional adenocarcinoma (Figs. 15.13 and 15.14) but can also display a marked cribriform pattern (Fig. 15.15A and B); identification of this pattern of growth should prompt ordering stains for prostate-specific antigen and prostate-specific acid phosphatase to rule out prostate cancer.[43] Rarely, metastatic prostate cancer can be negative for prostate-specific antigen and prostate-specific acid phosphatase; under these circumstances and particularly if there is a well-established history of prostate cancer, a few more recently available markers can be used, which are strongly positive in a high percentage of these tumors, including

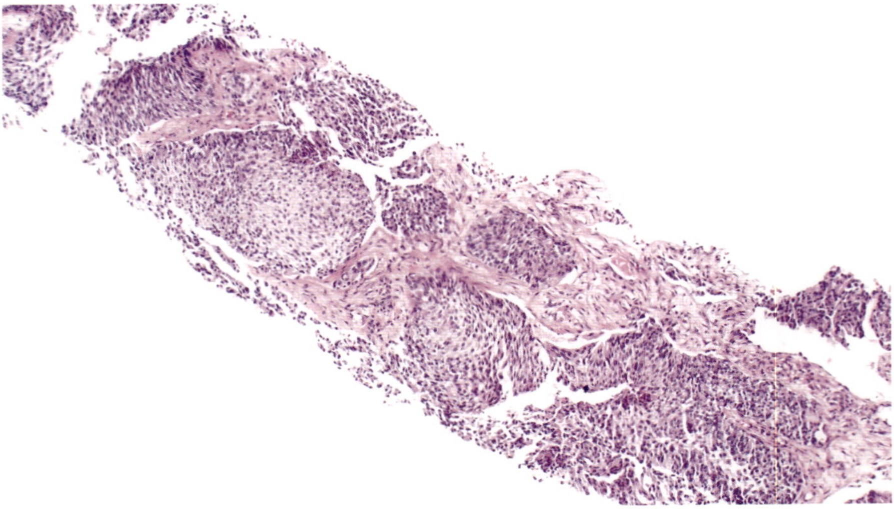

FIGURE 15.12 **Core needle biopsy demonstrating metastatic urothelial carcinoma.** The tumor shows a nested pattern of growth of squamoid appearing cells that can easily be confused with squamous cell carcinoma of the lung.

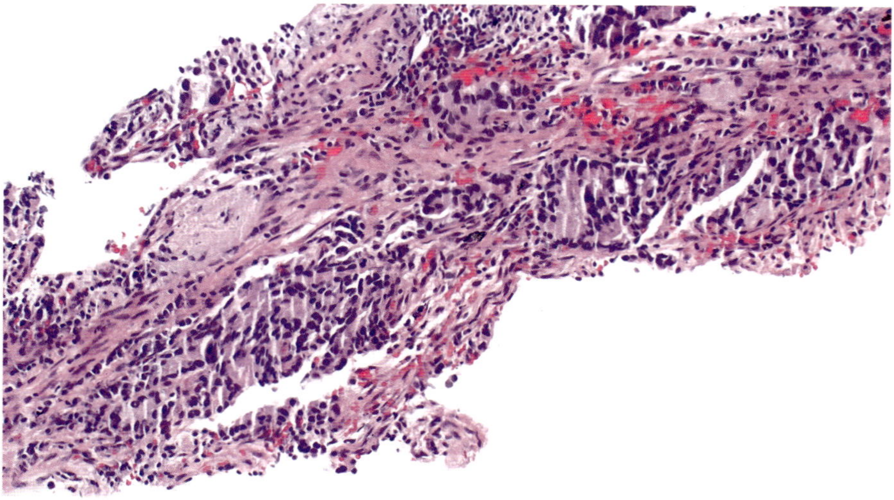

FIGURE 15.13 **Core needle biopsy demonstrating metastatic prostatic adenocarcinoma to the lung.** The tumor shows glandular formation, including compressed cribriform growth, and is difficult to differentiate from an adenocarcinoma of the lung by microscopy alone.

androgen receptor, prostate-specific membrane antigen (PSMA), P501S, and NKX3.1 (Fig. 15.16).[44,45] Metastases to the lungs from testicular cancer occur with frequency, particularly with malignant germ cell tumors.[46,47] It has been shown that metastasectomy plays a role in the management of these patients.[48,49] A peculiar phenomenon observed in these tumors at the metastatic site is maturation of the tumor, where the metastatic

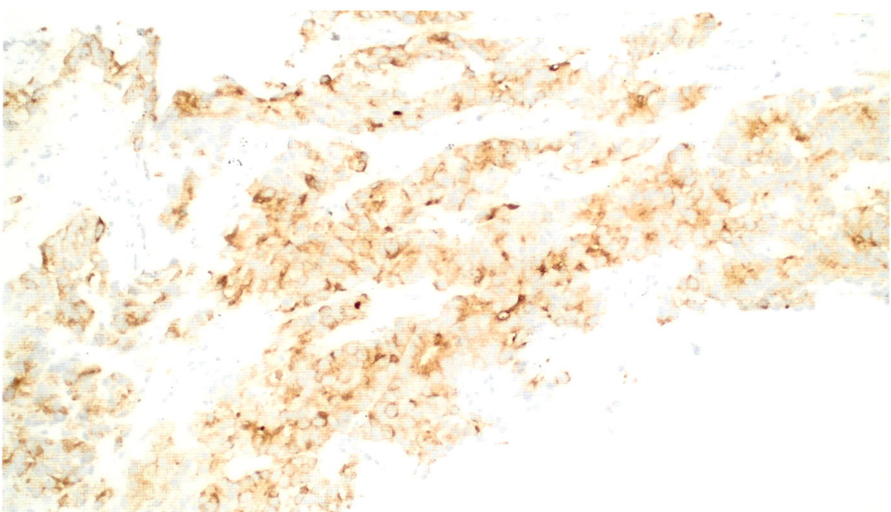

FIGURE 15.14 **An immunostain for prostate-specific antigen shows strong cytoplasmic positivity in metastatic prostate adenocarcinoma.**

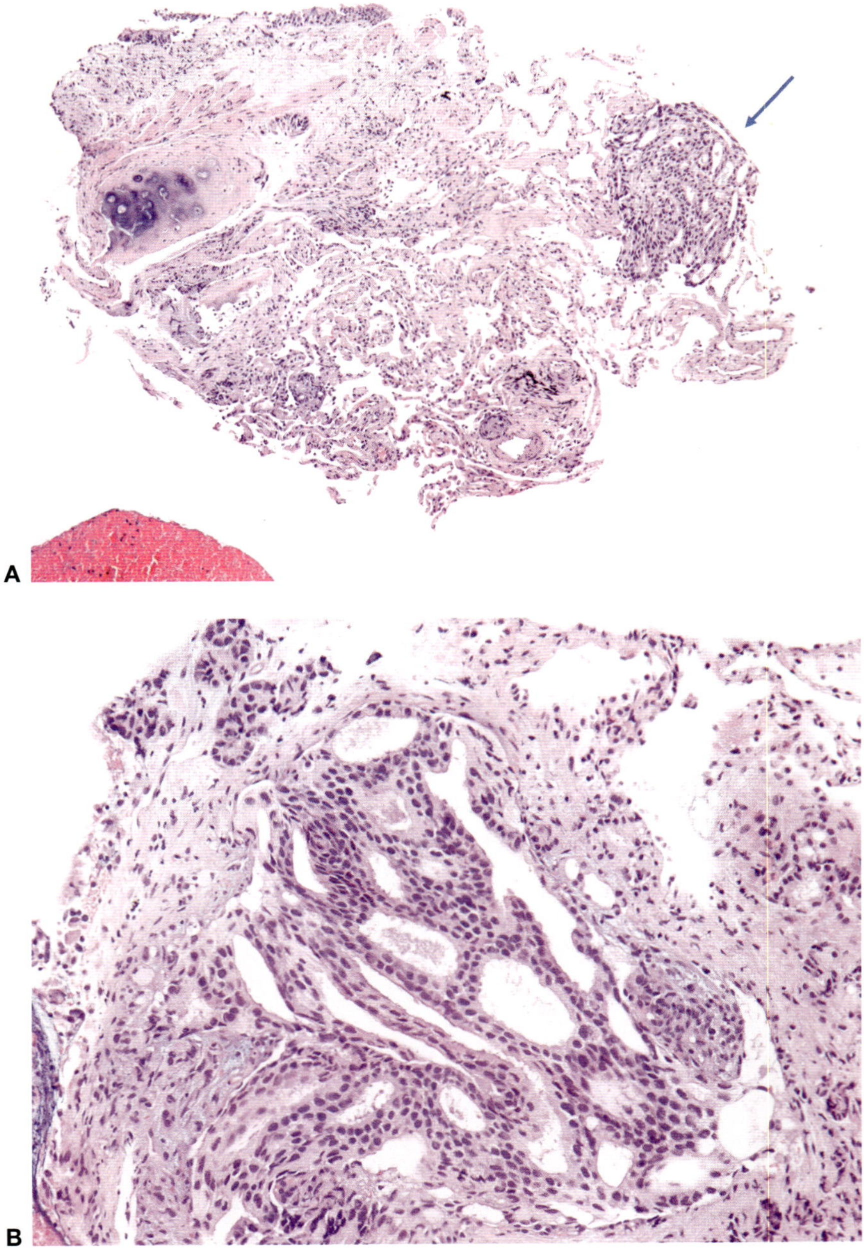

FIGURE 15.15 **A.** Transbronchial biopsy showing normal bronchial mucosa and cartilaginous plate and a minute focus of adenocarcinoma within alveolated parenchyma (*arrow*). **B.** Higher magnification showing cribriform glandular spaces lined by atypical cells with hyperchromatic nuclei characteristic of prostate carcinoma.

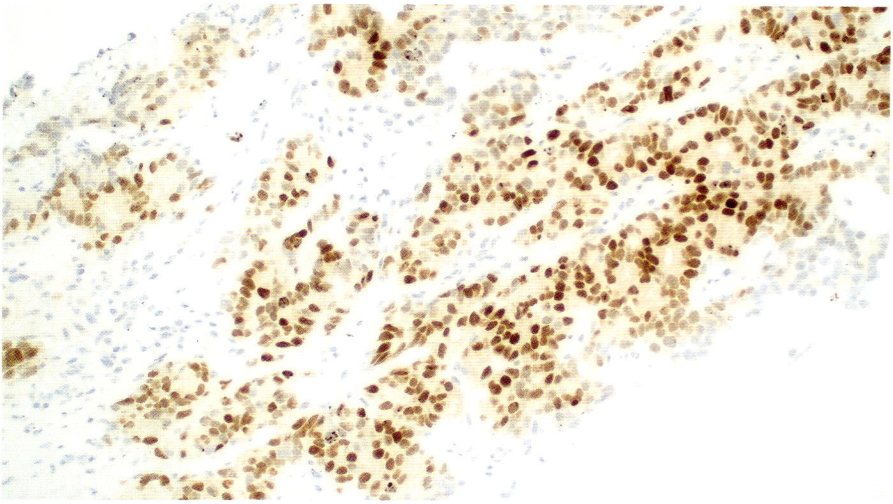

FIGURE 15.16 Immunohistochemistry for NKX3.1 shows strong nuclear positivity in metastatic prostate carcinoma.

deposits will contain only mature teratomatous elements (Fig. 15.17).[50] The lung is also a favored site of metastasis for testicular and uterine choriocarcinoma characterized by large, hemorrhagic tumor masses, although disseminated disease may also occur. The lesions will usually show bizarre

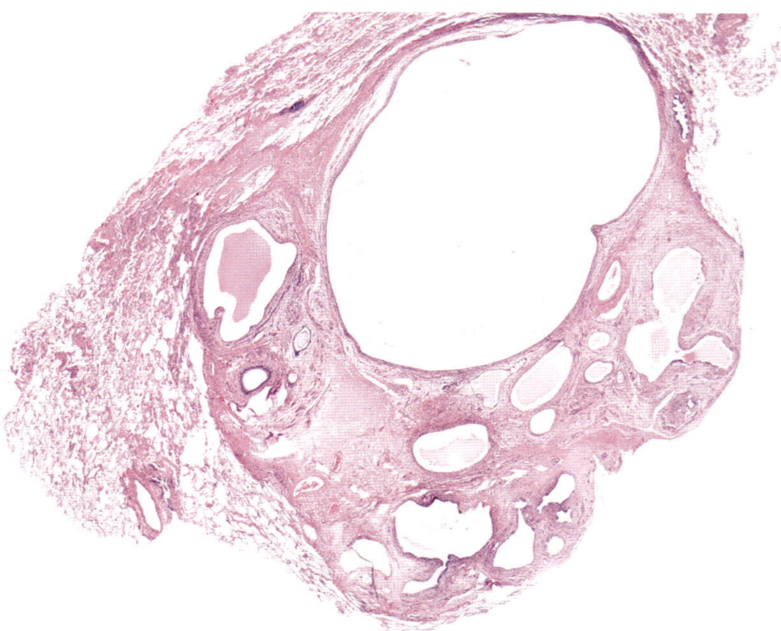

FIGURE 15.17 Lung metastasis from testicular teratocarcinoma showing "maturation" phenomenon, whereby only mature teratomatous elements are present at the metastatic site.

nuclear pleomorphism owing to the syncytiotrophoblastic component, with prominent interstitial hemorrhage; less frequently, only the cytotrophoblastic component may be evident. The tumors need to be distinguished from anaplastic large cell carcinoma, pleomorphic sarcomas, and large cell carcinoma of the lung that can occasionally contain a trophoblastic giant cell component. The latter tumors will display focal positivity for β-human chorionic gonadotropin, making the use of this stain of limited value for separating the two. Clinicopathologic correlation and a detailed clinical history are indispensable for diagnosis under these circumstances.

Tumors of the female reproductive tract can also be a common source of metastases to the lungs, mainly from carcinoma of the uterus and cervix.[51-53] Metastases of endometrioid adenocarcinoma of the uterus and ovary can show a back-to-back cribriform arrangement of glands with prominent subnuclear vacuolization; the latter will be helpful for distinguishing it from primary lung adenocarcinoma (Fig. 15.18). The tumors must be distinguished, however, from the fetal adenocarcinoma of the lung, which can closely resemble a metastatic endometrioid adenocarcinoma. Fetal lung adenocarcinoma will show positivity of the tumor cells for TTF-1 and β-catenin, unlike endometrioid adenocarcinoma that is usually negative for those markers. Papillary serous carcinomas of the ovary or uterus also metastasize to the lung. They can be recognized by their high-grade

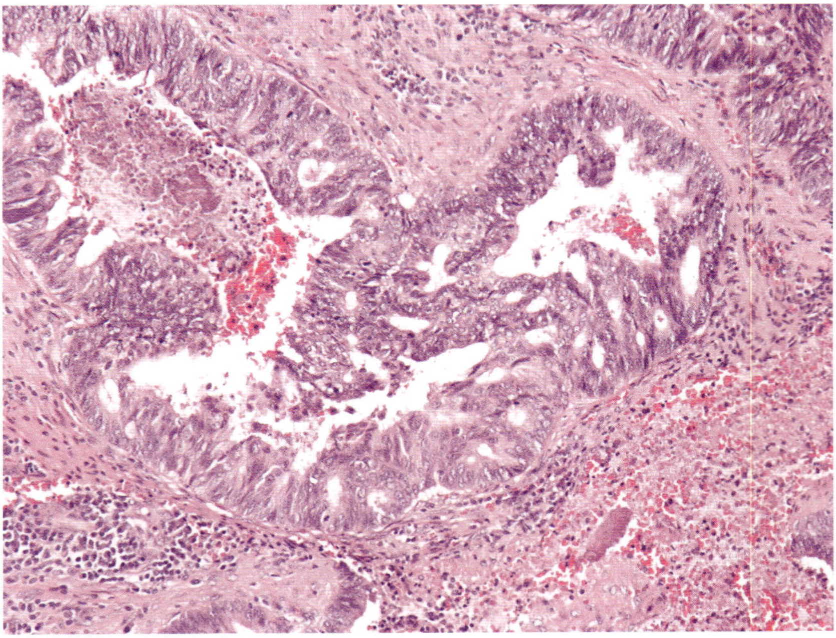

FIGURE 15.18 Metastasis to the lung from endometrioid adenocarcinoma shows back-to-back cribriform arrangement of glands.

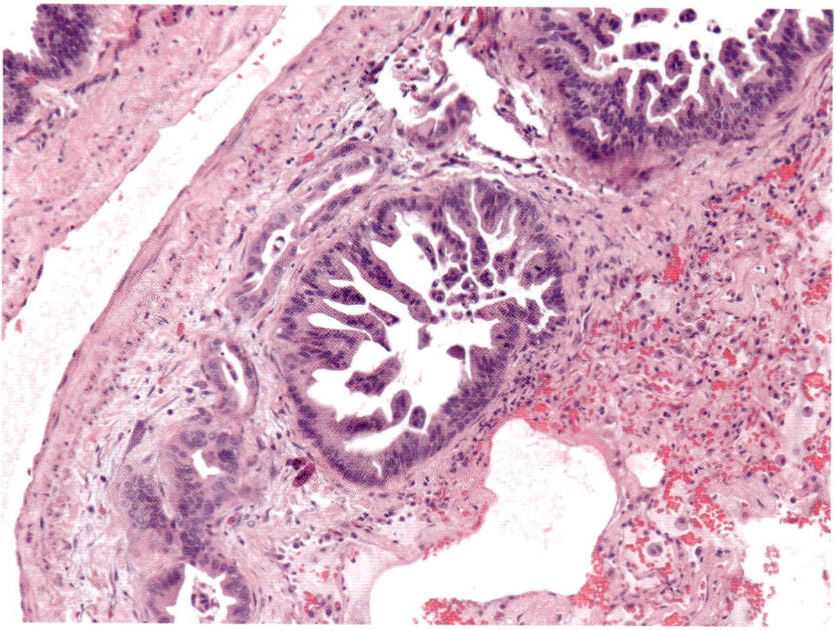

FIGURE 15.19 Metastasis of papillary serous carcinoma of the ovary to the lung shows plugging of lymphatics by tumor.

cytology and papillary architecture; however, clinical correlation is always indicated to separate them from primary papillary carcinoma of the lung (Fig. 15.19). In equivocal cases, positive staining for estrogen and progesterone receptors, PAX8, and WT1 will favor a metastasis from gynecologic cancer.[54] Metastases to the lung from cervical squamous cell carcinoma can cause difficulties for diagnosis with primary squamous cell carcinoma of the lung in the absence of an appropriate clinical history. Detection of HPV by DNA in situ hybridization has been utilized to identify metastatic lesions from the cervix, and reverse transcriptase polymerase chain reaction can be used to demonstrate the presence of the viral RNA in the metastatic lesions.[55] The use of antibodies to p16 is of no value in this setting, given that p16 expression in lung squamous cell carcinoma is caused by a different oncogenic mechanism and not related to HPV.[56]

Metastases From Other Epithelial Malignancies

Breast carcinoma is a common source of lung metastases, and the lung can be a frequent site of initial relapse for these tumors.[57] Distinction from a second primary lung cancer can be problematic, especially if a long latency period has supervened since the removal of the primary tumor. Moreover, up to 23% of lung metastases from breast cancer can be solitary.[58] Breast cancer metastases to the lung can show a prominent lymphangitic pattern of spread (Fig. 15.20A and B); it can adopt a miliary pattern of

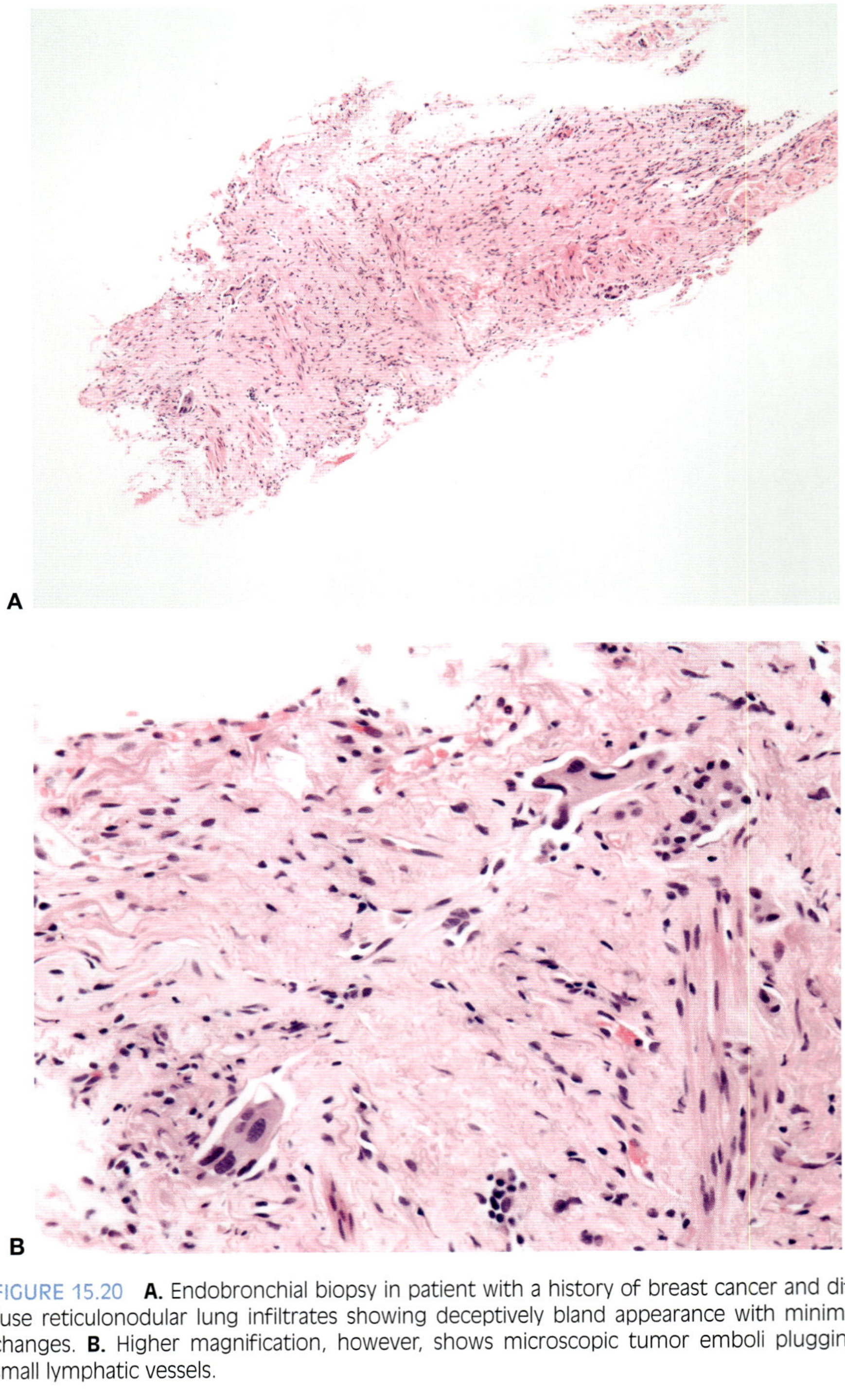

FIGURE 15.20 **A.** Endobronchial biopsy in patient with a history of breast cancer and diffuse reticulonodular lung infiltrates showing deceptively bland appearance with minimal changes. **B.** Higher magnification, however, shows microscopic tumor emboli plugging small lymphatic vessels.

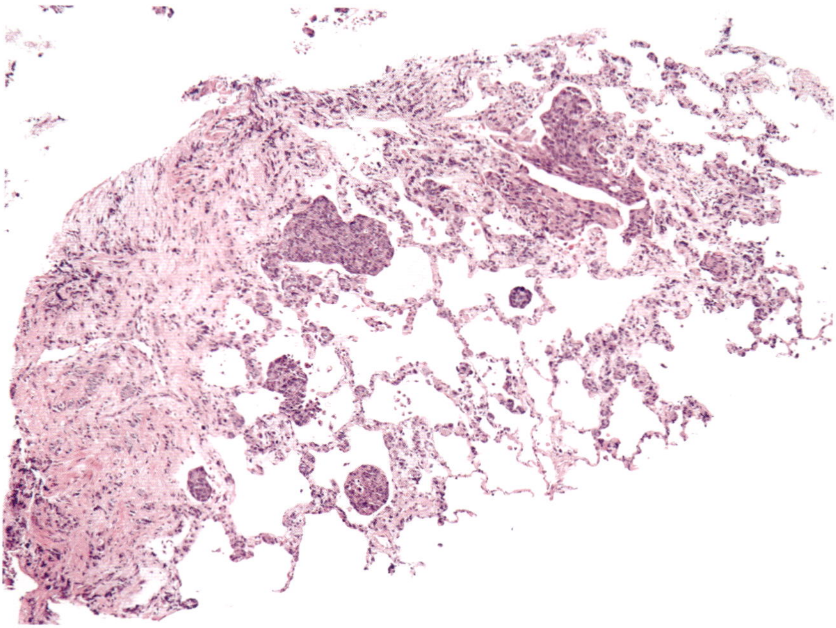

FIGURE 15.21 **Transbronchial biopsy showing metastatic breast carcinoma spreading through the airspaces.** Tumor plugs are seen within the alveolar lumens.

distribution with diffusely scattered microscopic nodules; it can show a tubular pattern of spread extending within the airspaces; or it can adopt a lepidic pattern of growth, resembling lepidic pulmonary adenocarcinoma (Fig. 15.21; eFigs. 15.9 and 15.10).[59] These tumors can also display a variety of morphologic appearances that can mimic other primary and metastatic lung tumors. Metastatic ductal carcinomas of the breast to the lung can display an acinar growth pattern as well as a single-file configuration reminiscent of metastatic anaplastic carcinoma of the stomach or invasive lobular carcinoma of the breast (Fig. 15.22A-C). It can also present with cribriform architecture that recapitulates ductal carcinoma in situ of the breast (Fig. 15.23), or it can grow as sheets of poorly differentiated tumor cells without any specific architecture (Fig. 15.24). Without a proper clinical history, it may be impossible to recognize the tumor as coming from the breast. Lung metastases from breast ductal carcinoma usually stain positive for CK5/6, CK7, estrogen and progesterone receptors, GATA3, E-cadherin, GCDFP-15, and mammaglobin. They are negative for TTF-1, napsin A, and p63.

Another type of epithelial neoplasm that can metastasize to the lungs is adnexal carcinomas of the skin (squamous cell carcinoma, basal cell carcinoma, basosquamous carcinoma, and other malignant adnexal tumors). Adnexal carcinomas are almost universally positive for p63; care must be

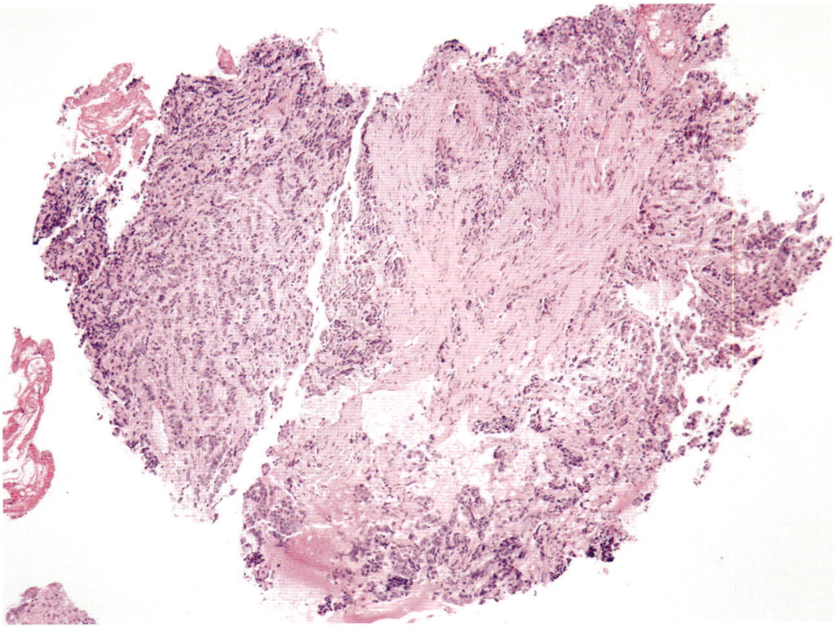

A

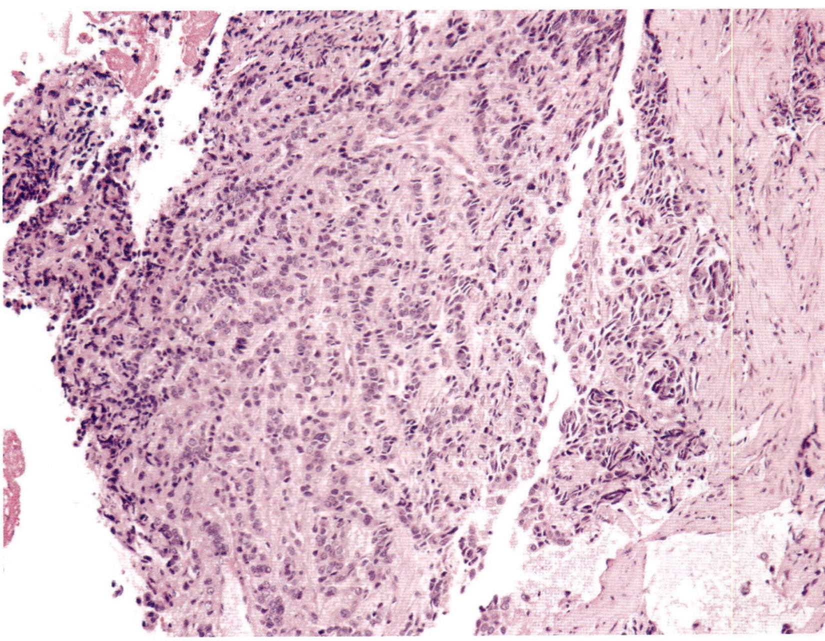

B

FIGURE 15.22 **A.** Endobronchial biopsy in patient with metastasis of breast carcinoma showing replacement of the lung by invasive tumor. **B.** Higher magnification showing atypical tumor cells infiltrating connective tissue in a single-file arrangement.

C
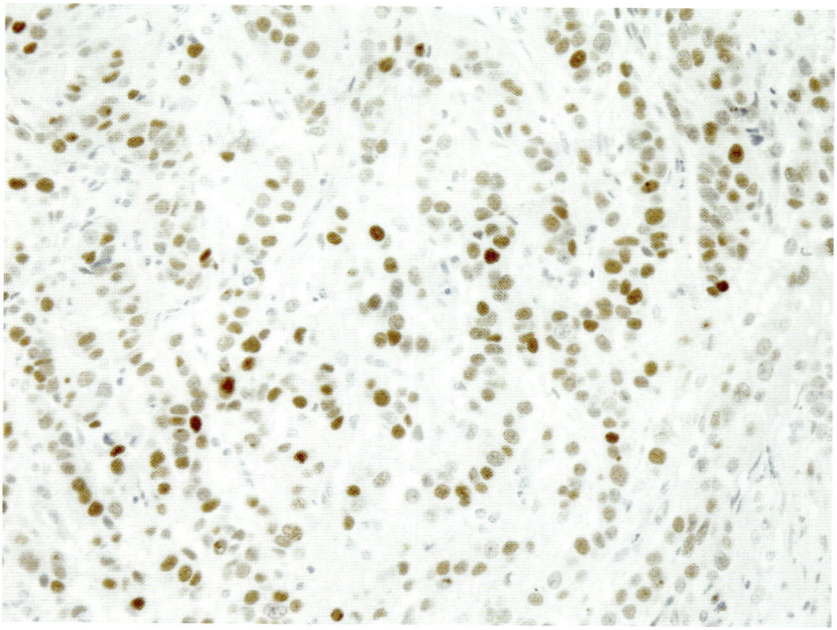

FIGURE 15.22 (*continued*) **C.** Immunohistochemical stain for estrogen receptor showing positive nuclear staining of the tumor cells.

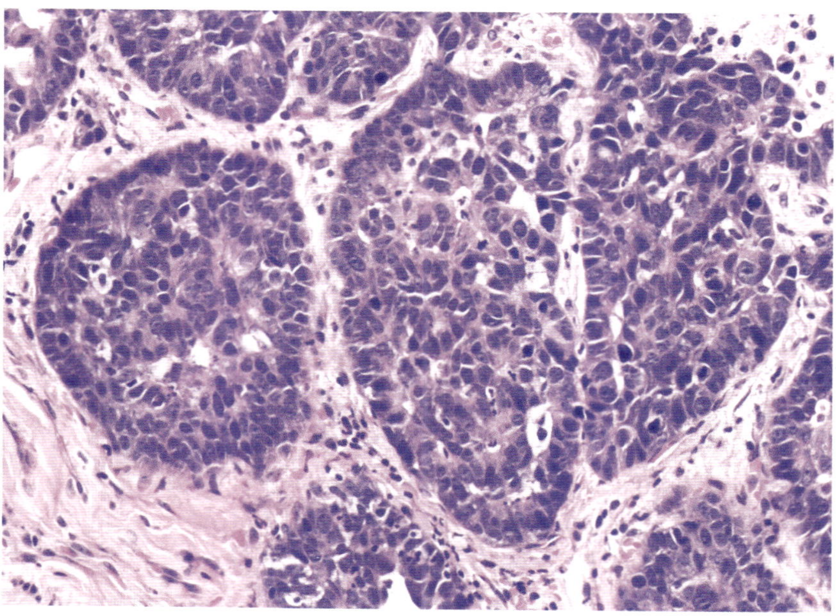

FIGURE 15.23 **Metastasis to the lung from invasive ductal carcinoma of the breast showing islands of tumor cells with a vague cribriform architecture resembling breast ductal carcinoma in situ.**

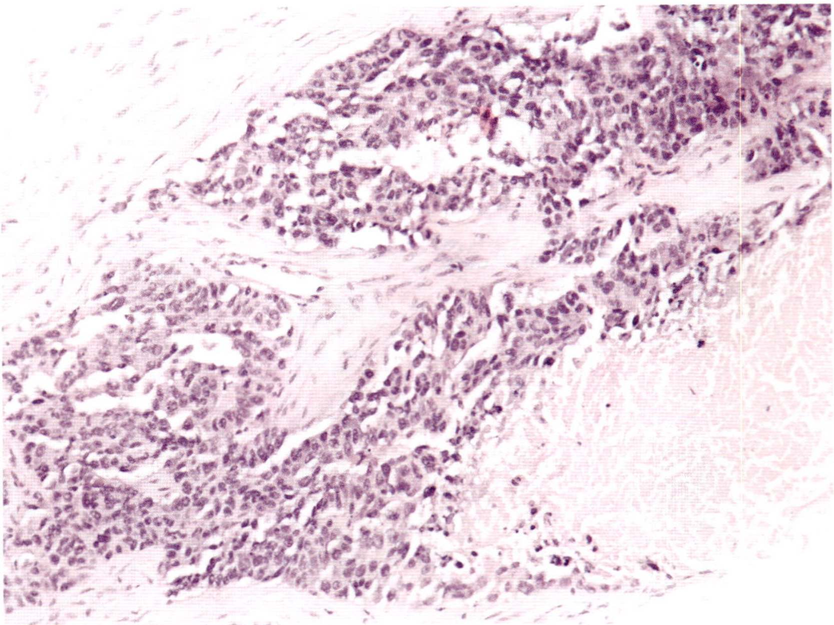

FIGURE 15.24 Metastasis to the lung of invasive ductal carcinoma of the breast showing sheets of poorly differentiated tumor cells without any particular architecture.

taken not to mistake them on small biopsies for squamous cell carcinoma of the lung. Thymic tumors may also rarely metastasize to the lung from the mediastinal compartment.[60] Thymomas of all subtypes as well as thymic carcinomas will be strongly positive for p63 and p40, which may potentially lead to confusion with squamous cell carcinoma of the lung.[61] As with all other metastases to the lung, an adequate clinical history will be indispensable for proper interpretation. The use of CD5 and CD117 stains has been proposed as a diagnostic tool for thymic carcinomas;[62,63] however, positivity for these markers in this context must be approached with caution as a substantial subset of non–small cell lung carcinomas have been demonstrated to react with these markers too, particularly CD117.[64]

METASTASES FROM BONE AND SOFT TISSUE SARCOMAS

Bone and soft tissue sarcomas are a frequent source of metastases to the lungs; the lung is, in fact, the most common site of metastases for malignant bone and soft tissue sarcomas.[65] Histologic distinction between a primary and a secondary tumor may not be possible based on histologic examination alone; clinicopathologic correlation is required to make this determination. Metastases of sarcoma to the lung significantly outnumber primary mesenchymal tumors of the lung. Establishing a correct diagnosis of metastatic sarcoma to the lung is of clinical importance because resection of the metastatic lesions has been associated with improved survival.[47,66,67] Metastases to the lung from sarcomas are most often peripheral and subpleural and well demarcated from the surrounding lung parenchyma. Endobronchial metastases simulating a bronchogenic neoplasm, however, have also been described.[68]

Metastases From Bone Tumors

Osteogenic sarcoma is the most common malignant bone tumor to metastasize to the lungs (Fig. 15.25). Although, in the past, the lungs were the first site of relapse for patients with osteosarcoma, the incidence of isolated pulmonary metastases from osteosarcoma has been reduced significantly since the introduction of modern chemotherapy protocols. Metastases from osteosarcoma occurring in children and young adults are most often multiple and peripheral but may also be single and more centrally located.[69] Metastatic deposits of osteosarcoma in the lung generally show similar features to the primary lesions (Fig. 15.26); however, they may show a maturation phenomenon with massive chondroid differentiation simulating chondrosarcoma or with massive collagenization leaving behind only minimal viable malignant elements. The malignant components may, thus, not be sampled in limited biopsy material precluding an accurate diagnosis. Clinical correlation is indispensable under such circumstances.

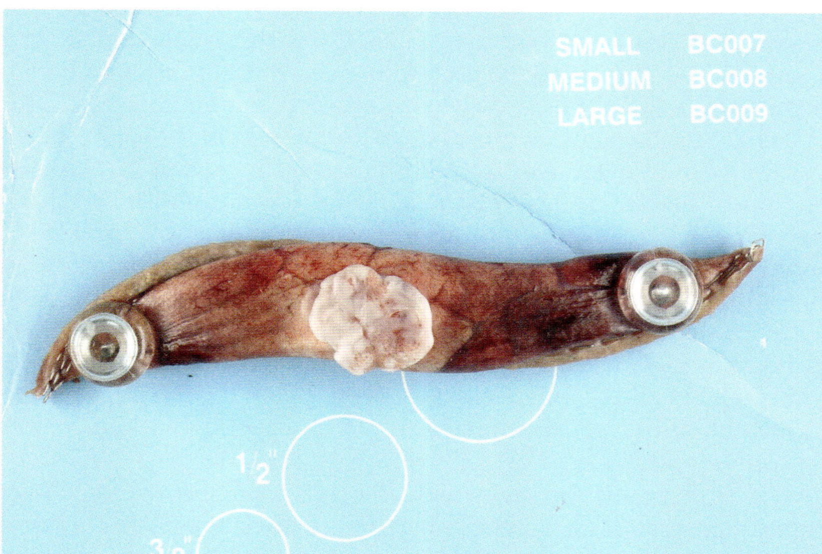

FIGURE 15.25 A Gross photograph demonstrating a small wedge biopsy with metastatic osteosarcoma composed of a centrally located bony white surface nodule stuck to the visceral pleura.

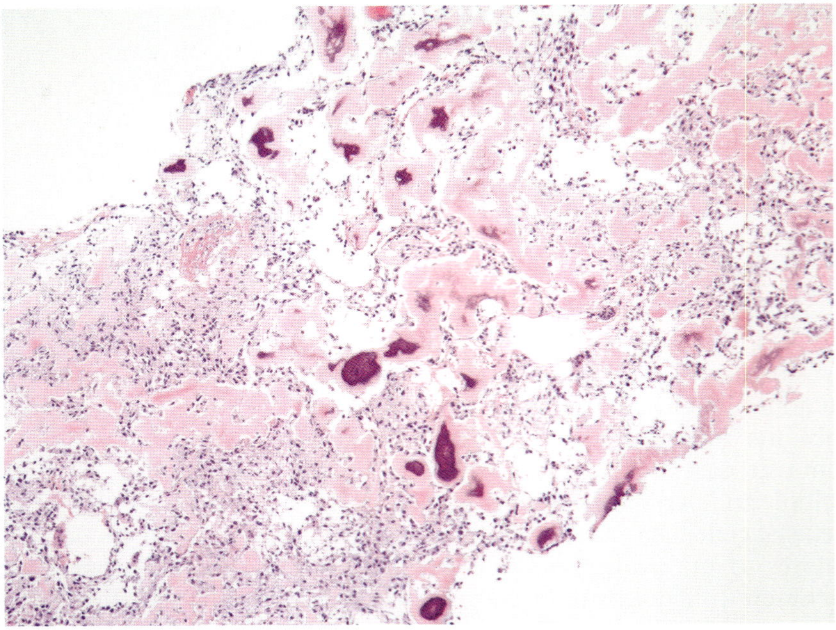

FIGURE 15.26 Core biopsy of peripheral lung nodule with metastatic osteosarcoma showing abundant osteoid flanked by an atypical spindle cell proliferation.

Another common bone tumor in the pediatric age group that metastasizes to the lungs is Ewing sarcoma (Fig. 15.27). The tumor can be confused histologically for other small round blue cell tumors in this age group, such as rhabdomyosarcoma, neuroblastoma, lymphoblastic leukemia, and desmoplastic small round cell tumor. Strong positivity for CD99, to the exclusion of other markers, will be of value for arriving at the correct diagnosis. An additional tool in equivocal cases is the detection of the *EWSR1::FLI1* translocation on chromosome 22q12 by molecular testing. Tumors will also generally be positive for FLI-1 immunohistochemistry; however, it should be remembered that FLI-1 is an entirely nonspecific marker and may be positive in many other tumor types.[70] Evaluation of pediatric small round blue cell tumors should thus be carried out using a panel of immunohistochemical stains that includes CD99, FLI-1, GLI-1, ETV, WT1, BCOR, CD20, CD3, CD43, TdT, cytokeratins, neuroendocrine, and myogenic markers (desmin, myogenin, etc.).

Less commonly, the lungs will be a site of metastasis for chondrosarcoma.[71] Metastases are usually from grade II or grade III chondrosarcomas; metastasis from grade I chondrosarcoma in general is exceedingly rare.[72] Histologically, the metastatic lesions usually present as solitary or multiple well-circumscribed pulmonary nodules. The histology recapitulates that of the primary tumor in the bone, with atypical chondrocytes

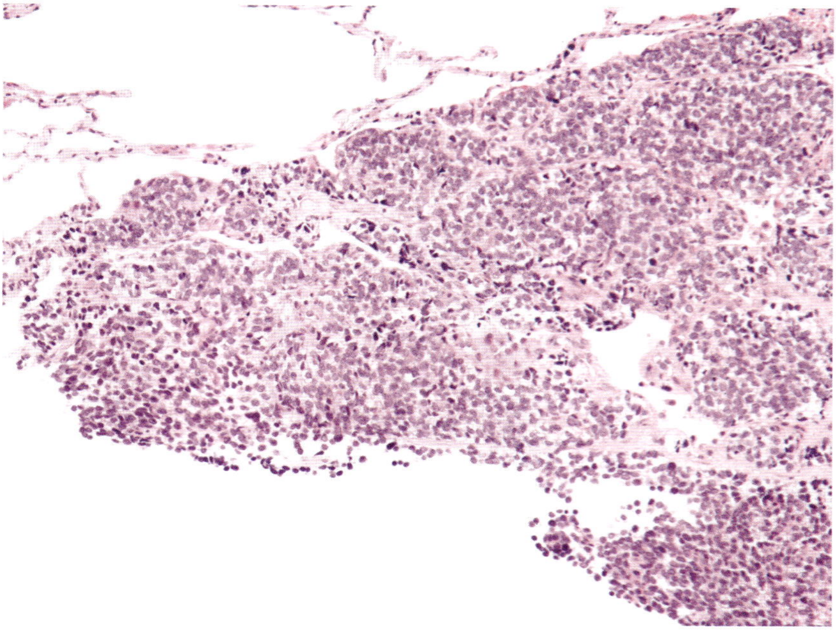

FIGURE 15.27 Lung metastasis of Ewing sarcoma showing sheets of small round blue cells; the tumor cells were strongly positive for CD99 and negative for other differentiation markers.

embedded in a chondromyxoid stroma (Fig. 15.28A). In cases in which biopsy material is limited, it may be difficult to differentiate a metastasis of chondrosarcoma from other myxoid neoplasms, including myoepithelial carcinoma and extraskeletal myxoid chondrosarcoma (Fig. 15.28B). In the extremely rare case of a metastasis of a low-grade lesion, it may be difficult to histologically distinguish a biopsy of metastatic chondrosarcoma from a cartilaginous hamartoma. Immunohistochemistry is rarely helpful in these situations, and a detailed clinical history is needed to arrive at the proper diagnosis.

Metastases From Soft Tissue Sarcomas

The lung is a favored site of metastases for soft tissue sarcomas. Virtually, any type of sarcoma can metastasize to the lung. Because a large variety of sarcomas can also arise as primary tumors in the lung, it may be impossible to differentiate a primary from a metastatic lesion without supportive clinical data. The histologic differential diagnosis for sarcomas metastatic to the lung includes pulmonary carcinosarcoma, sarcomatoid (spindle cell) carcinoma, and pulmonary blastoma.[67] Making this distinction on a small biopsy may be impossible unless very distinctive or clearly diagnostic areas for these tumors are present in the sample. In many instances, the best diagnosis that can be offered will be that of "spindle cell

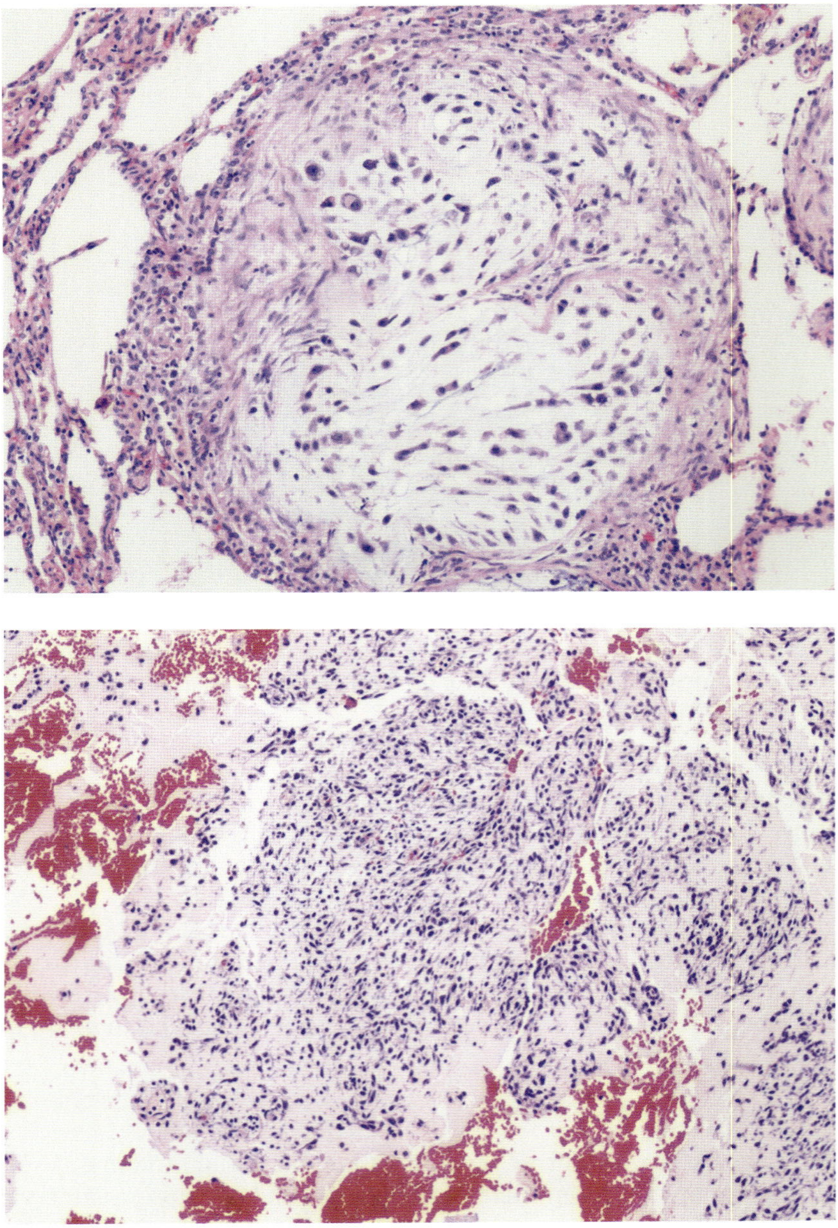

A

B

FIGURE 15.28 **A.** Lung metastasis from a patient with a prior history of a grade II chondrosarcoma. Notice the well-circumscribed nodule showing atypical chondrocytes embedded in a myxoid stroma. **B.** Lung metastasis from an extraskeletal myxoid chondrosarcoma. The wedge biopsy showed groups of spindled to ovoid cells embedded in a myxoid stroma. This lesion may be difficult to differentiate from a chondrosarcoma metastasis without appropriate clinical history.

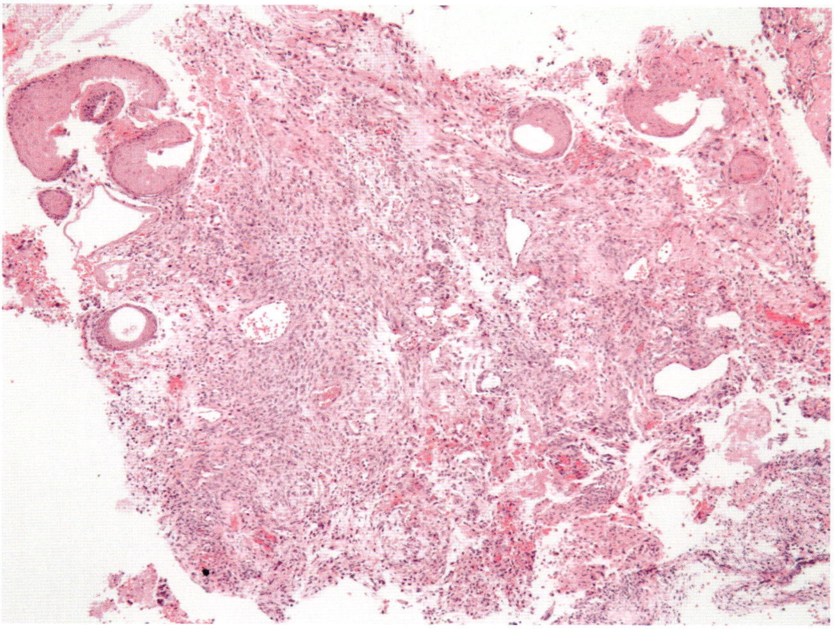

FIGURE 15.29 **Endobronchial metastasis of synovial sarcoma showing monotonous population of spindle cells entrapping bronchial glands.** The patient had a known history of synovial sarcoma of the ankle.

malignant neoplasm, not otherwise specified" or "high-grade sarcoma, not otherwise specified." In general, metastases from soft tissue sarcomas can predominantly comprise spindle cells, epithelioid cells, pleomorphic cells, or an admixture in varying proportions of the above. Tumors comprised predominantly or exclusively of spindle cells include synovial sarcoma, malignant peripheral nerve sheath tumor, leiomyosarcoma, and myofibroblastic sarcomas (Fig. 15.29). Tumors composed of epithelioid cells include epithelioid sarcoma, alveolar soft part sarcoma, epithelioid malignant peripheral nerve sheath tumor, epithelioid leiomyosarcoma, and others (Fig. 15.30). Tumors characterized by pleomorphic tumor cells include pleomorphic liposarcoma, dedifferentiated liposarcoma, and undifferentiated pleomorphic sarcoma. Many of these lesions can display areas exhibiting "rhabdoid" morphology; that is, tumor cells with globular, densely eosinophilic cytoplasmic inclusions that displace the nuclei to the periphery because of cytoplasmic accumulations of intermediate filaments. The presence of "rhabdoid" features generally portends a more aggressive behavior. A peculiar phenomenon observed in pulmonary metastases from soft tissue sarcomas is a change in morphology from the original lesion.[5] Some tumors may show a maturation phenomenon, whereby the tumor cells adopt a better differentiated morphology or undergo cartilaginous, smooth muscle, or other types of differentiation; others may undergo a

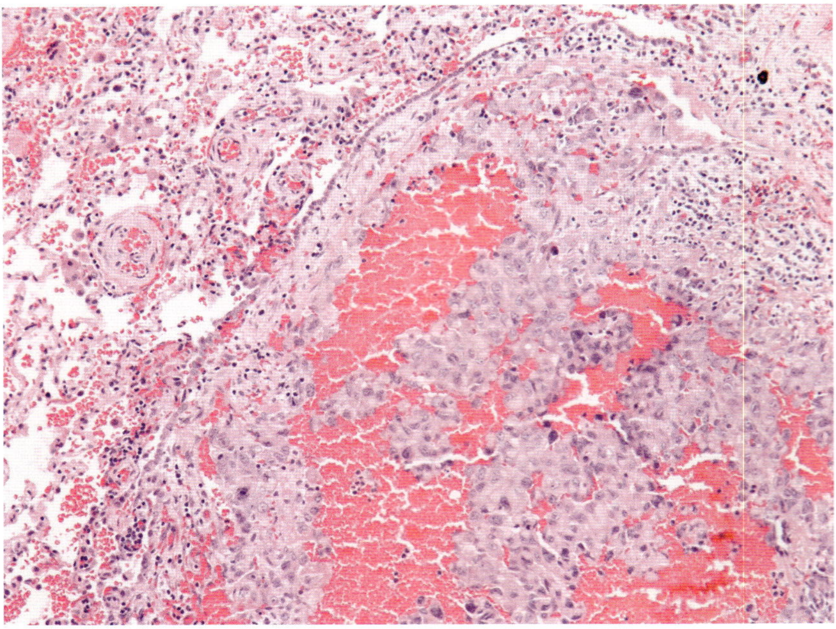

FIGURE 15.30 **Metastasis to the lung from epithelioid sarcoma of the hand; notice the cluster of round, epithelioid cells with abundant cytoplasm.** Some of the cells display homogeneous eosinophilic "rhabdoid" inclusions in the cytoplasm.

regressive process in which they will revert to a more primitive phenotype, reminiscent of a primitive fibroblastic tumor. Another feature of metastases of soft tissue sarcoma to the lungs is the tendency for the tumor to entrap normal airspaces at the periphery in the advancing border of the lesions simulating a biphasic neoplasm, a pitfall that can be averted by noticing the normal, benign appearance of the epithelial structures and by demonstration of TTF-1 or napsin A positivity in those cells.

Immunohistochemistry and molecular pathology can play a major role in identifying the specific type of sarcoma (Table 15.1); however, strict clinicopathologic correlation will be indispensable to establish whether the lesion represents a primary or metastatic tumor.

Sarcomas of the Female Genital Tract

Uterine leiomyosarcoma is the commonest type of sarcoma of the female genital tract to metastasize to the lungs. Metastases to the lung from uterine leiomyosarcoma are generally a late event, and the metastases may appear very well differentiated and of low-grade histology, leading to confusion with a benign smooth muscle proliferation.[73] Metastatic leiomyosarcoma shows immunoreactivity with smooth muscle–associated markers, including smooth muscle actin, smooth muscle myosin, and h-caldesmon, but the use of these markers will not permit a distinction between a tumor

TABLE 15.1 Most Characteristic Genetic Alterations and Immunohistochemistry in Select Soft Tissue Sarcomas

Tumor Type	Genetic Abnormality	Gene Fusion or Amplification Product	Immuno Profile
Synovial sarcoma	t(X;18)	*SS18::SSX*	Keratin, EMA, bcl-2, CD99, calponin, TLE-1, S-100 protein, SS18-SSX, SSX-C terminus
Low-grade fibromyxoid sarcoma	t(7;16)	*FUS::CREB3L2*	MUC4
Well-differentiated liposarcoma and dedifferentiated liposarcoma	Supernumerary ring and giant marker chromosomes	Amplification of 12q13–15, including *MDM2* and *CDK4*	S-100 protein, MDM2, CDK4, p16
Myxoid/round cell liposarcoma	t(12;16)	*FUS::DDIT3*	S-100 protein
Clear cell sarcoma of tendons and aponeuroses	t(12;22)	*EWSR1::ATF1*	S-100 protein, HMB45, Melan-A, vimentin
Extraskeletal myxoid chondrosarcoma	t(9;22)	*EWSR1::NR4A3*	Vimentin, CD99, INSM1
	t(9;17)	*TAF2N::NR4A3*	
	t(9;15)	*TCF12::NR4A3*	
Alveolar soft part sarcoma	(X;17)	*ASPCR1::TFE3*	TFE3, PAS
Extrarenal rhabdoid tumor	Loss of *SMARCB1*	None	Loss of INI1
Ewing sarcoma/PNET	t(11;22)	*EWSR1::FLI1*	CD99
	t(21;22)	*EWSR1::ETV*	
CIC-rearranged sarcoma	t(4;19)	*CIC::DUX4*	Variable CD99, WT1, ETV4, DUX4
	t(10;19)		

(*continued*)

TABLE 15.1 Most Characteristic Genetic Alterations and Immunohistochemistry in Select Soft Tissue Sarcomas (*continued*)

Tumor Type	Genetic Abnormality	Gene Fusion or Amplification Product	Immuno Profile
BCOR-rearranged sarcoma	Inv(X)	*BCOR::CCNB3*	Variable CD99, BCOR
Desmoplastic small round cell tumor	t(11;22)	*EWSR1::WT1*	Keratin, desmin, chromogranin, synaptophysin, vimentin
Alveolar rhabdomyosarcoma	t(2;13)	*PAX3::FOX01*	Desmin, myoglobin, myogenin, myo-D1
	t(1;13)	*PAX7::FOX01*	
Leiomyosarcoma	Complex karyotype with numerous gains and losses, but no consistent recurrent aberration at the chromosomal level	None	SMA, SMMS, desmin, calponin, h-caldesmon
Endometrial stromal sarcoma	t(7;17)	*JAZF1::SUZ12*	Vimentin, desmin, CD10, ER/PR
Epithelioid sarcoma	Loss of *SMARCB1*	None	Keratin, vimentin, CD34, loss of INI1
Fibrosarcoma	None	None	Vimentin, CD34, bcl-2, CD99

SMA, smooth muscle actin; SMMS, smooth muscle myosin; ER/PR, estrogen receptor/progesterone receptor.

originating in the lung, uterus, or soft tissue. A helpful adjunct for diagnosis in such cases is the use of bcl-2, an oncofetal protein involved in the regulation of apoptosis that is strongly expressed in müllerian-derived (female genital) smooth muscle but not in smooth muscle tumors arising from extragenital soft tissue.[74] Strong positivity of the tumor cells for bcl-2 will strongly point in the direction of a metastasis from the female genital tract. Likewise, strong nuclear expression for WT1 will also favor a primary tumor originating from the uterus. Stains for estrogen and progesterone receptor are also more likely to be expressed in metastatic smooth muscle lesions from the female genital tract than in primary lung tumors. Metastases of high-grade uterine leiomyosarcoma may occur synchronously with the primary tumor and will show a bizarre morphology reminiscent of a high-grade undifferentiated pleomorphic sarcoma ("malignant fibrous histiocytoma").

Endometrial stromal sarcoma is another uterine tumor that shows a propensity to metastasize to the lungs, particularly in the late stages of low-grade lesions. A solitary lung metastasis may occasionally be the first manifestation of the tumor.[75] Metastases of endometrial stromal sarcoma can be easily mistaken for a variety of other mesenchymal neoplasms and usually present as a monotonous proliferation of uniform small round or oval cells that may adopt a striking hemangiopericytomatous growth pattern. A distinctive feature that should bring to mind the possibility of endometrial stromal sarcoma is the identification of small spiral arterioles scattered in the stroma (Fig. 15.31A). Another rare manifestation of metastatic endometrial stromal sarcoma to the lung is that of cystic lesions; tumors with these features were originally described as "mesenchymal cystic hamartoma of lung" only to be later demonstrated to represent metastases from endometrial stromal sarcomas. The lesions are characterized by cystic spaces lined by respiratory epithelium showing clusters or sheets of small spindle cells.[76] Immunohistochemical stains will play a role in the diagnosis because the tumors are strongly positive for CD10, a marker that is not commonly expressed in other tumors bearing similar morphologic features (Fig. 15.31B). The tumors are also characterized by positivity for estrogen receptor, progesterone receptor, and desmin. More recently, specific molecular genetic abnormalities have been demonstrated in these tumors, including a t(7,17) translocation with involvement of chromosome arms 6p and 7p resulting in a fusion protein, *JAZF1::SUZ12*, which can be identified in paraffin sections by fluorescence in situ hybridization.[77] Numerous other fusions have also been identified in these tumors, including rearrangements of the *BCOR*, *YWHAE*, *MEAF6*, and *MTBD1* genes, which may be of use in the diagnosis of difficult cases.[78] There needs to be a high level of suspicion, however, for the proper recognition of this tumor at metastatic sites. Confirmation of the existence of a previous uterine endometrial stromal sarcoma through a proper clinical history will be helpful for definitive diagnosis.

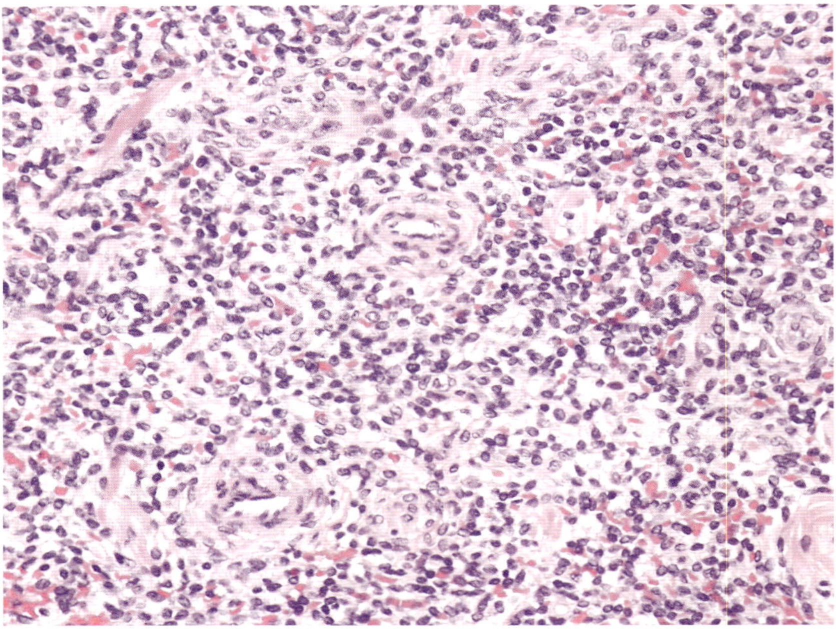

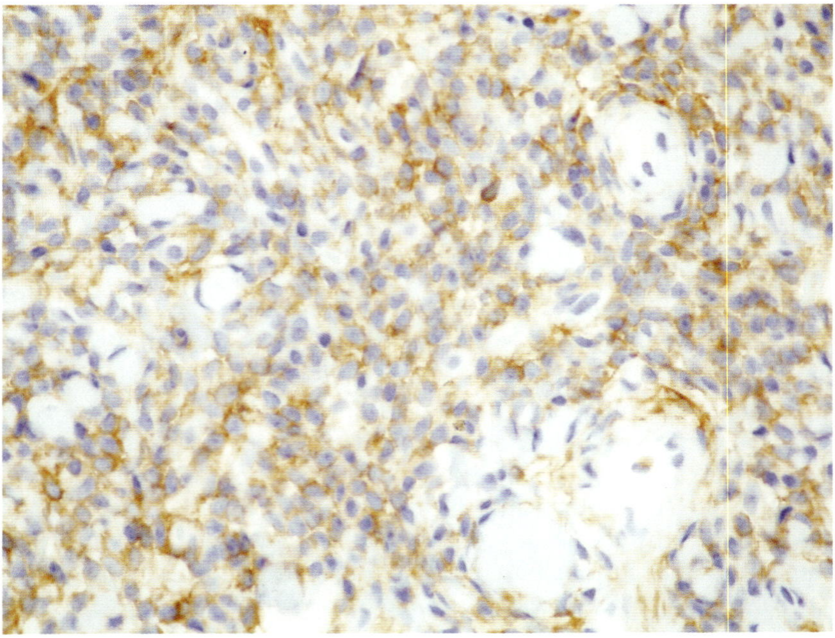

FIGURE 15.31 **A.** Pulmonary metastasis from endometrial stromal sarcoma showing a monotonous population of small to oval cells containing a few spiral arterioles in the stroma. **B.** Immunohistochemical staining for CD10 is seen in an endometrial stromal sarcoma metastasis.

METASTASES FROM MALIGNANT MELANOMA

The lung is the second most frequent site of metastases from malignant melanoma and the first site of relapse for the disease.[79,80] In a large autopsy series, the lungs were involved with metastases of melanoma second only to lymph nodes.[81] The presence of lung metastases in melanoma generally portends a poor prognosis. Metastases of malignant melanoma are most often multiple and bilateral; however, solitary metastases may also occur. Endobronchial metastases of malignant melanoma present with symptoms of bronchial obstruction owing to an endobronchial polypoid mass. Because malignant melanoma can have a protean morphologic appearance, metastases of melanoma can be difficult to diagnose and may simulate many other tumors. Identification of melanin pigment in the tumor cells facilitates the diagnosis (Fig. 15.32); however, pulmonary metastases from malignant melanoma are often amelanotic and will contain no identifiable pigment (Fig. 15.33A and B). Malignant melanomas can show a wide spectrum of cytologic appearances, including epithelioid, spindle, balloon, granular, signet ring, rhabdoid, small lymphocyte like, and bizarre anaplastic tumor cells. In addition, the tumor cells can adopt varied growth patterns, including fascicular, nested, sheetlike, trabecular, myxoid, and sclerosing.[5] The use of immunohistochemical stains will be necessary for arriving at a definitive diagnosis in many instances. Most metastatic

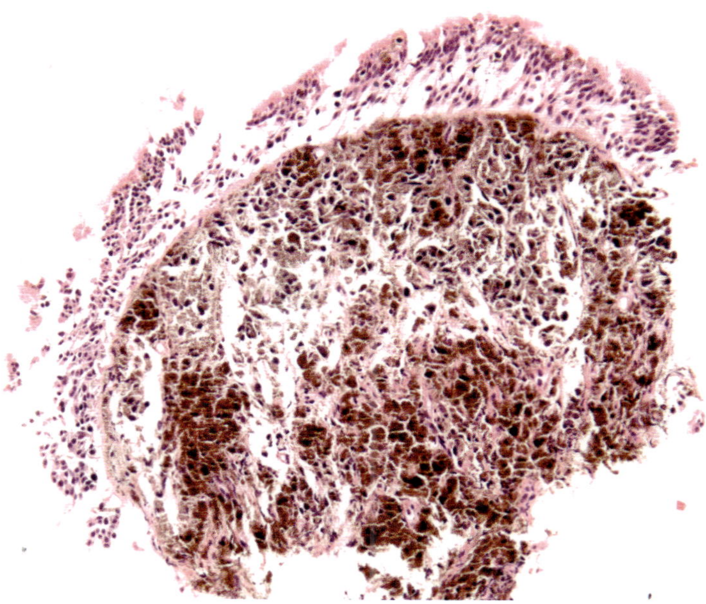

FIGURE 15.32 Endobronchial biopsy in patient with metastatic malignant melanoma showing a heavily pigmented atypical cell population underlying the bronchial mucosa.

A

B

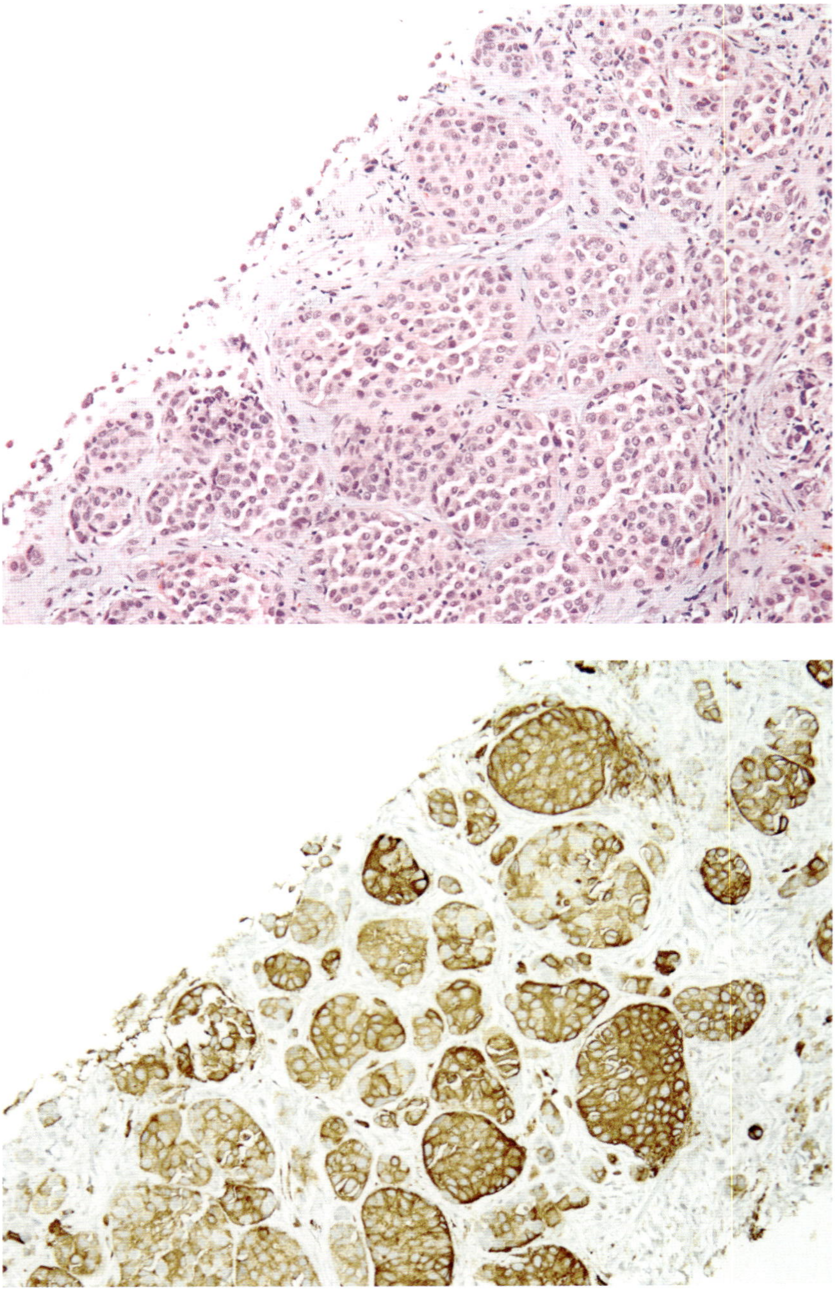

FIGURE 15.33 **A.** Core biopsy of peripheral lung nodule in patient with a history of malignant melanoma showing nests of epithelioid tumor cells devoid of melanin pigment. **B.** Immunohistochemical stain with HMB45 showing cytoplasmic staining of the tumor cells supporting the diagnosis of metastatic malignant melanoma.

malignant melanomas stain positive for S-100 protein and will react with one or more melanocyte-associated markers, such as HMB45, Melan-A, SOX10, and tyrosinase. Rare cases may lose their reactivity for S-100 protein or for some of the other melanocyte-associated markers. Moreover, a few melanoma metastases will express epithelium-associated markers, such as CEA and epithelial membrane antigen, introducing a major pitfall for diagnosis in these tumors. The use of a panel of antibodies that includes epithelial and melanocytic markers is, therefore, recommended in the evaluation of poorly differentiated tumors suspected of being malignant melanoma. Comparison of the pulmonary lesion with prior biopsies from the primary tumor may also be of assistance in defining whether the two lesions correspond to the same neoplasm. It should be kept in mind, however, that malignant melanoma may also show a tendency to undergo changes in morphologic appearances at metastatic sites and that metastasis may occur in the setting of an occult or regressed primary.[5] Changes in antigenic expression of markers in metastatic lesions of melanoma have also been documented that can introduce difficulties when comparing metastases with the original lesion.[82] Another consideration is that so-called undifferentiated and dedifferentiated melanomas may metastasize to the lungs and bear little resemblance to conventional melanoma; in this scenario, use of ancillary molecular diagnostics is likely required to identify melanoma-associated mutational signatures.[83]

METASTASES FROM "BENIGN" TUMORS

Metastases to the lungs from tumors that are generally regarded as benign ("benign metastasizing tumors") have been recorded in a number of instances. The commonest example is the condition known as "benign metastasizing leiomyoma."

Benign Metastasizing Leiomyoma

This term is used to describe single or multiple lung nodules comprising benign-appearing smooth muscle occurring in women of reproductive age or older with a history of prior or concurrent benign uterine leiomyomas. Another term used for the condition is leiomyomatous hamartoma, because of the tendency for the lesions to entrap normal respiratory glandular epithelium at their periphery creating the impression of a biphasic epithelial-mesenchymal neoplasm. The lesions appear to be hormonally dependent and contain estrogen and progesterone receptors. The exact nature of these lesions is still debatable; some believe them to be hamartomatous, whereas others contend that they represent actual metastases from low-grade, well-differentiated uterine leiomyosarcomas.[73] A more recent study using micro-RNA analysis in these tumors found that the lesions did not express micro-RNAs regarded as translational inhibitors in any of the 10 cases studied, compared with high expression in all cases of leiomyosarcoma tested.[84] The authors concluded that benign metastasizing

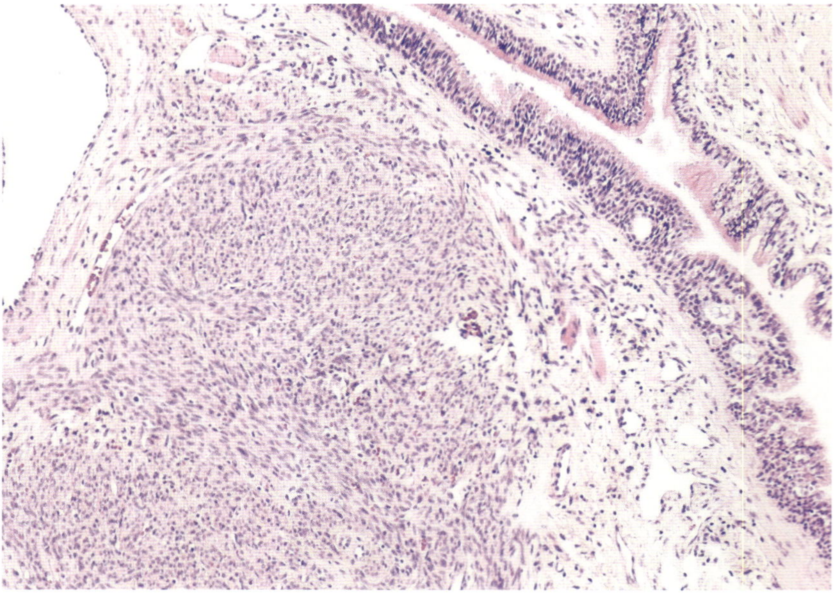

FIGURE 15.34 **Example of a benign metastasizing leiomyoma showing a small nodule of bland-appearing spindled myoid cells embedded in the pulmonary parenchyma.** No mitotic activity or features of malignancy are present.

leiomyoma is, indeed, a benign process. Another distinguishing feature was the strong expression of bcl-2, which helps to separate them from primary smooth muscle tumors of the lung that are negative for this marker. Histologically, these tumors resemble benign uterine leiomyomas with a population of bland-appearing spindle cells (Fig. 15.34). Because of their small size and peripheral location, the lesions are seldom biopsied and are most often examined in resection specimens or removed by wedge biopsy.

Other "Benign" Metastases to the Lung

Some of the other tumors that can show metastatic deposits in the lung after a considerable latency period include intracranial meningioma and giant cell tumor of bone.

Benign metastasizing meningioma is a term that refers to a benign-appearing pulmonary nodule with features of meningioma that develops after a long latency period in a patient with a history of intracranial meningioma.[85,86] The lesions are well circumscribed and show the characteristic features of meningioma, with spindle or oval cells devoid of nuclear atypia or mitotic activity that tend to adopt a whorling configuration (Fig. 15.35). The main differential diagnosis is with minute meningothelial nodules, which, by contrast, are microscopic and usually seen as an incidental finding in patients whose lungs were resected for other causes. Minute meningothelial nodules are generally not associated with a history of meningioma.

Benign metastasizing giant cell tumor of bone refers to an analogous situation in which a pulmonary metastasis showing the features

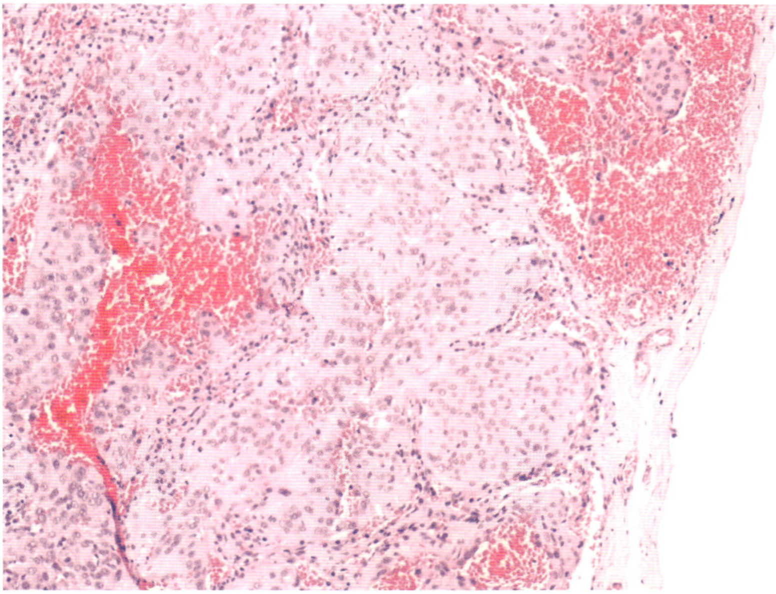

FIGURE 15.35 **Benign metastasizing meningioma identified within the lung in a patient with a prior history of cranial meningioma that had been resected.**

of a conventional giant cell tumor of bone develops in a patient with a prior history of giant cell tumor of bone.[87,88] Histologically, the lesions are identical to conventional giant cell tumor of bone (Fig. 15.36). A clinical history is required for proper diagnosis.

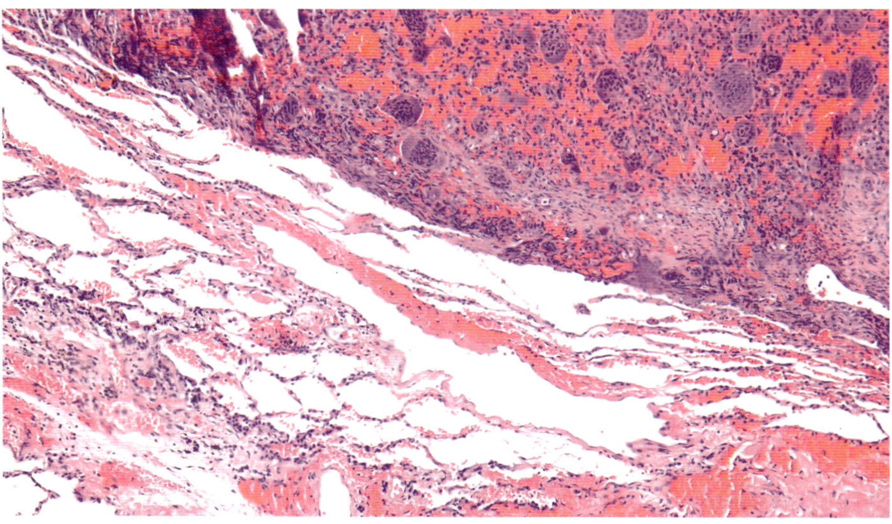

FIGURE 15.36 **Wedge biopsy resection specimen demonstrating a case of metastatic giant cell tumor of bone.** The tumor shows multiple large multinucleated giant cells but does not show any overt evidence of malignant transformation.

REFERENCES

1. Suster S. Pulmonary metastases of extrapulmonary tumors. In: Saldana M, ed. *Pathology of Pulmonary Disease*. J.B. Lippincott; 1994:701-710.
2. Davis EW, Peabody JW, Katz S. The solitary pulmonary nodule. A ten year study based on 215 cases. *J Thorac Surg*. 1956;32:728-771.
3. Toomes H, Delphendahl A, Manke HG, Vogt-Moykopf I. The coin lesion of the lung. A review of 995 resected coin lesions. *Cancer*. 1983;51:534-537.
4. Barnett J, Belsey J, Tavare AN, et al. Pre-surgical lung biopsy in management of solitary pulmonary nodules: a cost effectiveness analysis. *J Med Econ*. 2019;22(12):1307-1311.
5. Suster S, Moran CA. Unusual manifestations of metastatic tumors to the lungs. *Semin Diagn Pathol*. 1995;12:193-206.
6. Rosenblatt MB, Lisa JR, Collier F. Primary and metastatic bronchioloalveolar carcinoma. *Dis Chest*. 1967;52:147-153.
7. Sheperd MP. Endobronchial metastatic disease. *Thorax*. 1982;37:362-369.
8. Pena GNM, Jiang C. Endobronchial, laryngeal and mediastinal melanoma: a rare constellation of metastatic disease. *BMJ Case Rep*. 2019;12(5):e228957.
9. Viadora E, Brass IDJ, Pickren JW. Cascade spread of blood-borne metastases in solid and non-solid cancers of humans. In: Weiss L, Gilbert HA, eds. *Pulmonary Metastases*. GK Hall; 1978.
10. Papac RJ. Distant metastases from head and neck tumors. *Cancer*. 1984;53:342-346.
11. Lu HJ, Hsieh CC, Yeh CC, et al. Clinical, pathophysiologic, and genomic analysis of the outcomes of primary head and neck malignancy after pulmonary metastasectomy. *Sci Rep*. 2019;9(1):12913.
12. Zhou Y, Höti N, Ao M, et al. Expression of p16 and p53 in non-small-cell lung cancer: clinicopathological correlation and potential prognostic impact. *Biomark Med*. 2019;13(9):761-771.
13. El-Salem F, Mansour M, Gitman M, et al. Real-time PCR HPV genotyping in fine needle aspirations of metastatic head and neck squamous cell carcinoma: exposing the limitations of conventional p16 immunostaining. *Oral Oncol*. 2019;90:74-79.
14. Gatta LB, Balzarini P, Tironi A, et al. Human papillomavirus DNA and p16 gene in squamous cell lung carcinoma. *Anticancer Res*. 2012;32(8):3085-3089.
15. Spiro RH, Huvos AG, Strong EW. Adenoid cystic carcinoma of salivary origin. A clinicopathologic study of 242 cases. *Am J Surg*. 1974;128:512-518.
16. Sidhu GS, Forrester EM. Acinic cell carcinoma: long-term survival after pulmonary metastases. *Cancer*. 1977;40:756-759.
17. Luevano A, Rao N, Mackinnon A, et al. Cribriform adenocarcinoma of the lung: clinicopathologic, immunohistochemical and molecular study of 15 cases. *Mod Pathol*. 2012;25:483A.
18. Suster DI, Ronen N, Mejbel HA, Harada S, Mackinnon AC, Suster S. Non-small cell lung carcinoma with clear cell features: a clinicopathologic, immunohistochemical, and molecular study of 31 cases. *Virchows Arch*. 2024;485:83-96.
19. Suster D, Mackinnon AC, Ronen N, Mejbel HA, Harada S, Suster S. Non-small cell lung carcinoma with clear cell features and FGFR3::TACC3 gene rearrangement: clinicopathologic and next generation sequencing study of 7 cases. *Am J Surg Pathol*. 2024;48:284-291.
20. Crombé A, Buy X, Godbert Y, et al. 23 lung metastases treated by radiofrequency ablation over 10 years in a single patient: successful oncological outcome of a metastatic cancer without altered respiratory function. *Cardiovasc Intervent Radiol*. 2016;39(12):1779-1784.
21. Rozhinskaya L, Pigarova E, Sabanova E, et al. Diagnosis and treatment challenges of parathyroid carcinoma in a 27-year-old woman with multiple lung metastases. *Endocrinol Diabetes Metab Case Rep*. 2017;2017:16-0113. doi:10.1530/EDM-16-0113

22. Pyo JS, Cho WJ. Diagnostic and prognostic implications of parafibromin immunohistochemistry in parathyroid carcinoma. *Biosci Rep*. 2019;39(4):BSR20181778.
23. Juhlin CC, Nilsson IL, Lagerstedt-Robinson K, et al. Parafibromin immunostainings of parathyroid tumors in clinical routine: a near-decade experience from a tertiary center. *Mod Pathol*. 2019;32(8):1082-1094.
24. Yousem SA. Pulmonary intestinal-type adenocarcinoma does not show enteric differentiation by immunohistochemical study. *Mod Pathol*. 2005;18:816-821.
25. Inamura K, Satoh Y, Okumura S, et al. Pulmonary adenocarcinomas with enteric differentiation: histologic and immunohistochemical characteristics compared with metastatic colorectal cancers and usual pulmonary adenocarcinomas. *Am J Surg Pathol*. 2005;29:660-665.
26. Canney A, Sheahan K, Keegan D, Tolan M, Hyland J, Green A. Synchronous lung tumors in a patient with metachronous colorectal carcinoma and a germline MSH2 mutation. *J Clin Pathol*. 2009;62:471-473.
27. Moran CA, Hochholzer L, Fishback NL, Travis WD, Koss MN. Mucinous (so-called "colloid") adenocarcinoma of the lung. *Mod Pathol*. 1992;5:634-638.
28. Castro CY, Moran CA, Flieder DG, Suster S. Primary signet-ring cell adenocarcinoma of the lung: a clinicopathologic study of 15 cases. *Histopathology*. 2001;39:397-401.
29. Cassiere SG, McLain DA, Emory WB, Hatch HB Jr. Metastatic carcinoma of the pancreas simulating primary bronchogenic carcinomas. *Cancer*. 1980;46:2319-2321.
30. Krasinskas AM, Chiosea SI, Pal T, Dacic S. KRAS mutational analysis and immunohistochemical studies can help distinguish pancreatic metastases from primary lung adenocarcinomas. *Mod Pathol*. 2014;27(2):262-270.
31. Park SY, Kim BH, Kim JH, Lee S, Kang GH. Panels of immunohistochemical markers help determine primary sites of metastatic adenocarcinoma. *Arch Pathol Lab Med*. 2007;131(10):1561-1567.
32. Malmros K, Lindholm A, Vidarsdottir H, et al. Diagnostic gastrointestinal markers in primary lung cancer and pulmonary metastases. *Virchows Arch*. 2024;485:347-357.
33. Agaimy A, Fuchs F, Moskalev EA, Sirbu H, Hartmann A, Haller F. SMARCA4-deficient pulmonary adenocarcinoma: clinicopathological, immunohistochemical, and molecular characteristics of a novel aggressive neoplasm with a consistent TTF1^{neg}/CK7^{pos}/HepPar-1^{pos} immunophenotype. *Virchows Arch*. 2017;471:599-609.
34. Nguyen T, Phillips D, Jain D, et al. Comparison of 5 Immunohistochemical markers of hepatocellular differentiation for the diagnosis of hepatocellular carcinoma. *Arch Pathol Lab Med*. 2015;139(8):1028-1034.
35. Katzenstein AL, Purvis R Jr, Gmelich J, Askin F. Pulmonary resection for metastatic renal adenocarcinomas. Pathologic findings and therapeutic value. *Cancer*. 1978;41:712-723.
36. Trinidad S, Lisa JR, Rosenblatt MB. Bronchogenic carcinoma simulated by metastatic tumors. *Cancer*. 1963;16:1521-1529.
37. Lin S, Zheng Y, Qin Z, et al. Surgical intervention in renal cell carcinoma patients with lung and bronchus metastasis is associated with longer survival time: a population-based analysis. *Ann Transl Med*. 2019;7(14):323.
38. Procházková K, Vodička J, Fichtl J, et al. Outcomes for patients after resection of pulmonary metastases from clear cell renal cell carcinoma: 18 years of experience. *Urol Int*. 2019;103(3):397-302. doi:10.1159/000502493
39. Eichelberg C, Minner S, Isbarn H, et al. Prognostic value of alpha-methyl CoA racemase (AMACR) expression in renal cell carcinoma. *World J Urol*. 2011;31(4):847-853.
40. Mete O, Asa SL, Giordano TJ, Papotti M, Sasano H, Volante M. Immunohistochemical biomarkers of adrenal cortical neoplasms. *Endocr Pathol*. 2018;29(2):137-149.
41. Chang A, Amin A, Gabrielson E, et al. Utility of GATA3 immunohistochemistry in differentiating urothelial carcinoma from prostate adenocarcinoma and squamous cell carcinomas of the uterine cervix, anus and lung. *Am J Surg Pathol*. 2012;36:1472-1476.

42. Gentile PS, Carlon HW, Huang TY, Yam LT, Lam WK. Disseminated prostatic carcinoma simulating primary lung cancer. Indications for immunodiagnostic studies. *Cancer*. 1998;62:711-715.

43. Copeland JN, Amin MB, Humphrey PA, Tamboli P, Ro JY, Gal AA. The morphologic spectrum of metastatic prostatic adenocarcinoma to the lung: special emphasis on histologic features overlapping with other pulmonary neoplasms. *Am J Clin Pathol*. 2002;117:552-557.

44. Sheridan T, Herawi M, Epstein JL. The role of P501S and PSA in the diagnosis of metastatic adenocarcinoma of the prostate. *Am J Surg Pathol*. 2007;31:1351-1355.

45. Gurel B, Ali TZ, Montgomery EA, et al. NKX3.1 as a marker of prostatic origin in metastatic tumors. *Am J Surg Pathol*. 2010;34:1097-1105.

46. Morrow CE, Vassilopolous PP, Grage TB. Surgical resection for metastatic neoplasms of the lung: experience at the university of Minnesota Hospitals. *Cancer*. 1980;45:2981-2992.

47. Mountain CF, McMurtrey MJ, Hermes KE. Surgery for pulmonary metastases: a 20-year experience. *Ann Thorac Surg*. 1984;38:323-327.

48. Liu D, Abolhoda A, Burt ME, et al. Pulmonary metastasectomy for testicular germ cell tumors: a 28-year experience. *Ann Thorac Surg*. 1998;66(5):1709-1714.

49. Xiao H, Liu D, Bajorin DF, Burt M, Bosl GW. Medical and surgical management of pulmonary metastases from germ cell tumors. *Chest Surg Clin N Am*. 1998;8(1):131-143.

50. Moran CA, Travis WD, Carter D, Koss MN. Metastatic mature teratomas in lung following testicular embryonal carcinoma and teratocarcinoma. *Arch Pathol Lab Med*. 1993;117:641-644.

51. Mountain CF, Khalil KG, Hermes KE, Frazier OH. The contribution of surgery to the management of carcinomatous pulmonary metastases. *Cancer*. 1978;41:833-841.

52. Ki EY, Lee KH, Park JS, Hur SY. A clinicopathological review of pulmonary metastasis from uterine cervical cancer. *Cancer Res Treat*. 2016;48(1):266-272.

53. Hacker NF, Rao A. Surgical management of lung, liver and brain metastases from gynecological cancers: a literature review. *Gynecol Oncol Res Pract*. 2016;3(1):7.

54. Ramalingam P. Morphologic, immunophenotypic, and molecular features of epithelial ovarian cancer. *Oncology (Williston Park)*. 2016;30(2):166-176.

55. Plaza JA, Ramirez N, Nuovo GJ. Utility of HPV analysis for evaluation of possible metastatic disease in women with cervical cancer. *Int J Gynecol Pathol*. 2004;23:7-12.

56. Sterlacci W, Tzankov A, Veits L, et al. A comprehensive analysis of p16 expression, gene status, and promoter hypermethylation in surgically resected non-small cell lung carcinomas. *J Thorac Oncol*. 2011;6:1649-1657.

57. Minn AJ, Gupta GP, Siegel PM, et al. Genes that mediate breast cancer metastasis to lung. *Nature*. 2005;436(7050):518-524.

58. Schlappack OK, Baur M, Steger G, Dittrich C, Moser K. The clinical course of lung metastases from breast cancer. *Klin Wochenschr*. 1988;66:790-795.

59. Rossmann P, Vortel V. Pulmonary metastases imitating alveolar cell carcinoma. *J Pathol Bacteriol*. 1961;81:313-317.

60. Hirono M, Nonaka M, Himuro N, Tomita Y, Kataoka D, Kadokura M. Two cases of thymoma with pulmonary metastasis: a case report. *World J Surg Oncol*. 2014;12:114.

61. Suster D, Pihan G, Mackinnon AC, Suster S. Poorly differentiated nonkeratinizing squamous cell carcinoma of the thymus: clinicopathologic and molecular genetic study of 25 cases. *Am J Surg Pathol*. 2018;42(9):1224-1236.

62. Pan CC, Chen PC, Chiang H. Kit (CD117) is frequently overexpressed in thymic carcinomas but is absent in thymomas. *J Pathol*. 2004;202:375-381.

63. Nakagawa K, Matsuno Y, Kunitoh H, Maeshima A, Asamura H, Tsuchiya R. Immunohistochemical Kit (CD117) expression in thymic epithelial tumors. *Chest*. 2005;128:140-144.

64. Kriegsman M, Muley T, Harms A, et al. Differential diagnostic value of CD5 and CD117 expression in thoracic tumors: a large scale study of 1465 non-small cell lung cancer cases. *Diagn Pathol*. 2015;10:210.

65. Chao C, Goldberg M. Surgical treatment of metastatic pulmonary soft-tissue sarcoma. *Oncology (Williston Park)*. 2000;14(6):835-841.

66. Predina JD, Puc MM, Bergey MR, et al. Improved survival after pulmonary metastasectomy for soft tissue sarcoma. *J Thorac Oncol*. 2011;6:913-919.

67. Digesu CS, Wiesel O, Vaporciyan AA, Colson YL. Management of sarcoma metastases to the lung. *Surg Oncol Clin N Am*. 2016;25(4):721.

68. Udelsman R, Roth JA, Lees D, Jelenich SE, Pass HI. Endobronchial metastases from soft tissue sarcomas. *J Thorac Cardiovasc Surg*. 1984;87:260-269.

69. Rasalkar DD, Chu WC, Lee V, Paunipagar BK, Cheng FWT, Li CK. Pulmonary metastases in children with osteosarcoma: characteristics and impact on patient survival. *Pediatr Radiol*. 2011;41:227-236.

70. Lin O, Fillipa DA, Teruya-Feldstein J. Immunohistochemical evaluation of FLI-1 in acute lymphoblastic lymphoma (ALL): a potential diagnostic pitfall. *Appl Immunohistochem Mol Morphol*. 2009;17:409-412.

71. Canals RMI, Fuentes RE, Plaza AR, et al. Metastatic pulmonary chondrosarcoma: clinical description and literature review. *Arch Bronconeumol*. 2015;51(1):52.

72. Nakamura T, Matsumine A, Yamada S, et al. Oncological outcome after lung metastasis in patients presenting with localized chondrosarcoma at extremities: Tokai Musculoskeletal Oncology Consortium Study. *Onco Targets Ther*. 2016;9:4747-4751.

73. Wolff M, Kaye G, Silva F. Pulmonary metastases (with admixed epithelial elements) from smooth muscle neoplasms. Report of nine cases, including three males. *Am J Surg Pathol*. 1979;3:325-331.

74. Suster S, Fisher C, Moran CA. The spectrum of bcl-2 oncoprotein reactivity in benign and malignant spindle cell tumors of soft tissue, skin, serosal surfaces, and gastrointestinal tract. An immunohistochemical study of 380 cases. *Am J Surg Pathol*. 1998;22:863-872.

75. Abrams J, Talcott J, Corson JM. Pulmonary metastases in patients with low-grade endometrial stromal sarcoma. Clinicopathologic findings and immunohistochemical characterization. *Am J Surg Pathol*. 1989;13:133-139.

76. Abrams J, Talcott J, Corson JM. Pulmonary metastases in patients with low-grade endometrial stromal sarcoma. Clinicopathologic findings with immunohistochemical characterization. *Am J Surg Pathol*. 1989;13:133-140.

77. Micci F, Walter CU, Teixeira MR, et al. Cytogenetic and molecular genetic analyses of endometrial stromal sarcoma: nonrandom involvement of chromosome arms 6p and 7p and confirmation of JAZF1/JJAZ1 gene fusion in t(7,17). *Cancer Genet Cytogenet*. 2003;144:119-124.

78. Hrzenjak A. JAZF1/SUZ12 gene fusion in endometrial stromal sarcomas. *Orphanet J Rare Dis*. 2011;11:15.

79. Tas F. Metastatic behavior in melanoma: timing, pattern, survival, and influencing factors. *J Oncol*. 2012;2012:647684.

80. Velu PP, Cao C, Yan TD. Current surgical management of melanoma metastases to the lung. *J Thorac Dis*. 2013;5(Suppl 3):S274-S276.

81. Patel JK, Didolkar MS, Pickren JW, Moore RH. Metastatic patterns of malignant melanoma. A study of 216 autopsy cases. *Am J Surg*. 1978;135:807-812.

82. Plaza JA, Suster D, Perez-Montiel D. Expression of immunohistochemical markers in primary and metastatic malignant melanoma: a comparative study in 70 patients using a tissue microarray technique. *Appl Immunohistochem Mol Morphol*. 2007;15:421-425.

83. Kasago IS, Chatila WK, Lezcano CM, et al. Undifferentiated and dedifferentiated metastatic melanomas masquerading as soft tissue sarcomas: mutational signature analysis and immunotherapy response. *Mod Pathol*. 2023;36:100165.

84. Nuovo GJ, Schmittgen TD. Benign metastasizing leiomyoma of the lung: clinicopathologic, immunohistochemical, and micro-RNA analyses. *Diagn Mol Pathol.* 2008;17:145-150.
85. Miller DC, Ojemann RG, Proppe KH, McGinnis BD, Grillo HC. Benign metastasizing meningioma. *J Neurosurg.* 1985;62:763-769.
86. Pramesh CS, Saklani AP, Pantvaidya GH, et al. Benign metastasizing meningioma. *Jpn J Clin Oncol.* 2003;33(2):86-88.
87. Bertoni F, Present D, Sudanese A, Baldini N, Bacchini P, Campanacci M. Giant cell tumor of bone with pulmonary metastases. Six case reports and review of the literature. *Clin Orthop Relat Res.* 1988;237:275-282.
88. Muheremu A, Huang Z, Niu X. Treatment for giant cell tumor of the spine metastasizing to the lung: a report of two cases and a literature review. *Oncol Lett.* 2015;9(3):1321-1326.

INDEX

Note: Page numbers followed by *f* indicate figures; those followed by *t* indicate tables respectively.

F

G

M

R